Comprehensive Health Insurance
Billing, Coding, and Reimbursement

Comprehensive Health Insurance
Billing, Coding, and Reimbursement

Deborah Vines
Ann Braceland
Elizabeth Rollins
Susan Miller

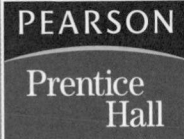

PEARSON
Prentice
Hall

Upper Saddle River, New Jersey 07458

Library of Congress Cataloging-in-Publication Data

Comprehensive health insurance : billing, coding, and reimbursement / Deborah Vines . . . [et al.].
  p.; cm.
  Includes index.
  ISBN-13: 978-0-13-236815-5
  ISBN-10: 0-13-236815-3
  1. Medical fees. 2. Nosology—Code numbers. 3. Health insurance claims—Code numbers.
4. Health insurance claims processing industry. I. Vines, Deborah. II. Braceland, Ann III. Rollins,
Elizabeth.
  [DNLM: 1. Forms and Records Control—methods. 2. Insurance Claim Reporting. 3. Insurance,
Health, Reimbursement. 4. Patient Credit and Collection—methods. W 80 C737 2009]
  R728.5.C67 2009
  616.8900719 1—dc22

                                                                        2007043994

Publisher: Julie Levin Alexander
Publisher's Assistant: Regina Bruno
Executive Editor: Joan Gill
Associate Editor: Bronwen Glowacki
Editorial Assistant: Mary Ellen Ruitenberg
Project Manager: Triple SSS Press Media
  Development
Director of Marketing: Karen Allman
Senior Marketing Manager: Harper Coles
Senior Marketing Manager: Francisco Del
  Castillo
Marketing Specialist: Michael Sirinides
Marketing Assistant: Lauren Castellano
Managing Production Editor: Patrick Walsh
Production Liaison: Julie Li

Production Editor: Puneet Lamba
Media Product Manager: John Jordan
Manager of Media Production: Amy Peltier
New Media Project Manager: Stephen J.
  Hartner
Manufacturing Manager: Ilene Sanford
Manufacturing Buyer: Pat Brown
Senior Design Coordinator: Christopher
  Weigand
Interior Designer: Karen Quigley
Cover Designer: Karen Quigley
Cover Image: Jupiter Images/Vincent Alessi
Composition: Aptara
Printing and Binding: Quad/Graphics
Cover Printer: Phoenix Color Corporation

Pearson Education LTD. London
Pearson Education Singapore, Pte. Ltd
Pearson Education, Canada, Ltd
Pearson Education—Japan
Pearson Education Australia PTY, Limited

Pearson Education North Asia Ltd
Pearson Educación de Mexico, S.A. de C.V.
Pearson Education Malaysia, Pte. Ltd
Pearson Education, Upper Saddle River,
  New Jersey

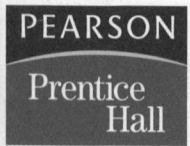

10 9
ISBN-10:   0-13-236815-3
ISBN-13: 978-0-13-236815-5

Over the years I have had the privilege of watching students choose to be trained and seek employment in the healthcare industry. It brings such gratification to watch students complete their training, find employment, and be proud of their accomplishments. I want to express my gratitude to my students for letting me share this experience. Current students have shared with me their opinions and provided input regarding what they feel would provide a better training environment. Graduates have returned and talked about which parts of the training they received were beneficial and which needed to be revised for future students. I have benefited greatly from this input not only professionally, but personally.

I wish to say thank you to my children, Tessa and Sean, my three sisters, and my parents for always encouraging me. With their sacrifices, support, and encouragement I was able to see the end results of my aspirations.

—Deborah Vines

During the past 30 years I have seen and learned how "medicine" has become a "business." Being raised in a medical family, I have had hands-on experience and teachings. I would like to give special thanks to my father, the late Francis J. Bonner, M.D., who was a professor at Jefferson Medical College in Philadelphia, Pennsylvania. Through working with him, I obtained an appreciation for quality patient care and instructional guidance. To my husband "Buzz" there are no words that can express the gratitude I have for your unconditional support and love during this experience. Without your daily support and understanding, deadlines would not have been met; you are appreciated! To my wonderful children, Lisa, Robert, and Chris, who heard me discuss this project for the past 3 years, I thank you for your listening, encouragement, and support. Thanks also to my brothers, Dr. Frank, Dr. Charles, Dr. James, and Dr. Dennis, for their support and encouragement.

In particular, I would also like to thank William F. Bonner, M.D., the medical director of Physical Medicine and Rehabilitation at St. Mary's Hospital in Langhorne, Pennsylvania, for his informative discussions on workers' compensation throughout this project.

Last but not least, I want to thank all of the students and graduates of Allied Career Center. You have enriched my life with your thoughts, questions, and comments. Without you there would be no publication!

—Ann Braceland

First, I would like to thank my family and especially my father, David R. Stager, Sr., M.D. Without his faith and unwavering support throughout the years, I would not be writing this today. Thank you to my husband Chris, who supports and encourages me every day and makes me laugh when I am frustrated. I have been blessed with excellent role models and mentors who guided and encouraged me to succeed in every endeavor. I have been very fortunate through the years to meet and educate many wonderful people who have changed my life. Alumni and present students of Allied Career Center have pushed me to learn even more with their insightful questions and feedback. Without our students, we wouldn't have been able to fulfill this dream. Last, I would like to acknowledge and thank my coauthors and friends for their dedication in making this dream a reality.

—Elizabeth Rollins

I would like to express my thanks and appreciation to my family for their never-ending support. And especially to my children, Abe, Aleisha, and Aaron, for always believing in me and encouraging me. I could not have done this without your ongoing support. Looking back over the past 20 years I have spent in the medical field, there is no other career more rewarding and satisfying than giving back to others what you have learned in the medical field and seeing students grow and achieve their goals.

—Susan Miller

Contents

Chapter 3

Understanding Managed Care: Medical Contracts and Ethics   44

Section III   Medical Coding

Chapter 4   ICD-9-CM Medical Coding   62

Chapter 5   Introduction to CPT® and Place of Service Coding   106

Chapter 6   Coding Procedures and Services   130

CPT is a registered trademark of the American Medical Association.

Chapter 7   HCPCS and Coding Compliance   160

Section V   Government Medical Billing

Chapter 11   Medicare Medical Billing   314

Chapter 12

Medicaid Medical Billing   358

Chapter 13   TRICARE Medical Billing   390

Section VI   Accounts Receivable

Chapter 14   Explanation of Benefits and Payment Adjudication   412

Chapter 15   Refunds and Appeals   462

Section VII   Injured Employee Medical Claim

Chapter 16   Workers' Compensation   496

Section VIII   Use of Medical Practice Management Software

Chapter 17   Electronic Medical Claims Processing   528

This textbook was written to provide students with the knowledge and skills necessary to work in a variety of billing and coding positions in the medical field. Many textbooks have been written in the past on this subject matter; however, daily feedback from students using this material and learning to become medical office specialists has allowed the authors to make the material in this text particularly current and relevant. The student will learn the process of billing and how to handle a patient from the initial appointment through the collection process. In addition to submitting claims to insurance carriers, the process of billing may include reviewing medical records, verifying patient benefits, submitting a secondary claim, posting payments, and appealing the insurance carrier's decision.

This book has been written so that it is easy to read and comprehend. It is designed for students who have not previously worked in the medical field as well as students who have worked in the field but have only been exposed to certain aspects of the billing process. An ideal employee at a medical practice has a clear understanding of how each element in the process affects all other steps, which is the underlying concept of this textbook. Practice exercises presented throughout the text allow students to test their knowledge of the concepts presented. This hands-on practice supplements lecture content and allows for better understanding of the skills presented.

Medical facilities are rapidly becoming more automated with each passing year. Historically, however, physician practices and hospitals have invested more funds in patient care equipment than in administrative equipment. According to the National Center for Health Statistics, only about 31% of hospital emergency departments, 29% of outpatient departments, and 17% of doctors' offices have electronic medical records to support patient care. The use of electronic records in health care lags far behind the computerization of information in other sectors of the economy. Although computerization of patient clinical records has been slow, electronic healthcare billing systems are used in three-quarters of physician office practices. Hence, this text reviews both automated and nonautomated procedures.

The Development of This Text

This book originated 5 years ago and was written by educational instructors who worked in the healthcare field for 10+ years prior to teaching. The authors' students routinely expressed dismay that the required textbooks did not provide a clear understanding of the order of the steps involved from the time a patient was scheduled for an appointment to the resolution of the patient's account. As a result of that feedback, the authors developed "workbooks" for each course in addition to the required reading materials. The workbooks ultimately became the chapters of this textbook. Students also stated that the required reading in their textbooks was outdated. Therefore, this textbook has a companion website that will provide the student and instructor with updated information and URLs where they can review current changes in the health-care industry.

Organization of the Text

The authors spent a great deal of time researching the material in this text in order to address the most frequently asked student questions and to clearly illustrate the key concepts of the medical billing and coding processes. The accumulated experience of the authors allows for a unique presentation of content, exercises, examples, and professional tips within each chapter.

Features of the Text

The following special features appear in this text:

Chapter Objectives: Each chapter begins with a list of key learning objectives that students should master on completion of the chapter.

Key Terms: A list of key terms appears at the beginning of each chapter, and the terms are highlighted where they are first introduced in the text. A comprehensive glossary is provided at the end of the text.

Case Studies with Critical Thinking Questions: A thought-provoking case study is presented at the beginning of each chapter along with critical thinking questions. Students must rely on the content in the text and their own critical thinking skills to answer the questions.

Introduction: Each chapter includes introductory material that explains to readers what they will encounter within the chapter.

Examples: Numerous examples are provided throughout the text to stress the correct use of the billing and coding guidelines being discussed.

Professional Tips: Professional Tips appear throughout the text and provide additional information related to billing and coding processes the student might use on the job.

Practice Exercises: Practice Exercises appear in most of the chapters to allow for student practice and mastery of skills.

HIPAA Icon: Any material within the text that is related to the Health Insurance Portability and Accountability Act (HIPAA) is flagged with an icon so that students can identify the "need to know" law. Appendix H also provides valuable information on HIPAA regulations.

Chapter Summary: The chapter summary serves as a review of the chapter content.

Chapter Review: End-of-chapter questions are provided in true/false, multiple choice, and completion formats and help reinforce learning. The review questions measure the students' understanding of the material presented in the chapter. These tools are available for use by the student or by the instructor as an outcomes assessment.

For Additional Practice: These additional case studies and billing and coding exercises allow for additional student practice and mastery of skills.

Resources: This listing provides additional information (organization contact information, websites, etc.) related to the chapter content.

The Learning Package

The Student Package

- Textbook
- CD-ROM: The interactive CD-ROM will provide students with more than 60 cases with which they can practice what they have learned. Students will be given a case study and access to the proper forms to use in either a guided practice or a test environment. To get started, students are presented with an interactive tutorial that will guide them through the billing process. The tutorial shows students how to move through the program and provides examples of the different information required by different providers on the various billing forms. Also offered on the CD-ROM are short, chapter-specific quizzes and HIPAA guidelines along with a full audio glossary. All of the tools on the CD-ROM will help students get the practice they may not have had the opportunity to receive during their internships.
- Student Workbook: The Student Workbook contains key terms, chapter objectives, chapter outlines, critical thinking questions, practice exercises, review questions, and end-of-workbook tests/case study-type problems that test student knowledge of the key concepts presented in the core textbook.
- Companion Website: Every student will have open access to our online study guide which contains helpful links, self test questions, and an online glossary. Students will be able to submit their results for a score that can be sent to a professor or themselves for further evaluation. This resource, combined with the Student CD, will give students the opportunity to put into practice those skills they are being taught in the classroom.
- Medical software: Medisoft coverage is provided in an appendix, and a Medisoft tutorial of 25 case studies is available for separate purchase.

The Instructional Package

- Instructor's resource manual: The Instructor's Resource contains chapter learning objectives, lesson plans for each learning objective with a customizable section for instructor notes, teaching tips, concepts for lecture, PowerPoint lecture slides that correspond to each concept for lecture, and suggestions for classroom activities.
- CD-ROM: The instructor's CD-ROM has a test generator and more than 1,500 test questions.
- PowerPoint slides: The slides can be used during daily lectures.
- Transition guides: These guides help make text implementation easy.

Deborah Vines has worked extensively for more than 20 years in the healthcare industry as a practice administrator and manager in physical therapy, dermatopathology, and pediatrics. She has also held management positions in the hospital setting. As director of operations for a national healthcare staffing corporation, she has traveled across the United States, working directly with physicians and medical human resources personnel to secure jobs for individuals in the medical billing, coding, and collection fields. A mentionable achievement of Ms. Vines' is that in one fiscal year she assisted 300 recruits to find employment in the medical billing industry through mentoring and training. This achievement led her to open Allied Career Center in Dallas, Texas, a successful vocational school specializing in medical office specialist training.

Ann Braceland, NCICS, has been working in the medical field since graduating from Gwynedd Mercy College with an associate's degree in nursing science. As a practice manager, her extensive work in the field of managed care and medical billing and coding allowed her to research and find means to inform others through her teaching of the changes and challenges that arise in the medical field. Mrs. Braceland has established and managed satellite offices in physical and occupational medicine. She is a Medicare representative with a vast spectrum of knowledge that she uses to train staff and physicians in compliance coding and billing. As director of training for the instructors of Allied Career Center in Dallas, Texas, her presentation of the material for students led to the publication of this book. Mrs. Braceland is a National Certified Insurance and Coding Specialist.

Elizabeth Rollins, NCICS, began her career in a nationally renowned, multiple-office pediatric ophthalmology practice. She worked in every position, from medical receptionist and appointment scheduling, to medical records and insurance claims submission, before being promoted to insurance/collection manager. She completed insurance claims by hand and typed the patient billing statements for 4 years until the practice became computerized. As a certified account manager for a national healthcare staffing corporation, Mrs. Rollins met with hospitals, physicians, clinics, and CBOs to assess their employment needs and showcase her roster of employees ready for hire. Elizabeth is a National Certified Insurance and Coding Specialist and enjoys instructing, writing courses, and helping students.

Susan Miller, NCICS, has 20 years of experience in the medical field and currently specializes in dialysis billing. She was previously a lead instructor at Allied Career Center in Dallas, Texas, preparing students for a career in the medical field as medical office specialists. She has acted as a supervisor at insurance companies and worked one on one with policyholders to assist them in better understanding their health insurance policies. In 2004 she obtained the title of National Certified Insurance and Coding Specialist. She also holds certificates from Career Colleges and Schools of Texas and Brookhaven College for interactive leadership skills for educators.

We would all like to thank our publisher, Prentice Hall; our editors, Joan Gill, executive editor, and Alexis Breen Ferraro, developmental editor; and the following reviewers, who used their personal time to provide feedback for our project. Without your hard work and guidance, none of this would have been possible:

Vanessa Armor, RHIT
Instructor
Ivy Tech Community College,
Michigan City Campus, Indiana

Dr. Robin Berenson
Spartanburg Community College,
South Carolina

Dorothy Burney
Adjunct Professor Allied Health/
Certified Coding Specialist
City College, Florida

Barbara Dahl, CMA, CPC
Medical Assisting Program Coordinator
and Department Chair
Whatcom Community College,
Washington

Susan DeGirolamo, RMA, NCPT, NCICS
Instructor
Pennsylvania Institute of Technology,
Pennsylvania

Annette Derks, CPC, CHI
Instructor
Canyon College, Florida

Shirley Jelmo, CMA, RMA
Medical Assisting Instructor
PIMA Medical Institute, Colorado

Kathy Kneifel
Instructor
Everett Community College, Washington

Tiffany Rosta, CMA
Medical Instructor
Kaplan Career Institute, Pennsylvania

Lorraine M. Smith
Instructor
Fresno City College, California

Teresa Williamson
Medical Coding and Billing Professor
Chaffey Community College, California

Chapter Opener Features

Chapter Objectives

Each chapter opens with a list of learning objectives, which can be used to identify the material and skills the student should know upon successful completion of the chapter.

▶

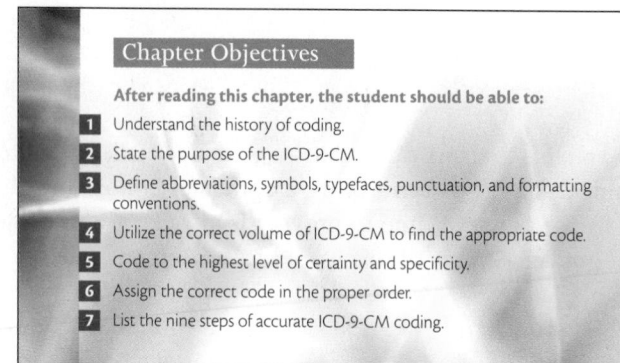

◀ Key Terms

The Key Terms section appears at the beginning of each chapter. The terms are listed in alphabetical order and the terminology appears in boldface on first introduction in the text. All terms are defined in the comprehensive glossary that appears at the back of the book.

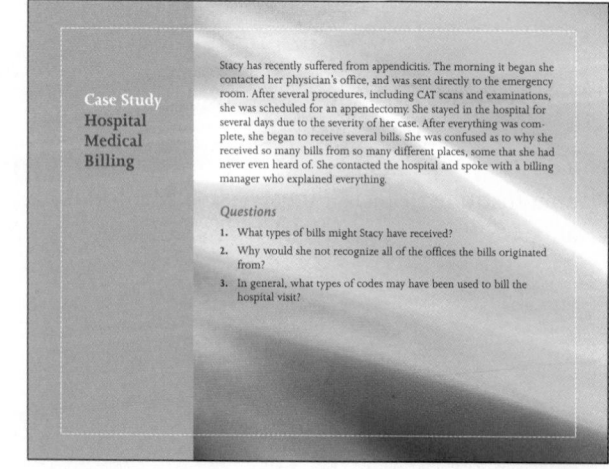

Case Study with Critical Thinking Questions

Thought-provoking case studies provide scenarios that help students understand how the material presented in the chapter relates to the medical billing and coding profession. Critical thinking questions appear after each case study, and students must rely on the content in the text and their own critical thinking skills to answer the questions.

▶

Additional Features

Professional Tips

Helpful billing and coding tips are interspersed throughout the text and provide additional information the student might use on the job.

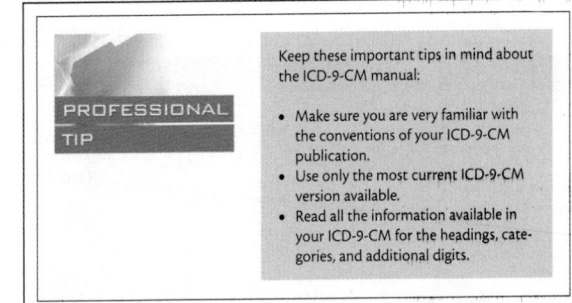

PROFESSIONAL TIP

Keep these important tips in mind about the ICD-9-CM manual:

- Make sure you are very familiar with the conventions of your ICD-9-CM publication.
- Use only the most current ICD-9-CM version available.
- Read all the information available in your ICD-9-CM for the headings, categories, and additional digits.

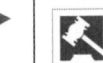

Example

An orthopedic surgeon has performed a knee replacement and during the postop follow-up, the patient presents with a sprained wrist due to a fall. The physician reports an E/M code with the 24 modifier appended to it for the management of the sprained wrist. 99024 is used for the normal postoperative visit. The "-24" appended to the E/M code, 99024-24, informs the payer that this is separate from the visit for the knee replacement.

Examples

Numerous examples are provided throughout the text to stress the correct billing and coding guidelines.

HIPAA Information

Any material within the text that is related to HIPAA is flagged with an icon so that students can identify the "need to know" law.

For electronic billing, the Health Insurance Portability and Accountability Act of 1996 (HIPAA) developed standards and regulations that the health industry must follow in order to standardize patient care. The law that regulates electronic billing is known as the Administrative Simplification Subsection of HIPAA, which covers entities such as health plans, clearinghouses, and healthcare providers. HIPAA refers to these entities as *covered entities*, which encompasses the medical practice or health plan and all of its employees. These regulations govern your job and behavior. When people working with billing in the medical field refer to HIPAA, they are generally referring to this subsection. The Administrative Simplification Subsection has four distinct components:

PRACTICE EXERCISE 9.2

Completion of CMS-1500 (Section I)

Fill out form locators 1 through 13 on the CMS-1500 form based on the information given here. To complete this exercise, copy the CMS-1500 form provided in Appendix D or download it from the CD-ROM that accompanies this text.

Liz Mary Smith is a patient in the medical office where you work. This information appears on her patient information form:

Name:	Liz Mary Smith
Gender:	Female
Birth Date:	July 1, 1996
Marital Status:	Single
Phone:	214-555-2984
Address:	4591 Explorer Drive
	Plano, TX 12345
Responsible Person:	Harry L. Smith (father)
Insured's DOB:	August 5, 1950
Insured's Gender:	Male
Insured's Home Address:	5419 W. 8th Street, Apt. 306
	Norman, OK 12345
Insured's Employer Address:	Vines Lumber Co.
	6840 Judy Street
	Norman, OK 12345
Social Security number:	425-68-3030
Insurance Carrier:	BMA
	P.O. Box 7459
	Memphis, TN 12345
Insurance Certificate Number:	78815-080-07-000
Insurance Group Number:	G123456

Treatment and progress notes in the patient medical record indicate diagnosis of left acute otitis media (382.9), on January 13, 20XX. The medical office collects only the coinsurance and waits for payment directly from the insurance carrier. Guarantor's signature on file for charges to be paid directly to provider, FORM SIGNED January 13, 20XX.

Authorization to release medical information on file.

Check the accuracy of your work by comparing your claim form to the completed claim form in Appendix J.

Practice Exercises

Practice Exercises provide students with the opportunity to practice and master skills presented in the text.

Informational Tables and Forms

These appear throughout the text and summarize pertinent information. They provide students with visuals and comparisons to reinforce the lesson.

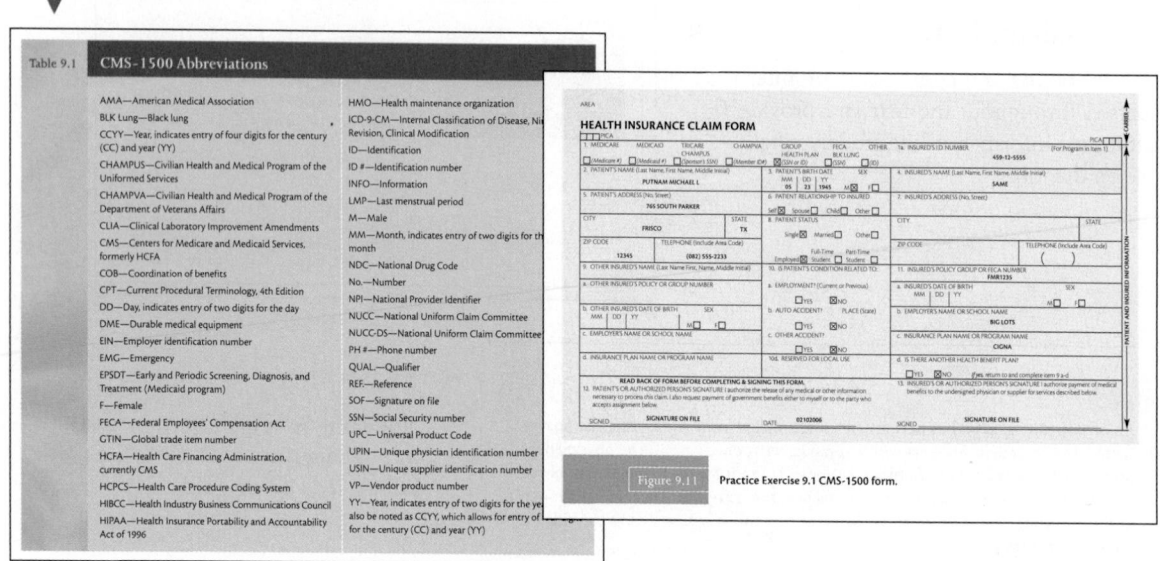

Table 9.1 CMS-1500 Abbreviations

AMA—American Medical Association
BLK Lung—Black lung
CCYY—Year, indicates entry of four digits for the century (CC) and year (YY)
CHAMPUS—Civilian Health and Medical Program of the Uniformed Services
CHAMPVA—Civilian Health and Medical Program of the Department of Veterans Affairs
CLIA—Clinical Laboratory Improvement Amendments
CMS—Centers for Medicare and Medicaid Services, formerly HCFA
COB—Coordination of benefits
CPT—Current Procedural Terminology, 4th Edition
DD—Day, indicates entry of two digits for the day
DME—Durable medical equipment
EIN—Employer identification number
EMG—Emergency
EPSDT—Early and Periodic Screening, Diagnosis, and Treatment (Medicaid program)
F—Female
FECA—Federal Employees' Compensation Act
GTIN—Global trade item number
HCFA—Health Care Financing Administration, currently CMS
HCPCS—Health Care Procedure Coding System
HIBCC—Health Industry Business Communications Council
HIPAA—Health Insurance Portability and Accountability Act of 1996

HMO—Health maintenance organization
ICD-9-CM—Internal Classification of Disease, Ninth Revision, Clinical Modification
ID—Identification
ID #—Identification number
INFO—Information
LMP—Last menstrual period
M—Male
MM—Month, indicates entry of two digits for the month
NDC—National Drug Code
No.—Number
NPI—National Provider Identifier
NUCC—National Uniform Claim Committee
NUCC-DS—National Uniform Claim Committee
PH #—Phone number
QUAL—Qualifier
REF—Reference
SOF—Signature on file
SSN—Social Security number
UPC—Universal Product Code
UPIN—Unique physician identification number
USIN—Unique supplier identification number
VP—Vendor product number
YY—Year, indicates entry of two digits for the year, also be noted as CCYY, which allows for entry of four digits for the century (CC) and year (YY)

Figure 9.11 — Practice Exercise 9.1 CMS-1500 form.

Chapter Review

Chapter Summary

Each Chapter Summary is an excellent review of the chapter content.

Chapter Summary

- Medicare is divided into two main programs: Medicare Part A, which is hospital insurance, and Medicare Part B, which is medical insurance.
- The fee-for-service method is a method of charging for healthcare services under which each procedure is based on a specific amount of reimbursement. Medicare determines their fees for service using the resource-based relative value scale reimbursement method.
- Recording the information from the Medicare card accurately is extremely important because that information will be used on many claims forms and medical documentation materials throughout the patient's history with the facility.
- A provider may choose to participate or not participate in the Medicare program. Medicare reimbursement depends on participation and non-participation.
- Medigap is a supplemental insurance sponsored by Medicare. It is an optional policy available to individuals who qualify for Medicare.
- For Medicare Part A the UB-04 is used for filing claims. The CMS-1500 is used for Medicare Part B.
- Medicare Fraud is knowingly and willfully executing, or attempting to execute a scheme to defraud any health care benefit program. Medicare abuse involves payment for items or services when there is no legal entitlement.

Chapter Review Questions

End-of-chapter questions are provided in true/false, multiple-choice, and completion formats, and help reinforce learning. The review questions measure the student's understanding of the material presented in each chapter. These tools are available for use by the student or can be used by the instructor as an outcome assessment.

> **4.** *Consultations:* Before coding a consultation, ask and answer questions about the service. If the answer is "no" to any of the following questions, do not report the service as a consultation:
> - Did you receive a request for an opinion from another physician?
> - Does the documentation of the service clearly demonstrate who made the request and the nature of the opinion requested?
> - Has the provider provided a written report of his or her opinion/advice to the referring physician?

Chapter Review

True/False

Identify the statement as true (T) or false (F).

_____ 1. There are four types of audits.

_____ 2. An accreditation audit is performed by the facility prior to claims submission.

_____ 3. Code edits are conducted by the medical coder.

_____ 4. When conducting an internal audit the three key elements reviewed are history, examination, and medical decision making.

_____ 5. Code edits screen for improperly or incorrectly reported procedure codes.

_____ 6. Compliance plans focus on training of physicians to use the AMA documentation guidelines for E/M services.

_____ 7. *Downcoding* refers to a coding method in which lower level codes are selected to avoid government investigation.

_____ 8. The term *external audit* may refer to an audit conducted by a consultant that the medical practice has hired.

For Additional Practice

Use the following information to complete a CMS-1500 form.

Physician Information:	Charles H. Borden, M.D.
	980 Frederick Road
	Dallas, TX 12345
Phone:	899-555-2276
EIN:	22-9872767
Professional License:	TX2056
UPIN:	3468923
Medicaid PIN:	K00J879
NPI:	1234568901
Patient Information:	Katherine Becker
	254 Pleasure Avenue
	Dallas TX 12345
	999-555-3457
DOB:	06/23/1954
Social Security number:	968-34-0025
Patient Account:	12358
Status:	Married
Sex:	Female
Patient's Insurance Information:	Medicaid ID# 5555211106
	1123 High Point
	Dallas, TX 12345
	800-973-1123

◀ For Additional Practice

These coding exercises and case scenarios provide students with additional opportunity to practice skills and reinforce concepts presented in the chapter. These tools are available for use by the student or can be used by the instructor as an outcome assessment.

Resources ▶

This listing provides additional information (organization contact information, websites, etc.) related to chapter content.

Resources

Alliance of Claims Assistance Professionals (ACAP)
873 Brentwood Drive
West Chicago, IL 60185-3743
www.claims.org; askacap@charter.net

American Academy of Professional Coders (AAPC)
2480 South 3850 West, Suite B
Salt Lake City, Utah 84120
Phone: 800-626-CODE
www.aapc.com; info@aapc.com

Certification information and other extensive information for coders, office managers, claims examiners, hospital outpatient coders, experienced reimbursement specialists, and coding educators. The website job ad section lets you post your résumé and receive job alerts by e-mail.

American Association for Medical Transcription (AAMT)
100 Sycamore Avenue, Suite M
Modesto, CA 95354
Phone: 800-982-2182
www.aamt.org

Provides career information, employment opportunities, networking, local association information, and approved education programs. You can post your résumé online and receive e-mail job alerts.

American Health Information Management Association (AHIMA)
233 North Michigan Avenue, 21st Floor
Chicago, IL 60601
www.ahima.org

Comprehensive Health Insurance
Billing, Coding, and Reimbursement

A Career in Health Care

1 Introduction to Professional Billing and Coding Careers

The content presented in this section will help the student understand the career opportunities available for the professional medical office specialist. Chapter 1 presents important information on professional billing and coding careers, including employment demands and trends, job descriptions, professional memberships, and the medical billing and coding certifications that are valuable to career advancement.

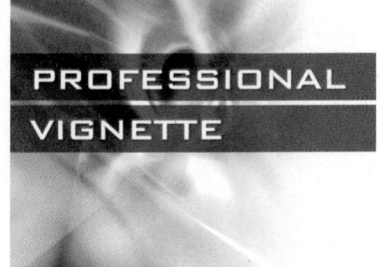

PROFESSIONAL VIGNETTE

My name is Gene Simon, RHIA, RMD (Risk Manager Designee). Having gone back to college later in life, and not wanting to be in a clinical position, I decided to enter the field of Health Information Management (HIM). It was a fascination of mine to be educated in the hugely diversified field of analyzing, abstracting and disseminating health data. I first thought the field consisted of only reading a medical record, but soon found out how wrong I was!

Through years of practice one becomes what the title suggests; a Registered Health Information Administrator. We work with, and must have a thorough knowledge of EVERY department and EVERY aspect of the medical facility. As I learned, practiced, climbed the ladder of success, and obtained positions beyond my wildest imagination, it dawned on me, "Why can't I pass on this invaluable information to the younger generation?".

I decided to become an instructor and then to become Supervisor of the Coding/Billing and HIM departments as well as "Educator of the year". But something was still missing from my goals; helping others to achieve "their" goals.

At this point in my life I have had hundreds of students in the hallways, in my classes and especially at graduation ceremonies step up and say with a big smile on their face and tears in their eyes, "Mr. Simon, you have changed my life, and for that I will be forever grateful". This is what being an instructor is all about; changing other people's lives for the better!

Chapter 1

Introduction to Professional Billing and Coding Careers

Chapter Objectives

After reading this chapter, the student should be able to:

1. Recognize different types of facilities that would employ allied health personnel.

2. Define job descriptions pertaining to a position.

3. Discuss options available for certification.

Key Terms

admitting clerk
centralized billing office
   (CBO)
certifications
insurance verification
   representative

medical biller
medical coder
patient account services
   (PAS)

registered health
   information technician
   (RHIT)

Case Study
Introduction to Professional Billing and Coding Careers

Elizabeth had nearly completed her course on medical billing and coding. As much as she had enjoyed the class, she was now concerned that she would only have one job choice. She discussed this matter with her instructor.

The instructor explained that with the training Elizabeth had received, she would have opportunities for diverse positions in a variety of medical facilities. Continuing her education by attending seminars in order to be aware of the ever-changing aspects of medical billing would increase her marketability and potential for advancement.

Questions

1. Make a list of the pros and cons of possible career options as you currently see them. Later in the course, reevaluate the issues you listed.

2. What medical facilities in your area would be potential employers of medical coders and billers?

3. How would joining professional organizations help you advance your career?

Introduction

In this textbook, the student will learn the process of submitting, coding, and resolving medical claims. There are many steps to this process. Procedures are dictated not only by the facility in which the medical office specialist works, but also by state and federal government regulations. To launch your new career, it is important that you understand the career opportunities that are available, the job titles and responsibilities for which you are qualified, and the certifications that are valuable for career advancement.

Employment Demand

Before the 1970s, it was common for a physician on receipt of his or her license to open a solo/private practice. The physician would practice independently, depending on advertising and referrals for the practice to grow. The staff consisted of a receptionist, a nurse, and possibly one or two support staff. As more and more patients began to use managed care, however, physicians faced financial difficulties. Clients had previously paid for services at the time they were rendered, but with managed care contracts it became the physician's responsibility to file claims and wait 30 days or longer for payment.

The delay in payment changed the way physicians' practices were managed. Physicians were forced to add additional staff to handle the processing of claims, and if claims forms were not submitted correctly or in a timely fashion, the financial health of the practice suffered—it is difficult to pay expenses with uncollected funds. The physician's increased staff needs created a demand for trained and certified medical billers, medical office assistants, and medical coders. Physicians and nurses comprise only 40% of all healthcare providers. The other 60% are allied health employees. Allied health employees are those members of the clinical healthcare profession whose positions are distinct from the medical and nursing professions. As the name implies, they are all allies in the healthcare team, working together to make the healthcare system function.

Facilities

Physician's Practice

The size of a physician's practice is generally categorized as solo/private practice, small group (3 to 9 physicians), or large group (10 or more physicians).

Solo/Private Practice

In the solo/private practice setting, the staff may consist of a nurse, a receptionist, and a medical biller and/or office manager. The receptionist and medical biller are often cross trained for coverage purposes.

Small-Group Practice

In a small-group practice, the physicians may have the same specialty, for instance, the group may consist of four or five general practitioners. Small-group practices frequently contract out their billing and accounts receivable. In addition to the medical receptionist, they may have a staff member who verifies insurance and one who assists with scheduling and checking patients in or out. These responsibilities fall under the title of medical office assistant. A medical records clerk or medical assistant may also be employed.

Large-Group Practice

An excellent example of a large group is a specialized practice, such as a back institute, which might consist of an orthopedic surgeon, neurosurgeon, internist, chiropractor, physiatrist, pain specialist, exercise physiologist, and a team of physical and occupational therapists. Large-group practices commonly handle claims and account receivables in house. Depending on how many physicians are in the group and what their specialties are, the large group may employ several people.

Hospital

Hospitals were also affected by managed care. It is very rare today to find a privately owned hospital; most are owned by corporations. In a large metropolitan area it is not uncommon for three or more hospitals with different names to actually be under one corporation. Examples of these corporations include Hospital Corporation of America (HCA) and Tenet Health Care Corporation. As an allied health employee, you may work in the admissions, outpatient, inpatient, or emergency departments. You could be employed as a patient access specialist in Patient Services or a scheduler in the Radiology Department.

Patient Account Services Facility

Previously, hospital facilities usually had a billing or financial department located on site that a patient could physically visit to address any billing concerns or make payments. Today there may still be a department such as this, but the staff's responsibilities are limited to answering basic questions. The actual handling and processing of data and claims is most often accomplished off-site. HCA, for example, refers to their off-site locations as **patient account services (PAS)**.

A PAS facility handles hospitals' claims and account receivables for the state in which the PAS facility is located and possibly for surrounding states. As many as 500 employees may work in one PAS facility. The patients, physicians, or hospital staff will never have contact with these individuals other than via telephone or computer. A PAS facility has multiple departments, such as Government Billing, Insurance Verification, Appeals, Correspondence, and so forth. Each department involves a variety of jobs. If you want a career with opportunities to advance, working in a PAS may be the ideal choice.

Centralized Billing Office

If a physician chooses not to handle claims within her facility, a contract will be signed with a **centralized billing office (CBO)**. CBOs contract with physicians to handle their claims and/or accounts receivable. A CBO can employ 2 to 3 people or well over 200. A CBO is similar to a PAS office except that it specializes in physicians' practices rather than hospitals. It is a separate entity from the physician's practice with different ownership.

Job Titles and Responsibilities

After completion of a course of study the medical office specialist is qualified for entry-level positions such as medical biller, government medical biller, payment poster, medical collector, refund specialist, insurance verification representative, medical records technician, admitting clerk and apprentice coder, medical receptionist, patient information clerk, medical secretary, medical records technician, or admitting clerk. Each facility will have its own specific job description and/or job title for each of the positions just listed. Knowledge of medical billing and coding is imperative to perform well in all of these positions because, even though medical billing may not be the primary responsibility of certain positions, every staff member influences the accuracy of information submitted on a medical claim such as the patient data, documentation of the procedure and diagnosis, and medical coding.

Medical Office Assistant

In some facilities, this position is also referred to as a medical, administrative medical assistant, secretary or medical receptionist. Medical office assistants usually work in physicians' offices. They are considered front office staff and primarily handle administrative duties. Responsibilities include organization and the ability to make the office function smoothly. In this position one might perform duties such as scheduling and confirming patients' diagnostic appointments, surgeries, and medical consultations. The medical office assistant might compile and record medical charts, reports, and correspondence; answer telephones; and direct calls to appropriate staff. He might also receive and route messages and documents such as laboratory results to appropriate staff as well as greet visitors, ascertain the purpose of the visit, and direct them to appropriate staff.

Medical Biller

Other job titles for a **medical biller** are billing specialist, patient account representative, claims processor, electronic claims processor, reimbursement specialist, and billing coordinator. Responsibilities may include submitting insurance claims, entering all patient data and charge information, and contacting the insurance carrier on outstanding or incorrectly paid claims.

Medical Coder

Healthcare professionals who manage the coding of medical records have job titles such as **medical coder**, health information coder, medical coding specialist, coding specialist, or health information technician. The duties and responsibilities may include research and reference checking of medical records and accurately coding the primary/secondary diagnoses and procedures using the International Classification of Diseases, Ninth Revision, Clinical Modification (ICD-9-CM) and the American Medical Association's Current Procedural Terminology (CPT®) coding books. They abstract and compile data from medical records for appropriate optimal reimbursement for physicians, hospitals, or professional charges.

Registered Health Information Technician (RHIT)

The **registered health information technician (RHIT)** position may also be referred to as coder, file clerk, health information clerk, health information systems technician, medical records analyst, medical records clerk, medical records director, medical records technician, or office manager. Job responsibilities may include compiling, processing, and maintaining medical records of physician and hospital patients in a manner consistent with the medical, administrative, ethical, legal, and regulatory requirements

CPT is a registered trademark of the American Medical Association.

of the healthcare system. The job involves reviewing records for completeness, accuracy, and compliance with regulations and the release of information to persons and agencies according to regulations.

Payment Poster

A *payment poster* generally reads the Explanation of Benefits documents issued by insurance carriers and posts the payments or contractual adjustments to the appropriate patient account. This requires excellent data entry skills, math skills, and a good working knowledge of insurance contracts.

Medical Collector

A *medical collector* contacts patients and insurance carriers to collect money owed to the medical facility. This position requires a great deal of patience and tact. Most of this job is performed on the telephone; however, after contacting an insurance carrier, it may be necessary to gather and send additional information before a claim can be processed. A medical collector may also be required to send patient billing statements.

Refund Specialist

A *refund specialist* analyzes patient accounts to discern whether or not a refund is required and, if so, to whom the money should be returned. This position requires researching and analytical skills.

Insurance Verification Representative

An **insurance verification representative** contacts insurance carriers to verify benefit information for patients. This individual may also perform precertification and/or prior authorization of services duties. Determining a patient's financial responsibility prior to services being rendered is often required.

Admitting Clerk or Front Desk Representative

The **admitting clerk** or front desk representative has face-to-face contact with patients. Registering and greeting patients, having patients complete paperwork, answering questions, data entry of patient demographic and insurance information, and requesting information and payment are the general duties of the admitting clerk position. Dealing with patients who may be upset or irritable is also required. In some facilities, the admitting clerk is responsible for appointment scheduling; in other facilities, the scheduler is a separate position.

Patient Information Clerk

The patient information clerk is responsible for answering questions about and explaining Health Insurance Portability and Accountability Act (HIPAA) privacy regulations, living wills, do-not-resuscitate (DNR) orders, other information and to patients and their family members. This position may also require data entry of patient demographics and/or appointment scheduling.

Professional Memberships

Professional memberships help you stay current in your field. They can offer information about upcoming conferences and professional development opportunities. As a member, you will be eligible to attend the group's conferences. Whether at the state, regional, or national level, professional conferences offer excellent opportunities to build your network of professionals in the field, learn the latest developments in your field, and take professional courses and seminars. Professional membership is an excellent addition to your résumé. It shows you are involved and dedicated to your particular field. Professional associations publish journals and/or newsletters that are helpful for keeping you up to date on issues and developments in your field. When you are interviewing for a position, this can be invaluable information. You can read about companies or individuals with whom you would like to work.

With your membership, you will often have access to member information. Contacting someone in your field about possible employment as a fellow member of the association may open a door. It is recommended that you join at least one professional organization, but research them beforehand to find the appropriate one for your career goals. These organizations may have a local chapter as well, so check your local telephone directory for local groups.

Certifications

Medical billing and coding **certifications** are valuable to your career advancement. Medical billing and coding certificates are available at every level of expertise. Certification for medical coding and billing is not a requirement for employment, but having a few billing and coding certifications will definitely help you to advance your medical billing or medical coding career. Examples of certification agencies are the American Health Information Management Association (AHIMA), American Academy of Professional Coders (AAPC), National Center for Competency Testing (NCCT), and the National Healthcareer Association (NHA). General and contact information for these agencies are listed at the end of this chapter in the Resources section.

Medical Office Assistant Certification

National Certified Medical Office Assistant

To achieve certification as a National Certified Medical Office Assistant (NCMOA), you must have a high school diploma or equivalent. You must have graduated from an approved program of study as a medical office assistant or provide documentation of 1 year of experience as a medical office assistant. The exam requires areas of study in computer literacy, business communication, medical terminology, law and ethics, patient control, insurance, office procedures, and Occupational Safety and Health Administration (OSHA) regulations. The NCMOA certification is awarded through the NCCT.

Certified Medical Administrative Assistant

To qualify as a certified medical administrative assistant (CMAA), you must be a graduate of a healthcare training program or have one or more years of full-time job experience. The CMAA certification is awarded through the NHA.

Medical Billing Certifications

Certified Medical Billing Specialist

A candidate for Certified Medical Billing Specialist (CMBS) certification is an individual who is motivated to improve her medical billing knowledge and develop new skills to assist providers in maximizing their reimbursement through proper coding and documentation. To achieve certification, an individual must successfully complete a series of six courses and provide the Medical Association of Billers (MAB) with a supervisor's, provider's, or instructor's evaluation of billing performance. The CMBS certification is awarded by MAB.

Medical Coding Certifications

Certified Coding Associate

Coders who earn the Certified Coding Associate (CCA) certification, awarded by AHIMA, can immediately demonstrate their competency in the field, even if they don't have much job experience. Earning a CCA demonstrates a commitment to coding even for those who are new in the field. The CCA should be viewed as a starting point for an individual starting a new career as a coder.

Certified Professional Coder

The Certified Professional Coder (CPC) certification is designed to evaluate a medical coder's knowledge of medical terminology, human anatomy, ICD-9-CM concepts, the Health Care Procedure Coding System (HCPCS) concepts, coding concepts, surgery and modifiers, evaluation and management concepts, anesthesia coding, radiology, laboratory and pathology concepts, and medicine. To receive the CPC certification, you must have 2 years of work experience and pass the certification exam. Those applicants who are successful in passing the certification examination, but have not met the required coding work experience, will be awarded the initial designation Certified Professional Coder–Apprentice (CPC-A). The CPC certification is awarded through the AAPC.

Certified Professional Coder–Hospital

Because there are distinct differences in CPT coding for physician services versus outpatient facility services, the AAPC has a separate examination and certification for outpatient facility coding titled Certified Professional Coder–Hospital (CPC-H). To receive the CPC-H certification, you must have 2 years of work experience and pass the certification exam. Those applicants who are successful in passing the certification examination, but have not met the required coding work experience, will be awarded the initial designation Certified Professional Coder–Hospital–Apprentice (CPC-H-A).

Certified Coding Specialist

Coding accuracy is very important to healthcare organizations because funding cannot be received without accurate coding. Accordingly, the Certified Coding Specialist (CCS) demonstrates tested skills in medical coding. The CCS certification exam assesses mastery or proficiency in coding rather than entry-level skills. The CCS certification is awarded through AHIMA.

Certified Coding Specialist–Physician

The Certified Coding Specialist–Physician (CCS-P) certification demonstrates expertise in physician-based settings such as physicians' offices, group practices, and specialty clinics. The CCS-P certification exam assesses mastery or proficiency in coding rather than entry-level skills. If you perform coding in a doctor's office, clinic, or similar setting, you should consider obtaining the CCS-P certification to demonstrate or validate your ability. The CCS-P certification is awarded through AHIMA.

Medical Records Certification

Registered Health Information Technician

Registered health information technicians are health information technicians who ensure the quality of medical records by verifying their completeness, accuracy, and proper entry into computer systems. RHIT certification proves proficiency and ability in accurate patient record maintenance, management, and analysis. The RHIT certification is awarded through AHIMA.

Chapter Summary

- Changes in the way health care is paid for created a demand for allied health personnel trained in medical billing and coding.
- An allied health employee can find employment in a variety of medical settings.
- After completion of a course of study, the student is qualified for entry-level positions such as medical biller, insurance verification representative, admitting clerk, and medical collector.
- Certification demonstrates dedication to advancement and competency.

Chapter Review

True/False

Identify the statement as true (T) or false (F).

 1. PAS is an abbreviation for patient account services facility.

 2. The medical office assistant might compile and record medical charts, reports, and correspondence.

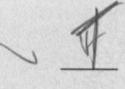 3. HIPAA is an abbreviation for Hospital Information Per American Medical Association.

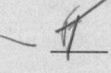 4. Certification is not required in most states.

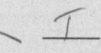 5. Math skills are important when working with refunds and posting of payments.

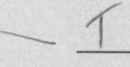 6. Coding accuracy is very important to healthcare organizations because funding cannot be received without accurate coding.

T   **7.** Registered health information technicians are health information technicians who ensure billing of medical records by verifying their completeness, accuracy, and proper entry into computer systems.

T   **8.** An admitting clerk may be responsible for appointment scheduling.

I   **9.** A collector may be required to send out patient billing statements.

I   **10.** A medical office assistant is considered front office staff and primarily handles administrative duties.

Multiple Choice

Identify the letter of the choice that best completes the statement or answers the question.

B   **1.** A business that contracts with physicians to handle their claims and/or accounts receivable is referred to as a(n):
   a. physician billing office.   c. accounts receivable corporation.
   b. centralized billing office.   d. billing and coding facilitator.

D   **2.** A person who is considered front office staff and primarily handles administrative duties is called a(n):
   a. medical secretary.   c. medical receptionist.
   b. medical office assistant.   d. all of the above.

C   **3.** A health information technician has the responsibility to:
   a. contact patients about their outstanding balance.
   b. assist the physician in surgery.
   c. research and code medical records.
   d. provide patients with information about their software.

b   **4.** What job description requires excellent data entry skills, math skills, and a good working knowledge of insurance contracts?
   a. medical records technician   c. insurance verifier
   b. payment poster   d. contract reviewer

D   **5.** A medical collector will contact most patients by:
   a. mail.   c. in person.
   b. during appointments.   d. telephone.

A   **6.** A refund specialist position requires:
   a. researching and analytical skills.   c. data entry and math skills.
   b. patience and tact.   d. organization and telephone skills.

D   **7.** What job description routinely requires face-to-face contact with the patient?
   a. medical biller   c. medical collector
   b. insurance verifier   d. admitting clerk

_A_ **8.** Professional memberships help their members by:
  a. providing current information in their field.
  b. organizing social events.
  c. providing legal services.
  d. assisting with verifying benefits.

_A_ **9.** An example of a certification agency is:
  a. American Health Information Management Association.
  b. American Academy of Professional Workers.
  c. National Center for Coding Testing.
  d. National Heart Association.

_D_ **10.** What abbreviation stands for a coder who specializes in hospital coding?
  a. HPC-C
  b. CHC-P
  c. CPC-P
  d. CPC-H

Completion

Complete each sentence or statement.

1. What are the three common sizes of physician practices? __Individual__, __3-9__, __10 ⇁__.

2. __PSR__ and __Billing Spec__ are other job titles for a medical biller.

3. As a medical collector it is important to have __patience__ and __tact__.

4. The knowledge of medical __billing__ and __Coding__ is imperative to perform well in all medical administrative positions.

5. A medical office assistant may be also referred to as a medical __secr.__ or medical __adminsitrato__

6. The payment poster generally reads the __ICD-9__ from insurance carriers and posts the payments or contractual adjustments to the appropriate patient account.

7. An insurance verification representative will determine the patient's financial responsibility __prior__ to services being rendered.

8. Professional membership is an excellent addition to your __Resume__.

9. To receive the CPC-H certification, you must have __2__ years of work experience and pass the certification exam.

10. The registered health information technician certification is awarded through the __AHIMA Health employees__

Resources

Alliance of Claims Assistance Professionals (ACAP)
873 Brentwood Drive
West Chicago, IL 60185-3743
www.claims.org; askacap@charter.net

American Academy of Professional Coders (AAPC)
2480 South 3850 West, Suite B
Salt Lake City, Utah 84120
Phone: 800-626-CODE
www.aapc.com; info@aapc.com

Certification information and other extensive information for coders, office managers, claims examiners, hospital outpatient coders, experienced reimbursement specialists, and coding educators. The website job ad section lets you post your résumé and receive job alerts by e-mail.

American Association for Medical Transcription (AAMT)
100 Sycamore Avenue, Suite M
Modesto, CA 95354
Phone: 800-982-2182
www.aamt.org

Provides career information, employment opportunities, networking, local association information, and approved education programs. You can post your résumé online and receive e-mail job alerts.

American Health Information Management Association (AHIMA)
233 North Michigan Avenue, 21st Floor
Chicago, IL 60601
www.ahima.org

AHIMA is an association of health information management (HIM) professionals. Members are dedicated to the effective management of the personal health information needed to deliver quality health care to the public. Founded in 1928 to improve the quality of medical records, AHIMA is committed to advancing the HIM profession in an increasingly electronic and global environment through leadership in advocacy, education, and certification.

American Medical Billing Association (AMBA)
4297 Forrest Drive
Sulphur, OK 73086
Phone: 580-622-2624
www.ambanet.net/AMBA.htm

The AMBA website presents information about online courses, networking opportunities, and information on preparing for the examination to become a certified medical reimbursement specialist.

Health Professions Institute (HPI)
P.O. Box 801
Modesto, CA 95355-0801
Phone: 209-551-2112
www.hpisum.com

This organization publishes many books and periodicals and conducts seminars for the medical transcription community. HPI has a free Student Network and information on medical transcription courses. *Perspectives* magazine, an electronic magazine, is free to medical transcription professionals.

Healthcare Information and Management Systems Society (HIMSS)
230 East Ohio, Suite 500
Chicago, IL 60611-3269
Phone: 312-664-4467
www.himss.org

The HIMSS website includes a membership directory, résumé posting, and job alerts, and allows you to research potential employers and career development resources with résumé and interviewing advice and more. Members only.

Medical Association of Billers
2701 North Tenaya Way, Suite 190
Las Vegas, NV 89128
www.physicianswebsites.com

The Medical Association of Billers is an internationally recognized billing and coding support organization created in 1995 in Las Vegas, Nevada. Their purpose is to provide medical billing and coding specialists with a reliable source for procedural and diagnostic coding information.

Medical Coding and Billing
Information about coding and billing careers can be accessed at *www.medicalcodingandbilling.com*. This site includes certification, education, and medical office management career information.

Medical Group Management Association (MGMA)
104 Inverness Terrace East
Englewood, CO 80012
Phone: 303-799-1111 or 877-275-6462
www.mgma.com

This organization is designed for supervisors of medical group practices. The website lists job ads, networking and internship information, and a Core Learning Series for education. Job ads are compiled in a monthly publication titled *MGMA Connections*.

Medical Records Institute
425 Boylston Street, 4th Floor
Boston, MA 02116
Phone: 617-964-3923
www.medrecinst.com; cust_service@medrecinst.com

This organization promotes electronic and mobile health records, among others.

MT Jobs
www.mtjobs.com

Sponsored by MT Daily, this site provides free job searches, résumé posting, e-mail job alerts, and employer profiles.

MT Monthly
106 Norway Lane
Oak Ridge, TN 37830
Phone: 800-951-5559 or 865-387-5555
www.mtmonthly.com

MT Monthly is a national newsletter for medical transcriptionists. *MT Monthly* currently offers the book entitled *Working as a Medical Transcriptionist at Home*. The website has links to placement services, products, and related websites.

National Center for Competency Testing (NCCT)
7007 College Boulevard, Suite 705
Overland Park, KS 66211
www.NCCTinc.com

Established in 1989, NCCT is able to work as an independent certifying agency in order to avoid any allegiance to a specific organization or association. In this way, NCCT is able to work with many organizations, but can remain independent of any outside allegiances, bias, or agenda. Every applicant interested in sitting for a certification exam must meet NCCT requirements and must pass a criterion-referenced examination.

National Healthcareer Association (NHA)
134 Evergreen Place, Ninth Floor
East Orange, NJ 07018
Phone: 800-499-9092 or 973-678-9100
www.nha2000.com

The NHA offers education, training, and certification for many healthcare jobs, including Certified Medical Transcriptionist and Certified Billing and Coding Specialist.

Professional Association of Health Care Office Managers (PAHCOM)
461 East Ten Mile Road
Pensacola, FL 32534-9714
Phone: 800-451-9311
www.pahcom.com

The PAHCOM website has information on education, local chapters, and the Certified Medical Manager exam. The benefits page of the website posts job openings.

The Relationship between the Patient, Provider, and Carrier

The chapters in this section will provide the student with the knowledge of the history of health care in America, the different types of insurance plans and insurance plan coverage, and the types of managed care organizations and alternative healthcare plans available to patients. Because the majority of payments received in a medical facility come from insurance carriers, it is necessary for the medical office specialist to understand the complexities of the different insurance plans. This section will outline the different job responsibilities of the medical office specialist, such as contacting insurance carriers for benefits information, estimating patient financial responsibility, and filing insurance claims.

This section also presents information on managed care and medical contracts, the importance of ethics in managed care, and outlines the roles of the medical office specialist in reviewing MCO contracts.

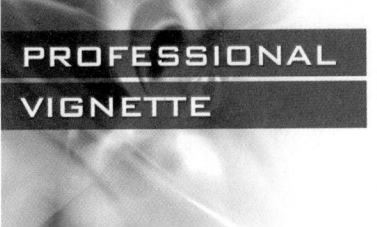

PROFESSIONAL VIGNETTE

My name is Susan DeGirolamo, RMA, NCPT, NCICS. I started in this field because I needed a career in which I was able to support my two boys as a single mother. At the age of 32 I returned to school full-time. This meager leap became a major stepping-stone for me. I began as a medical assistant for a surgeon where I learned much more than any school could simulate. It was at this facility that I inherited the job of billing—by hand. This tedious assignment, lead me to continue my education and earn my certification as a biller and coder. Thanks to my experiences in the field and continued education I went into teaching so that I can help students be able to take that first step that may also lead them anywhere. I have been presented with the opportunity to write curriculum and also review medical textbooks that are used in the same type of school from which I graduated. Education is a powerful tool, and I am still learning as I write this notation. I am pursuing my Associates Degree in the Allied Health field, not knowing the expanse of possibilities that lies before me, but knowing that I will become even more empowered.

Chapter 2 | Understanding Managed Care: Insurance Plans

Chapter Objectives

After reading this chapter, the student should be able to:

1 Understand the history and impact of managed care.

2 Be able to discuss the organization of managed care and how it affects the provider, employee, and policyholder.

3 Calculate the financial responsibility of the patient.

4 Identify the type of managed care plan in which a patient is enrolled.

5 Recognize various types of insurance coverage.

Key Terms

assignment of benefits
carriers
coinsurance
commercial health
   insurance
copayment
deductible
enrollee
group Insurance
health maintenance
   organization (HMO)

inpatient
insured
managed care
managed care
   organization (MCO)
outpatient
point-of-service (POS)
policyholder
preauthorizations
preexisting condition

preferred provider
   organization (PPO)
premiums
primary care physician
   (PCP)
providers
referral
special risk insurance
subscribers
utilization

Case Study
Managed Care
Terminology

Upon arriving at Dr. Brown's Office, Mary was asked for her insurance card. As she handed the card over, Rebecca, the medical office specialist, noted that it was an HMO plan. After Mary's appointment, Rebecca was asked to schedule the patient to meet with Dr. Thomas, a general surgeon. Rebecca remembered that Mary was on an HMO plan and checked to see if the plan would allow Mary to see Dr. Thomas. He was listed as a participating provider. She scheduled the appointment and placed a referral on file with the HMO. A copy of the referral was given to Mary to take with her.

Questions

1. What does it mean that Mary is on an HMO plan?
2. Why was it important that Rebecca checked to see if Mary could see Dr. Thomas?
3. What is the purpose of the referral, and why did Rebecca give the patient a copy?

Introduction

Because the majority of payments received in a medical facility come from insurance carriers, the medical office specialist must understand the complexities of the different types of insurance plans. Understanding insurance plans and how the changes in our healthcare system came about is important for being able to explain the system to patients who have questions. Other responsibilities of the medical office specialist include contacting insurance carriers for benefits information, estimating patient financial responsibility, and filing insurance claims. The patient's benefits are also referred to as their schedule of benefits. The schedule of benefits list what procedures will and will not be covered by the health plan. This chapter helps medical office specialists meet those responsibilities by explaining the intricacies of various types of health plans.

The History of Health Care in America

A medical office specialist serves patients from diverse generations and ethnic groups. The medical office specialist must take this into consideration when responding to questions and remarks made by patients. Knowledge of the history of health care in America will assist the medical office specialist when communicating with patients.

Twenty years ago the majority of the population paid doctors directly for their services or purchased health insurance policies sold by companies who based their cost of doing business on their expenditures plus a reasonable added profit. In the past, private insurers or **carriers** did not have to advertise, lobby, or contribute to political causes. Patients could choose any doctor they wished to provide care. The population was content with this arrangement until the cost of health care began to rise and gave birth to the idea of managed care.

Prior to managed care, the American health care system financially rewarded healthcare **providers** (the individual or facility providing medical care) for giving more care, and patients paid directly for that care. The employer would select a healthcare policy for its employees and pay all **premiums** (the costs of purchasing the insurance policy). The employee could accept or decline and find insurance through his spouse or independently. Usually the employee would not decline because the only expense to him would be the annual **deductible** (the amount employees had to pay out of their pockets before insurance began paying) that had to be met. Once the employee reached his deductible, he did not have a financial reason or concern if medical costs increased.

Medical costs continued to escalate due to an aging population and the development of high-technology procedures and pharmaceuticals. Society began excessively suing providers and, to protect themselves, providers practiced "defensive" medicine to avoid malpractice suits and jury awards. Defensive medicine resulted in tests and drugs being ordered or prescribed that may not have been necessary. Insurance companies continued to pay the providers increased fees to cover the providers' rising costs of making more services available, and the insurance companies charged higher premiums to the employers. Employers were no longer financially able to pay the full premium for their employees and began requiring the employee to contribute monetarily. Employers began having their employees contribute a percentage of the premium, such as 20% or 30%. When employees saw their take-home pay decreasing, in addition to having to meet a deductible each year, they began to protest the cost of medical care. This also happened to government-funded programs, except instead of raising premiums, the federal and state governments raised taxes. The unchecked expense of the health care continued. The government could not ignore the outcries of the public.

The healthcare crisis meant that, despite the high quality of care available to many Americans, the cost of health care had grown so rapidly that many people were uninsured or underinsured. Traditional ways to control costs had not proven successful. As a result, employers had chosen not to extend health insurance to a number of employees and, if necessary, to hire temporary employees who were not eligible for health insurance benefits to avoid the high costs of purchasing the insurance.

Likewise, the federal and state governments faced a continuing budget crisis caused in large part by the rise in healthcare expenditures as a total portion of the budget. Budget cuts and deficits continued at the state and federal levels, while policy makers struggle with how to control healthcare costs. Although the answers are not easy, the question the nation asked was "How do we lower healthcare costs without jeopardizing the quality of and access to care?"

As in most financial disputes, each party considered the other party responsible for the cost of health care. Employers pressured insurance companies to control premiums. Insurance companies pressured providers to control costs. Employees wanted the employer to provide them with insurance options in order to feel ownership of the money spent for their care. The government felt it necessary to intervene. The government's solution was **managed care**. Managed care is a method of controlling healthcare costs and ensuring that medical care is available to everyone.

The idea of managed care has been a long-standing concept, but one that was only offered to those who were employed or associated with a few visionaries, such as Henry Kaiser, an American industrialist and shipbuilder. The timeline in Table 2.1 shows the progress of managed care through its inception to today.

Table 2.1	Managed Care Timeline
1917	Western Clinic in Tacoma provides prepaid physician services for the lumber industry.
1929	Dr. Justin Ford Kimball at Baylor Hospital in Texas establishes the Baylor Plan, a prepaid hospitalization plan that first uses the Blue Cross logo.
	Ross-Loss prepaid medical clinic is started by Drs. Donald Ross and H. Clifford Loss under contract with the Los Angeles Department of Water and Power for its employees.
	Rural Farmers' Cooperative Health Plan is started by Michael Shadid in Elk City, Oklahoma.
1933	Dr. Sidney Garfield establishes prepaid plan to fund care for his Contractors General Hospital, which provided care to workers on the Los Angeles aqueduct.
1937	The Group Health Association (GHA) is started in Washington, D.C., to serve employees of the Federal Home Loan Bank.
1938	Henry J. Kaiser recruits Dr. Garfield to establish a prepaid clinic and hospital care for his Grand Coulee Dam project in Washington State.
1939	The Blue Shield program is adopted for participating prepaid physician plans.
1942	At the request of Henry Kaiser, Dr. Garfield expands the Grand Coulee program to Kaiser-managed shipyards and the Kaiser steel mill.
1945	Group Health Cooperative of Puget Sound is established in Seattle, Washington.
	Permanente Health Plans opens to the public in California, in addition to serving Kaiser employees.

(continued)

Table 2.1	Managed Care Timeline (continued)

1947	The American Medical Association (AMA) is indicted and convicted of antitrust violations due to organized efforts to curb physician participation in group health plans.
	Health Insurance Plan (HIP) of Greater New York is established to serve New York City employees.
1949	Eighty-one Blue Cross hospital plans and 44 Blue Shield medical plans cover 24 million Americans.
1952	Permanente Health Plans changes name to Kaiser, while medical group retains Permanente name. Kaiser membership grows to 250,000.
1954	First individual practice association (IPA) is formed, the San Joaquin Medical Foundation, in California.
1955	Kaiser expands to Oregon and total membership reaches 500,000.
1958	Kaiser expands to Hawaii.
1959	Blue Cross companies cover 52 million Americans and Blue Shield plans cover 40 million.
1963	Kaiser membership reaches 1 million.
1968	Kaiser expands to Colorado and Ohio.
1970	Paul Ellwood coins the term *health maintenance organization* (HMO).
1973	The HMO Act of 1973 is signed into law by President Nixon, using federal funds and policy to promote HMOs.
1976	Kaiser membership reaches 3 million.
1979	Blue Cross Blue Shield collectively covers 87.4 million Americans.
1980	Kaiser expands to the Mid-Atlantic region.
1981	Kaiser membership reaches 4 million.
1982	California legislation is enacted that allows selective contracting for Medicaid and private insurance, paving the way for other states to enact similar laws facilitating preferred provider organizations (PPOs).
	The Tax Equity and Fiscal Responsibility Act (TEFRA) makes it easier and more attractive for HMOs to contract with the Medicare program.
1985	National total HMO enrollment reaches 19.1 million.
1990	National total HMO enrollment reaches 33.3 million.
	National PPO enrollment surpasses HMO enrollment with 38.1 million members.
	The National Committee for Quality Assurance (NCQA) is established.
1991	HEDIS is released. HEDIS is a set of standardized performance measures designed to ensure that purchasers and consumers have the information they need to reliably compare the performance of managed health care plans.
1994	Blue Cross Blue Shield Association eliminates requirement that all member plans must maintain not-for-profit status.
1995	National total HMO enrollment reaches 50.6 million.
1996	The Health Insurance Portability and Accountability Act of 1996 (HIPAA) includes patient privacy compliance and health plan portability provisions.
1999	NCQA initiates accreditation of PPOs, which now cover 89 million Americans.
2000	National total HMO enrollment is 80.9 million, declining for the first time from the previous year's level of 81.3 million in 1999.
2003	The Medicare Prescription Drug Improvement and Modernization Act establishes a Part D drug benefit, establishes health savings accounts (HSAs), renames the Medicare+Choice program to Medicare Advantage, and increases payment rates to Medicare Advantage plans.
2004	National total HMO enrollment is 68.8, and national PPO enrollment is 109 million.
2006	National total HMO enrollment is 67.7, and national PPO enrollment is 108 million.
	Medicare Part D prescription benefit becomes effective.

Medical Reform

Medical reform has been in existence for many decades. Historically, any changes to the provision of health benefits to the public affected the employer, employee, and insurer—the changes rarely affected the provider. In reading this chapter, however, it will become evident that in the last decade the provider and medical facilities have been required to revamp the way they operate their businesses and provide patient care. Providers have not succumbed easily to these changes.

Managing and Controlling Healthcare Costs

Managed care is a system that, in theory, controls the cost and delivery of health services to members who are enrolled in a specific type of healthcare plan.

The goals of managed health care were and still are to ensure that:

- Providers deliver high-quality care in a facility that manages or controls costs.
- Medical care or procedures are medically necessary and appropriate for the patient's condition or diagnosis.
- Medical care is rendered by the most appropriate provider.
- Medical care is rendered in the most appropriate, least-restrictive setting.

The way in which the managed care systems ensure delivery of high-quality care while managing and controlling costs is through networks and discounted fees for services.

When a **managed care organization (MCO)** contracts with a physician or medical facility, reimbursement for each procedure is paid at a discounted fee. The discounted fee is determined by the MCO, which views the fee as the usual and customary fee. The provider has a standard or usual fee that she charges each patient per a procedure code. The provider's standard fee is on the insurance claim when submitted to the MCO. The MCO will reimburse the provider according to the agreed-on discounted fee ("contract fee"), which is a component of the contract. Because the discounted fee is lower than the

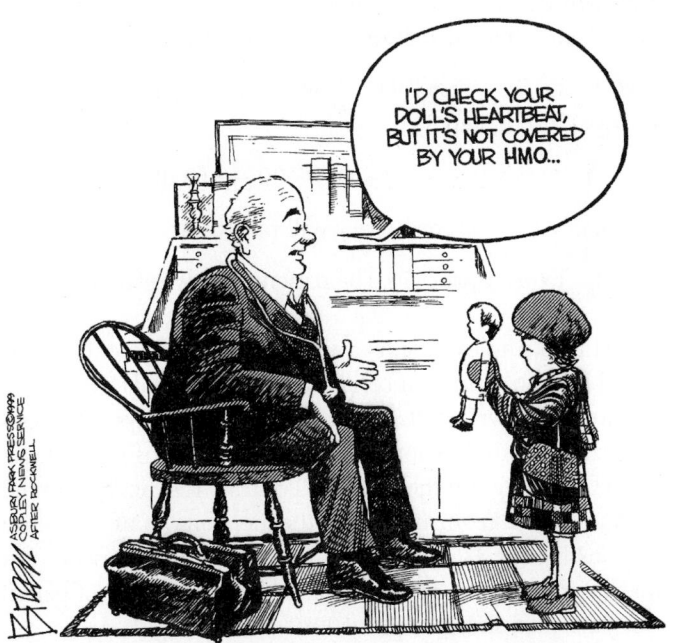

Reprinted by permission of Copley News Service and Steve Breen.

provider's standard fee, the provider will write off the difference between the standard fee and contract fee. The provider accepting the lower reimbursement reduces medical costs.

Discounted Fees for Services

An insurance carrier can state in an insurance contract that it will pay "reasonable and customary fees" or "usual, customary, and reasonable fees." These may be referred to as "R and C fees" or "UCR fees," respectively.

A *usual fee* is an individual provider's average charge for a certain procedure (that is, the standard fee). For example, a general practitioner may consistently charge $30.00 for brief office visits. Such charges would be shown on the doctor's fee schedule and charge slip.

A *customary fee* is determined by what doctors with similar training and experience in a certain geographic location typically charge for a procedure. For example, the range for an appendectomy performed by surgeons in a certain metropolitan area might range from $875.00 to $1000.00. Therefore, a surgeon's charge of $900.00 would be considered a customary fee and would be covered by insurance. Another surgeon who charges $1200.00 for the same procedure would only receive $900.00 in payment from the insurance carrier.

As a medical office specialist, you may need to estimate the amount due from a patient prior to services being rendered. For accounting purposes, knowing the expected payment from the carrier and the write-off (adjusted amount) is also necessary. The following explanation and Practice Exercise 2.1 will help the medical office specialist in determining dollar amounts. To determine the amount paid by the carrier, any adjustment or write-off, and the amount due from the patient (or paid at the time of service by the patient), use the following steps:

Billed Amount	$400.00	No deductible
Allowed Amount	$275.00	$10.00
		copay

STEP 1   *Contractual adjustment or write-off amount.* Subtract allowed amount from billed amount:

$$\$400.00 - \$275.00 = \$125.00$$

This will be the write-off amount or contractual adjustment. Once it has been determined, all other calculations will deal with the $275.00 allowed amount.

STEP 2   *Carrier's responsibility.* Subtract any unpaid deductible or copay (if no deductible or copay, go to Step 3):

$$\$275.00 - \$10.00 = \$265.00$$

This is the portion the carrier will pay toward the medically necessary procedure.

STEP 3   *Patient responsibility.* The patient is only responsible for the copay in this example.

This example presents a very simple scenario. On claims that involve unpaid deductibles and coinsurance, further math calculations are required. Determining discounted fees, write-offs, coinsurance, and copays requires knowledge of basic algebra including addition, subtraction, and figuring of percentages.

The carrier and the provider contract for the discounted fee, which is the "allowed amount." The co-insurance is the percentage of the allowed amount the patient is responsible for. As an example, if the insurance carrier's rate of benefit is 75%, the remaining 25% is the patient's coinsurance. Total rate of benefits after the patient and carrier have paid should equal 100%.

Calculate the financial responsibility of the carrier and the amount the physician must write off.

1. Ginger Smith was seen in Dr. Sampson's office today for an allergic reaction to a prescribed drug. Total charges today are $100.00. Allowed amount is $77.00.

   $23⁰⁰ _____ $ 77 _____

   Discount amount   Carrier pays provider

2. Wesley Camp is having outpatient surgery at the Day Surgery Center. Mr. Camp is on a PPO plan. His benefits pay at 80%. Total charges today are $2400.56. Allowed amount is $1976.23.

   424.33 _____   1976.23 _____

   Discount amount   Carrier pays provider

3. Scott Snyder is being seen in Dr. Eveready's office today for hypertension. Mr. Snyder is on an HMO plan. Dr. Eveready is an endocrinologist. Scott does not have a referral. Total charges today are $166.00. Allowed amount is $110.00.

   56 _____   110 _____

   Discount amount   Carrier pays provider

4. Andrew Payne is having outpatient surgery at the Carrollton Surgery Center. Total charges are $2225.00. Allowed amount is $2000.00. Benefits pay at 40%.

   225.00 _____   800 _____

   Discount amount   Carrier pays provider

5. Robin Hughes is being seen in Dr. Barry's office today to have a toothpick removed from his toe. Total charges today are $125.00. Allowed amount is $95.00.

   30 _____   95 _____

   Discount amount   Carrier pays provider

6. Douglas Jackson was seen in the doctor's office today to remove a mole from his left cheek. Total charges today are $377.00. The allowed amount is $217.00. Benefits pay at 75%.

   377
   217 = 160.00 _____   162.75 _____   → discount amt (217.00)
                                                          x
   Discount amount   Carrier pays provider   x benefit (.75%)

On completion of this exercise, refer to Appendix J to check the accuracy of your work.

Medically Necessary Patient Care

When doctors and medical facilities sign contracts with managed care organizations, they are, in theory, improving the care they are providing to patients. However, under a managed care contract, a physician or facility has guidelines to which they must adhere for medically necessary procedures. These policies and guidelines are not public information. Therefore, patients are not aware of these guidelines, which restrict a provider from ordering extensive tests or procedures to pinpoint the actual diagnosis.

Requiring the provider to justify what services are being provided to the patient emphasizes the question of medical necessity. In rendering a service to a patient, the provider must determine if the service is medically necessary. The diagnosis may be warranted; however, the treatment provided may not.

The definition of *medical necessity* is written into each contract a physician signs with an MCO. For instance, HMO contracts are stricter than PPO contracts. Therefore, physicians have to approach the services they choose to provide to their patients based on the type of policy the patient has.

MCOs have grown and with this growth they have developed more stringent utilization services that providers must follow when ordering tests or surgery. **Utilization** refers to the pattern of care for a medical service. Utilization guidelines help the MCO determine if a service, whether it is a procedure or test, is medically necessary. These guidelines are used by MCOs to deny medical services to patients, so providers must determine the necessity of tests and services prior to providing them. They must assess the care they feel is required to accurately diagnose or treat the patient based on the MCO contract they have with the patient's insurance company.

At times, patients are forced to be discharged from hospitals when the MCO case manager has determined that the length of hospital stay they are being provided is not medically necessary. For example, a physician may schedule inpatient surgery, but the MCO case manager may override an inpatient stay because, according to the MCO utilization guidelines, the patient's care is best suited for outpatient care.

Care Rendered by Appropriate Provider

One goal of managed care is for patient care to be provided by the most appropriate provider. This goes hand in hand with providing cost-efficient, quality services to patients. This goal has been attained in several ways.

Managed care utilizes a network of providers. This is true in HMOs, PPOs, and **point-of-service (POS)** plans. Each MCO provides a wide array of physicians and hospital services from which an **enrollee** (person enrolled in a contract with the insurance plan) can choose. They also contract with independent laboratory and diagnostic facilities. In doing so, each enrollee has the ability to choose his provider (depending on which managed care plan he is enrolled in) and receive services.

An MCO enrollee may be required to choose a **primary care physician (PCP)**. HMOs utilize PCPs most often. The PCP, also referred to as a *gatekeeper*, is the provider who coordinates a patient's care. Commonly, a general practitioner, family medicine physician, obstetrician/gynecologist (OB/GYN), or internal medicine doctor acts as the patient's PCP. If the PCP cannot provide care, the PCP will refer the patient to the appropriate specialist within the network who can provide the needed medical care. If a patient wishes to see a specialist, the patient must first schedule a visit with her primary care physician. If the PCP feels an appointment with a specialist is warranted, he will authorize the visit to the specialist. Use of a primary care physician cuts down on unnecessary visits to specialists and unnecessary tests. The PCP is required to make every attempt to diagnose and treat the patient prior to referring her to a specialist.

Appropriate Medical Care in Least Restrictive Setting

A goal of all MCOs is for the patient to receive care in the most appropriate and least restrictive setting. These restrictive settings are important to the efficiency and delivery of health care in the provider's facility. The PCP or the specialist within the network has requirements to meet as to where the patient is sent for radiology, laboratory, mammography, and other types of services.

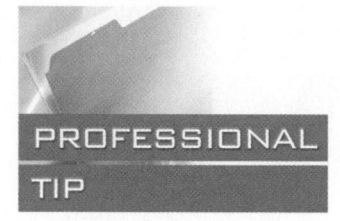

The medical office specialist needs to be familiar with the patient's MCO plan with regard to where services can be obtained. In order for the insurance carrier to pay, the patient may only seek services from a facility within his plan network.

Withholding Providers' Funds

An MCO may have a *withhold program*, now known as *pay for performance*. A withhold program refers to a provision in an MCO contract, which states that the MCO will withhold a percentage of the physician's revenue until year-end. This allows the MCO to evaluate the physician's medical management in terms of its cost effectiveness. If the physician has not sent the patients for numerous diagnostic tests, procedures, etc., the amount withheld will be paid to the provider. If the physician has ordered several expensive tests, the MCO may keep the amount withheld. This type of verbiage is an incentive for the provider not to order tests. The purpose of withholding programs is to encourage providers to utilize cost-effective services and procedures. The pay for performance program is aimed at allowing providers to give good quality care within the networks' facilities while reducing costs.

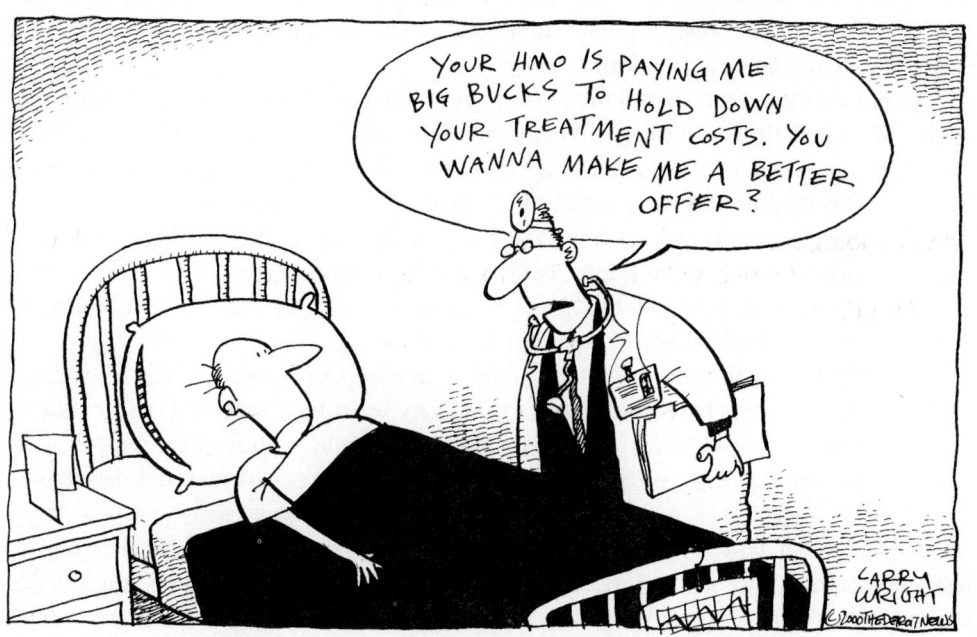

Reprinted by permission of Larry Wright.

Types of Managed Care Organizations

The major types of managed care plans are:

- Health maintenance organizations
- Preferred provider organizations
- Point-of-service plans.

Each of these plans has distinctive features or characteristics.

Health Maintenance Organization (HMO)

A popular alternative to traditional insurance programs is the **health maintenance organization (HMO)**, which is a medical center or a designated group of providers that provides medical services to **subscribers** (persons who are covered on the insurance policy) for a fixed monthly or annual premium. The **policyholder**, interchangeably called the *insured, subscriber,* or *member,* usually has a very small (or no) copayment when he needs services.

A **copayment** is a fixed dollar amount the member pays for each office visit or hospital encounter. The plans have various rules for copayment, coinsurance, and deductible amounts. **Coinsurance** is the portion of the provider's fees that the patient has to pay. The subscriber to an HMO plan is able to obtain health care on a regular basis with unlimited medical attention. Thus, HMOs encourage subscribers to take advantage of preventive healthcare services in an attempt to make healthcare coverage more cost efficient. HMOs do tend to cover more preventive procedures such as annual physicals, prostate cancer testing, and mammography.

- A distinctive feature of an HMO is that the subscriber chooses a primary care physician, who is sometimes known as a gatekeeper. The PCP arranges, provides, coordinates, and authorizes all aspects of a member's health care. PCPs are usually family doctors, internal medicine doctors, general practitioners, or OB/GYNs.
- An HMO enters into contractual arrangements with healthcare providers (e.g., physicians, hospitals, and other healthcare professionals) and together form a provider network.
- Members are required to see only providers within this network if they are to have their health care paid for by the HMO. If the member receives care from a provider who isn't in the network, the HMO will not pay for care unless it was preauthorized by the HMO or deemed an emergency.
- Members can only see a specialist (e.g., cardiologist, dermatologist, rheumatologist) if they are referred and the PCP authorizes the service. The **referral** must be approved by the HMO. If the member sees a specialist without a referral, the HMO will not pay for the service.
- HMOs are the most restrictive type of health plan because of the restrictions the members have in selecting a healthcare provider. However, HMOs typically provide members with a greater range of health benefits for the lowest out-of-pocket expenses, such as either no or a very low copayment and deductible.

As mentioned, HMOs greatly restrict whom a patient may see for medical services. This restriction significantly reduces members' premiums. HMOs have generated considerable controversy; as in many plans doctors receive financial incentives for reducing the amount of medical services provided to patients. One method of doing this has been to pay doctors a fixed monthly fee for each patient. Another method is to have physicians on staff. The physician works for the HMO medical center and receives an annual salary and benefits just like any employee.

The four main types of HMOs, discussed next, vary in the way they link providers in order to create a healthcare delivery system.

Group Model HMO

A group model HMO is an organization that contracts with a multispecialty physicians' group to provide physician services to an enrolled group. Physicians are employees of the group practice and generally are limited to providing care only to the HMO's members.

Individual Practice Association HMO

Individual practice association (IPA) HMOs are the most decentralized and involve contracting with individual physicians to create a healthcare delivery system. The HMO contracts with community hospitals and providers of services such as laboratories and diagnostics. Pharmacy services are provided through a contracted network of independent and chain community pharmacies and mail order service.

Network Model HMO

Network HMOs contract with more than one community-based multispecialty group to provide wider geographical coverage. The group practices under contract with one HMO vary from large to small, from primary care to multispecialty practice.

Staff Model HMO

The staff model HMOs employ salaried physicians who treat members in facilities owned and operated by the HMO. Most services, including diagnostic, laboratory, and pharmacy services, are provided on-site. A team of health professionals delivers the care.

Preferred Provider Organization (PPO)

The **preferred provider organization (PPO)** contracts with physicians and facilities to perform services for PPO members at specified rates. These rates, or fees, are contractually adjusted so that the PPO member is charged less than nonmembers. The PPO gives subscribers a list of PPO member-providers from which subscribers can receive health care at PPO rates. If a patient chooses to receive treatment from a provider who is not in the PPO network, the patient has to pay any difference between the PPO's rate and the outside provider's rate. PPOs generally require preauthorization for major medical services.

Each physician in a practice may be a member of more than one PPO, and all the doctors in the practice may not necessarily belong to the same PPO. Some of the main features of PPOs include the following:

- PPOs are similar to HMOs in that they enter into contractual arrangements with healthcare providers (e.g., physicians, hospitals, and other healthcare professionals) and together form a provider network.
- Unlike an HMO, members don't have a PCP (gatekeeper) nor do they have to use an in-network provider for their care. However, PPOs offer members higher benefits as financial incentives to use network providers. The incentives may include lower deductibles, lower copayments, and higher reimbursements. For example, if the subscriber sees an in-network family physician for a routine visit, she may only have a small copayment or deductible. If she

sees a non-network family physician for a routine visit, she may have to pay as much as 50% of the total bill.

■ PPO members typically do not have to get a referral to see a specialist. However, as mentioned earlier, there's a financial incentive to use a specialist who is a member of PPO's provider network.

■ PPOs are less restrictive than HMOs in the choice of healthcare provider. However, they tend to require greater out-of-pocket payments from their members.

Point-of-Service (POS) Options

Because many patients do not wish to accept services from only their HMO providers, some HMO plans add a point-of-service option. Patients who choose this option do not have to use only the HMO's physicians. However, if they choose to see physicians outside the network, they must pay increased deductibles and coinsurance. This option makes the HMO more like a PPO, in terms of choices available to the patients.

■ The reason it is called a *point-of-service* option is because members choose which option—HMO or PPO—they will use each time they seek health care.

■ Like an HMO and a PPO, a POS plan has a contracted provider network.

■ POS plans encourage, but do not require, members to choose a primary care physician. As in a traditional HMO, the PCP acts as a "gatekeeper" when making referrals. Members who choose not to use their PCPs for referrals (but still seek care from an in-network provider) still receive benefits but will pay higher copays and/or deductibles than members who use their PCPs.

■ POS members also may opt to visit an out-of-network provider at their discretion. If that happens, the member's copayments, coinsurance, and deductibles will be substantially higher.

■ POS plans are becoming more popular because they offer more flexibility and freedom of choice than standard HMOs.

Criticism of MCO

Managed care has not been without its trouble or criticism. Some of the major issues that face HMOs, prepaid medical groups, and government-sponsored managed care plans are providing necessary care in emergency situations and providing long-term care for the chronically ill. MCOs are criticized for not offering patients the ability to appeal or hold liable the MCO with regard to procedures and even surgeries the MCO has denied on the basis of them not being medically necessary.

MCOs will contract with hospitals to provide care for their enrollees. When an enrollee suffers a medical emergency, she must go to an in-network hospital or emergency clinic in order for the service to be covered under the MCO's policy. In addition, policies require that the MCO be notified within 48 hours after admission; however, calling an MCO is often the last thing a patient thinks about during an emergency. An enrollee should not assume that all physicians in the hospital network are participating in the managed care plan.

For example, Kaiser HMO has facilities throughout the United States that are structured as staff model HMOs. The patient must go to that one facility for all medical care, including the hospital. In an emergency this can be very risky. Consider the situation in which a woman who lived in Dallas, Texas, began having labor contractions. She called an ambulance and the baby was delivered while en route. The Kaiser hospital was located in central Dallas, miles away and the roads were heavy with traffic. If she had admitted herself, or if the ambulance had taken her to any other hospital, the medical cost would not have been covered by her Kaiser HMO policy. Many MCO contracts have been modified and addendums added to accommodate emergency situations, but sometimes it takes many phone calls and appeals to the MCO by the patient and provider to receive reimbursement. Table 2.2 outlines the advantages and disadvantages of managed care organizations.

Patients diagnosed with hypertension, diabetes, cancer, renal disease, or other diseases requiring ongoing treatment may run into problems with their MCO. These patients' treatments are often costly and require services from many providers. Some managed care plans' requirements, such as referrals and **preauthorizations** (written approval) for treatment, actually add a layer of bureaucracy and cost to the delivery of care and sometimes lead to delays in necessary care. The most progressive managed care plans identify these patients and provide case managers to ensure efficient delivery of services and patient compliance with treatment plans to provide high-quality service and to avoid the catastrophic costs associated with long and avoidable hospital stays.

Many health plans have also been criticized for not allowing patients to appeal treatment decisions other than through the MCO-governed arbitration process. A sample of a *treatment decision* would be the MCO denying a procedure or diagnostic test because it claims it is not medically necessary. For the toughest cases involving the potential use of costly, experimental treatments, progressive HMOs are adding impartial panels of medical experts to determine what care is medically appropriate. The health plans that are not addressing the concerns of their enrollees, particularly if they are for-profit plans, face an enormous backlash of public criticism for not balancing the need to control costs while preserving access to high-quality services.

Alternative Healthcare Plans

In recent years, several different types of alternative healthcare plans have emerged, giving patients a broader choice in the type of insurance coverage they can carry.

Exclusive Provider Organization

Exclusive provider organizations (EPOs) are a type of managed care plan that combines features of HMOs (e.g., enrolled members, limited providers' network, gatekeepers, utilization management, preauthorization system), and PPOs (e.g., flexible benefit design, negotiated fees, and fee-for-service payments). An EPO is referred to as *exclusive* because employers agree not to contract with any other plan. Members are eligible for benefits only when they use the services of the network of providers with certain exceptions for emergency or out-of-area services. If a patient decides to seek care outside the network, generally he is not reimbursed for the cost of treatment. Technically many HMOs can be considered EPOs except that EPOs are regulated under insurance statutes rather than federal and state HMO regulations. As a result, the EPO is priced lower than a PPO to the employer, but an EPO's premiums are usually more expensive than an HMO's premiums.

Independent Physician Association

A group model HMO, such as an *independent physician association (IPA)*, sometimes referred to as an *individual physician alliance*, represents providers who have formed an organization

Table 2.2	Advantages and Disadvantages of Managed Care Organizations

Advantages of Managed Care	Disadvantages of Managed Care
MCOs help to restrain the overall growth of healthcare costs by demanding discounted prices from doctors and hospitals for care.	When an enrollee suffers a medical emergency, he must go to an in-network hospital or emergency clinic in order for the service to be covered under his policy.
Hospitals and physicians are acting more efficiently in order to attract MCOs. MCOs contract with large companies and enroll a significant number of members, which forces providers to lower their own costs and to strive to improve the quality of their care. This means reducing overhead costs and the number of unnecessary tests they perform.	A managed care plan typically restricts the physician's latitude in caring for patients. The utilization guidelines of a managed care company may strongly suggest a plan of treatment different from the plan preferred by the treating physician. This situation could increase the likelihood of a malpractice suit being brought against that provider.
The MCOs collect and analyze data on how well they deliver care, such as identifying what percentage of children in an HMO are immunized. This information is combined with outcomes data to help document how well the HMO is meeting its needs. This helps consumers choose the best managed care plan for their families.	The physician runs the risk of obtaining unfavorable or undesirable results by enrollees of the managed care company. This can have a financial impact on the physician's practice. These members can require an extraordinary amount of the physician's time because of their age group or medical conditions.
The data the managed care plan gathers is analyzed for clinical services. This tells how well a patient does when she receives a particular service, such as cataract surgery. The outcome data measures how much difference the MCO's intervention made in the consumer's health and quality of life. This data helps providers understand if a procedure or test is necessary for treatment.	Managed care companies can create an increased administrative burden on a physician's office because of incompatible claims systems, the need for authorization before providing care, required physician interaction with utilization review departments, and required quality assurance reporting.
Managed care plans are creating disease management programs and care pathways. For example, an HMO could design and implement a disease management program for patients with diabetes that combines health education, routine blood sugar testing, doctor visits, and drug therapy. HMOs develop their disease management programs with the help of experts, in particular medical specialties, and they rely heavily on the latest studies of what works best for particular types of patients.	A participating provider may experience additional financial burdens if the managed care company requires participating physicians to carry additional malpractice insurance.
Plans make extensive use of healthcare professionals, such as physicians' assistants, nurse practitioners, and certified nurse midwives. These practitioners, who have less training than physicians, work with doctors to provide many basic healthcare services to consumers and are less costly than physicians for MCOs to employ. They can also perform many of the primary case tasks that physicians do and provide very high-quality care for a wide range of illnesses at a lower cost.	MCOs negotiate fees with providers that are lower than the providers' usual fees. If the negotiated fees are too low this could cause the provider "to make up the difference" by seeing more patients. Seeing more patients per day may result in not enough time being spent with each patient; thus, resulting in patient dissatisfaction.
Plans are continuously studying new medical technologies and drugs in order to keep abreast of new medical products and services and to determine what is safe and most effective for consumers and under what conditions these services or products should be made available. They are assessing everything from what prescription drugs to offer to what kinds of surgical implants MCO members should be receiving.	

to provide prepaid health care to individuals and/or groups who purchase the coverage. Subscribers must exclusively use the affiliated members of the IPAs, such as designated doctors, pharmacies, and hospitals. Physicians in a group model HMO are not employees of the plan. Instead, they remain self-employed and see both members of the HMO and nonmember patients.

Physician-Hospital Organization

A *physician-hospital organization* (PHO) is another approach to coordinating services for patients. Physicians join with hospitals to create an integrated medical care delivery system. Surgery centers, nursing homes, laboratories, and other facilities may also be connected with the PHO. This union then makes arrangements for insurance with a commercial carrier or an HMO.

Self-Insured Employers

A *self-insured plan* is one in which the payer is an employer or other group, such as a labor union. Assuming the full risk for the payment of healthcare services, the employer or labor union uses the premium it would have paid an insurance carrier to establish a fund to provide benefits for its employees or group members.

The employer may contract with an organization to manage and pay the claims for the employees' medical services. The "health plans" will be administered by an insurance company (known as a third-party administrator or TPA).

The medical office specialist needs to know if the **insured** person's plan is self-insured by the patient's employer. Self-insured plans are regulated by the Employee Retirement Income Security Act (ERISA). This law regulates all MCOs that have been contracted as third-party administrators for a self-insured employer. ERISA is regulated by the U.S. Department of Labor and does not abide by state insurance rules and regulations. A medical office specialist who finds it necessary to file a complaint with such a carrier on an issue such as a denied claim or an incorrect payment will be appealing to federal courts.

A medical office specialist will need to recognize the type of MCO policy a patient has and the characteristics of the policy. Table 2.3 summarizes the different MCOs and their characteristics.

Insurance Plans

To provide protection for hospitalization and medical expenses, various prepaid medical care plans have been established. Some are private, such as Blue Cross Blue Shield, and some are government sponsored, such as Medicare, Medicaid, Tricare, and CHAMPVA.

Commercial Health Insurance

Commercial health insurance is a general term for policies offered through for-profit companies such as Aetna, Prudential, and United Healthcare. The policy can be fee-for-service policy or a managed care one. Such policies are licensed and regulated by a State Board of Insurance according to the state in which the companies are located or the state in which they are incorporated.

Table 2.3	Various Types of MCOs and Their Characteristics

HMO	PPO	POS	EPO
■ State licensed ■ Most stringent guidelines ■ Limited network of providers ■ Members assigned to PCPs ■ Members must use network except in emergencies or pay a penalty ■ Usually there is a financial reward to providers for managing the cost of care	■ Limited network of providers but larger than HMO ■ Members may be assigned to PCPs but restrictions on accessing other physicians not as tight as in HMO ■ Financial penalty for accessing non-network providers less severe than in an HMO ■ Usually there is no reward to providers for managing the cost of care	■ Hybrid of HMO and PPO networks ■ Members may choose from a primary or secondary network ■ Primary network is HMO-like ■ Secondary network is often a PPO network ■ Out-of-pocket expenses are lower within the primary network and higher when using the secondary network ■ Members have more choices with less expense than with a PPO	■ Doesn't have an HMO license ■ Members are eligible for benefits only when they use network providers ■ Financial penalties for members leaving the network are similar to those of HMO ■ Priced lower than a PPO but higher than an HMO
IPA Model HMO	**Staff Model HMO**	**Network Model HMO**	**Group Model HMO**
■ An association formed by physicians with separately owned practices (solo or small group) ■ HMO may contract with physicians separately or through the IPA	■ HMO hires the physicians and pays them salaries ■ HMO owns the network ■ HMO owns the clinic sites and health centers	■ HMO uses two or more group practices or a group practice plus a combination of staff physicians and contracted independent physicians to form a network of providers ■ Allow members to choose their providers	■ HMO contracts with multi-specialty groups. ■ May be open-panel or closed-panel

Types of Insurance Coverage

Insurance can be classified as either **group insurance** or individual insurance. With group insurance, one master policy is issued to an organization or employer and covers the eligible members or employees and their dependents. Thus, all the members or employees have similar healthcare coverage. Group insurance plans provide better benefits with lower premiums than individual insurance plans. Individual insurance applies only to the person taking out the policy and to that person's dependents. Because it is not obtained at a group rate, the premiums are higher than for group insurance.

Descriptions of the major types of health insurance coverage follow. A basic health insurance policy might include hospital, medical, and surgical insurance. A comprehensive insurance package would include several of the major types of insurance listed next.

Indemnity/Fee for Service

An indemnity plan provides coverage for all medically necessary services. The policy-holder and/or patient may receive medical services from the provider they choose. The provider is reimbursed for his services if it is the usual and customary fee. No fee discounts are taken. The provider does not have to request preauthorization for services.

Hospital

Hospital insurance provides protection against the costs of hospital care. It generally provides a room allowance (a stated amount per day for a semiprivate room) with a maximum number of days per year. Special provisions are made for operating room charges, x-rays, laboratory work, drugs, and other medically necessary items while the insured person is an **inpatient**. An inpatient is a person who is admitted to the hospital for a minimum of 24 hours.

Hospital Indemnity Insurance

This insurance offers limited coverage. There are two different methods by which a patient may receive benefits. The policy may pay a "per diem" or fixed amount for each day the patient is in the hospital and states a maximum number of days it will pay. The payment goes directly to the patient who may use it for medical services or other expenses such as prescriptions. Usually, the amount the patient receives is less than the cost of the hospital stay. The other method of payment will pay a portion of the patient's medical expenses after another policy has paid. This is considered a supplemental policy.

Medical

Medical insurance covers benefits for **outpatient** medical care including physicians' fees for hospital visits and nonsurgical procedures. The term *medical* refers to physicians' costs. Special provisions are made for diagnostic services such as laboratory, x-ray, and pathology costs. An outpatient is a person who receives medical care at a hospital or other medical facility but who is not admitted for more than 24 hours.

Surgical

Surgical insurance provides protection for the cost of a physician's fee for surgery, whether it is performed in a hospital, in a doctor's office, or elsewhere, such as a surgical center. Charges for anesthesia generally are covered by surgical insurance.

Outpatient

Outpatient insurance usually provides protection for emergency department visits and other outpatient divisions in a hospital or medical facility such as x-ray, pathology, and psychological services.

Major Medical

Major medical insurance offers protection for large medical expenses established by a regular health insurance policy. There is usually an added cost for this type of insurance coverage.

Special Risk

A person can also obtain protection against a certain type of accident (for example, an airplane crash) or illness (for example, cancer) through **special risk insurance**.

Catastrophic Health Insurance

This insurance is among the least expensive forms of health insurance. Deductibles are generally large for these types of policies. There may also be caps on the amount the policy will pay in case of illness. These policies are only suitable for individuals with the financial means to handle routine illnesses and hospitalizations.

Short-Term Health Insurance

Short-term life insurance can only be purchased for a specific period of time. Coverage provided by such policies ranges from catastrophic to comprehensive, with the latter being considerably more expensive. Short-term health insurance often comes with strict qualifying procedures and may not cover preexisting medical conditions. A **preexisting condition** is a diagnosis that the insured has previously been treated for. In particular, pregnancy and childbirth are not usually covered by these policies.

COBRA Insurance

A federal law makes it possible for most people to continue their group health coverage for a period of time. Called COBRA (for the Consolidated Omnibus Budget Reconciliation Act of 1985), the law requires that if the insured works for a business of 20 or more employees and leaves his job or is laid off, he can continue to get health coverage for at least 18 months. However, the person will have to pay the entire premium, including the employer's portion, rather than just the portion of it he paid when he was working.

People are also able to get insurance under COBRA if their spouses were covered but they are now widowed or divorced. Also, if somebody was covered under her parents' group plan while in school, she can continue in the plan for up to 18 months under COBRA until she finds a job that offers her health insurance.

Full-Service Health Insurance

These policies cover all illnesses, allow treatment virtually anywhere, and come with deductibles as high or as low as policyholders are willing to pay for. At the other end of the health insurance spectrum, Medicare/Medicaid is a form of public health insurance available to retirees and low-income individuals.

Long-Term Care

This insurance covers both medical and custodial services. These services can range from at-home care, including assisting someone with daily personal and household chores, to day care services at a facility, to assisted living residences, to nursing home care. The degree of care is based on the current requirements and condition of the person who is in need of long-term care.

Supplemental Insurance

Supplemental insurance is purchased to cover expenses, such as coinsurance, that are not covered by the primary insurance policy. An example is a Medigap policy, which is a supplemental health insurance policy sold by private insurance companies to fill the "gaps" in the original Medicare plan coverage. If a patient has a commercial policy, however, he cannot use a Medigap policy.

The Provider's View of Managed Care

Managed care has its pros and cons (as discussed earlier in Table 2.2). Providers are required to follow contractual agreements with the carriers in order to receive payment for services provided. Some physicians or providers see these agreements as restrictions on their way of providing medical care and managing their facilities. The standard length of a contract between an MCO and a provider is 1 year. If a physician discovers that there are too many restrictions, she has to give a written 30- or 60-day notice before she can close the practice to members of the MCO plan. (This is why a provider is sometimes listed in a directory but is no longer participating in the network.)

Patient Care

HMOs, PPOs, and fee-for-service plans often share certain features, including preauthorization, utilization review, and discharge planning.

A patient may be required to get preauthorization from their plan or insurer before admission to a hospital for certain types of surgery. If preauthorization is not obtained, then the cost of the procedure will not be covered. Utilization review is the process by which a plan determines whether a specific medical or surgical service is appropriate or medically necessary. Discharge planning is an approach that facilitates the transfer of a patient to a more cost-effective facility if the patient no longer needs to stay in the hospital. For example, if, following surgery, a patient no longer needs hospitalization but cannot be cared for at home, the person may be transferred to a skilled nursing facility.

Facility Operations

Contracting with an MCO requires that the provider implement changes in the operation of their facilities, staff, and methods of treating patients. Providers have to reduce inefficiency and waste in their own operations. As a result, physicians are joining larger groups of doctors that can provide a wide range of primary care and specialty services. This makes it easier to refer patients from one doctor to another. By joining a larger group, the doctors can share expenses by sharing office space, staff, utilities, etc.

Some providers are doing less testing before surgery. Hospitals are developing care pathways to help move consumers through their hospital stays as efficiently as possible. In a care pathway, the hospital studies the services the patient needs and plans the entire treatment program for the whole stay.

Verifying Insurance Coverage

The administrative staff or medical office specialist must obtain complete and accurate information on a patient who comes into the doctor's office or hospital. Not only is this information helpful in facilitating the care of the patient, but it is also necessary for the processing of insurance claims. Most facilities maintain this information in the computer database. If the information is kept in the patient's chart, it must be separated from the patient's medical records with regard to any clinical component. All patient demographics and insurance information must be updated on a regular basis.

If a patient has a health insurance plan, the medical office specialist should ask to see the identification (ID) card. This card states the name of the insurance policy, the subscriber's name, and the insurance policy number. The front and back of the card should be photocopied and a current copy kept in the patient's file.

After receiving the insurance information, whether via phone, fax, mail or when the patient completes information at the time of the visit, the insurance must be verified. The medical office specialist should call the insurance company and verify the information on the card. The following questions should be asked after establishing what type of plan the patient has: the amount of the deductible and whether it has been met, coinsurance or copay amounts, any exclusions, limitations, or riders on the policy, any preexisting conditions, lifetime maximum, referrals needed, and effective coverage date. The type of facility or specialty will determine what types of questions to verify. An example would be verifying a long hospital stay versus a physical examination at a family practice office. All information received should be documented and end with the insurance company's contact person's name and phone number and the date and time the medical office specialist spoke with them. The medical office specialist's name and date should also be noted. This is very important in case there is a denial of the claim or collection problems after services are provided.

Complete Practice Exercise 2.2 by documenting the action you would take for each situation or calculate the coinsurance.

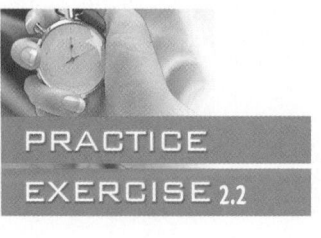

PRACTICE EXERCISE 2.2

Document the action you would take for each situation or calculate the coinsurance.

1. You are the medical office specialist at the Allied Medical Clinic. Peggy Miller is being seen today. You call her insurance carrier to verify benefits. The carrier's customer services representative informs you that the patient's insurance was canceled 2 months ago.

    What action would you take?

    _____

    _____

    _____

2. You are the medical office specialist at the Allied Medical Clinic. Your supervisor has asked you to go up to the front desk and explain to a patient what her estimated coinsurance will be for the procedure she plans to have on October 19. The total charges are $475.00. The allowed amount is $326.00. Her benefits pay at 90%.

    What is the patient's coinsurance: _____?

On completion of this exercise, refer to Appendix J to check the accuracy of your work.

Collecting Insurance Payments

With managed care organizations, the healthcare provider also experiences changes in the way he receives payment for services rendered. The medical office specialist must be well informed on this subject, because duties will include many phases of health insurance. Patients ask many questions about health insurance and expect the medical office specialist to know the answers. Many patients do not pay doctors directly; instead insurance companies pay the doctors. It is the medical office specialist's responsibility to see that the doctor receives compensation for services. This responsibility is partly fulfilled by the processing of insurance claim forms.

Assignment of Benefits

Providers may receive payment directly from the patient or accept an **assignment of benefits**. When a provider accepts an assignment of benefits, the provider agrees to receive payment directly from the patient's insurance carrier. In this case, the patient signs an assignment of benefits statement. This statement authorizes the insurance company to send payments directly to the provider. If the provider does not accept assignment, the patient must pay at the time of service. The patient bills her insurance carrier and receives reimbursement.

When the patient does not sign the assignment of benefits, it is sometimes very difficult to receive payment in full from the patient. Providers should have a statement in their policy and procedures manual that instructs the medical office specialist not to file the claim for the patient and to instead ask for payment in full at the time of service if the patient refuses to assign benefits.

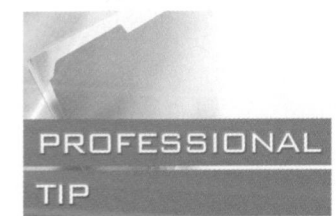

The medical office specialist must be aware that some insurance carriers will not honor an assignment of benefits form if the provider has not contracted with the carrier (referred to as a non-network or nonparticipating provider). Even though the patient assigns the benefits and the provider accepts assignment, the payment for the services will be sent directly to the patient/subscriber.

Chapter Summary

- Managed care is a system that in theory controls the cost and delivery of health services to members who are enrolled in a specific type of healthcare plan.
- The goals of managed health care were and still are to ensure that providers deliver high-quality care in a facility that manages or controls costs, and that all medical care or procedures are medically necessary and appropriate for the patient's condition or diagnosis.
- Managed care utilizes a network of providers. This is true in HMOs, PPOs, and POS plans. Each MCO provides a wide array of physicians and hospital services from which enrollees can choose.
- A managed care plan typically restricts the physician's latitude in caring for patients. The utilization protocol of a managed care company may strongly suggest a plan of treatment different from the plan preferred by the treating physician.

■ The administrative staff or medical office specialist must obtain complete and accurate information on a patient who comes into the doctor's office or hospital. Not only is this information helpful in facilitating the care of the patient, but it is also necessary for the processing of insurance claims.

Chapter Review

True/False

Identify the statement as true (T) or false (F).

_____ 1. Coinsurance is paid by the provider.

_____ 2. The deductible is the amount the insured must pay for each healthcare encounter, such as an office visit.

_____ 3. Under a discounted fee-for-service arrangement, a provider and a payer negotiate the provider's fees.

_____ 4. Fee-for-service contracts establish coinsurance payments for patients' charges.

_____ 5. HMO members are usually allowed to receive medical services from any provider that they choose without additional cost.

_____ 6. Under an indemnity plan, an insurance company agrees to cover the financial losses of a medical practice.

_____ 7. A managed care system combines the financing and the delivery of healthcare services.

_____ 8. Under a POS option, HMO members can receive services from any provider, but they must pay a greater amount for encounters with non-network providers.

_____ 9. A policyholder is a person who buys an insurance plan.

_____ 10. Indemnity plans usually require preauthorization for many services.

_____ 11. PPO is the abbreviation for plan/provider options.

_____ 12. Under a PPO, healthcare providers perform services for plan members at discounted fees.

_____ 13. The role of a PCP is to coordinate a patient's overall care.

_____ 14. A healthcare provider is an individual, group, or organization that provides medical or other healthcare services.

_____ 15. A referral to a specialist by a PCP is usually required under fee-for-service plans.

_____ **16.** HMOs are usually licensed by local city or town governments.

_____ **17.** A PPO is the same as an HMO.

_____ **18.** Fee-for-service plans typically have an annual deductible.

_____ **19.** The amount of freedom offered in different managed care programs (HMO, PPO, EPO) is basically the same.

_____ **20.** If a patient goes to a network hospital for services, he can always assume all of the physicians are in network as well.

_____ **21.** If a patient needs to receive emergency care at a hospital, she should notify her insurance company within 1 week of admission.

_____ **22.** If a provider is listed in the MCO provider directory, it can be assumed they are participating in the network.

_____ **23.** One incentive for an insured to use a network provider is reduced out-of-pocket costs.

_____ **24.** PPO plans do not have an annual deductible.

_____ **25.** A group model HMO contracts with multispecialty physicians' groups to provide physician services to an enrolled group.

Multiple Choice

Identify the letter of the choice that best completes the statement or answers the question.

_____ **1.** In the United States, rising medical costs are a result of:
a. increased spending on drugs.
b. increased use of alternative treatments.
c. advances in technology.
d. all of the above.

_____ **2.** Under a written insurance contract, the policyholder pays a premium and the insurance company provides:
a. surgery.
b. copayments.
c. payment for medical services.
d. preventive medical services.

_____ **3.** An indemnity plan covers:
a. all medical services.
b. medically necessary services.
c. the episode of care.
d. all members' premiums.

_____ **4.** Which of the following conditions must be met before payment is made by the insurer?
a. payment of premium, deductible, and coinsurance
b. payment of the copayment
c. payment of the premium and coinsurance
d. payment of the deductible

_____ 5. Under an indemnity plan a patient may use the services of:
   a. only HMO network providers.   c. any affiliated provider.
   b. any provider.   d. only out-of-network providers.

_____ 6. Patients who enroll in an HMO may use the services of:
   a. only HMO network providers.   c. any affiliated provider.
   b. only out-of-network providers.   d. any provider.

_____ 7. Patients who enroll in a point-of-service type of HMO may use the services of:
   a. only HMO network providers.   c. any provider.
   b. only out-of-network providers.   d. any affiliated provider.

_____ 8. In a PPO plan, referrals to specialists are:
   a. required.   c. not required.
   b. more expensive.   d. none of the above.

_____ 9. Four models of health maintenance organizations are:
   a. staff, group, IPA, and POS.   c. staff, group, IPA, and PCP.
   b. staff, group, IPA, and PPO.   d. staff, group, network, and IPA.

_____ 10. In the staff HMO model, physicians are:
   a. federal employees.   c. independent contractors.
   b. state employees.   d. employees of the HMO.

_____ 11. When a POS operation is elected under a health maintenance organization, the patient may:
   a. choose providers only from the HMO's network.
   b. choose providers who are not in the HMO's network.
   c. choose any provider without additional expenses.
   d. choose providers only from the IPA's network.

_____ 12. Which of the following is required when a HMO patient is admitted to the hospital?
   a. referral   c. coinsurance
   b. preauthorization   d. utilization

_____ 13. Health maintenance organizations are regulated:
   a. only by federal law.   c. only by state law.
   b. only by local law.   d. by both federal and state law.

Completion

Complete each sentence or statement.

1. Annual physical examinations and routine screening procedures are referred to as _____.

2. A policyholder's _____ includes the spouse and children.

3. _____ plans are regulated by the Employee Retirement Income Security Act (ERISA).

4. The _____ is the percentage of each claim that the insured must pay.

5. In managed care, patients often pay a specified amount called a(n) _____ for an office visit to a provider.

6. A member of an HMO must get a(n) _____ from the primary care physician before seeing a specialist.

7. The healthcare delivery system that is like an HMO but does not require the patient to get referrals from a PCP is a(n) _____.

8. The schedule of _____ lists the medical services that are covered by an insurance plan.

9. The physician who coordinates a patient's care in a health maintenance organization is called the _____.

Resources

Glossary of Managed Care Terminology: *www.pohly.com/terms.html*
Managed Care Museum: *www.managedcaremuseum.com*

Chapter 3 Understanding Managed Care: Medical Contracts and Ethics

Chapter Objectives

After reading this chapter, the student should be able to:

1 Understand the key elements of a managed care contract that dictates the provider's compensation for services.

2 Identify covered services for patients, which can include preventive medical services and type of office visits.

3 Recognize the obligation of a medical office specialist to uphold a standard of ethics.

4 Know definitions that are utilized in a managed care contract in order to understand the contract and discuss claims issues with the patient and carrier.

5 Conduct discussions with the patient regarding accounts, following the Patient's Bill of Rights.

Key Terms

National Committee for
   Quality Assurance
   (NCQA)
network

nonparticipating provider
   (non-PAR)
participating provider
   (PAR)

policyholders
schedule of benefits

Case Study
Understanding Managed Care: Medical Contracts and Ethics

Evelyn has been going to Dr. Darow's Office for 15 years. On her most recent visit Dr. Darow requested that Jane, the front office manager, waive the copay. Jane informed Dr. Darow that it was not allowed. Dr. Darow was upset and stated that it was his office and if he wanted to waive a copay for a patient, that it was his choice. Jane then allowed the patient to be seen without collecting a copay. Later the office manager came to Jane and informed her that per the doctor's contract with the insurance company, they are required to take the copay, and she requested that Jane call the patient and inform her of the situation.

Questions

1. Did Jane do the right thing in allowing the patient to be seen without collecting the copay?

2. Why is the physician not allowed to waive a copay for a patient?

3. What would be the best way to approach the call to the patient letting her know that she would still have to pay the copay?

Introduction

In order for a provider to be reimbursed for treatment of a patient who is a member of a managed care plan, that provider must sign a contract with the plan. The contract outlines what is expected of the provider, reimbursement amounts, time limits for submitting insurance claims, and other details. The medical office specialist may be asked to review a managed care organization (MCO) contract to determine if it would be a financially rewarding arrangement between the insurance carrier and the provider. Within a managed care contract, the medical office specialist may be required to refer to the contract to determine the compensation and billing guidelines and the covered medical expenses for the particular MCO, as discussed in this chapter. In working with patients and their insurance carriers, medical office specialists are entrusted with patients' personal information. This chapter discusses the standards of ethics that a medical office specialist is expected to uphold.

Purpose of a Contract

Many patients and providers are affected on a daily basis by the use of managed care. Will all of the services a physician provides be covered by the managed care contract? Will the reimbursement for services be adequate? Will the physician be able to provide the necessary services to the patients he will be treating?

Contracts between the physician or healthcare facility are generally negotiated by the physician(s) or upper management. The contract will affect all staff members. In certain facilities, especially in a medical central billing office, a medical office specialist may be responsible for posting payments received from the insurance carrier, appealing denials, or explaining nonpayment to the contracted physician.

A physician or facility may find it necessary to contract with outside services or hire additional personnel to ensure that all accounts receivable are received and paid to the fullest amount.

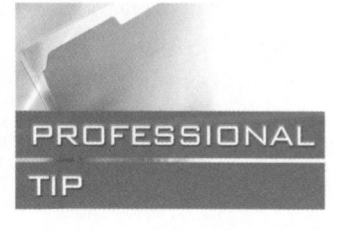

PROFESSIONAL TIP

A centralized billing office (CBO) will contract with a physician or facility to handle all claims submissions. Responsibilities will vary, but normally the CBO will take control of the account after a patient visit, from submission of the claim to resolution of the claim and anything that happens in between. The CBO representative's title is account manager. The account manager may be responsible for anywhere between two and five accounts.

A Legal Agreement

A managed care contract is a legal agreement or document between a healthcare provider (physician, hospital, and clinic or outpatient center) and an insurer, health maintenance organization (HMO) or other network, whereby the provider agrees to discount her usual and customary charges in exchange for an increase in patient load.

By contracting with a provider to deliver care to the **policyholders** (also called *members* and *enrollees*) of a managed care plan the MCO develops a **network** for its members. The provider must contract with the managed care organization to be in the MCO's network.

MCOs contract with physicians, facilities, pharmacies, and laboratories to offer a full-service network of providers who have agreed to discount their fees for members of the managed care plan. These network providers have also agreed to utilize other providers in the network when the patient needs to be referred outside of their respective offices. This keeps costs down for the patient and insurance carrier, and benefits the providers by bringing in more patients who are plan members. The provider who signs an MCO contract is classified as a **participating provider (PAR)**. When a patient is seen by a provider who is not under contract with the MCO, the provider is a **nonparticipating provider (non-PAR)**.

Compensation and Billing Guidelines

A key element of any managed care contract is the provider's compensation for services. The contract and its related documents contain detailed requirements for claims submission and reimbursement requirements.

First, the contract should clearly state how and when the provider is to be paid. On reading the contract, the medical office specialist should clearly understand the administrative requirements of submitting claims and the timing of receiving payment. For example, the time period within which a provider must submit claims must be clearly stated on the contract. Second, the particular forms used to submit claims must be identified by name. Third, all arrangements with regard to the coordination of benefits and late payments must be carefully spelled out in the contract. Finally, because providers do not contract directly with the various payers and plans administered by the MCO, language must be added to the contract that requires the MCO to use its "best efforts" to ensure timely payments by these third-party payers and plans.

A managed care contract may offer different types of payment. Common types of payments include discounted fee-for-service, per diem, per case, percentage of premiums, and capitation arrangements. Any of these payment methods can be satisfactory, but each may pose problems as well. In today's managed care environment, the most common compensation options for licensed professionals are the discounted fee-for-service, per case charges, and capitation arrangements.

Under a discounted fee-for-service arrangement, covered services are compensated at a discount of the provider's usual and customary charges. The provider's discounted fee is negotiated by the provider and the payer. Providers are inclined to accept these discounts in return for the increased patient volume that results from an arrangement of this type with the payers. Under a per case or per visit charge arrangement, the payer compensates the provider at a predetermined rate for each episode of care provided. Because discounted fee-for-service and per case charges can arguably encourage a provider to increase the level of services provided, payers often implement strict rules or incentives to restrain any such resulting increases. Under a capitation arrangement, the provider, typically a primary care provider, is compensated for covered services based on a fixed pre-paid monthly payment that is often referred to as a per-member-per-month (PMPM) amount. Unlike the discounted fee-for-service or per case payment methods, a capitation arrangement typically presents a heightened case management or "gatekeeper" obligation and an increased financial risk to the provider.

In reviewing any managed care contract, be alert for any provisions that allow the MCO to "rebundle," or add to the covered services included in a single bundled fee, or

PRACTICE

EXERCISE 3.1

In the compensation and billing section of an MCO contract, what three things will pertain to the job responsibilities of a medical office specialist?

1. _____

2. _____

3. _____

On completion of this exercise, refer to Appendix J to check the accuracy of your work.

to amend any terms of the compensation arrangement at will. To accommodate the provider's fiscal planning, all material terms of the agreement, particularly those having to do with compensation and payment, should only be modified at the time the contract is renewed, or with the prior express consent of both parties to the contract.

Managed care contracts often prohibit, or otherwise limit, the provider from seeking payment directly from members of the MCO and related plans. The medical office specialist should be aware of the applicable rules that control when, how, and under what circumstances the provider may seek particular payments from either members or the MCO when the provider is not otherwise reimbursed for services rendered. Complete Practice Exercise 3.1 to test your knowledge.

Covered Medical Expenses

All managed care contracts should have a section that lists all services that are considered "covered" services for patients. The list of medical services covered under the insured's policy is called the **schedule of benefits**. This schedule includes preventive medical services and lists types of office visits. If a plan is capitated, this section should discuss which office procedures are covered in the capitated plan and which are not. This will allow the medical office specialist to determine which of the provided services should be billed to the insurer and which to the patient. This list should include the procedure code (CPT®)* and the rate for each service.

The type of plan that is being contracted for is also listed in this section. If it is a preferred provider organization (PPO), HMO, or exclusive provider organization (EPO), this section should list the guidelines of the prospective plan.

Payment

With a fee-for-service plan, the medical office specialist should check the time limit for submitting claims. This is usually a 6- to 12-month period. What billing form will be used? (Do not automatically assume that it is the CMS-1500 form.) What billing requirements must be met to allow for processing and payment of claims? Does the MCO provide ongoing staff training as billing requirements change? Does the contract provide for payment to physicians within a specified period? What penalty or interest charge will be paid to the practice if payment is delayed? When are late charges paid to the practice? Some providers negotiate for language in the contract that specifies that the MCO will reimburse the practice at its usual and customary fee—not at the discounted fee-for-service rate stipulated in the contract—if payment is not made in the specified period.

*CPT is a registered trademark of the American Medical Association.

Another consideration is that if a plan is truly a capitated plan, does it pay at the beginning of the month? Many MCOs pay on the 15th or 30th of the month and can thus hinder a practice's cash flow.

When a plan has problems paying providers on a timely basis, this may indicate inefficient claims processing, insufficient enrollees, or a lack of the required start-up funds.

Who handles the coordination of benefits? The ability to request payment from another insurer for the amount due should be specifically delegated through the managed care contract. Can the fee schedule be changed without prior notice or agreement by the practice? Are periodic reviews of charges and changes made in the fee schedule? What are the changes based on? An increasing number of managed care plans are looking at a resource-based relative value scale (RBRVS), using the Medicare RBRVS with a different conversion factor. A medical office specialist should beware of language stipulating that a fee schedule can be derived using other value scales that are generally accepted in the community.

Ethics in Managed Care

The healthcare reform debate in 1992–1993 during President Bill Clinton's administration made clear the inevitability of fundamental changes in the financing and delivery of health care. The necessity of such changes is widely accepted. The shape and scope of the changes are the subject of intense disagreement. The demise of the Clinton proposals, which advocated a strong role for government, left the field of healthcare reform wide open to the private sector. Insurance companies and other healthcare corporations responded rapidly and aggressively, developing and marketing new models of healthcare delivery. The evolution of these models, collectively referred to as *managed care*, is changing the American healthcare system.

As transformation of this industry continues, corporate business values, such as efficiency, cost reduction, inventory management, competition, and profit, are influencing the traditional medical ethics and values of the solo practitioner: the one-on-one doctor–patient relationship and fee-for-service payment. The shift in values and structure of the healthcare system is inherently neither bad nor good. In fact, in a system where demand seems infinite and resources are finite, such shifts are both necessary and desirable.

The healthcare system can no longer accommodate unlimited demand for medical services. Healthcare providers can no longer pretend to offer the maximum benefits of technology to all comers. It is time to accept that cost matters as much as access and quality. Managed care organizations of various sizes and types are bringing the principles and values of business into the front ranks of healthcare delivery. The MCOs are reducing costs by standardizing, regulating, and streamlining the supply side (providers), and by reducing demand and controlling access on the buyer's side (patients).

Medicine and business have always been somewhat uneasy partners. Most physicians have also been, to one degree or another, businesspersons who were well paid for their professional services. Now, however, business and health are intertwined in new ways. Instead of the business aspects being controlled by physicians, now managers, accountants, and actuaries often control the business aspects. The values and ethical principles of business and medicine have evolved largely separately and distinct from each other. Now that the lines of distinction are blurring, conflicts are inevitable.

Changes in Healthcare Delivery

The comingling of business and medical values is changing the types of services offered and the way in which they are delivered. This merger is changing the very roots of the system, including the fundamental relationships between patient, provider, and third-party payer, and even the motivation for providing (or not providing) a particular service. We discuss next some of the more significant of these fundamental changes.

In many cases the vendor of health care is no longer a private physician or group of providers, but rather a large, usually for-profit, corporation. In a system based on managed care, the patient's choice of provider usually is much more limited than under a traditional fee-for-service structure. In fee-for-service systems, patients could choose nearly any provider or self-refer to specialists if they wished. Now many coverage arrangements are negotiated between employers or unions and MCOs. Patients must choose from a list of providers who have contracted with the new "vendor" (MCO) and agreed to a predetermined payment rate. In most managed care plans, if a patient needs to see a specialist, she must be referred by the primary care provider or the visit is not covered by the plan.

MCO and Provider Credentialing

To ensure that providers are adhering to the MCO's ethics in providing patient care, the managed care organization evaluates the provider through a credentialing process designed to check the provider's medical credentials, service fees, and workplace environment. The **National Committee for Quality Assurance (NCQA)**, which is an accrediting agency for MCOs, requires that an MCO plan being reviewed for accreditation itself demonstrate that it has a thorough credentialing process for its providers. The MCO's provider credentialing process must examine each physician's background for evidence of fraud, criminal activity, disciplinary actions, and malpractice history.

Although this is an admirable standard, not all managed care plans are accredited, nor have they all asked to be accredited, so not all provider credentialing processes are as good as they could be. If an MCO examines a doctor's background, it may still elect to contract with a doctor with a questionable record. Sometimes this is the only doctor in the area with a specialty that the managed care plan needs to include in its network in order to be competitive.

Also, the MCOs credentialing process does not guarantee that a doctor who is a member of an MCO is better than one who is not. Despite what the managed care plan learns about physicians during the credentialing process, the plan provides limited information to consumers about the qualifications of doctors in contracts. The amount of physician information provided to consumers varies from plan to plan.

After the provider credentialing process, the managed care organization will decide whether or not to extend an invitation or "contract" to the provider. The written contract states, among many other things, that the provider will provide medically appropriate care at a discounted rate for plan enrollees. Providers who sign these contracts are considered part of a network.

Medical management components are being focused on and the services that are being provided are being looked at more carefully today than they have been in the past decade. MCOs want their policyholders to be satisfied with the care they are receiving from the physicians within the network. To ensure this, MCOs are grading these physicians on the services that they render to their patients.

Ethics of the Medical Office Specialist

A medical office specialist has an obligation to uphold a standard of ethics. Ethics are the rules or standards governing conduct of a person or the members of a profession. Working as a liaison between the provider and patient, and between the provider and carrier, it is difficult at times to determine where the specialist's loyalty lies. As long as a medical office specialist follows the MCO contractual guidelines and is knowledgeable about the

Patient's Bill of Rights that is discussed later in this chapter, no ethics conflicts should arise.

Occasions have arisen when a medical office specialist has been asked to perform job assignments that do not follow legal guidelines. Some of the new laws that have been implemented state that a medical office specialist can and will be held liable for fraudulent billing. Historically, all legal burdens fell on the provider, but today the medical office specialist can be prosecuted. Consider this example of fraudulent billing:

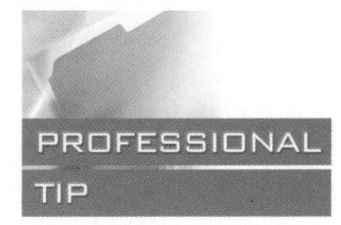

A medical office specialist should always document, sign, and date all conversations regarding patients' accounts whether the conversation is with the provider, patient, or carrier.

PROFESSIONAL TIP

> From approximately late 2003 into 2005, at various back pain clinics within the state of Georgia, the TOPELS engaged in insurance fraud scams that together sought to deprive Blue Cross and Blue Shield of Georgia ("Blue Cross"), based in Columbus, Georgia, of almost $2 million. The scheme involved false billing for a non-surgical back pain procedure known as Vertebral Axial Decompression or "VAX-D." Blue Cross considers VAX-D to be investigational and not medically necessary, and has made clear to health care providers that it does not cover the procedure. However, the TOPELS sought and received reimbursement from Blue Cross for this non-covered procedure anyway, by misleading Blue Cross into believing they were instead performing other services that were covered. Specifically, the TOPELS used an inapplicable medical billing code on their insurance claims that pertained only to surgical nerve decompression procedures, rather than the medical billing code for VAX-D. The TOPELS also instructed their employees not to call the procedure "VAX-D" when speaking to Blue Cross representatives, and to conceal references to "VAX-D" in the patient files.

As noted in the preceding extract, the staff was instructed not to call the procedure by its appropriate name. A medical office specialist has the responsibility to question and decline this type of request. If it is mandatory, then it is time to find another job.

Contract Definitions

The following definitions are utilized in MCO contracts. A medical office specialist should be familiar with these terms in order to review the contract and discuss claims issues with the patient and carrier.

- *Benefit plan:* The contract issued by a payer, the plan document, or any other legally enforceable instrument under which a covered person may be entitled to covered services and which is in force with respect to such covered person.

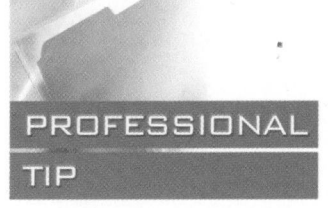

The medical office specialist should always keep in mind when discussing claims issues with a patient that the patient may not be familiar with these terms, so layman terms may be needed.

PROFESSIONAL TIP

- *Contracted services:* Those covered services provided by a physician that are consistent with the physician's training, licensure, and scope of practice.
- *Coordination of benefits (COB):* The determination of which of two or more health benefit plans will provide health benefits for a covered person as primary or secondary payers.

■ *Copayment:* The charge, as determined by the benefit plan, a covered person is required to pay at the time covered services are provided.

■ *Covered person:* An individual who is an insured, enrolled participant or enrolled dependent under a benefit plan.

■ *Covered services:* Those healthcare services provided to covered persons under the terms of the benefit plan.

■ *Emergency services:* Those services provided after the sudden onset of a medical condition manifesting itself by acute symptoms of sufficient severity, including severe pain, such that the absence of immediate medical attention reasonably could be expected to result in:

1. Placing the covered person's health in serious jeopardy;
2. Serious impairment to bodily functions; or
3. Serious dysfunction of any bodily organ or part.

■ *Fee maximum:* The maximum allowable fee payable by the corporation or payer for the provision of a given contracted service by a physician to a covered person; such fee is determined by the corporation in accordance with corporation policies and procedures.

■ *Medical director:* The physician specified by the corporation as its medical director.

■ *Medically necessary:* Refers to the use of services or supplies, or both, as determined by the corporation's medical director, or his designee, that:

1. Are accepted by the healthcare profession as appropriate and effective for the condition being treated;
2. Are based on recognized standards of the healthcare specialty involved;
3. Are not experimental, investigative, or unproven;
4. Are not solely for the convenience of a covered person or a healthcare provider; and
5. Do not involve the use of greater resources than are required for adequate medical care.

Benefit plans may use the term *medically efficient* and other terms rather than, or in addition to, the term *medically necessary.*

■ *Participating hospital:* A state-licensed hospital that has been designated by the corporation as a hospital to which a participating provider may authorize the admission of covered persons for covered services; provided, however, that covered persons may be admitted to any appropriate hospital for the provision of emergency services.

■ *Participating provider:* A licensed healthcare professional, including the physician, a facility, or an entity that has entered into a participation agreement to provide covered services to covered persons.

■ *Payer:* An insurance company, third-party administrator, or self-insured health benefit plan that is contractually obligated to indemnify or make payment on behalf of covered persons with respect to covered services and that has contracted directly or indirectly with the corporation to arrange for the provision of covered services to covered person.

Compensation for Services

Each MCO contract has a section that addresses the compensation of the provider for services rendered to the patient. Figure 3.1 is based on an actual managed care contract. The compensation section is one that a medical office specialist will need to be familiar with for future reference.

Billing

With respect to all Contracted Services provided by Physician to Covered Person pursuant to this Agreement, Physician shall bill Corporation or Payer, as applicable, on a form mutually agreed to, at Physician's usual and customary rate that is charged by Physician without regard to whether a particular person has health plan benefits. Billing information provided by Physician shall include Covered Person identification information and an itemization of all services and charges provided as Contracted Services hereunder.

COB Recoveries

After Physician has billed Corporation or Payer as Provided in Section IV(A) of this Agreement and has collected applicable co-payments, coinsurance, and deductibles. Physician shall seek recovery from Payers having primary payment responsibility according to the COB rules of the applicable Benefit Plan. In the event that Corporation or Payer is not the initial Payer, Corporation or Payer shall pay in accordance with Section IV(D) of this Agreement and will take as credits against such payment amounts any payment Physician has received from the initial Payer(s). In the event Physician subsequently receives any payment from initial Payer(s) after Corporation or Payer has paid for such services, Physician shall promptly pay to Corporation or Payer the amount of the overpayment.

Third-Party Liability Recoveries and Subrogation

As applicable, Physician, Corporation, or Payer shall also seek payment from applicable third-party Payers who have payment responsibility other than as health benefit plan Payers. Except that Physician agrees to allow Corporation or Payer to acquire and exercise full and exclusive rights of subrogation whenever a third party, other than health benefit plan Payer, is liable for payment for services that are provided by Physician for which Corporation or Payer would otherwise be responsible hereunder.

Payment

In connection with Contracted Services provided by Physician hereunder, Corporation or Payer shall pay to Physician an amount equal to the lesser of Physician's usual and customary charge or the Fee maximum, less all coinsurance, co-payments, deductibles, and recoveries described above. Payment shall be remitted to Physician generally within thirty (30) days of the later of (1) receipt of a fully completed, uncontested claim submitted in accordance with the billing procedures of Corporation, or (2) the resolution of all applicable recovery issues. Any portion of such payment that is not remitted to Physician within such period shall be subject to an interest penalty at the rate of eighteen percent (18%) per annum, with interest accruing from the first calendar day following the end of such period, and with such penalty being payable by Corporation or Payer, as applicable, to Physician. Corporation or Payer shall not make payment in an amount that, when added to the coinsurance, co-payments, deductibles, and recoveries described in this Section, exceeds the amount payable under this Agreement. Corporation or Payer shall not be required to make payment under this Agreement pursuant to billings received later than ninety (90) days from the date Contracted Services were provided unless Physician notifies Corporation within such period that a claim for such services has been presented to another Payer for payment.

(continued)

Figure 3.1

Sample contents based on a managed care contract's compensation section.

Figure 3.1

(continued)

No Balance Bill

The combination of applicable co-payments, deductibles, coinsurance, third-party recoveries described in this section, and amounts payable hereunder shall constitute payment in full for Contracted Services. Physician may not balance bill or impose any surcharge upon the Covered Person or individuals responsible for their care. Nor shall Physician seek payment from Covered Persons or such individuals for later billings denied by Corporation or Payer in accordance with paragraph D of this Section IV.

Limitations Regarding Payment

To the extent that Corporation compensates Physician's services through payment to a participating Hospital for the professional component of hospital-based Physician services, Physician shall seek payment for such services solely from the Participating Hospital and shall not bill Corporation, Payer, or a Covered Person for such services.

Hold Harmless Provision for Utilization Review Decision

With respect to compensation for Contracted Services provided by Physician hereunder, Physician agrees that in no event shall Physician bill, charge, seek compensation, remuneration, or reimbursement from, or have any recourse against a Covered Person, persons, or entities other than Corporation or Payer for any benefit penalties that have been applied to such compensation subsequent to utilization review decisions over which such Covered Person has no control, provided that such covered Person has fulfilled the notification responsibilities for contacting the applicable utilization review entity as such responsibilities are set forth in the Benefit Plan. Except that, this Section shall not apply with respect to Contracted Services provided hereunder if such benefit penalties apply according to the terms of a Benefit Plan of a self-insured Payer.

Patient's Bill of Rights

Along with MCO contracts between the managed care plan and the provider, patients are provided with protection and should be made aware of their rights. Although there is no written contract between the provider and the patient, all providers and managed care organizations ethically must abide by the patient's bill of rights. Many health plans have adopted the principles outlined in Figure 3.2.

Reprinted by permission of Bob Englehart.

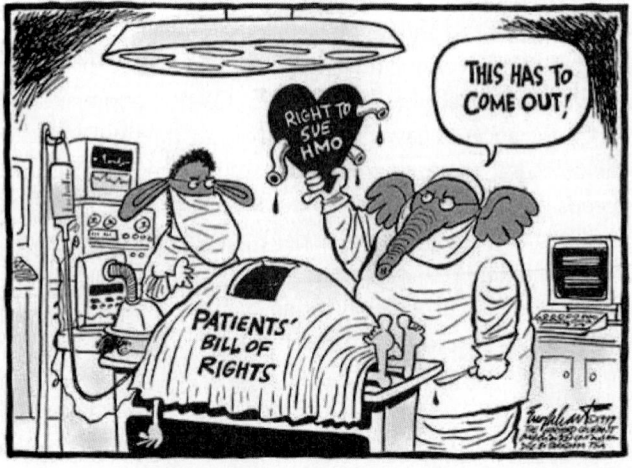

The following was adopted by the U.S. Advisory Commission on Consumer Protection and Quality in the Health Care Industry in 1998. Many health plans have adopted these principles.

Information Disclosure. You have the right to accurate and easily understood information about your health plan, health care professionals, and health care facilities. If you speak another language, have a physical or mental disability, or just don't understand something, assistance will be provided so you can make informed health care decisions.

Choice of Providers and Plans. You have the right to a choice of health care providers that is sufficient to provide you with access to appropriate high-quality health care.

Access to Emergency Services. If you have severe pain, an injury, or sudden illness that convinces you that your health is in serious jeopardy, you have the right to receive screening and stabilization emergency services whenever and wherever needed, without prior authorization or financial penalty.

Participation in Treatment Decisions. You have the right to know your treatment options and to participate in decisions about your care. Parents, guardians, family members, or other individuals that you designate can represent you if you cannot make your own decisions.

Respect and Nondiscrimination. You have a right to considerate, respectful, and nondiscriminatory care from your doctors, health plan representatives, and other health care providers.

Confidentiality of Health Information. You have the right to talk in confidence with health care providers and to have your health care information protected. You also have the right to review and copy your own medical record and request that your physician change your record if it is not accurate, relevant, or complete.

Complaints and Appeals. You have the right to a fair, fast, and objective review of any complaint you have against your health plan, doctors, hospitals, or other health care personnel. This includes complaints about waiting times, operating hours, the conduct of health care personnel, and the adequacy of health care facilities.

Figure 3.2

Patient's bill of rights.

Chapter Summary

- The medical office specialist should be familiar with the billing guidelines in a contract. The contract should list all covered services and state when the provider will be paid.
- A managed care contract is a legal agreement between a healthcare provider (physician, hospital, and clinic or outpatient center) and an insurer, HMO, or other network.
- Managed care contracts often prohibit, or otherwise limit, the provider from seeking payment directly from members of the MCO and related plans.
- Managed care is undoubtedly changing how healthcare providers work. In many areas, managed care is creating fierce competition among healthcare providers for managed care plan contracts.
- A medical office specialist has the responsibility to decline if requested to act unethically.

■ The patient has a bill of rights that protects his or her right to accurate and easily under-stood information about his or her health plan, healthcare professionals, and healthcare facilities.

■ A medical office specialist should be familiar with the terms in order to review the contract and discuss claim issues with the patient and carrier.

Chapter Review

True/False

Identify the statement as true (T) or false (F).

_____   **1.** A capitated payment is pre-paid to a provider to cover a plan member's health services for a specified period.

_____   **2.** It is mandatory for all managed care organizations to be accredited.

_____   **3.** The amount that an insured person must pay for each office visit is called the copayment.

_____   **4.** Credentialing refers to the process of verifying that providers and work-place meet certain professional standards.

_____   **5.** Under a discounted fee-for-service arrangement, a provider and a payer negotiate the provider's fees.

_____   **6.** Ethics are standards of behavior for licensed medical staff and other em-ployees of medical practices.

_____   **7.** Medical professional etiquette includes the respectful and courteous treat-ment of patients.

_____   **8.** Fee-for-service contracts establish capitated payments for patients' charges.

_____   **9.** A key element of any managed care contract is the provider's compensa-tion for services.

_____   **10.** A licensed healthcare professional that is entered into a participation agreement with an MCO is called a non-participating provider.

Multiple Choice

Identify the letter of the choice that best completes the statement or answers the question.

_____   **1.** Under a written insurance contract, the participating provider agrees to pro-vide covered services to covered persons and the insurance carrier provides:
a. payments for medical services.   c. surgery.
b. preventive medical services.   d. copayments.

_____   **2.** Payment on a capitated plan is:
a. paid after claim is received by carrier.
b. paid by the patient.
c. a retroactive payment.
d. pre-paid.

_____   **3.** Under a capitated rate for each plan member, which of the following does a provider share with the third-party payer?
a. payments   c. services
b. risk   d. the premium

_____   **4.** The capitated rate per-member-per-month amount covers:
a. all medical services .
b. services listed on the schedule of benefits.
c. the episode of care.
d. all members' premiums.

_____   **5.** PMPM is the abbreviation for:
a. premenstrual after midnight.
b. provider membership per management.
c. per member per month.
d. provider management by provider manual.

_____   **6.** The Patient's Bill of Rights consists of this principle:
a. respect and non-discrimination
b. information disclosure
c. confidentiality of health information
d. all of the above

_____   **7.** COB is defined as:
a. Contract of Benefits.   c. Contract of Business.
b. Claim of Benefits.   d. Coordination of Benefits.

_____   **8.** The list of medical services covered under the insured's policy is called the:
a. plan of treatment.   c. fee schedule.
b. schedule of benefits.   d. policy plan provisions.

_____   **9.** The term _medically necessary_ refers to the use of services or supplies, or both, as determined by the corporation's medical director, or his designee, that:
a. are accepted by the healthcare profession as appropriate and effective for the condition being treated.
b. are based on unrecognized standards of the healthcare specialty involved.
c. are experimental, investigative, or unproven.
d. are for the convenience of a covered person.

_____   **10.** A No Balance Bill provision in an MCO contract prohibits the provider from:
a. collecting the copayment prior to the appointment.
b. waiving the deductible in an emergency situation.

    c. allows the patient to wait 60 days prior to paying coinsurance.

    d. from seeking payment from the patient for contractual adjustments.

Completion

Complete each sentence or statement.

1. Managed care organizations evaluate the provider through a(n) _____ process.

2. Under a capitation arrangement, the provider is compensated for covered services based on a fixed pre-paid monthly payment that is often referred to as a(n) _____ amount.

3. The provider must _____ with the managed care organization to be in the MCO's network.

4. The charge, as determined by the Benefit Plan, a Covered Person is required to pay at the time covered services are provided is called a(n) _____ .

5. A managed care contract is a(n) _____ agreement between a healthcare provider an insurance carrier.

6. Network providers agree to utilize other providers in the _____ when the patient needs to be referred outside of their respective offices.

7. The schedule of _____ lists the medical services that are covered by an insurance policy.

8. The _____ bill clause prohibits the provider from billing the patient for amounts the carrier has contractually adjusted from the physician's fees.

Resources

Advisory Commission on Consumer Protection and Quality in the Health Care Industry: **www.consumer.gov**

American Hospital Association (AHA), *The Patient Care Partnership: Understanding Expectations, Rights and Responsibilities* is a valuable brochure that is available at the AHA website: **www.aha.org**

U.S. Department of Health and Human Services, Office of Inspector General. This website is a resource that can be consulted for ways to identify and prevent fraudulent billing as defined by the Attorney General: **http://oig.hhs.gov**

Medical Coding

Medical Coding

Diagnosis coding is a critical part of medical billing. Chapter 4 presents an understanding of diagnosis coding that begins with an understanding of the three volumes of the ICD-9-CM and how to use each of them. This chapter presents the student with the knowledge to properly use the ICD-9-CM and key coding guidelines.

Chapter 5 presents an introduction to the CPT® book and place of service coding. Understanding the use of procedure codes and the correct use of modifiers is the most important aspect of coding. This chapter discusses how evaluation and management codes are used to report office visits, hospital visits, nursing home visits, rehabilitation center visits, and home visits.

Chapter 6 presents the organization of the CPT index, instructions for using the CPT codes, the format of the terminology, and important coding steps. It presents the knowledge needed to locate the appropriate code for reporting the procedures and/or services performed.

Competent coding is part of the overall effort being made by medical practices to comply with regulations in many areas. For instance, the diagnosis code chosen must match the procedure performed. In addition, medical office specialists who work with patient records as they code must be knowledgeable about patient privacy regulations and how to keep patient data secure. Chapter 7 discusses the uniform method used by healthcare providers and medical suppliers to report professional services, procedures, and supplies.

CPT is a registered trademark of the American Medical Association.

Audits, whether performed in the office or by an external auditor, are formal examinations or reviews of documentation to determine whether the documentation adequately substantiates the service billed and shows medical necessity. Chapter 8 discusses the purpose of an audit, the different types of auditing, key elements of service, the correct coding of evaluation and management (E/M) services based on medical necessity, and how to prevent coding errors with specific E/M codes.

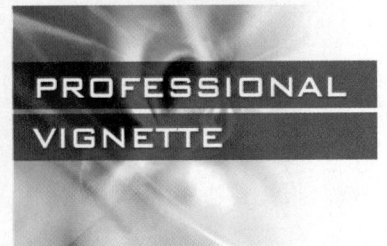

PROFESSIONAL VIGNETTE

My name is Judy Murray and I am a Certified Medical Assistant. After my two children entered high school, I went to a local adult education school for medical assisting. I found the classes fun, exciting and discovered that I was smarter than I thought. I decided to continue on at the local community college, and received an Associates Degree in Medical Assisting and then the CMA title.

I began my career doing clinical work, but soon after began to perform administrative responsibilities as well. As time went on I spent more time doing billing and less time working in the back office. Eventually, I was specializing in billing. I was able to fill in at the front desk or in the back drawing blood, performing EKG, etc,.

While I was employed in the medical office I was asked to teach bookkeeping and insurance classes at an adult education program. I found teaching at the adult level very rewarding as well as challenging. My past experience helped instill confidence that the students would be able to follow their dreams and that the profession would welcome their talents and abilities. Eventually, I taught classes at the college level, which offered me the opportunity to once again further my education and professional career. I sat for the national certification exam for Certified Professional Coders through the American Association of Professional Coders. I am now Judy Murray CMA (AAMA), CPC.

Billing is really a team effort; everyone in the office must do their part in order for the system to function efficiently. I love billing; it is very challenging and rewarding. It is amazing to look back to the beginning of my professional career and see how far I have grown professionally and personally in twenty years. I recently retired from teaching and am currently working two days a week for a plastic surgeon. The flexibility of, and opportunities in this profession are numerous and very rewarding.

Chapter 4 ICD-9-CM Medical Coding

Chapter Objectives

After reading this chapter, the student should be able to:

1. Understand the history of coding.
2. State the purpose of the ICD-9-CM.
3. Define abbreviations, symbols, typefaces, punctuation, and formatting conventions.
4. Utilize the correct volume of ICD-9-CM to find the appropriate code.
5. Code to the highest level of certainty and specificity.
6. Assign the correct code in the proper order.
7. List the nine steps of accurate ICD-9-CM coding.

Key Terms

addenda
adverse effect
combination code
complication code
conventions
crosswalk
diagnosis
diagnostic statement
eponym
etiology

ICD-9-CM
late effect
main term
manifestation
morphology
NEC (not elsewhere classified)
NOS (not otherwise specified)
primary diagnosis

principal diagnosis
residual effect
rule out
secondary
sign
subterms
supplementary terms
symbols
symptom

Donte was a medical coding extern. Still new to the practice, he was given a few medical cases to code. The first case that he received was that of a diabetic patient. The physician has listed diabetes mellitus as the primary code and migraine headaches as the secondary code. Upon looking up the code for diabetes in the coding index, he uses 250.0, and for the headaches he uses 784.0. When checking his work, the manager found a couple of mistakes. She explained that the code for diabetes was not complete and the code for a migraine headache was incorrect.

Questions

1. What common mistake did Donte make in coding?
2. What is the appropriate code for migraine headache? *346.8*
3. What is the appropriate code for diabetes mellitus? *250.t*

249.6

Introduction

Diagnostic coding is a critical part of medical billing. If the correct diagnostic code is not selected, a claim may be denied. The **diagnosis** establishes the medical necessity of the procedure or services performed for the patient. If the insurance claim is not coded to the highest level of specificity and recorded in the proper order, the claim may be reimbursed at a reduced dollar amount. Understanding diagnostic coding begins with understanding the three volumes of the International Classification of Diseases, Ninth Revision, Clinical Modification, known as **ICD-9-CM**, and how to use each of them.

Definition of Diagnosis Coding

Healthcare professionals have long used coding systems to describe procedures, services, and supplies. However, most described the reason for the procedure, service, or supply with a diagnostic written statement, rather than an official diagnostic code. Of those healthcare professionals who used diagnostic codes, either due to a requirement for a computer billing system or for electronic claims filing, many did not code accurately. With the passage of the Medicare Catastrophic Coverage Act of 1988, diagnostic coding using the ICD-9-CM became mandatory for Medicare claims. In the area of healthcare reimbursement and rules and regulations, the typical progression is that changes required for Medicare are followed shortly by similar changes for Medicaid and private insurance carriers (third-party payers).

Proper diagnosis coding involves using the ICD-9-CM volumes to identify the appropriate codes for medical conditions that pertain to the patient's health (as recorded in the patient record) and entering those codes correctly on medical claims forms. Knowledge of medical terminology is a must to be able to read and understand the physician's documentation. This is the first step in the reimbursement process. Each service or procedure performed must be submitted with a diagnosis that will accurately link the patient's encounter to the service or procedure performed. Medical necessity must be established before the insurance carrier will make a payment to the provider of services.

The ICD-9-CM codes submitted on the CMS-1500 and UB-04 are generally used to determine medical necessity for coverage. The ICD-9-CM codes are also used by outside agencies or organizations to forecast healthcare needs, evaluate facilities and services, review costs, and conduct studies of trends in diseases over the years.

History of Diagnosis Coding

Some forms of medical diagnostic coding date back to 16th-century England and are found in the London bills of mortality. The London bills of mortality were introduced in the early 16th century, mainly as a way of warning about plague epidemics. The information was collected by parish clerks and published every week. In 1629 the cause of death was given, and by the early 18th century, the age at death was also being included.

Most of the information on the bills of mortality was supplied by searchers. A searcher is a person who would research the cause of death. Their lack of medical knowledge meant that the causes of death listed were vague or hopelessly wrong. Causes of death listed over the years include being affrighted, bladder in the throat,

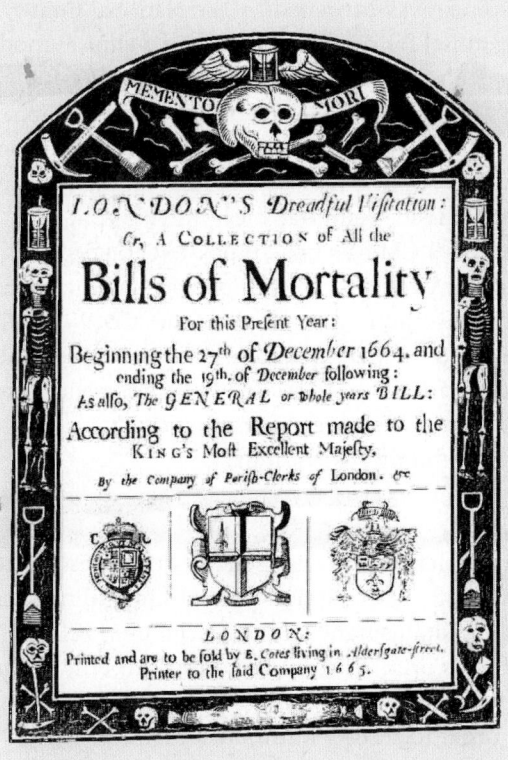

Figure 4.1

Annual return of the Bills of Mortality for 1665; the front cover and the statistics for the period of the plague.

breakbone fever, canine madness, commotion, eel think, frog, gathering, grocer's itch, hectic fever, kink, milk leg, screws, stranguary, stuffing, rag picker's disease, St. Anthony's fire, tympany, worm fit, wolf, and being planet struck. Figure 4.1 shows the cover of the annual Bills of Mortality for 1665 and the statistics for the period of the plague.

The ongoing statistical study of disease and death evolved in 1937 into the International List of Causes of Death. Over the years, revisions were made and the title was changed to the International Classification of Causes of Death (ICD).

In 1948 the ICD came under the direction of the World Health Organization (WHO), which used this information to assist in tracking mortality (death) and morbidity (sickness) in order to make statistical assessments of international health and disease trends. The name of the classification was changed to the International Classification of Diseases and the ICD acronym was retained.

In 1977 a committee was convened by the National Center for Health Statistics to provide advice and counsel for the development of a clinical modification of the ICD-9. The resulting ICD-9-CM is a clinical modification of the WHO's International Classification of Diseases, Ninth Revision. The term *clinical* is used to emphasize the modification's intent; namely, to serve as a useful tool in the area of classification of morbidity data for indexing of medical records, medical care review, ambulatory and other medical care programs, as well as for basic health statistics.

Since 1979, the ICD-9-CM has made it possible to encode, computerize, store, and retrieve large volumes of information from patients' medical records. Hospitals, physician offices, and other healthcare providers use the ICD-9-CM to code and report clinical information required for participation in various government programs, such as Medicare and Medicaid, and for professional standards review organizations. As important as diagnosis coding is to the reimbursement process, it is equally important for tracking disease and compiling statistical data.

Until the passage of the Medicare Catastrophic Coverage Act of 1988, healthcare professionals were not required to report ICD-9-CM codes when billing government or private insurance carriers for reimbursement. Most healthcare professionals simply included the text or written description of the injury, illness, sign, or symptom that was the reason for the visit. Insurance carriers who used ICD-9-CM coding had to code the diagnostic statements prior to inputting claims into their computer systems for reimbursement. The passage of the act required providers to submit a diagnostic code on insurance claims in order to receive reimbursement.

To comply with the regulations, healthcare professionals must convert the reason for the procedures, services, or supplies performed or issued from written diagnostic statements that may include specific diagnoses, signs, symptoms, and/or complaints into ICD-9-CM diagnostic codes.

Purpose of ICD-9-CM Coding

ICD-9-CM coding is used by physicians' offices, hospitals, clinics, home healthcare agencies, and other healthcare providers to substantiate the need for patient care or treatment and to provide statistics for morbidity and mortality rates. The ICD-9-CM coding serves the following purposes:

- Establishes medical necessity
- Translates written terminology or descriptions into a universal, common language
- Provides data for statistical analysis.

The clinical modification (CM) allowed the data to be used to:

- Classify morbidity data for reporting
- Compile and compare healthcare data
- Assist in evaluating the appropriateness and timeliness of medical care for review purposes
- Assist in planning healthcare delivery systems
- Establish patterns of patient care among healthcare providers
- Analyze payments for health care
- Conduct epidemiologic and clinical research.

Addenda

In the ICD-9-CM coding book an addenda or addition is added annually. Diagnosis coding changes, or **addenda**, for Volumes 1 and 2 are approved by a federal committee. The changes take effect each year on October 1. Volume 3 is revised annually by the Centers for Medicare and Medicaid Services (CMS). Annual updates to Volume 1 and 2 include changes such as:

- Addition of new codes
- Deletion of old ICD-9-CM codes
- Revisions to descriptors.

As soon as the new addendum is available in October it is necessary to use the updated diagnostic codes. CMS has made it mandatory that all claims submitted be updated with the correct diagnosis.

The Future of Diagnosis Coding: ICD-10-CM

In 1992, the WHO finished its 10th revision to the International Classification of Diseases. The National Center for Health Statistics has developed a clinical modification of the classification for morbidity purposes. The ICD-10-CM is planned as the replacement for ICD-9-CM, Volumes 1 and 2. But until implementation of the ICD-10-CM, the ICD-9-CM remains the diagnosis coding standard required by government and private payers across the country.

The ICD-10-CM is much more detailed than the ICD-9-CM with roughly 8,000 possible categories of death. For the first time, the ICD-10-CM uses alphanumeric codes. Some coding rules have also been changed. There will be a **crosswalk**, which will assist the coder to go from one version to another. A crosswalk is a comparison for the same or similar classifications under two coding systems. The crosswalk will be used with the ICD-9-CM and ICD-10-CM to establish the new alphanumeric code.

Notable improvements in the content and format of the 10th edition include the addition of information relevant to ambulatory and managed care encounters; expanded injury codes; the creation of combination diagnosis/symptom codes to reduce the number of codes needed to fully describe a condition; the addition of a sixth character; incorporation of common fourth- and fifth-digit subclassifications; laterality; and greater specificity in code assignment. The new structure will allow further expansion than was possible with the ICD-9-CM. No implementation date has been set yet for the ICD-10-CM. Implementation will be based on the process for adoption of standards under the Health Insurance Portability and Accountability Act of 1996 (HIPAA).

The Three Volumes of the ICD-9-CM

The ICD-9-CM is made up of three main volumes:

- Volume 1: Tabular/Numerical List of Diseases
- Volume 2: Alphabetic Index of Disease
- Volume 3: Tabular and Alphabetic Index of Procedures.

Volumes 1 and 2 are used for physician billing and contain diagnostic codes and symptoms. Volume 3 is used for hospital and skilled nursing facility billing, and contains codes for both surgical and nonsurgical procedures.

Table 4.1	Chapters in Volume 1's Classification of Diseases and Injuries
Chapter 1	Infectious and Parasitic Diseases (001–139)
Chapter 2	Neoplasms (140–239)
Chapter 3	Endocrine, Nutritional and Metabolic Diseases, and Immunity Disorders (240–279)
Chapter 4	Diseases of the Blood and Blood-Forming Organs (280–289)
Chapter 5	Mental Disorders (290–319)
Chapter 6	Diseases of the Nervous System and Sense Organs (320–389)
Chapter 7	Diseases of the Circulatory System (390–459)
Chapter 8	Diseases of the Respiratory System (460–519)
Chapter 9	Diseases of the Digestive System (520–579)
Chapter 10	Diseases of the Genitourinary System (580–629)
Chapter 11	Complications of Pregnancy, Childbirth, and the Puerperium (630–677)
Chapter 12	Diseases of the Skin and Subcutaneous Tissue (680–709)
Chapter 13	Diseases of the Musculoskeletal System and Connective Tissue (710–739)
Chapter 14	Congenital Anomalies (740–759)
Chapter 15	Certain Conditions Originating in the Perinatal Period (760–779)
Chapter 16	Symptoms, Signs, and Ill-Defined Conditions (780–799)
Chapter 17	Injury and Poisoning (800–999)

Volume 1: Tabular/Numerical List of Diseases

The tabular list is a numeric listing of diagnostic codes and descriptions consisting of 17 chapters that classify diseases and injuries, two sections containing supplementary codes (V and E codes), and five appendixes.

Classification of Disease and Injuries

The main part of Volume 1 is used to find codes for use on medical forms and documents. It contains 17 chapters with disorders grouped by body systems or condition, as listed in Table 4.1. Each chapter contains:

- Chapter headings
- Categories—three-digit code numbers
- Subcategories—four-digit code numbers
- Subheadings
- Fifth-digit subcategories—five-digit code numbers (subclassifications).

Supplementary Classifications (V and E Codes)

Two supplementary classifications included in Volume 1's tabular list:

- *V Codes*: Supplementary Classification of Factors Influencing Health Status and Contact with Health Services (V01–V83)
- *E Codes*: Supplementary Classification of External Causes of Injury and Poisoning (E800–E999)

Appendixes

The tabular list includes the five appendixes listed in Table 4.2.

Table 4.2	Five Appendices Included in the Tabular
Appendix 1	Morphology of Neoplasms
Appendix 2	Classification of Drugs by American Hospital Formulary Services
Appendix 3	Classification of Industrial Accidents According to Agency
Appendix 4	List of Three-Digit Categories
Appendix 5	Supplementary Classifications of External Causes of Injury and Poisoning (E Codes)

Volume 2: Alphabetic Index of Diseases

This volume contains the *Alphabetic Index to Diseases*, which is used to look up main terms listed in Volume 1. It also contains menu terms and modifiers; a table of drugs and chemicals; an index of external causes of injury and poisoning; and two special tables on hypertension and neoplasms. Volume 2 should *not* be used as a source to code in most cases. This volume is used to begin the initial diagnosis search. (The hypertension and neoplasm tables are the exception. Both are discussed later in this chapter.)

Table of Drugs and Chemicals

Figure 4.2 shows a sample of Volume 2's classification of drugs and other chemical substances to identify poisoning states and external causes of adverse effects.

Index to External Causes of Injury and Poisoning

This section contains the index to the codes that classify environmental events, circumstances, and other conditions as the cause of injury and other adverse effects.

Special Tables

The two special tables, located within the alphabetic index and found under the main terms are the hypertension table and the neoplasm table, both of which are discussed later.

Volume 3: Tabular and Alphabetic Index of Procedures

Volume 3 consists of two sections: a tabular list of codes and an alphabetic index. These codes define *procedures* instead of diagnoses. Frequently used incorrectly by healthcare professionals, codes from Volume 3 are intended only for use by hospitals and skilled nursing facilities.

ICD-9-CM Table of Drugs and Chemicals Addenda (FY08)
Effective October 1, 2007

Substance	Poisoning	Accident	Therapeutic Use	Suicide Attempt	Assault	Undetermined
Alpha-1 blockers	971.3	E855.6	E941.3	E950.4	E962.0	E980.4
Bisphosphonates						
intravenous	963.1	E858.1	E933.7	E950.4	E962.0	E980.4
oral	963.1	E858.1	E933.6	E950.4	E962.0	E980.4
Flomax	971.3	E855.6	E941.3	E950.4	E962.0	E980.4
Tamsulosin	971.3	E855.6	E941.3	E950.4	E962.0	E980.4

Figure 4.2

Excerpt from the "Classification of Drugs and Other Chemical Substances to Identify Poisoning States and External Causes of Adverse Effects" table in Volume 2 of the ICD-9-CM.

Source: International Classification of Diseases, Ninth Revision, Clinical Modification (2007). Reprinted by permission of Practice Management Information Corporation.

ICD-9-CM Conventions

Many abbreviations, symbols, typefaces, punctuation, and formatting **conventions** are used in the ICD-9-CM. The formatting conventions or typographic conventions used in the ICD-9-CM are fairly exclusive to each volume.

Some typographic conventions are also specific to a publisher. For example, many publishers of the latest versions indicate somehow that a code needs a fifth digit in order to be coded correctly, but the symbol used to indicate the need may be different for each publisher.

The term *encounter* is used to refer to all settings, including hospital admissions. In the context of these guidelines, the term *provider* is used throughout the guidelines to mean physician or any qualified healthcare practitioner who is legally accountable for establishing the patient's diagnosis.

The medical term describing the condition for which a patient is receiving care is located in the physician's diagnostic statement. For each encounter the **diagnostic statement** includes the main reason for the patient encounter. It may also provide the descriptions of additional conditions or symptoms that have been treated or are related to the patient's current illness.

The physician must give a primary diagnosis each time a patient is seen. The **primary diagnosis** is the patient's main reason for the visit or encounter. A patient that is admitted to the hospital is given two diagnoses, the admitting diagnosis and the principal diagnosis. The admitting diagnosis is the reason for admission; the **principal diagnosis** is the final diagnosis after examination or tests have been performed in the hospital.

Use of the Two Main Volumes

Volumes 1 and 2 are related like chapters in a book. To locate a diagnostic code or patient's condition, a specific process must be followed:

1. The *alphabetic index (Volume 2) is used* first to find the code or the condition. The medical office specialist uses this index to do the initial search for the correct code.
2. After a code is found in the alphabetic index, the tabular list (Volume 1) is used next to research the specific code.

(As mentioned earlier, Volume 3 covers procedures and is not discussed further in this chapter.)

Use the Alphabetic Index (Volume 2) First

The ailment, **manifestation** (a sign or symptom of a disease), or diagnosis is looked up under the condition. Examples of chart notes and the main term/primary diagnosis follow.

> **Example**
>
> Patient comes in for a physical examination (checkup). The *primary diagnosis* would be Physical Examination. The *main term* would be *Examination* and the anatomic site or body part is Physical.

Example

Patient comes in for a blood pressure check because of hypertension. The *primary diagnosis* is Hypertension. The *main term* is Hypertension.

Example

Patient presents with the chief complaint of foot pain. If the physician is unable to diagnose the condition at the time of the visit/encounter the chief complaint is used. The *main term* would be Pain, which would be located in the index, and then the anatomic site or body part is chosen, in this case Foot. The *primary diagnosis* is Foot Pain.

Example

The physician gives a diagnosis of Gastric Ulcer. The *main term* would be Ulcer and the anatomic site, Gastric. The *primary diagnosis* is Gastric Ulcer.

When researching for the diagnosis, condition, or symptom the **main term** will be in **boldface** type and followed by a code (numerical number).

Patients often have more than one chief complaint at the time of their visit or additional illnesses that may affect their present condition and/or treatment. Thus, the primary diagnosis is always listed first as the main reason for the visit/encounter, followed by any other conditions, symptoms, or illnesses.

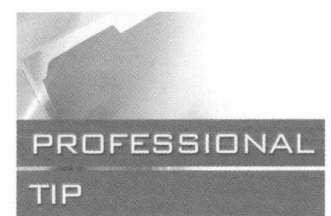

PROFESSIONAL TIP

Example

Patient presents with the chief complaint of foot pain. The *main term* is **Pain 780.96.**

Subterms are always indented two spaces to the right under main terms. **Subterms** may show the **etiology** of the disease (its cause or origin) or describe a particular type or body site for the main term, as shown in the following example.

Example

Pain(s)

    abdominal 789.0
    adnexa (uteri) 625.9
    alimentary, due to vascular
      insufficiency 557.9

    anginoid (see also Pain,
      precordial) 786.51
    anus 569.42
    arch 729.5

Supplementary terms are not essential to the selection of the correct code but aid the coder in finding the correct term. Supplementary terms are in parentheses or brackets as shown in Figure 4.3.

Figure 4.3

Supplementary terms help the coder find the correct subterm.

Syndrome
    Bernard-Sergent (acute adrenocortical insufficiency)

Swelling 782.3
Syndrome—see also Disease
    Addisonian 255.41
    Batten-Steinert 359.21
    Bernard-Sergent (acute adrenocortical insufficiency) 255.41
    Cricopharyngeal 787.20
    Curschmann (-Batten) (-Steinert) 359.21
    Diabetic amyotrophy 250.6 [353.1]

Source: International Classification of Diseases, Ninth Revision, Clinical Modification (2008). Reprinted from National Center for Health Statistics, http://www.cdc.gov/nchs/datawh/ftpserv/ftpicd9/ftpicd9.htm#guidlines.

Example

Pain(s)

   back (postural)

Carryover lines, or turnover lines, are always indented more than two spaces from the level of the preceding line. If the main term or subterm is too long to fit on one line, as is often the case carryover or turnover lines are used. It is important for the coder to read carefully to distinguish between carryover lines and subterms.

Example

Pain(s)   **psychogenic 307.89**

   back (postural) 724.5
   low 724.2

Instructional Terms
The alphabetical index also includes a number of instructional terms that can help the coder. These terms are discussed next.

See   The "*see*" instruction following a main term in the alphabetic index indicates that another term must be referenced. It is necessary to go to the main term referenced by the "*see*" note to locate the correct code. The coder has no other choice.

Example

Infection, infected, infective

   purulent—*see* Abscess

See Also   A "*see also*" instruction following a main term in the index indicates that there is another main term that may also be referenced that may provide additional useful index entries. It is not necessary to follow the *"see also"* note when the original main term provides the necessary code.

Example

Infection, infected, infective

Nasal sinus (chronic) (*see also* **Sinusitis**) 473.9

See Category   This is a variation on the instructional term *see.* This refers the coder to a specific category. *The coder must always follow this instructional term.*

See Also Category   This variation on the instructional term *see also* refers the coder to a reference elsewhere if the main term or sub term is not sufficient to reference the correct code.

Additional Terms

Eponyms   An **eponym** is a term for diseases, syndromes, and procedures that are named after people and locales. Some eponyms are named after the physician who developed the procedure and some after the patient who has the disease. Examples of eponyms are Lou Gehrig's disease, Legionnaire's disease, Lyme disease, and Hodgkin's disease. The diagnostic statement may list the eponym or medical term(s) for the condition. For example, amyotrophic lateral sclerosis may be documented instead of Lou Gehrig's disease. Either the medical term or the eponym may be used to locate the main term in the Alphabetic Index.

NEC   The acronym **NEC (not elsewhere classified)** is used with ill-defined terms to alert the coder that a specified form of the condition is classified differently. The category number for a term including NEC is to be used only when the coder lacks the information necessary to code the term to a more specific category.

Use the Tabular List (Volume 1) Next

Volume 2 has shown the coder the place where the search for the correct code begins. When the correct code/main term has been located, Volume 1 is then researched for the specific code to assign.

Punctuation

In Volume 1, the way in which punctuation is used has meaning. The medical office specialist should familiarize herself with these various meanings:

:   Colons are used after an incomplete phrase or term that requires one or more of the modifiers indented under it to make it assignable to a given category. The exception to this rule pertains to the abbreviation NOS, which is discussed in the next section.

[ ]   Square brackets are used to enclose synonyms, alternate wordings, or explanatory phrases.

Example

460 Acute nasopharyngitis [common cold]

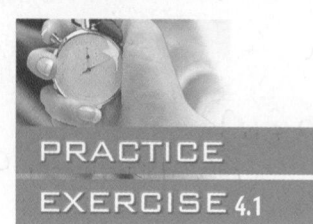

PRACTICE

EXERCISE 4.1

Use your ICD-9-CM to select the correct diagnosis codes for the following sample narrative description:

Indicate whether the following three statements are true or false about Volume 2, the alphabetic index:

1. Contains alphabetic index of main terms.

2. Volume in which initial diagnosis search should begin.

3. Eponyms can be found in this volume by using only one method.

Place a double underline below the main terms and a single underline below any subterms in each of the following statements. Then determine the correct codes in the alphabetic index only:

1. Restless leg syndrome   *333.94*

2. Rheumatoid arthritis   *714.0*

3. Spasmodic asthma with status asthmaticus   *493.9*

4. Acute serous otitis media   *381.01*

5. Congenital stenosis of the aortic valve   *396.0   746.3*

6. Narrowing of the vertebral artery with cerebral infarction   *433.2/434.91*

7. Bone marrow donor   *V59.3*

8. Gastrointestinal disorder   *536.9*

9. Pregnancy test with positive result

10. Ulcer with gangrene

11. Follow-up examination

12. Pneumopathy due to dust

13. Sclerosing keratitis

14. Malocclusion due to missing teeth

15. Organic sleep apnea

On completion of this exercise, refer to Appendix J to check the accuracy of your work.

( )   Parentheses are used to enclose supplementary words that may be present or absent in a statement of disease without affecting the code assignment.

Example

470 Deviated nasal septum

Deflected septum (**nasal**) (**acquired**)

711.0 Pyogenic arthritis [0-9]

Arthritis or polyarthritis (due to):

coliform [Escherichia coli]
Hemophilus influenzae [H. influenzae]
pneumococcal
Pseudomonas
staphylococcal
streptococcal
Pyarthrosis

Use additional code to identify infectious organism (041.0-041.8

Figure 4.4

An example of the "Use additional code" instructional note.

Source: International Classification of Diseases, Ninth Revision, Clinical Modification (2008). Reprinted from National Center for Health Statistics, http://www.cdc.gov/nchs/datawh/ftpserv/ftpicd9/ftpicd9.htm#guidlines.

Instructional Notes

Instructional notes are used to define terms, provide coding instructions, and provide fifth-digit information.

Use Additional Code   The "Use additional code" instruction is placed in the tabular list in those categories where the coder may wish to add further information, by means of an additional code, to give a more complete picture of the diagnosis or procedure. "*Code also:*" is the same as "Use additional code." An example of "Use additional code" is shown in Figure 4.4.

Code First Underlying Disease As   The "Code first underlying disease as" instruction is used for those codes not intended to be used as the principal diagnosis. These codes are for symptoms only (manifestation) and never for causes. The codes and their descriptions are in italic type, meaning that the code cannot be listed first, even if the diagnostic statement is written that way. Some publishers code this in blue to alert the coder that this is a manifestation.

Example

711.3 *Postdysentric arthropathy*
    Code first underlying disease as:

dysentery (009.0)
enteritis, infectious (008.0-009.3)

paratyphoid fever (002.1-002.9)
typhoid fever (002.0)

As shown in the previous example, the primary code is given as to the underlying disease. The order of the codes is as follows: The etiology comes first, followed by the manifestation code. The term *postdysentric arthropathy* refers to a manifestation of the disease (as listed in the example), so the correct code here would be 009.3, 711.3 (fifth digit required).

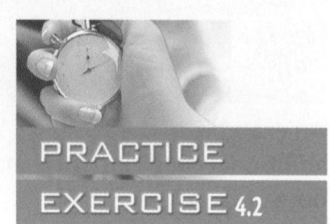

Use your ICD-9-CM to select the correct diagnosis codes for the following sample narrative description. Code the following:

1. Cerebral degeneration in generalized lipidoses _____

2. Curvature of spine associated with other conditions _____

3. Cryptococcal meningitis _____

On completion of this exercise, refer to Appendix J to check the accuracy of your work.

Additional Terms

Includes   Indicates separate terms, such as modifying adjectives, sites, conditions entered under a subdivision (such as a category), to further define or give examples of the content of the category.

Example

461 Acute sinusitis
   Includes:

   abscess acute, of sinus (accessory) (nasal)
   empyema acute, of sinus (accessory) (nasal)
   infection acute, of sinus (accessory) (nasal)

Excludes   Exclusion terms are enclosed in a box and are printed in italics to draw attention to their presence. The importance of this instructional term is its use as a guideline to direct the coder to the proper code assignment. In other words, all terms following the word *Excludes:* are to be coded elsewhere as indicated in each instance.

Example

461 Acute sinusitis

   Excludes: Chronic or Unspecified Sinusitis (473.0-473.9)

NOS   **NOS (not otherwise specified)** means unspecified. This acronym refers to a lack of sufficient detail in the diagnostic statement to be able to assign it to a more specific subdivision within the classification.

> **Example**
>
> **841.9 Unspecified site of elbow and forearm**
>
> **Elbow NOS**

NEC   As in Volume 2, NEC (not elsewhere classified) is used with ill-defined terms to alert the coder that a specified form of the condition is classified differently. The category number for the term including NEC is to be used only when the coder lacks the information necessary to code the term to a more specific category.

Symbols   **Symbols** are used to alert the coder that something is different with the code.

▲   means that there is a revision to the text of the existing code.
●   means that the code is new to this revision.
④ ⑤   a number within a circle (4 or 5) means that the code must be coded either to the fourth level or the fifth level of specificity.

Chapters in Volume 1

As discussed previously, the tabular list is organized by chapter according to the etiology, or body system. Each tabular list chapter is divided into sections with titles that indicate the types of related illnesses, diseases, or conditions. Within each section the codes are tabulated by their numbers:

■ The *category* is a three-digit number that represents the main section of the chapter:

> **Example**
>
> **250 Diabetes Mellitus**

■ The *subcategory* is a four-digit number that is listed under the category:

> **Example**
>
> **250.0 Diabetes Mellitus without mention of complication.**

■ The *subclassification* is a five-digit number that is listed under the subcategory:

> **Example**
>
> **250.00 Diabetes Mellitus without mention of complication, type II, not stated as uncontrolled.**

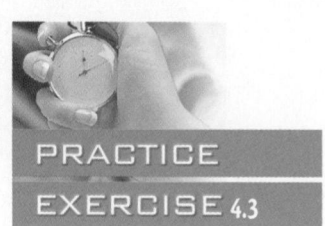

PRACTICE
EXERCISE 4.3

Use your ICD-9-CM to select the correct diagnosis codes for the following sample narrative description.

Why is it important to use the alphabetic index and then the tabular list to find the correct code? Work through this coding process and then comment on your result.

1. Double underline the main term and underline the subterm in the following statement: "Patient complains of abdominal cramps."

2. Find the term from the preceding statement in the alphabetic index and list its code.

3. Verify the code in the tabular list, reading all instructions. List the code you have determined to be correct.

4. Did the result of your research in the tabular list match the main term's code in the alphabetic index?

5. Why or why not?

On completion of this exercise, refer to Appendix J to check the accuracy of your work.

How to Code

A joint effort between the provider and the coder is essential to achieve complete and accurate documentation, code assignment, and reporting of diagnoses and procedures. Guidelines have been developed to assist both the provider and the coder in identifying those diagnoses and procedures that are to be reported. The importance of consistent, complete documentation in the medical record cannot be overemphasized. Without such documentation, accurate coding cannot be achieved. Three steps need to be followed for obtaining the most specific and accurate code:

1. **Determine the reason for the encounter.**   The reason in the physician's statement or medical documentation as to why the patient sought care, together with the medical examination, is the *primary diagnosis*. The primary diagnosis, whether it is a manifestation, condition, or disease, is the main term that should first be located in the alphabetic index.

2. **Locate the term in the alphabetic index (Volume 2).**   The main term for the primary diagnosis is located in the alphabetic index. These guidelines should be followed for choosing the correct term:

    Use any supplementary terms in the diagnostic statement to help locate the main term.

    Read and follow any notes below the main term.

    Review the subterms to find the most specific match to the diagnosis.

    Read and follow any cross-references.

    Make note of a two-code (etiology and/or manifestation) indication.

3. **Verify the code in the tabular list (Volume 1).**   The code for the main term is located in the tabular list. These guidelines are observed to verify the selection of the correct code:

Read any *include* or *exclude* notes, checking back to see if any apply to the code's
   category, section, or chapter. The medical office specialist often will have
   to research backward to the category, section, or chapter.
Observe fifth-digit requirements.
Follow any instructions requiring the selection of additional codes (such as
   "Code also," or "Code first underlying disease as").
List multiple codes in the correct order.

Key Coding Guidelines

Three key coding guidelines will help medical office specialists as they code insurance
claims:

1. Code the primary diagnosis first, followed by current coexisting conditions.
2. Code to the highest level of certainty.
3. Code to the highest level of specificity.

Primary Diagnosis First, Followed by Current Coexisting Conditions

The ICD-9-CM code for the diagnosis, condition, problem, or other reason for the encounter documented in the medical record as the main reason for the procedure, service, or supply provided should be listed first. Additional ICD-9-CM codes that describe
any current coexisting conditions are then listed. This means that any conditions that
may affect the patient's treatment for the specific visit should be coded. Do *not* code
conditions that were previously treated and no longer exist.

   If the patient presents with no complaints of illness or injury, a V code will be used
for the primary diagnosis. (V codes are discussed later in this chapter.)

> **Example**
> **Patient presents for an annual physical examination. V70.0.**

Code to the Highest Level of Certainty

Often the physician has not determined the diagnosis at the time of the encounter.
The medical office specialist should code the condition for the encounter, such as
describing symptoms, signs, abnormal test results, or other reasons for the encounter. Chapter 16 in Volume 1, Symptoms, Signs, and Ill-Defined Conditions, will
be used for this purpose. The alphabetic index is first researched for the symptom or
sign and then verified in the tabular list. A **sign** is an objective indication that can be
evaluated by the physician, such as weight loss, blood pressure, and respirations. A
symptom is a subjective statement by the patient that cannot be confirmed by an examination, such as the patient's complaint of headache. This is referred to as *coding to
the highest degree of certainty.*

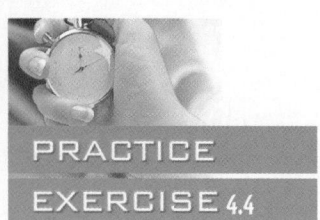

Use your ICD-9-CM to select the correct diagnosis codes for the following sample narrative description. Code the following:

Patient presents with severe headache; rule out brain tumor _____

On completion of this exercise, refer to Appendix J to check the accuracy of your work.

Example

Patient presents with high blood pressure. The physician wants to further evaluate the patient before diagnosing hypertension. The code for this encounter is High Blood Pressure: 796.2.

Diagnoses documented in the patient's chart as "probable," "suspected," "questionable", or **rule out** should not be coded. The only encounter for which "probable," "suspected," "questionable," or "rule out" is accepted is for the UB-04 claims form for the admitting diagnosis (inpatient) only.

Code to the Highest Level of Specificity

Assign three digit codes only if there are no four-digit codes within the coding category.
Assign four-digit codes only if there is no fifth-digit subclassification for that category.
Assign the fifth-digit subclassification codes for those categories where it exists.
Claims submitted with three- or four-digit codes where four- or five-digit codes are available may be returned to you for proper coding. It is recognized that a very specific diagnosis may not be known at the time of the initial encounter. However, that is not an acceptable reason to submit a three-digit code when four or five digits are available. An example follows.

Example

If the patient has chronic bronchitis, ICD-9-CM code 491, and the physician has not yet documented whether the bronchitis is simple, mucopurulent, or obstructive, the code for unspecified chronic bronchitis, ICD-9-CM code 491.9, should be listed.

When coding to the highest level of specificity, the coder often will have to research backward to the category to find the subclassification:

Example

Stenosis of carotid artery
With cerebral infarction (5th digit)
433.11

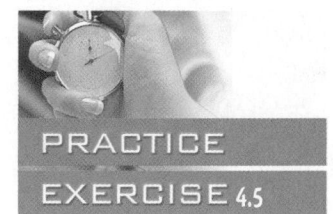

PRACTICE
EXERCISE 4.5

Use your ICD-9-CM to select the correct diagnosis codes for the following sample narrative description. Code the following:

1.   Outlet dysfunction constipation _____

2.   Sleep disturbance _____

3.   Generalized convulsive epilepsy _____

4.   Chronic obstructive asthma with an acute exacerbation _____

5.   Decubitus ulcer of the hip _____

On completion of this exercise, refer to Appendix J to check the accuracy of your work.

Surgical Coding

For surgical procedures, use the ICD-9-CM code for the diagnosis for which the surgery was performed. If the postoperative diagnosis is known to be different than the preoperative diagnosis at the time the claim is filed, use the ICD-9-CM code for the postoperative diagnosis. Before coding, the medical office specialist should check the operative report to verify whether the postoperative diagnosis is different than the preoperative diagnosis.

Coding Late Effects

A **late effect**, also referred to as a **residual effect**, is a condition that remains after a patient's acute illness or injury. There is no time limit on when a late effect can be used. The residual may be apparent early, such as in stroke cases, or it may occur months or years later. The diagnostic statement may say "Late, due to an old . . ." or "Due to a previous. . . ." Thus, coding of late effects generally requires two codes sequenced in the following order:

Requires 2 codes sequenced [handwritten]

1.   The condition or nature of the late effect is sequenced first.
2.   The late effect code is sequenced second.

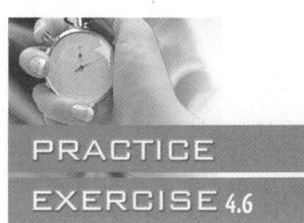

Use your ICD-9-CM to select the correct diagnosis codes for the following sample narrative description.

PRACTICE
EXERCISE 4.6

1.   Code the following diagnoses:
     OPERATIVE REPORT
     PREOPERATIVE DIAGNOSIS: Lump in right breast ___ 611.72 [handwritten]
     POSTOPERATIVE DIAGNOSIS: Right-breast cancer ___ ~~174.81~~ 174.9 [handwritten]

2.   Which diagnosis is reported on the claim form? ___ ~~174.81~~ To be reported [handwritten]

On completion of this exercise, refer to Appendix J to check the accuracy of your work.

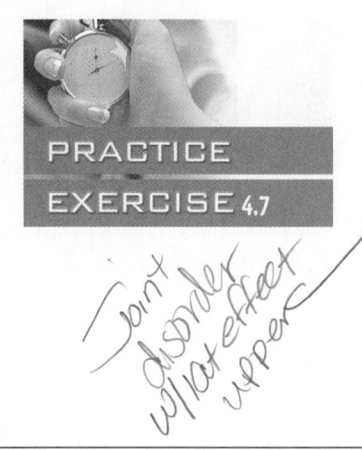

Use your ICD-9-CM to select the correct diagnosis codes for the following sample narrative description. Code the following:

1. Dysphagia from a CVA _____ 187.2 / 438.82

2. Swelling due to an old fracture of the shoulder _____ 719.07 / 905.2

3. Nausea as a late effect of radiation sickness _____ 787.02 / 909.2

4. Muscle weakness due to an old sprain and strain of the ankle _____ 728 / 87
905.4

Joint disorder w/ late effect upper

On completion of this exercise, refer to Appendix J to check the accuracy of your work.

effects 980

The diagnosis will require two codes: The first code will be the late effect, followed by the code for the cause or etiology. Go to "Late effect" in the alphabetic index.

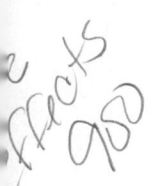

Example

Muscle weakness due to poliomyelitis.
   Correct Coding Order: 728.87, 138

Acute and Chronic Conditions

If the same condition is described as both acute (subacute) and chronic, and separate subentries exist in the alphabetic index at the same indentation level, code both and sequence the acute (subacute) code first. A sudden flare-up or exacerbation of a patient's chronic condition may be characterized as acute.

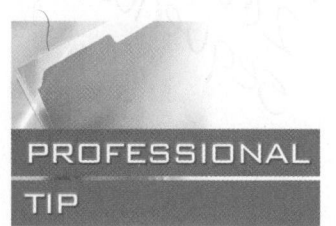

If the encounter is for an illness for which the alphabetical index gives a choice of acute versus chronic, code the acute first.

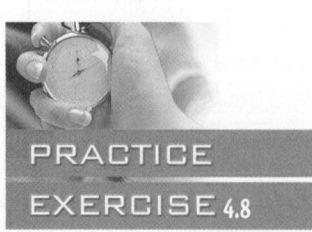

Use your ICD-9-CM to select the correct diagnosis codes for the following sample narrative description. Code the following:

1. Acute renal failure _____ 584.9

2. Chronic renal failure _____ 585.9

On completion of this exercise, refer to Appendix J to check the accuracy of your work.

Use your ICD-9-CM to select the correct diagnosis codes for the following sample narrative description. Answer the following questions:

PRACTICE EXERCISE 4.9

1. What does code 536 exclude? _functional disorders of stomach specified as psychogenic (306.4)_

2. What does code 244 include? _athyrodism, hypothyradism, myexdena (Adult, Juvenile) thyroid gland insufficiency } acquired_

3. What is the main term and supplementary term for code 460? _acute respiratory infections / naso phargynitis (comonon cold)_

4. The note under 653 instructs the coder to do what? _code 1st any associated obstructed labor (660.1)_

5. When coding diabetic nephropathy, which code is listed first? _250.4 (583.81) diabetes melitus code 1st then neuropathy_

On completion of this exercise, refer to Appendix J to check the accuracy of your work.

Combination Codes: Multiple Coding

In addition to difficult coding situations, there are also cases where you will need to recognize the need for "multiple" or "combination" codes. Multiple coding means that two or more codes are used together to accurately identify a diagnosis. Multiple codes are necessary whenever you see that the ICD-9-CM notes "Use additional code" or "Code also underlying disease."

A **combination code** is one code that describes conditions that frequently occur together. Combination terms are often listed as subterms in the alphabetic index. A combination code is a single code used to classify two diagnoses or a diagnosis (etiology) with an associated secondary process (manifestation) or a diagnosis with an associated complication. Combination codes are identified by referring to subterm entries in the alphabetic index and by reading the inclusion and exclusion notes in the tabular list.

Some key words that indicate a combination term are:

associated with	complicated by
due to	following
secondary to	with
without	

_829_

_719.01_
_905.2_

Example

Subdural hemorrhage with concussion 852.29

V Codes

V codes can be used in many different ways. Depending on the encounter, the V code could be primary or supplemental. Usually, if the V code is primary, the reason for this encounter was not due to an injury or illness. That is, V codes are mainly used for encounters other than disease or injury such as annual checkups, physical exams, and immunizations. The V code would be the primary reason for the encounter since there is no chief complaint at these types of visits. These visits are also referred to as a *well checkups*. There are three exceptions in which the V Code *is* used as the primary code when there is a disease:

(handwritten: lot for disease or injury)

1. Chemotherapy
2. Radiation
3. Rehabilitation.

(handwritten: 3 exceptions for V codes)

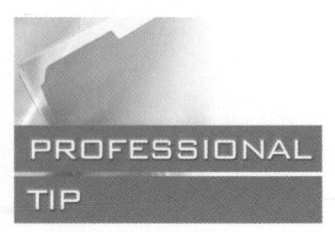

PROFESSIONAL TIP

HIV/AIDS—the code must distinguish between exposure and/or testing positive for the presence of the acquired immunodeficiency syndrome (AIDS) virus.

The question that must be asked is "Why is the patient here today?" Although the patient may have cancer for which he is receiving chemotherapy or radiation, the encounter today is not for the disease but for the treatment. In this case, the V code is primary and the disease is **secondary**.

V codes fall into one of three categories: problems, services, or factual.

1. **Problems:**   V codes identify a problem that could affect a patient's overall health status but is not itself a current illness or injury. The V code in this example is supplemental.

Example

Allergy to drug

2. **Services:**   As mentioned, a V code can be used to describe circumstances other than an illness or injury that prompted the patient's visit. This is an exception to the rule for coding V codes. Although there is a disease, the V code is coded primary because it is the main reason for the encounter. The disease would be coded supplemental to the V code.

Example

Chemotherapy
Radiation
Rehabilitation

3. **Factual:**   V codes are used to describe certain facts that do not fall into the "problem" or "service" categories. For example, coding the type of birth, look under "Outcome of Delivery."

Admission for	Dialysis	Maladjustment
Aftercare (of)	Donor	Observation
Attention to	Examination	Problem (with)
Care (of)	Fitting of	Prophylactic
Carrier	Follow-up	Replacement (by) (of)
Checking/checkup	Health or healthy	Screening
Contact	History (of)	Transplant
Contraception	Maintenance	Vaccination
Counseling		

Figure 4.5

Key words in diagnostic statements that may result in selection of a V code.

Example

Single liveborn to indicate birth status.

V codes indicate a reason for an encounter—*they are not procedure codes*. A corresponding procedure code must accompany a V code to describe the procedure performed. Key words found in diagnostic statements that may result in selection of a V code are shown in Figure 4.5.

Examples of V code chart notes and the correct order of codes are shown here:

Example

A patient has strep throat (034.0) that is resistant to penicillin.

> **Alphabetic index: Resistance to Drugs by microorganisms Penicillin**
> **Tabular list: V09.0 Infection with drug resistant microorganisms to Penicillin**
> **Correct code: V09.0**
> **Correct code sequence: 034.0 (strep throat), V09.0**

Example

A patient who has a family history of colon cancer presents with rectal bleeding (569.3).

> **Alphabetic index: History (personal) of Family malignant neoplasm (of) colon**
> **Tabular List: V16.0**
> **Correct code: V16.0**
> **Correct code sequence: 569.3, V16.0**

Example

A patient presents to a healthcare facility for care after having unprotected sex with a partner who has tested positive for human immunodeficiency virus (HIV).

> **Alphabetic index: Exposure to HIV**
> **Tabular list: V01.7, contact with or exposure to other viral diseases**
> **Correct code: V01.79**

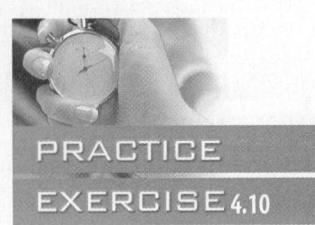

Use your ICD-9-CM to select the correct diagnosis codes for the following sample narrative description. Select the correct V code for each of the following scenarios:

1. Encounter for occupational therapy _____V57.21_____

2. Routine adult medical examination (doctor's office) _____V70.0_____

3. Exposure to severe acute respiratory syndrome (SARS)-associated coronavirus _____

On completion of this exercise, refer to Appendix J to check the accuracy of your work.

Example

A child presents for routine childhood immunizations and is given an MMR vaccination.

> **Alphabetic index: Vaccination Prophylactic Measles-mumps-rubella (MMR)**
> **Tabular list: V06.4, Need for prophylactic vaccination and inoculation against measles, mumps-rubella**
> **Correct code: V06.4**

Example

A patient presents for antepartum care at the end of her seventh month of pregnancy. She has not sought medical care of any type during the pregnancy and, other than insufficient weight gain, does not appear to have any complications or problems at this time.

> **Primary diagnosis: Pregnancy, insufficient prenatal care (Supervision of high risk pregnancy because of lack of prenatal care) V23.7**
> **Secondary diagnosis: Insufficient weight gain during pregnancy 646.83**

E CODES: Supplemental Classifications of External Causes of Injury and Poisoning

E codes permit the classification of environmental events, circumstances, and conditions as the cause of injury, poisoning, or other adverse effects. The use of E-codes, together with the code identifying the injury or condition, provides additional information of particular concern to industrial medicine, insurance carriers, national safety programs, and public health agencies. Codes that document external causes of injury and poisoning are intended to provide data for injury research and evaluation of injury prevention strategies. E codes capture how the injury or poisoning happened (cause), the intent (unintentional or accidental; or intentional, such as suicide or assault), and the place where the event occurred.

Some major categories of E codes include those shown in Figure 4.6.

Transport accidents	Poisoning and adverse effects of drugs or medicinal substances	Figure 4.6
Accidental falls	Accidents cause by fire and flames	
Accidents due to natural and environmental factors (hurricanes and tsunami)	Late effects of accidents or self-injury	
Assaults or purposely inflicted injury	Suicide or self-inflicted injury	

Major categories of E codes.

E codes are located in Volume 1 in a section immediately following the V codes. Notice that the E codes have three digits before the decimal point with an "E" preceding the number. Locating E codes is a little different from locating V codes. E codes have their own alphabetical index, which is located in Volume 2, Section 3 (after Drugs and Chemicals), Index to External Causes. E codes are *always* supplemental to the primary code because they describe how the injury occurred, not the injury itself.

Metabolic VBt

Example

A woman fell off a horse she was riding and injured her back.

> E code index: Accident Caused by, due to Animal, being ridden
> Tabular list: E 828, Accident involving animal being ridden; injured person is the rider of the animal. Indicates the coder needs to code with a fourth digit to indicate who was injured (in this case, the rider)—E828.2
> Correct code: E828.2

Example

The driver of a car was seriously injured when he was involved in a head-on collision with another car.

> E code index: Accident Motor Vehicle Collision
> Tabular list: E812, Other motor vehicle traffic accident involving collision with motor vehicle; injured individual was the driver. Indicates a fourth digit to indicate who was injured (in this case, the driver)—E812.0
> Correct code: E812.0

Use your ICD-9-CM to select the correct diagnosis codes for the following sample narrative description. Select the correct E code for the following scenarios:

1. Injured by hurricane _____

2. Electric shock from broken power line _____

3. Accidental injury caused by farm tractor _____

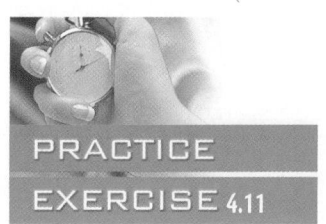

PRACTICE EXERCISE 4.11

On completion of this exercise, refer to Appendix J to check the accuracy of your work.

Table 4.3	Neoplasms	
A. Malignant	B. Benign
1. Primary	C. Uncertain behavior
2. Secondary	D. Unspecified
3. Ca *in situ*	

Neoplasm Table

Neoplasm is the medical term for any abnormal growth, commonly referred to as a tumor. Benign and or malignant lesions are called neoplasms. They are classified into four sections, as listed in Table 4.3.

Morphology refers to the form and structure of tumor cells. The morphology codes identify and classify a neoplasm by tissue origin. They are normally not used for insurance reporting. Morphology codes are primarily used in pathology and tumor registry indexes, not as a diagnosis. Morphology codes begin with "M" followed by five numerical digits. The first four digits identify the histologic type of the neoplasm and the fifth indicates its behavior. Morphology codes are used primarily by pathologists.

The Fifth-Digit Behavior Codes

The fifth digit of a morphology code indicates the behavior of the neoplasm. Fifth-digit codes are listed in Figure 4.7.

Malignant neoplasms are composed of tumor cells that can invade surrounding structures or distant organs. Their growth is more rapid than that of benign neoplasms. ICD-9-CM classifies malignant neoplasms as primary, secondary, and carcinoma *in situ* (preinvasive): *Ca* is an abbreviation for carcinoma, malignant tumor, or cancer.

1. Primary identifies the site of origin of the neoplasm. The point of origin is determined through the study of morphology (form and structure) of the tumor cell. Determination of the point of origin and type of cells is important in establishing the severity of illness and in planning treatment.

Example

Primary lung cancer—site where cancer originates

Figure 4.7

Fifth-digit behavior codes.

/0	Benign
/1	Uncertain whether benign or malignant, borderline malignancy
/2	Carcinoma *in situ*, intraepithelial, noninfiltrating, noninvasive
/3	Malignant, primary site
/6	Malignant, metastatic site, secondary site
/9	Malignant, uncertain whether primary or metastatic site

2. *Secondary* identifies the site(s) to which the primary tumor has spread, or *metastasized*, by direct extension to surrounding tissues. The morphology of a metastatic neoplasm is the same as that of the primary neoplasm.

Example

Secondary brain cancer—site where cancer has metastasized to or spread to.

3. *Carcinoma* in *situ* is composed of tumor cells that are undergoing malignant changes; however, these changes do not extend beyond the point of origin or invade surrounding normal tissue. Also described as:
   - Noninfiltrating carcinoma
   - Noninvasive carcinoma
   - Preinvasive carcinoma.

Example

Carcinoma *in situ* of the skin

Benign neoplasms are tumors that do not invade adjacent structures or spread to distant sites. Their growth may displace or exert pressure on adjacent structures. Some benign neoplasms have no potential for malignancy. However, others, such as adenomatous gastric polyps, have a premalignant potential and removal is indicated. Fortunately, most benign tumors can be completely excised.

Example

Benign neoplasm of the liver.

The classification of *uncertain behavior* includes tumors that show features of both benign and malignant behavior. These tumors may require further study before a definitive diagnosis can be established. The codes in this category are only used when the pathologist clearly indicates that the behavior of the neoplasm cannot be identified.

Example

Neoplasm of skin, uncertain behavior

Unspecified behavior is to be used only when a diagnosis (behavior or morphology) cannot be clearly identified in the medical record. Many reasons for coding unspecified behavior exist. One reason could be that the patient has moved to a new location and the physician does not have access to the patient's previous medical

Ask the following questions when coding neoplasms:

Where did it originate?

Where is the neoplasm currently?

What has been its cause?

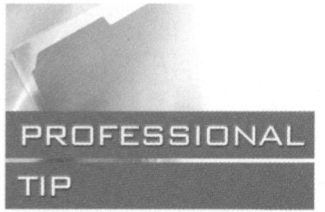

PROFESSIONAL TIP

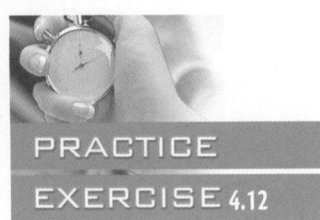

Use your ICD-9-CM to select the correct diagnosis codes for the following sample narrative description. Code the following:

1. Metastatic brain ca from the cervix _____

2. Secondary neoplasm on the auditory nerve _____

3. Primary tumor of the thyroid gland _____

On completion of this exercise, refer to Appendix J to check the accuracy of your work.

records, or the patient is sent to another facility for further study to determine the exact nature of the neoplasm.

Diseases of the Circulatory System

In order for the medical office specialist to code correctly for coronary conditions, it is imperative to have an understanding of the diseases and how they affect this body system. For example, the coder needs to be aware of chart documentation as to when a heart attack occurred, because myocardial infarctions are coded according to time. Following is a brief description of major coronary diseases.

Coronary Artery Disease

Coronary artery disease is a condition in which fatty deposits accumulate in the cells lining the wall of a coronary artery and obstruct blood flow. For the heart to contract and pump normally, the myocardium requires a continuous supply of oxygen-enriched blood from the coronary arteries. When the obstruction of a coronary artery worsens, ischemia to the heart muscle will develop, resulting in heart damage. The major cause of myocardial infarction and angina is coronary artery disease.

Ischemic Heart Disease

This category includes myocardial infarction (heart attack), angina pectoris, and all other forms (acute and chronic) of ischemic heart disease. Myocardial infarction is a medical emergency in which the blood supply is restricted or cut off, causing some of the heart's muscle (myocardium) to die from lack of oxygen. Myocardial infarction usually occurs when a blockage in a coronary artery restricts or cuts off the blood supply to a region of the heart. The heart's ability to keep pumping after a heart attack is related to the extent and location of the damaged tissue (infarction). Understanding common terms is important when coding this disease.

Listed here are common medical terms and their definitions related to coronary artery disease:

Angina: Spasmodic, choking or suffocative pain in the chest, due to lack of oxygen in the heart muscles.

Coronary occlusion: Complete obstruction of an artery of the heart, usually from progressive atherosclerosis, sometimes complicated by thrombosis.

Embolism: Clot that forms in the heart, breaks away, and lodges in the coronary artery.

Infarction: An area of coagulation necrosis in tissue due to local ischemia resulting from obstruction of circulation to the area, most commonly by a thrombus or embolus.

Ischemia: Deficiency of blood in a part, usually due to functional constriction or actual obstruction of a blood vessel.

Myocardial: Pertaining to the muscular tissue of the heart.

Thrombosis: An aggregation of blood factors frequently causing vascular obstruction at the point where it is formed.

Acute myocardial infarction (ICD-9-CM Category 410) is site specific. The documentation in the patient's chart should indicate what area of the heart muscle is affected. Under Category 410, note that a fifth-digit subclassification is required. A myocardial infarction is classified as acute if it is either specified as "acute" in the diagnostic statement or has a stated duration of 8 weeks or less. When a myocardial infarction is specified as "chronic" or with symptoms after 8 weeks from the date of onset, it should be coded to Subcategory 414.8, Other specified forms of chronic ischemic heart disease. If a myocardial infarction is specified as old or healed or has been diagnosed by special investigation (EKG) but is currently not presenting any symptoms, code using Category 412, Old myocardial infarction.

Example

Myocardial infarction 3 weeks ago (subsequent visit)
   410.92 Acute myocardial infarction, unspecified site (less than 8 weeks, subsequent episode of care)

Example

Chronic myocardial infarction with angina (after 8 weeks of infarction)

   414.8 Other specified forms of chronic ischemic heart disease
   413.9 Other and unspecified angina pectoris

Example

Myocardial infarction diagnoses by EKG, asymptomatic (or healed)
   412 Old myocardial infarction

Hypertension Table

Hypertension in medical terms refers to a condition of elevated blood pressure regardless of the cause. It has been called "the silent killer" because it usually does not cause symptoms for many years—often not until a vital organ has been damaged.

When blood pressure is checked, two values are recorded. The higher one occurs when the heart contracts (systole); the lower occurs when the heart relaxes between beats (diastole). Blood pressure is written as the systolic pressure followed by a slash and the diastolic pressure, for example, 120/80 mm Hg (millimeters of mercury).

Figure 4.8

Conditions due to or associated with hypertension.

ICD-9-CM Index to Diseases Addenda (FY08) Effective October 1, 2007

Hypertension Table	Malignant	Benign	Unspecified
Hypertension, hypertensive (arterial) (arteriolar) (crisis) (degeneration) (disease) (essential) (fluctuating) (idiopathic) (intermittent) (labile) (low renin) (orthostatic) (paroxysmal) (primary) (systemic) (uncontrolled) (vascular)	401.0	401.1	401.9
cardiorenal (disease)	404.00	404.10	404.90
with			
heart failure	404.01	404.11	404.91
and chronic kidney disease	404.01	404.11	404.91
stage I through stage IV or unspecified	404.01	404.11	404.91
venous, chronic (asymptomatic) (idiopathic)	—	—	459.30

Source: International Classification of Diseases, Ninth Revision, Clinical Modification (2008). Reprinted from National Center for Health Statistics, http://www.cdc.gov/nchs/datawh/ftpserv/ftpicd9/ftpicd9.htm#guidlines.

This reading would be referred to as "one twenty over eighty." Hypertension is defined in adults as 140 mm Hg systolic or 90 mm Hg diastolic on three separate readings recorded several weeks apart.

Figure 4.8 provides a complete listing of all conditions associated with hypertension. Four columns are shown:

- Condition (not titled as such in the excerpt)
- Malignant
- Benign
- Unspecified.

The first column identifies the hypertensive condition, such as:

Accelerated
Cardiovascular disease
Renal involvement
Heart involvement.

The last three columns identify the subcategories of the disease as malignant, benign, or unspecified. Do not select a code from the malignant or benign category unless the documentation indicates the specific type of hypertension. When the documentation does not indicate the type of hypertension, ask the physician to specify the type. If that alternative is not available, select "unspecified."

Example

Hypertension (arterial) (essential) (primary) (systemic) NOS to Category 401 with the appropriate fourth digit. Do not use either .0 (malignant) or .1 (benign) unless the medical record documentation supports it. Otherwise assign .9 (unspecified).

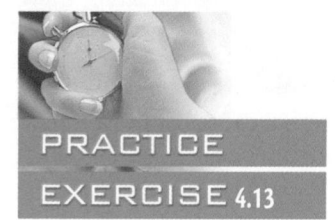

Use your ICD-9-CM to select the correct diagnosis codes for the following sample narrative description. Code the following:

1. Benign hypertension due to pyelonephritis _____

2. Unspecified hypertension due to a brain tumor _____

3. Essential hypertension _____

PRACTICE EXERCISE 4.13

On completion of this exercise, refer to Appendix J to check the accuracy of your work.

High blood pressure is a sign, not a disease. If the documentation states the patient has high blood pressure, assign the code from Chapter 16, Symptoms, Signs, and Ill-Defined Conditions:

Section 790-796 NONSPECIFIC ABNORMAL FINDINGS:

796.2 Elevated blood pressure reading without diagnosis of hypertension. This category is to be used to record an episode of elevated blood pressure in a patient in whom no formal diagnosis of hypertension has been made, or as an incidental finding.

Poisoning and Adverse Effects of Drugs

Two different sets of code numbers are used to differentiate between poisoning and adverse reactions to the correct substances properly administered. First, you must make the distinction between poisoning and adverse reaction.

A poisoning can occur in a variety of ways. An accidental poisoning occurs when an error was made in drug prescription or in the administration of the drug by physician, nurse, patient, or other person or self. An **adverse effect** is any response to a drug that is noxious and unintended and occurs with proper dosage. If an overdose of a drug was intentionally taken or administered and resulted in drug toxicity, this would be considered a poisoning. If a nonprescribed drug or medicinal agent was taken in combination with a correctly prescribed and properly administered drug, any drug toxicity or reaction from the interaction of the two drugs would be classified as a poisoning. In each instance, the appropriate code would be chosen. They are divided into six external causes, as shown in Figure 4.9.

The six causes of poisoning are differentiated from an adverse effect, which occurs when the drug was correctly prescribed and properly administered. These reactions are coded differently. Adverse effects of therapeutic substances correctly prescribed and

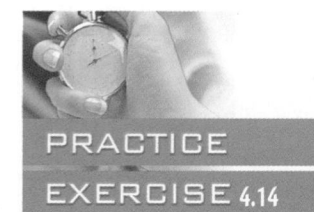

Use your ICD-9-CM to select the correct diagnosis codes for the following sample narrative description. Code the following:

Elevated blood pressure _____

PRACTICE EXERCISE 4.14

On completion of this exercise, refer to Appendix J to check the accuracy of your work.

Figure 4.9

| Poisoning | Accidental | Therapeutic use |
| Suicide attempt | Assault | Undetermined |

External causes of poisoning.

properly administered (toxicity, synergistic reaction, side effect, and idiosyncratic reaction) may be due to:

- Differences among patients such as age, sex, disease, and genetic factors
- Drug-related factors, such as type of drug, route of administration, duration of therapy, dosage, and bioavailability.

A poisoning is reported using at least three codes:

1. The first code from the Poisoning column of the Table of Drugs and Chemicals identifies the drug.
2. The second code indicates the condition(s) that resulted from the poisoning.
3. The E code from the Table of Drugs and Chemicals indicates the circumstance that caused the poisoning (accidental, suicide attempt, assault, or undetermined). See Practice Exercise 4.15.

Burns

Burns are classified by depth, extent, and by agent (E code). Burns are classified by depth as first degree (erythema), second degree (blistering), and third degree (full-thickness involvement).

Coding burns is unique because it is based on four basic elements:

1. Location of the burn
2. Degree of severity of the burn
3. Percentage of the total body burned
4. Percentage of the total body with third-degree burns (total body surface area, TBSA) is represented by the fifth digit.

These factors are used to determine the correct codes to use. Note that coding burns accurately always requires *at least two codes*. To code a burn, code it by location, followed by one code that covers the severity of the burn and the subclassification of the specific site of the burn. Always read the Note under the category to determine the subcategory and subclassification.

When coding multiple burns, assign separate codes for each burn site. Sequence burns from most severe to least severe. If the specific location of the burns is not documented use Category 946, Burns of multiple specified sites or Category 949, Burn, unspecified.

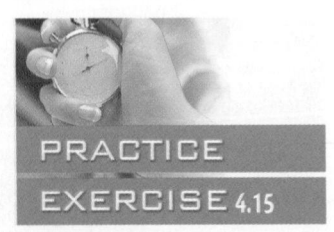

PRACTICE

EXERCISE 4.15

Use your ICD-9-CM to select the correct diagnosis codes for the following sample narrative description. Code the following:

Coma due to overdose of phenobarbital _____

On completion of this exercise, refer to Appendix J to check the accuracy of your work.

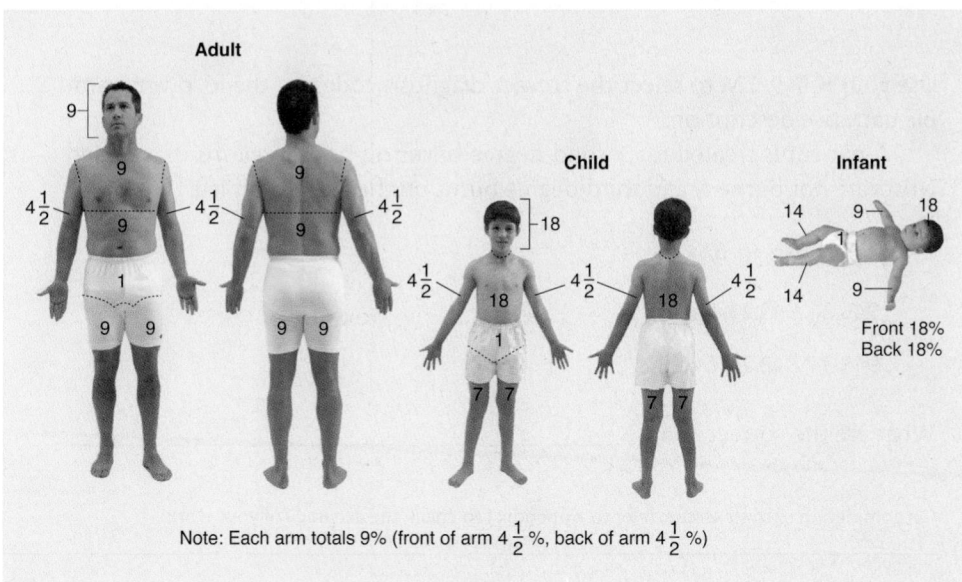

Adult

9

9

$4\frac{1}{2}$ 9 $4\frac{1}{2}$ $4\frac{1}{2}$ 9 $4\frac{1}{2}$

1

9   9   9   9

Child

18

$4\frac{1}{2}$ 18 $4\frac{1}{2}$ $4\frac{1}{2}$ 18 $4\frac{1}{2}$

1

7   7   7   7

Infant

14   9   18
1
14   9

Front 18%
Back 18%

Note: Each arm totals 9% (front of arm $4\frac{1}{2}$ %, back of arm $4\frac{1}{2}$ %)

Figure 4.10

The Rule of Nines.

Third degree burns present a challenge to the coder. Category 948, which deals with total body surface area, is to be used when the site of the burn is unspecified, or when you use categories 940 through 947 when the site is specified. Category 948 is used to report the extent of the total body surface burned. When using Category 948, the subcategory or fourth-digit codes are used to identify the percentage of TBSA involved in a burn (all degrees). The subclassification or fifth-digit category is assigned to identify the percentage of body surface involved in third-degree burns ONLY. Fifth-digit zero (0) is used when less than 10% or when no body surface is involved in a third-degree burn.

The Rule of Nines applies to Category 948 in estimating body surface involved. When determining the percentage of the whole body burned, the medical office specialist must think of the entire body as encompassing 100% of TBSA. This allows the coder to divide the body appropriately for the specific amount of the body.

The Rule of Nines

The Rule of Nines is as follows: The head and neck are assigned 9%; each arm, 9%; each leg, 18%; the anterior trunk, 18%; the posterior trunk, 18%; and genitalia, 1%.

Head and Neck	9
Each arm	18 (9 x 2)
Each leg	36 (18 x 2)
Anterior and posterior trunk	36 (18 x 2)
Genitalia	1 = 100

Figure 4.10 shows the percentages as they pertain to the Rule of Nines. Physicians may change these percentage assignments where necessary to accommodate infants and children who have proportionately larger heads than adults and patients who have large buttocks, thighs, or abdomens that involve burns. See Practice Exercise 4.16.

Diabetes

Diabetes presents a unique coding situation because the coding is based on the patient's diabetes type classification. Diabetes mellitus is a chronic metabolic disease of

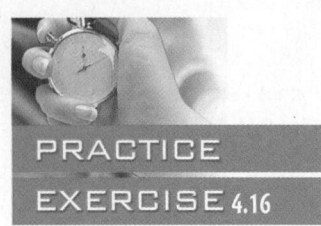

Use your ICD-9-CM to select the correct diagnosis codes for the following sample narrative description:

A patient is treated for second-degree burns on both forearms (hands and wrists are not burned) and third-degree burns on the right lower leg.

945.25, 943.30, 948.10

, 945.34, 943.21, 948.31

, 945.34, 943.21, 948.33

What are the correct codes? _____

On completion of this exercise, refer to Appendix J to check the accuracy of your work.

the pancreatic islet cells. Millions of people have this serious lifelong condition and more than 650,000 people are newly diagnosed with diabetes each year. Although it occurs most often in older adults, diabetes is also one of the most common chronic childhood diseases in the United States today.

To code claims for this disease correctly, it is critical that the coder understand the types of diabetes and underlying conditions related to diabetes mellitus. The three types of diabetes are:

- type I, insulin dependent
- type II, non-insulin dependent
- Gestational diabetes, which occurs during pregnancy.

Insulin-dependent diabetes mellitus (IDDM), or *type I diabetes*, usually results from damage or destruction of the pancreatic islets, leading to a reduction or absence of insulin secretion. Diabetes sometimes follows a viral infection, which suggests that the virus may have induced the disease by injuring or destroying the islets. Many patients with this type of diabetes have antibodies directed against their own islet cells, indicating that an abnormal immune response may also play a part in causing the disease. IDDM most often develops in children and young adults. For this reason, IDDM used to be known as "juvenile" diabetes. It is one of the most common chronic disorders in American children.

Type I diabetes mellitus indicates that:

- Insulin is not produced by the body or
- Production of insulin is decreased.

A patient with type I, insulin-dependent diabetes mellitus requires insulin to sustain life. The patient must be monitored carefully to identify complications of the disease, to monitor insulin levels, and to control diet.

Non-insulin-dependent diabetes mellitus (NIDDM), or *type II diabetes*, is the most common type of diabetes. It accounts for 90% to 95% of diagnosed diabetes. NIDDM usually develops in adults over age 40, also referred to as adult-onset, and is most common in overweight people. People with NIDDM usually produce some insulin, but their body's cells cannot use it efficiently because the cells are insulin resistant. The result is hyperglycemia and inability of the body to use its main source of fuel.

Gestational diabetes is demonstrated by abnormal glucose tolerance test results during pregnancy. It usually ends after delivery, but women with gestational diabetes may develop NIDDM later in life. Gestational diabetes results from the body's resistance to the action of insulin. Hormones produced by the placenta cause this resistance. Women with gestational diabetes require treatment for blood glucose control during pregnancy to prevent adverse effects to the fetus. Gestational diabetes is usually treated with dietary adjustments, although some women may need insulin. Gestational diabetes cannot be treated with oral hypoglycemic medications because these medicines can harm the fetus.

Coding subclassifications are based on the patient's insulin dependence rather than on a medical condition. The fourth digit in a diabetes code identifies the presence of any associated complication. The fifth-digit subclassification is based on the type classification and nature of the patient's diabetes management. The fifth digit is only assigned when the physician's documentation indicates the patient is insulin dependent. Also the statement "controlled or uncontrolled" helps further identify the condition.

0 type II or unspecified type, not stated as uncontrolled
1 type I [juvenile type], not stated as uncontrolled
2 type II or unspecified type, uncontrolled
3 type I [juvenile type], uncontrolled.

If the type of diabetes mellitus is not documented in the medical record, the default is type II.

Injuries, Complications, and Accidents

Situations involving injuries, complications, and accidents can be difficult because you must ask yourself a series of questions before you can determine how the problem or condition can be coded. Many details are needed about the circumstances of the condition or problem caused by an injury, complication, or accident in order to code accurately. Injuries are coded differently for:

- Internal versus external injuries
- Injuries to blood vessels.

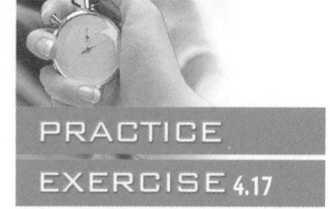

PRACTICE

EXERCISE 4.17

Use your ICD-9-CM to select the correct diagnosis codes for the following sample narrative description. Answer the following questions:

1. The patient has adult-onset diabetes being controlled by regular insulin shots. Which fifth digit would you code?

   0
   1
   2
   3
   The correct subclassification is: _____

2. If the patient has uncontrolled adult-onset diabetes with nephrosis, the code would be: _____

On completion of this exercise, refer to Appendix J to check the accuracy of your work.

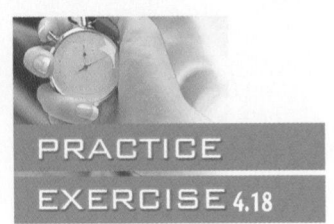

PRACTICE
EXERCISE 4.18

Use your ICD-9-CM to select the correct diagnosis codes for the following sample narrative description. Code the following:

1.   Fracture of three ribs _____

2.   Open Bennett's fracture _____

3.   Fracture of C1–C4 with anterior cord syndrome _____

On completion of this exercise, refer to Appendix J to check the accuracy of your work.

Fractures

Fractures are coded according to exact bone and whether the fracture is open or closed. An *open fracture* is a fracture of the bone with a skin wound. A *closed fracture* is a fracture of the bone with no skin wound. If the documentation does not state what type of fracture it is, always code closed.

Medical terminology for open fractures is as follows:

Compound	Puncture
Infected	With foreign body.
Missile	

Medical terminology for closed fractures is as follows:

Comminuted	Linear
Depressed	March
Elevated	Simple
Fissured	Slipped epiphysis
Greenstick	Spiral.
Impacted	

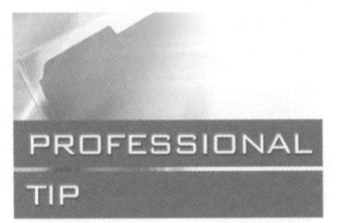

PROFESSIONAL
TIP

Know the definitions of open fractures; if it is not an open fracture or if the type of fracture is not stated, then code it as closed.

Complication Code

The **complication code** is usually the secondary code on the claim form since it was not the primary reason for the visit/encounter.

Accidents can be complex to code because you must use several codes to identify the injury and the circumstances of the injury. E codes are used to describe the circumstances, such as the location where the injury took place and any object that caused the accident. It usually takes more than one E code to code the situation accurately, but the place of occurrence is usually the most important and should be listed before the other E codes. Medicare Part B providers do not normally need to use E codes, but Medicare Part A providers are encouraged to use E codes.

There are many other situations for which coding can be difficult. Often it is the nature of the illness or injury itself that causes the complexity. Some difficult coding situations include:

Cardiac/circulatory system: These problems can occur over a long period of time and are coded based on the current state of the heart condition in many cases.

Late effects: This is a long-term effect from a previous illness or injury for which you must code what caused the late effect after the primary code.

Anomalies: Unique conditions in a patient for which you need to determine if the condition is congenital (present since birth) or acquired.

Example

During a routine tonsillectomy, the patient begins hemorrhaging.

474.00—chronic tonsillitis
998.11—hemorrhage complicating a procedure

Nine Steps of Accurate ICD-9-CM Coding

The following nine steps should be followed for accurate ICD-9-CM coding:

1. Locate the main term within the diagnostic statement.
2. Locate the main term in the alphabetic index (Volume 2). Keep in mind that the primary arrangement for main terms is by condition in Volume 2. Main terms can be referred to in outmoded, ill-defined, and lay terms as well as proper medical terms. They can also be expressed in broad or specific terms; as nouns, adjectives, or eponyms; and can be with or without modifiers. Certain conditions may be listed under more than one main term.
3. Remember to refer to all notes under the main term. Be guided by the instructions in any notes appearing in a box immediately after the main term.
4. Examine any modifiers appearing in parentheses next to the main term. See if any of these modifiers apply to any of the qualifying terms used in the diagnostic statement.
5. Take note of the subterms indented beneath the main term. Subterms differ from main terms in that they provide greater specificity, becoming more specific the further they are indented to the right of the main term in two-space increments. They also provide the anatomic sites affected by the disease or injury.
6. Be sure to follow any cross-reference instructions. These instructional terms ("*see*" or "*see also*") must be followed to locate the correct code.
7. Confirm the code selection in the tabular list (Volume 1). Make certain you have selected the appropriate classification in accordance with the diagnosis.
8. Follow instructional terms in Volume 1. Watch for exclusion terms, notes, and fifth-digit instructions that apply to the code number you are verifying. It is necessary to search not only the selected code number for instructions but also the category, section, and chapter. Many times the instructional information is located on one or more pages preceding the actual page on which you found the code number.
9. Finally, assign the code number you have determined to be correct.

Additional coding tips include:

- In an emergency situation, the coder should identify the acute conditions or symptom pathology for outpatient services.
- For inpatient services, list what the conditions are "due to."
- For multiple injuries, always sequence the most severe injury first.
- For causes of infections, code them as secondary.
- Limit use of unlisted diagnostic codes to situations where there is no definitive information available or where no other specific code is available.
- Distinguish between acute and chronic whenever the ICD-9-CM makes the distinction.

For inpatient coding on a UB-04, code each medical condition identified in the medical record. Use the medical record to get clarification, or go to the physician and ask questions. Be sure to only code those diagnoses, symptoms, conditions, or problems documented in the medical record. Do not read more into a diagnostic or procedural description than was intended by a physician.

Typically, the ICD-9-CM volumes guide you to the correct codes, but you need to take the time to read through information thoroughly once you have all the facts about the patient.

Oftentimes, the problem is not that coders cannot find the appropriate code in the manual, but that they have not been provided with enough information. When a treatment or diagnostic statement from a physician is too general or does not match the descriptions in the ICD-9-CM manual, the coder needs to investigate and get the information necessary to code correctly.

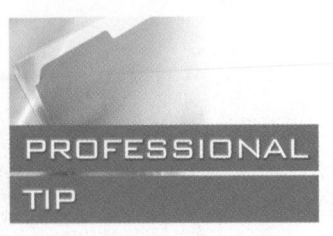

PROFESSIONAL TIP

Keep these important tips in mind about the ICD-9-CM manual:

- Make sure you are very familiar with the conventions of your ICD-9-CM publication.
- Use only the most current ICD-9-CM version available.
- Read all the information available in your ICD-9-CM for the headings, categories, and additional digits.

Chapter Summary

- ICD-9-CM coding is used by physicians' offices, hospitals, clinics, home healthcare agencies, and other healthcare providers to substantiate the need for patient care or treatment and to provide statistics for morbidity and mortality rates.
- The ICD-9-CM is made up of three main volumes:
  1. Volume 1: Tabular/Numerical List of Diseases
  2. Volume 2: Alphabetic Index to Diseases
  3. Volume 3: Tabular and Alphabetic Index of Procedures
- Proper diagnosis coding involves using the ICD-9-CM volumes to identify the appropriate codes for medical conditions that pertain to the patient's health (as recorded in the patient record), and entering those codes correctly on medical claims forms.

- Look up the main term in the alphabetic Index (Volume 2) first. The alphabetic index will point you to the correct area in which to begin your search in the tabular list (Volume 1).
- Locate the main term in the alphabetic index and read the subterms indented beneath it. Subterms differ from main terms in that they provide greater specificity and the anatomic site affected by the disease or injury.
- Use a three-digit category code only when no four-digit code exists. Use a four-digit subcategory code only when no fifth-digit subclassification code exists. This process is referred to as coding to the highest level of specificity.
- Physician practices do not code for "probable," "possible," or "rule out" diagnoses.
- Always read any notes such as "Use additional code," "Excludes," and "Includes" and follow the instructions.
- Always follow fourth- or fifth-digit instructions when coding.
- V-codes are used for non-related diseases or injuries.
- E-codes are always supplemental to the primary code, and they describe how the injury occurred.

Chapter Review

True/False

Identify the statement as true (T) or false (F).

_____ 1. A sudden flare-up of a patient's chronic condition may be characterized as acute.

_____ 2. The addenda to the ICD-9-CM are issued in June and take effect October 1 of each year.

_____ 3. An adverse effect is a harmful reaction caused by an overdose of a drug.

_____ 4. The alphabetic index of the ICD-9-CM is used first when locating a diagnostic code.

_____ 5. A coexisting condition is reported when it affects the patient's primary condition or is also treated during an encounter.

_____ 6. The etiology is the origin or cause of a disease.

_____ 7. A late effect occurs some period of time after the acute disease is resolved.

_____ 8. The manifestation is the cause or origin of an illness.

_____ 9. In the ICD-9-CM, NOS, or not otherwise specified, indicates a code to be used when too little information is available to assign another, more specific code.

_____ 10. The primary diagnosis represents the patient's most serious condition, regardless of the reason for the current encounter.

_____ 11. Subterms appear below the main term in the ICD-9-CM's alphabetic index.

_____ 12. Supplemental terms in the ICD-9-CM's alphabetic index are usually enclosed in parentheses or brackets.

_____ 13. V codes in the ICD-9-CM contain five numbers.

_____ 14. The ICD-9-CM diagnostic codes are made up of either three, four, or five digits and a description.

_____ 15. Codes in the tabular list of the ICD-9-CM are organized according to anatomic system or cause.

_____ 16. In the ICD-9-CM, parentheses are used around descriptions that are not essential parts of a term.

_____ 17. In the ICD-9-CM, a colon used with "Includes" or "Excludes" notes indicates a partial term that must be completed with one of the words following the colon.

_____ 18. The alphabetic index of the ICD-9-CM can be used alone to correctly locate a diagnostic code.

_____ 19. The guidelines for outpatient, or physician practice, diagnostic coding are the same as those which are followed to select codes for inpatients in hospitals.

_____ 20. A late effect usually requires two diagnosis codes, first the code for the specific late effect and second the code for the cause.

_____ 21. Signs and symptoms are reported when a patient's condition has not been diagnosed.

_____ 22. All of the patient's conditions, including diseases or illnesses no longer active or present, must be considered when selecting the correct diagnostic code for an encounter.

_____ 23. An annual preventive vaccination is reported using a V code from the ICD-9-CM.

_____ 24. A patient's chronic condition is reported each time it is treated during an encounter.

Multiple Choice

Identify the letter of the choice that best completes the statement or answers the question.

_____ 1. A combination code in the ICD-9-CM covers the:
a. coexisting condition.   c. chronic and acute illness.
b. etiology and manifestation.   d. none of the above.

_____ **2.** A comparison of two coding systems that shows which codes are used for similar classifications is a:
  a. convention.   c. crosswalk.
  b. category.   d. manifestation.

_____ **3.** A disease or procedure that is named for a person is a(n):
  a. eponym.   c. etiology.
  b. E code.   d. manifestation.

_____ **4.** A five-digit code in the ICD-9-CM is called a:
  a. category.   c. subcategory.
  b. subclassification.   d. V code.

_____ **5.** A personal history of cancer is reported with a(n):
  a. E code.   c. combination code.
  b. V code.   d. none of the above.

_____ **6.** The cross-reference _See also_ in the ICD-9-CM means that the coder:
  a. may look up the related term(s) that follows.
  b. must refer to the term that follows.
  c. either a or b.
  d. neither a nor b.

_____ **7.** An annual checkup is classified with a(n):
  a. combination code.   c. V code.
  b. E code.   d. five-digit code.

_____ **8.** The statement "patient has a family history of breast cancer" requires a(n):
  a. combination code.   c. V code.
  b. E code.   d. five-digit code.

_____ **9.** To find a code correctly in the ICD-9-CM, the first step is to locate the code in the:
  a. tabular list.   c. either a or b.
  b. alphabetic index.   d. neither a nor b.

_____ **10.** A condition that arises because of an injury or illness in the patient's medical history is called a(n):
  a. adverse effect.   c. comorbidity.
  b. manifestation.   d. late effect.

_____ **11.** Which section of the ICD-9-CM contains the code for a diagnostic statement of "elevated blood pressure"?
  a. V Codes.
  b. E Codes.
  c. Symptoms, Signs, and Ill-Defined Conditions.
  d. Diseases of the Circulatory System.

_____ **12.** In the ICD-9-CM, M codes (morphology codes) are used by:
  a. pathologists.   c. outpatient coders.
  b. nutritionists.   d. radiologists.

_____ **13.** In the ICD-9-CM's Neoplasm Table, a neoplasm is categorized as either:
a. malignant, benign, uncertain, or unspecified.
b. malignant, primary, secondary, or in situ.
c. primary, secondary, uncertain, or unspecified.
d. primary, secondary, in situ, or uncertain.

_____ **14.** In the ICD-9-CM, burns are classified according to the rule of:
a. inpatient coding.   c. TBSA.
b. nines.   d. first-degree burns.

_____ **15.** Which kind of fracture is indicated by the terms compound, infected, or puncture in the diagnostic statement?
a. closed   c. simple
b. open   d. unspecified

_____ **16.** An adverse effect is the result of:
a. intentional poisoning.   c. traffic accident.
b. unintentional poisoning.   d. signs and symptoms.

Completion

Complete each sentence or statement.

1. A physician's description of the main reason for a patient's encounter is called the diagnostic _____.

2. A(n) _____ effect remains after a patient's acute illness or injury.

3. If a fracture is not recorded as either closed or open, it is coded as _____.

4. When diagnostic codes are reported, the code for the _____ diagnosis is listed first, followed by the current coexisting conditions.

5. The guideline of not assigning diagnostic codes for suspected or probable conditions is referred to as "coding to the highest level of _____."

6. After surgery, the patient's diagnosis is different from the preoperative primary diagnosis. Which diagnosis is coded? _____

Code the Following

1. Abdominal pain of LLQ _____

2. Acute Bronchospasm _____

3. Herpes zoster myelitis _____

4. Smoking complicating pregnancy, childbirth, antepartum condition, or complication _____

5. Epilepsy complicating pregnancy, childbirth, or the puerperium _____

6. Uterine size date discrepancy, delivered _____

7. Encounter for removal of sutures _____

8. Papanicolaou smear of cervix with cytologic evidence of malignacy _____

9. Straining on urination _____

10. Postnasal drip _____

Resources

Private website of online diagnostic codes: ***http://icd9.chrisendres.com***
National Center for Health Statistics (NCHS): ***http://www.cdc.gov/nchs/***—website for
Department of Health and Human Services, Centers for Disease Control and Prevention

Chapter 5

Introduction to CPT® and Place of Service Coding

Chapter Objectives

After reading this chapter, the student should be able to:

1. Understand the history of CPT.
2. Understand evaluation and management (E/M) services.
3. Explain the three types of CPT categories.
4. Distinguish the need for modifiers.
5. Distinguish between a new and established patient.
6. Know the three key elements in choosing an E/M code.
7. Determine the correct E/M code.

Key Terms

American Medical Association (AMA)
Centers for Medicare and Medicaid Services (CMS)
chief complaint (CC)
consultation
counseling
Current Procedural Terminology (CPT)

E/M codes
established patient
examination
history
history of present illness (HPI)
medical decision making (MDM)

modifiers
nature of the presenting problem
new patient
nomenclature
past, family, and social history (PFSH)
review of systems (ROS)

CPT is a registered trademark of the American Medical Association.

**Case Study
Introduction
to CPT and
Place of
Service
Coding**

Mr. Leins had been a patient of Dr. Mitchell's previously but had moved out of the area 6 years ago. He recently moved back and was seeing the doctor for the first time since he returned. Dr Mitchell asked the billing supervisor whether he should bill Mr. Leins as a new or established patient.

She explained that the requirement for billing as a new or established patient was determined by the date the patient had last been seen by the provider. In this case, since it had been more than three years since the last date of service, Mr. Leins would be considered a new patient for billing purposes.

Questions

1. Why is there a differentiation made between a new and established patient even when the patient was seen by the doctor previously?

2. Do all E&M codes contain that differentiation?

3. What would be the result of an error in coding the patient as new when they were actually established?

4. What is the rule for determining when a patient is new or established for billing purposes?

Introduction

Understanding the use of procedure codes is the most important aspect of coding. If used correctly, the procedure codes determine the amount of reimbursement the provider will receive. Diagnostic codes show the reason for the procedure; the CPT codes determine whether the provider will be paid at the maximum or not.

The CPT is copyrighted and published by the American Medical Association and is updated annually. The first section of the CPT is known as Evaluation and Management (E/M) Services. These codes describe services provided by physicians to evaluate their patients and manage their care. This is the only section coded from which codes are used directly. The codes are widely used by physicians of all specialties and describe a very large portion of the medical care provided to patients of all ranges. This chapter will discuss how the **E/M codes** are used to report office visits, hospital visits, nursing home visits, rehabilitation center visits, and home visits. The classification of E/M services is important because the nature of physician activity and practice resource costs vary by the type of service, place of service, and patient's status and age.

CPT

The **American Medical Association (AMA)** first developed and published the **Current Procedural Terminology (CPT)** in 1966. The first edition helped encourage the use of standard terms and descriptors to document procedures in the medical record; helped communicate accurate information on procedures and services to agencies concerned with insurance claims; provided the basis for a computer-oriented system to evaluate operative procedures; and contributed basic information for actuarial and statistical purposes.

This first edition of the CPT contained primarily surgical procedures, with limited sections on medicine, radiology, and laboratory procedures. When first published, CPT coding used a four-digit system. The second edition, published in 1970, presented an expanded system of terms and codes to designate diagnostic and therapeutic procedures in surgery, medicine, and specialties. It was at this time that the five-digit codes were introduced, replacing the former four-digit system. Another significant change to the book was to list procedures related to internal medicine.

In the mid- to late 1970s, the third and fourth editions of the CPT were introduced. The fourth edition, published in 1977, represented significant updates in medical technology and a system of periodic updating was introduced to keep pace with the rapidly changing medical environment.

In 1983, CPT nomenclature was adopted for use by the **Centers for Medicare and Medicaid Services (CMS)**, formerly the Health Care Financing Administration (HCFA), as part of its Healthcare Procedure Coding System (HCPCS). With this adoption, CMS mandated the use of HCPCS (CPT) to report services for Part B of the Medicare program. In October 1986, as part of the Omnibus Budget Reconciliation Act, CMS also required state Medicaid agencies to use CPT codes for reporting outpatient hospital surgical procedures. Physicians may use procedure codes from any of the sections of the CPT.

In August 2000, the CPT code set was named as a national standard under the Health Insurance Portability and Accountability Act of 1996 (HIPAA).

Procedure codes are linked with diagnostic codes to establish the medical necessity of the procedure and the fee reimbursement to the providers. Medical office specialists should be aware of the importance of correct procedure coding. With a thorough knowledge of a third-party payer's policies, definition of "medical necessity," guidelines, and reporting requirements, the medical office specialist will be able to effectively submit "clean claims" (i.e., claims with no errors).

CPT Categories

The CPT has three categories: CPT Category I, CPT Category II, and CPT Category III.

CPT codes are implemented on January 1 of each year. All modifications and deletions are approved by the CPT Editorial Panel. The Editorial Panel consists of staff associated with national medical specialty societies, health insurance organizations and agencies, and individual physicians and other health professionals. The AMA prepares each annual update so that the new CPT Category I codes are available in the late fall of each year preceding their implementation. CPT Category II and CPT Category III codes are typically "early released" for reporting either January 1 or July 1 of a given CPT cycle. CPT Category I is a five digit numeric code with a descriptor. Category II is a four digit numeric-alpha code that ends with the letter F. CPT Category III is the same as CPT Category II except the code ends with the letter T.

CPT Category I

CPT Category I codes describe a procedure or service The descriptor in this category of CPT codes is generally based on the procedure being consistent with contemporary medical practice and being performed by many physicians in clinical practice in multiple locations. CPT Category I codes differ from ICD-9-CM codes, which are three to five digits with a decimal point after the third digit.

CPT Category I codes are subjected to a lengthy approval process conducted by the CPT Editorial Panel. In order for a procedure to be approved as a CPT Category I code, the CPT Editorial Panel at a minimum requires that many healthcare professionals perform the services across the country. In addition, FDA approval must be documented or imminent within a given CPT cycle, and the service must have proven clinical efficacy.

CPT Category I codes are restricted to clinically recognized and generally accepted services, not emerging technologies, services, and procedures (see CPT Category III discussion).

CPT Category II

CPT Category II codes are a set of optional tracking codes, developed principally for performance measurement. These codes are intended to facilitate data collection by coding certain services and/or test results that are agreed on as contributing to positive health outcomes and quality patient care. These codes may be services that are typically included in an E/M service or other component part of a service and are not appropriate for regular CPT Category I codes. Consequently, the CPT Category II codes do not have a relative value associated with them, as do CPT Category I codes.

The decision to develop CPT Category II codes for performance measures was based on a desire to standardize the collection of data for performance measurement. The current methods are based on detailed chart review or site surveys, which cost physicians time and money. By having coded data on services that are included as elements of performance measures, physicians have the option of supplying this information to plans through the administrative record. In this way, CPT Category II codes will ease the burden on physicians' offices to complete surveys and reduce the intrusion caused by chart review. Use of the administrative record for data on performance measures allow physicians to supply information without substantially adding to their paperwork, since this record is currently in use. CPT Category II codes concentrate on measurements that are developed and tested by national organizations, such as the National Committee for Quality Assurance, and those that are well established and currently used by large segments of the healthcare industry. The CPT Editorial Panel does not develop any measures. As with procedures, only CPT Category II codes with standardized language for existing performance measures will be established.

CPT Category II codes are assigned a numeric-alpha identifier with the letter "F" in the last field (e.g., 1234F) to distinguish them from CPT Category I codes. These codes are located in a separate section of the CPT book, following the Medicine section. Introductory language in this code section explains the purpose of these codes. The use of these codes is optional and not required for correct coding. To expedite reporting of CPT Category II codes, once the CPT Editorial Panel has approved these codes, the newly added codes are made available on a semiannual (twice a year) basis via electronic distribution on the AMA website.

CPT Category III

CPT Category III (Emerging Technology) codes are temporary codes for emerging technologies, services, and procedures. CPT Category III codes are intended to be used for data collection purposes to substantiate widespread use of new technologies, services, and procedures or those that are in the FDA approval process. Note that CPT Category III codes are not intended for use with services/procedures that have not been accepted by the CPT Editorial Panel because a proposal was incomplete, more information was needed, or the Federal Drug Administration (FDA) did not support the proposal. An important part of the reasoning behind the development of CPT Category III codes was the length and requirements of the CPT approval process for CPT Category I codes, which conflicted with the needs of researchers for coded data to track emerging technology services throughout the research process.

HIPAA's Final Rule supports the elimination of these local, temporary codes and the transition to national standard code sets. Many of the local, temporary codes were used by payers until services/procedures were more fully substantiated through research and received a CPT Category I code. Thus, CPT Category III codes can take the place of local, temporary codes used for this purpose.

As with CPT Category I codes, inclusion of a descriptor and its associated code number in CPT nomenclature does not represent endorsement by the AMA of any particular diagnostic or therapeutic procedure/service. Inclusion or exclusion of a procedure/service does not imply any health insurance coverage or reimbursement policy.

CPT Category III codes are assigned a numeric-alpha identifier with the "T" letter in the last field (e.g., 1234T). These codes are located in a separate section of the CPT book, following the CPT Category II code section. Introductory language in this code section explains the purpose of these codes. Once they have been approved by the CPT Editorial Panel, the newly added CPT Category III codes are made available on a semiannual basis via electronic distribution on the AMA website. The full set of CPT Category III codes is then included in the next published edition for that CPT cycle. These codes will be archived after 5 years if the code has not been accepted for placement in the CPT Category I section of the CPT book, unless it is demonstrated that a CPT Category III code is still needed. These archived codes are not reused.

Evaluation & Management	99201–99499
Anesthesia	00100–01999, 99100–99140
Surgery	10021–69990
Radiology	70010–79999
Pathology and Laboratory	80048–99199
Medicine	90281–99199, 99500–99600

Source: CPT only copyright 2007 American Medical Association. All rights reserved.

Figure 5.1

CPT Category I codes.

CPT Nomenclature

CPT **nomenclature** is a listing of descriptive terms, guidelines, and identifying codes for reporting medical services and procedures. Because the CPT nomenclature, a system of naming things, is not a strict classification system, some procedures may appear in sections other than in those in which they might ordinarily be "classified."

There are eight sections in the CPT code book. The first six sections pertain to CPT Category I codes (Figure 5.1).

The seventh and eighth sections pertain to the CPT Category II and CPT Category III codes, respectively. Their section names and sequences are as follows:

- CPT Category II Performance Measurement Codes 0001F–0011F
- CPT Category III New/Emerging Technology Codes 0001T–0060T

The procedures and services codes listed in the CPT nomenclature are presented in numeric order, with one exception: the E/M section appears at the beginning of the book. Because most physicians use the E/M codes in reporting a significant portion of their services, they were placed at the front of the book for ease of reference.

Symbols

To make CPT nomenclature more user friendly, over the years a number of code symbols have been incorporated into the book. On receipt of an updated CPT book, the medical coder should review the symbols. Some of the more frequently used symbols are these:

▲   *Revised code.* A triangle indicates that the code's descriptor has changed.
●   *New code.* This symbol indicates new to this edition.
►◄   *New or revised text.* These symbols enclose new or revised text other than the code's descriptor.
+   *Add-on code.* Describes secondary procedures only. Cannot be used as a primary code.

Guidelines

Specific guidelines are found at the beginning of each of the six sections of CPT Category I. The guidelines provide information that is necessary to appropriately interpret and report procedures and services found in that section. In addition to the guidelines that appear at the beginning of each section, several of the subheadings or subsections have special instructions unique to that section, resulting in guidelines and instructional notes appearing throughout the CPT book. Note that these guidelines and notes are critical to using CPT coding correctly.

CPT Modifiers

CPT **modifiers** are two-digit numeric indicators, with the exception of the physical status modifiers found in the guidelines of the Anesthesia section and Appendix A of the CPT book. The two-digit modifier, with a hyphen in front of it, is placed after the five-digit CPT code to indicate that the description of the service or procedure has been altered. The code and modifier are reported as a one-line entry on the claim form. Some modifiers apply only to certain sections, for example, the modifier "-25" is used only for E/M coding.

List of Modifiers for Evaluation and Management Coding

The following modifiers are used for evaluation and management coding:

21 Prolonged Evaluation and Management Service is used when the service provided is greater than the highest level described for the code range.

> **Example**
>
> **An established patient with multiple concurrent diseases requiring more than the highest level of office visit and other outpatient services. The physician examines the patient for emphysema, COPD, advanced diabetes, hypertension, and a gastric ulcer. After assessing the patient (90 minutes), all exceed the highest level of E/M service. Because the service exceeds the highest level of service, the modifier "-21" is appended to 99215: 99215-21.**

24 Unrelated Evaluation and Management Service by the Same Physician During a Postoperative Period is used when the E/M service is not related to the reason for surgery and is provided within the postoperative time period (global period) in the payer's reimbursement.

> **Example**
>
> **An orthopedic surgeon has performed a knee replacement and during the postop follow-up, the patient presents with a sprained wrist due to a fall. The physician reports an E/M code with the 24 modifier appended to it for the management of the sprained wrist. 99024 is used for the normal postoperative visit. The "-24" appended to the E/M code, 99024-24, informs the payer that this is separate from the visit for the knee replacement.**

25 Significant, Separately Identifiable Evaluation and Management Service by the Same Physician on the Same Day of the Procedure or Other Service is used when the physician provides an E/M service in addition to another E/M service or procedure on the same day.

> **Example**
>
> **A physician examines a patient for cervical radiculopathy. The modifier "-25" is appended to the 99214. An electromyography is reported as 95861. This shows the payer that a significant E/M service and a procedure were performed on the same day.**

32 Mandated Services is used when it is requested by the payer.

> **Example**
>
> **The patient's carrier requests a second opinion be performed prior to undergoing a surgical procedure. The consult is reported with the "-32" modifier attached.**

52 Reduced Service is used when an E/M service is less extensive than the descriptor indicates.

> **Example**
>
> **The physician began an initial gynecologic exam on the patient, but due to the patient's extreme discomfort, discontinued it. The modifier "-52" is appended to the E/M code.**

57 Decision for Surgery is used to indicate the visit was scheduled because a decision to have surgery was made and the patient was informed and counseled about the risks and outcomes.

> **Example**
>
> **At the request of his primary care physician (PCP), a patient consults a surgeon about his abdominal pain. The surgeon meets the requirements to report a consultation and the decision is made also to have surgery. The surgeon reports the consultation with the "-57" modifier attached.**

Coding to the Place of Service

The E/M section is divided into broad services such as office visits, hospital visits, and consultations. Most of the categories are again divided into subcategories of services, such as new patient, established patient; initial hospital care, subsequent hospital care; initial pediatric care, subsequent pediatric care; and initial neonatal critical care, subsequent neonatal critical care.

The CPT coding system makes specific distinctions for place of service in the evaluation and management codes. The place of service may have a considerable impact on reimbursement. Verify the correct place of service before choosing a code. The following are ranges of specific places of service:

Office (and Other Outpatient) Services	99201–99215
Hospital Observation Services	99217–99220
Hospital (Inpatient) Services	99221–99239
Consultations (Office)	99241–99245
Consultations (Inpatient)	99251–99255
Emergency Department Services	99281–99288
Pediatric Critical Care Patient Transport	99289, +99290
Critical Care Services	99291, +99292
Inpatient Pediatric and Neonatal Critical Care	99293–99300
Nursing Facility Services	99304–99318
Rest Home, Custodial Care, Domiciliary	99324–99337
Oversight Services for Domiciliary, Rest Home or Home	99339–99340
Home Services	99341–99350

Other Services Provided in the E/M Section

Services that also can be billed found in the Evaluation and Management Section include the following:

- Prolonged Services that are reported in addition to other physician services. For this reason these codes are add-on codes. These services can be provided either face to face (direct contact) with the patient or without direct contact with patient. The range of these codes is from 99354–99359.
- Physician Standby Services (99360) requires prolonged physician attendance without direct patient contact. This service is requested by another physician and is coded according to time for each 30 minutes. Second and subsequent periods of standby beyond the first 30 minutes must be met to bill each unit of time. Examples of standby services include operative standby, standby for cesarean/high risk delivery, standby for frozen section, and for monitoring an EEG.
- Other services found in this section that are not coded according to place of service are team conferences, telephone calls, anticoagulant management, disability and life insurance evaluations, and work related or medical disability evaluation services.

Office Versus Hospital Services

Office and other outpatient services are the most often reported E/M services. A patient is an *outpatient* unless admitted to a healthcare facility such as a hospital or skilled nursing facility for a 24-hour period or longer. When a patient is evaluated and then admitted to a healthcare facility, the service is reported using the codes for initial hospital care. An *inpatient* is a patient who has been admitted to the hospital and is expected to stay 24 hours or more.

Hospital observation service codes are used to report E/M services provided to patients designated as "observation status" in a hospital. These patients are there to be observed to determine whether they should be admitted to the hospital, transferred to another facility, or sent home. Not all hospitals have a specific area designated for observation patients. The patient does not have to be located in an observation area designated by the hospital, but rather designated as observation status.

The codes in this category of service are not used to report hospital observation services involving admission and discharge services provided on the same date. Hospital observation services involving admission and discharge are reported with codes 99234–99236.

Emergency Department Services

E/M services provided in the emergency department are reported with the codes in this series. These codes are not limited to use by emergency department physicians. No distinction is made between new and established patients. The reason for this is that many different physicians staff emergency departments and the services they provide are unscheduled and episodic. Time is not a factor in selecting the E/M service code.

Preventive Medicine Services

This is a specific category of E/M codes for reporting preventive medicine services. These services include the physical examination according to age, ordering of appropriate immunization(s), and laboratory/diagnostic procedures. The performance of immunizations and ancillary studies involving laboratory, radiology, and other procedures or screening tests identified with a specific CPT code is reported separately.

When reporting a preventive medicine E/M service and a problem-oriented E/M service on the same day, pay close attention to the diagnostic codes submitted on the claim. The diagnoses reported should justify the reason for reporting both services on the same day.

The initial preventive E/M codes are for reporting services provided to new patients. A common misconception is that the initial preventive medicine E/M service is reported for the first time the patient receives preventive medicine services, even if the patient has received problem-oriented services from the physician or another physician of the same specialty in the same group within the past 3 years.

Type of Patient

Once the place of service has been chosen, the type of patient must be identified. To determine if a patient is new or established, one must know the definitions of each.

New Patient

A **new patient** is one who has not received any professional services within the past 3 years from the physician or another physician of the same specialty who belongs to the same group practice.

Established Patient

An **established patient** is one who has received professional services within the past 3 years from the physician or another physician of the same specialty who belongs to the same group practice. Services that have been provided, such as telephone renewal of a prescription, if provided without a face-to-face encounter, are no longer considered when identifying patients as new or established.

Referral

A referral is the transfer of the total care or specific portion of care of a patient from one physician to another. A referral is not a request for consultation. If a patient is referred to the physician for total care or a portion of his care, use evaluation and management codes and other CPT codes if appropriate to report the services provided. If a patient is sent to the physician for a consultation, use E/M consultation codes to report the services provided.

Consultation

A **consultation** occurs when a second physician, at the request of the patient's physician or another appropriate source, examines the patient and renders an opinion. The patient must present with a written request for a consultation from the requesting physician (usually the PCP) or source, which should be filled in on the chart. The consultant must document her opinion in the patient's medical record as well as any services performed. The consultant must also render her opinion in writing to the requesting physician. The patient returns to the requesting physician. The consulting physician uses the E/M codes from the Consultations section. The definition of "another appropriate source" includes a physician assistant, nurse practitioner, doctor of chiropractic, physical therapist, occupational therapist, speech language therapist, psychologist, social worker, lawyer, or insurance company.

Level of E/M Service

With each category or subcategory of E/M services, three to five levels are available for reporting purposes. The number of levels within a category varies and is dependent on the types of services that might be provided.

The various levels describe the wide variations in skill, effort, time, and medical knowledge required for the prevention or diagnosis and treatment of illness or injury, and the promotion of optimal health.

The code descriptors for the level of service identify seven components, six of which are used in defining the levels of E/M services:

1. The extent of the history documented
2. The extent of the examination documented
3. The complexity of the medical decision making documented
4. Counseling
5. Coordination of care with other providers
6. Nature of the presenting problem
7. Time.

Specific steps must be taken to select the appropriate level of E/M service. Selection is based on the extent of three key components of the seven just listed:

1. The extent of the patient's history obtained
2. The extent of the examination documented
3. The complexity of the medical decision making.

These three components are discussed in more detail next. Figure 5.2 is an example of the range of E/M codes that can be used for a new patient.

New Patient

99201 **Office or other outpatient visit** for the evaluation and management of a new patient, which requires these three key components:

- a problem focused history;
- a problem focused examination;
- straightforward medical decision making.

Counseling and/or coordination of care with other providers or agencies are provided consistent with the nature of the problem(s) and the patient's and/or family's needs.

Usually, the presenting problem(s) are self limited or minor. Physicians typically spend 10 minutes face-to-face with the patient and/or family.

99202 **Office or other outpatient visit** for the evaluation and management of a new patient, which requires these three key components:

- an expanded problem focused history;
- an expanded problem focused examination;
- straightforward medical decision making.

Counseling and/or coordination of care with other providers or agencies are provided consistent with the nature of the problem(s) and the patient's and/or family's needs.

Usually, the presenting problem(s) are of low to moderate severity. Physicians typically spend 20 minutes face-to-face with the patient and/or family.

99203 **Office or other outpatient visit** for the evaluation and management of a new patient, which requires these three key components:

- a detailed history;
- a detailed examination;
- medical decision making of low complexity.

Counseling and/or coordination of care with other providers or agencies are provided consistent with the nature of the problem(s) and the patient's and/or family's needs.

Usually, the presenting problem(s) are of moderate severity. Physicians typically spend 30 minutes face-to-face with the patient and/or family.

99204 **Office or other outpatient visit** for the evaluation and management of a new patient, which requires these three key components:

- a comprehensive history;
- a comprehensive examination;
- medical decision making of moderate complexity.

Counseling and/or coordination of care with other providers or agencies are provided consistent with the nature of the problem(s) and the patient's and/or family's needs.

Usually, the presenting problem(s) are of moderate to high severity. Physicians typically spend 45 minutes face-to-face with the patient and/or family.

99205 **Office or other outpatient visit** for the evaluation and management of a new patient, which requires these three key components:

- a comprehensive history;
- a comprehensive examination;
- medical decision making of high complexity.

Counseling and/or coordination of care with other providers or agencies are provided consistent with the nature of the problem(s) and the patient's and/or family's needs.

Usually, the presenting problem(s) are of moderate to high severity. Physicians typically spend 60 minutes face-to-face with the patient and/or family.

Figure 5.2

Example of the range of E/M codes available for use with a new patient.

Extent of Patient's History

To determine the extent of the **history** documented, the following information must be obtained from the patient. If the patient is incapacitated, the physician may obtain the history from a family member. The history is documented as follows: (1) chief complaint, (2) history of present illness, (3) review of systems, and (4) past, family, and/or social history. These are discussed in the following subsections.

Chief Complaint

The **chief complaint (CC)** is a concise statement describing the symptom, problem, condition, diagnosis, or other factor that is the reason for the visit/encounter, usually stated in the patient's or guardian's words.

History of Present Illness

The **history of present illness (HPI)** is a chronological description of the development of the patient's present illness from the first sign and/or symptom to the present. Patients usually express their problems as symptoms (e.g., pain or discomfort) or signs (e.g., lump, cut, bruise, rash), with the exception of a newborn, whose presenting complaint may be related to his mother's complaint (e.g., maternal fever during labor). The further elaboration of any symptom requires attention to some or all of the dimensions of the HPI. Signs are better described by physical findings. Problems can also be described as the status of one or more chronic conditions.

CPT guidelines recognize eight dimensions of the HPI, including a description of:

1. Location (where in body the CC is occurring)
2. Quality (the character of the pain)
3. Severity (the rank of the symptoms or pain on a scale, such as 1 to 10)
4. Duration (how long the symptom or pain has been present or how long it lasts when it occurs)
5. Timing (when the symptom or pain occurs)
6. Context (the situation that is associated with the pain or symptom, such as eating dairy products)
7. Modifying factors (things done to make the pain or symptom change, such as using an ice pack)
8. Associated signs and symptoms (other things that happen when the symptom or pain happens, such as "When my chest pain occurs I have shortness of breath").

Review of Systems

The **review of systems (ROS)** is an inventory of body systems obtained through a series of questions asked by the physician. The physician seeks to identify signs and/or symptoms that the patient may be experiencing or has experienced. This helps define the problem, clarify the differential diagnosis, identify testing needed, or serve as baseline data on other systems that might be affected by any possible management (treatment) options. A ROS may be highly dependent on the age of the patient and irrelevant for newborns and young infants. The following elements of a system review have been identified in the CPT code set:

- Constitutional symptoms (fever, weight loss, etc.)
- Eyes
- Ears, nose, mouth, throat
- Cardiovascular

- Respiratory
- Gastrointestinal
- Genitourinary
- Musculoskeletal
- Integumentary (skin and/or breast)
- Neurologic
- Psychiatric
- Endocrine
- Hematologic/lymphatic
- Allergic/immunologic.

Past, Family, and Social History

The **past, family, and social history (PFSH)** includes a review of past medical experiences of the patient and the patient's family. Past history is dependent on the patient's age and not appropriate for a newborn infant.

The past history is a review of the patient's past experiences with illnesses, injuries, and treatments that includes significant information about:

- Prior major illnesses and injuries
- Prior operations
- Prior hospitalizations
- Current medications
- Allergies (e.g., drug, food)
- Age-appropriate immunization status
- Age-appropriate feeding/dietary status.

The family history is a review of medical events in the patient's family including significant information about:

- The health status or cause of death of parents, siblings, and children
- Specific diseases related to problems identified in the CC, HPI, and/or ROS
- Diseases of family members that may be hereditary or place the patient at risk.

The social history is an age-appropriate review of past and current activities that includes significant information about:

- Marital status and/or living arrangements
- Immunization history
- Current employment
- Developmental history
- School history
- Use of drugs, alcohol, and tobacco
- Levels of education
- Sexual history
- Other relevant social factors.

The levels of E/M services recognize four types of history as follows:

Problem focused	CC; brief HPI
Expanded problem focused	CC; brief HPI, problem-pertinent ROS

| Detailed | CC; extended HPI, problem-pertinent ROS, including review of a limited number of additional systems; pertinent PFSH (directly related to the patient's problems) |
| Comprehensive | CC; extended HPI; ROS directly related to problems identified in HPI plus review of all additional body systems; complete PFSH. Please now complete Practice Exercise 5.1. |

Extent of Examination

The extent of the **examination** performed depends on the clinical judgment of the physician and the nature of the patient's presenting problems. The levels of E/M services recognize four types of examinations:

Problem focused	A limited exam of the affected body area or organ system
Expanded problem focused	A limited exam of the affected body area or organ system and other symptomatic or related organ systems(s)
Detailed	An extended exam of the affected body area(s) and other symptomatic or related organ system(s)
Comprehensive	A general multisystem exam or a complete exam of a single organ system

The following body areas are recognized:

- Head, including the face
- Neck
- Chest, including breasts and axilla
- Abdomen

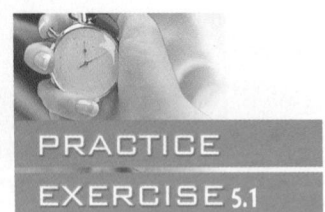

PRACTICE EXERCISE 5.1

Determine in which type of history category—Problem Focused, Expanded Problem Focused, Detailed, or Comprehensive—would you document these statements.

1. Patient presents with sore throat for 2 days. She has used saltwater gargle, which has not helped. She denies having any cough. Review of symptoms reveals no known allergies or family history of asthma.

2. Patient returns for follow-up visit for COPD. She states that the shortness of breath (SOB) has improved with Advair and Spiriva, which was prescribed at the last visit. Denies any chest pain. Patient takes Norvasc for hypertension. Lungs are clear to auscultation. Discussed the importance of diet and exercise. Return in 3 months.

On completion of this exercise, refer to Appendix J to check the accuracy of your work.

- Genitalia, groin, buttocks
- Back
- Each extremity.

The following organ systems are recognized:

- Eyes
- Ears, nose, mouth, and throat
- Cardiovascular
- Respiratory
- Gastrointestinal
- Genitourinary
- Musculoskeletal
- Skin
- Neurologic
- Psychiatric
- Hematologic/lymphatic/immunologic.

Complexity of Medical Decision Making

To determine the complexity of the **medical decision making (MDM)**, the physician must establish a diagnosis and/or select a management option as measured by the following:

1. The number of possible diagnoses and/or the number of management options that must be considered
2. The amount and /or complexity of medical records, diagnostic tests, and/or other information that must be obtained, reviewed, and analyzed
3. The risk of significant complications, morbidity, and/or mortality, as well as co-morbidities, associated with the patient's presenting problem.

Four types of medical decision making are recognized in the CPT nomenclature. Table 5.1 lists the types and the elements required to qualify for each type. To qualify for a given type of MDM, two of the three elements in Table 5.1 must be met or exceeded.

Table 5.1	The Four Types of Medical Decision Making		
Type of MDM	**Number of Diagnoses or Management Options**	**Amount and/or Complexity of Data to be Reviewed**	**Risk of Complications and/or Morbidity or Mortality**
Straightforward	Minimal	Minimal or none	Minimal
Low complexity	Limited	Limited	Limited
Moderate complexity	Multiple	Multiple	Multiple
High complexity	Extensive	Extensive	Extensive

> **Example**
>
> Low-complexity MBM is a limited number of diagnoses or management options, moderate amount and/or complexity of data to be reviewed, and low risk of complications and/or morbidity or mortality.

After determining the three key elements, the coder should analyze the requirements to report the service level.

1. The descriptor for each E/M code explains the standards for its use. For office visits and most other services to new patients, and for initial care visits, generally all three of the key component requirements must be met.

> **Example**
>
> 99203 Office or other outpatient visit for the evaluation and management of a new patient, which requires these three key components:
>
> - Detailed history
> - Detailed examination
> - Medical decision making of low complexity.

2. Most services for established patients and subsequent care require two of the three components.

> **Example**
>
> 99213 Office or other outpatient visit for the evaluation and management of an established patient, which requires at least two of these three key components:
>
> - Expanded problem focused history
> - Expanded problem focused examination
> - Medical decision making of low complexity.

Additional Components

Many descriptors mention additional components, as discussed next.

Counseling
In terms of E/M coding, **counseling** is a discussion with a patient and/or family for one of the following reasons:

- Diagnostic results, impressions, and recommended studies
- Prognosis
- Risks and benefits of treatment options
- Instructions and/or follow-up

Table 5.2	Types of Presenting Problems

Types	Definitions
Minimal	A problem that may not require the presence of a physician, but service is provided under the physician's supervision.
Self-limited or minor	A problem that runs a definite and prescribed course and is not likely to permanently alter the health status or has a good prognosis with management and compliance.
Low severity	A problem where the risk of morbidity without treatment is low; there is little to no risk of mortality without treatment; full recovery without functional impairment is expected.
Moderate severity	A problem where the risk of morbidity without treatment is moderate; there is moderate risk of mortality without treatment; uncertain prognosis or increased probability of prolonged functional impairment.
High severity	A problem where the risk of morbidity without treatment is high to extreme; there is a moderate to high risk of mortality without treatment or high probability of severe, prolonged functional impairment.

- Importance of compliance with chosen treatment options
- Risk factor reduction
- Patient and family education.

The Nature of the Presenting Problem

The **nature of the presenting problem** describes how severe the patient's condition is. A presenting problem is a disease, condition, illness, injury, symptom, sign, complaint, or other reason for a visit/encounter with or without a diagnosis being established at the time of the encounter. Presenting problems can be defined as shown in Table 5.2.

Time

One element of E/M coding is how much time the physician typically spends directly treating the patient. Typical times have been included in many of the code descriptors. The specific time in the visit codes are averages and therefore represent a range of times that may be higher or lower depending on the actual visit.

Example

This statement appears after the 99214 code for an established patient E/M service: Usually, the presenting problem(s) are of moderate to high severity. Physicians typically spend 25 minutes face-to-face with the patient and or family.

As mentioned earlier, counseling is a discussion with a patient regarding areas such as diagnostic results, instructions for follow-up treatment, and patient education. When counseling and/or coordination of care constitute more than 50% of the physician/patient and/or family encounter, then time may be considered the key or controlling factor to qualify for a particular level of E/M services. This includes time spent with those who have assumed responsibility for the care of the patient or decision making, whether or not they are family members (e.g., foster parents, person acting in

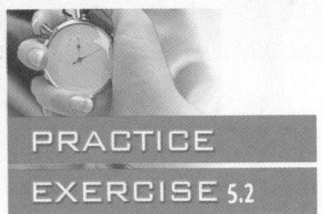

Read the following chart notes and choose the appropriate code.

1. For several years, Dr. Bonner has been treating Mrs. Henderson for type II diabetes, hypertension, and obesity. Three days before this appointment, blood work was performed to determine the status of her diabetes. She presents to the physician's office and the physician examines her for evidence of infection or circulatory problems. He then asks the patient about her compliance with the 1,200-calorie diet she has been on for the past 6 months.

    After reviewing these findings, the physician indicates to the patient that she will have to begin using insulin, because her diabetes is not responding to the current treatment. Mrs. Henderson begins to sob uncontrollably. She tells Dr. Bonner that this means she is going to die because her grandmother got gangrene from this kind of diabetes and died from it.

    After calming her, Dr. Bonner explains that using insulin is not a "death sentence." He discusses diet, insulin administration, and hypoglycemic reactions, as well as the symptoms of hyperglycemia. He instructs Mrs. Henderson as to proper foot and skin care and stresses the importance of seeing her ophthalmologist regularly. Mrs. Henderson is much calmer and feels that she will learn a lot from the booklets Dr. Bonner has given her.

    The total time Dr. Bonner spent with Mrs. Henderson is 25 minutes, with 20 of those minutes spent providing counseling and/or coordination of care. Because more than 50% of the encounter was spent providing counseling and/or coordination of care, the total face-to-face time between Mrs. Henderson and Dr. Bonner may be considered the key factor in selecting the level of E/M service. Therefore, because Mrs. Henderson is an established patient and 25 total minutes was spent with the patient it would be appropriate to report what code?

    Code _____

2. Chart note for an established patient: Office visit by established patient for monthly scheduled blood test to monitor Coumadin, which is an anticoagulant; nurse spends 5 minutes, reviews the test, confirms that the patient is doing well, and states that no change in the dosage is necessary.

    Code _____

3. A patient presents to Dr. B's office with complaints of fever, chills, malaise, and a cough. Dr. B obtains the history, performs an examination, and orders a chest x-ray. The patient is admitted to the hospital on the same day for intravenous antibiotic therapy for treatment of pneumonia. After completion of her office hours, Dr. B provides an E/M service to the patient in the hospital.

    Code _____

4. Home visit for established patient, straightforward case, problem-focused examination.

    Code _____

On completion of this exercise, refer to Appendix J to check the accuracy of your work.

locum, legal guardian). The extent of counseling and/or coordination of care must be documented in the medical record. When coordination of care is provided but the patient is not present, the case management and care plan oversight services subsections' codes are reported. These factors, although not the key components, help ensure that the correct service level is selected.

Assigning the Code

The code that has been selected is assigned. The need for any modifiers, based on the documentation of special circumstances, is also reviewed.

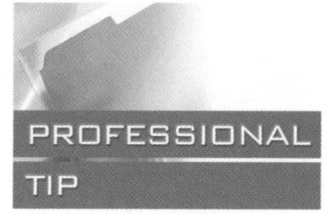

PROFESSIONAL TIP

When an E/M code is assigned, the patient's medical record must contain the clinical data to support it. The history, examination, and medical decision making must be sufficiently documented in the medical record so that the medical necessity and appropriateness of the service can be understood.

Chapter Summary

- The AMA first developed and published the CPT and updates it annually.
- The CPT has three categories: CPT Category I has six sections that refer to the CPT codes. CPT Category II contains performance measurement tracking codes and CPT Category III contains emerging technology codes.
- The CPT has specific guidelines located at the beginning of each section.
- Modifiers are two-digit numeric indicators which indicate that the description of the service or procedure has been altered.
- The CPT coding system makes specific distinctions for place of service in the E/M codes. The place of service may have a considerable impact on reimbursement.
- Reimbursement is also related to the type of patient: new, established, or consult.
- The three key components for determining an E/M code are the extent of the history documented, the extent of the examination documented, and the complexity of the medical decision making documented.

Chapter Review

True/False

Identify the statement as true (T) or false (F).

_____ 1. Physicians may use procedure codes from any of the sections of the CPT.

_____ 2. In performing an evaluation and management service, the physician often documents the HPI, which is an abbreviation for *history of previous illnesses*.

_____ 3. In the CPT, the term *consultation* describes services that a provider performs at the request of another provider after which the patient is returned to the requesting provider's care.

_____ 4. A new patient is one who has not received professional services within the past 2 years.

_____ 5. An established patient is one who has received professional services from the physician or another physician of the same specialty who belongs to the same group practice within the past 3 years.

_____ 6. Emergency department services distinguish between new and established patients.

_____ 7. Time is a factor when choosing an emergency department service.

_____ 8. An established patient receiving an annual exam for the first time is coded in the preventive medicine service as a new patient.

_____ 9. Hospital observation service codes are used to code for patients admitted to the hospital.

_____ 10. There are six categories of CPTs.

Multiple Choice

Identify the letter of the choice that best completes the statement or answers the question.

_____ 1. Of the four types of examinations that physicians perform, which level is the most complete?
   a. detailed
   b. expanded problem focused
   c. comprehensive
   d. problem focused

_____ 2. Routine annual physical examinations are reported using CPT's:
   a. consultation codes.
   b. office services codes.
   c. preventive medicine services codes.
   d. critical care services codes.

_____ 3. In selecting an evaluation and management code, three components are considered: the history, the examination, and the:
   a. family background.
   b. medical decision making.
   c. diagnoses options.
   d. interval history.

_____ 4. When choosing an E/M code, what is chosen first?
   a. alphabetic index
   b. medicine section
   c. place of service
   d. new patient

_____ 5. A CPT code can be distinguished from an ICD-9-CM code because it has:
   a. three digits with a decimal point.
   b. four digits.
   c. five digits with a modifier.
   d. five digits.

___ 6. In some billing cases it is necessary to add a two-digit modifier in order to:
a. indicate usual charges.
b. prevent miscoding.
c. give a more accurate description.
d. meet the payer's criteria.

___ 7. CPT codes, descriptions, and two-digit modifiers are copyrighted by the:
a. Blue Cross and Blue Shield Organization.
b. American Medical Association.
c. CPC coder.
d. World Health Organization.

___ 8. What is the number of the modifier for a Significant, Separately Identifiable Evaluation and Management Service by the Same Physician on the Same Day of the Procedure or Other Service that is used when the physician provides an E/M service in addition to another E/M service or procedure on the same day?
a. -25   c. -24
b. -26   d. -32

___ 9. The modifier for Decision for Surgery is:
a. -32.   c. -52.
b. -57.   d. -21.

___ 10. The CPT is revised:
a. every 2 years.   c. annually.
b. when necessary.   d. every 6 months.

___ 11. In the CPT, a round bullet symbol indicates a:
a. bundled code.   c. new code.
b. revised code.   d. deleted code.

___ 12. In the CPT, a triangle symbol indicates a(n):
a. new code.   c. decision for surgery.
b. descriptor has changed.   d. add-on code.

___ 13. The CPT Category I is divided into how many sections?
a. 4   c. 5
b. 6   d. 8

___ 14. Components of a medical history include all of the following except:
a. medical decision making.
b. chief complaint.
c. family history.
d. review of systems.

___ 15. A key component in coding medical decision making is the:
a. physician's level of education.
b. amount of time the physician spends with the patient.
c. level of complexity.
d. patient's childhood diseases.

Completion

Complete each sentence or statement, using your CPT manual.

1. In the CPT, E/M is the abbreviation for Evaluation and _____ Services.

2. Define the term *new patient.* _____
   _____
   _____

3. What subsection is used to code a physical annual examination? _____

4. What subsection is used for a consultation? _____

5. Is a patient who visits an emergency room coded as a new or an established patient?
   _____

6. Is critical care coded according to time? _____

7. What code is used for the annual assessment of a patient in a nursing facility
   whose condition could be stable, improving, or recovering? _____

8. What is the age of a neonate? _____

9. What is the age of an infant or young child? _____

For Additional Practice

Based on the description of the service, look up the appropriate CPT code and write it
in the space provided

1. Complex comprehensive initial consultation, office, medical decision of high
   complexity _____

2. Emergency department care, minimal care, straightforward medical decision,
   problem-focused history and exam _____

3. Admission to SNF, established patient, medical decision of low complexity,
   detailed history, comprehensive exam _____

4. The code for subsequent hospital care for a patient in a stable condition
   _____

5. Follow-up minimal consultation, office, straightforward medical decision making, problem-focused history and exam _____

6. Work-related medical disability evaluation by treating physician _____

7. Supervision of hospice patient care (25 minutes spent in 1 month) _____

8. Cardiothoracic surgeon provides a second opinion for the appropriateness of
   a mitral valve replacement; during the hour-long encounter, the physician

performs a comprehensive history and exam and follows up the visit with a written report to the PCP; MDM was moderate.

9. During an annual physical examination, a 45-year-old established patient complains of tiredness and shortness of breath during mild activity; physician performs a detailed cardiovascular assessment with additional detailed history; following complex MDM, the physician also schedules an immediate complete heart study. _____

10. Office visit for an established patient with a problem-focused history and examination _____

Resources

American Medical Association: *www.ama-assn.org/go/CPT*
The 2007 CPT Standard Edition, published by the American Medical Association: *www.cptnetwork.com*

Chapter 6 | Coding Procedures and Services

Chapter Objectives

After reading this chapter, the student should be able to:

1. Correctly use the CPT® index.
2. Understand the four primary classes of main entries in the CPT index.
3. Understand code ranges and conventions.
4. Discuss the purpose of each section and the guidelines.
5. Know how to use modifiers correctly.
6. Use add-on codes properly.
7. Review codes for accuracy.
8. Given procedural statements, apply coding guidelines to determine the correct CPT codes.

Key Terms

add-on codes
bundled code
Clinical Laboratory
   Improvement
   Amendment (CLIA)
cross-references
descriptor

fragmented billing
global period
global surgical concept
panel
physical status modifier
primary procedure
professional component

secondary procedure
separate procedure
special report
surgical package
technical component
unbundling
unlisted procedure

CPT is a registered trademark of the American Medical Association.

Case Study
Coding Procedures and Services

Sandy has recently been seeing Dr. Georgio for visits pertaining to a mastectomy. In the midst of seeing Dr. Georgio for the mastectomy that was performed four weeks ago, she also saw her for a vaginal infection. Sandy was confused when she received a bill for the visit. Up until now she had not received any bills from the physician. Upon contacting the billing office, they explained that all of the visits pertaining to the mastectomy were covered under a global charge, but that the most recent visit did not fall under that charge since it did not pertain to the mastectomy.

Questions

1. What does it mean that the mastectomy visits fall under a global charge?

2. Could there be a situation in which the vaginal infection could be tied to the global service?

3. Is there a universal time frame for all global services?

Introduction

Any procedure or service in any section of the Current Procedural Terminology (CPT) book may be used to report the services performed by any qualified physician or provider. The subsections are divided by type of service and body system. It is important that the coder become familiar with and develop an understanding of the general layout of the CPT book. Knowledge about how to use the CPT index will assist medical coders in locating the appropriate code for reporting the procedures and/or the services performed. The CPT index is not a substitute for the main text of the CPT. Even if only one code appears in the index, the user must refer to the main text to ensure that the code selection is accurate.

Organization of the CPT Index

When using the CPT index, it is important to understand how entries to the index have been made. It cannot be stressed enough that the CPT index is not a substitute for the main text of the CPT nomenclature. As just mentioned, even if only one code appears in the index, the user must refer to the main text of the CPT book to ensure that the code selection is accurate. The CPT index is located after the appendixes. The index is organized by main terms and it has four primary classes of main entries:

1. *Procedure or service:* Allergen Immunotherapy, Arthroscopy, Biopsy, Cardiac Catheterization, Debridement, Evaluation and Management, Laparoscopy, Osteopathic Manipulation, Physical Medicine/Therapy/Occupational Therapy, Vaccines, etc.
2. *Organ, or other anatomic site:* Abdomen, Bladder, Esophagus, Hip, Intestines, Malar Area, Olecranon Process, Prostate, etc.
3. *Condition:* Abscess, Blepharoptosis, Dislocation, Esophageal Varices, Hemorrhage, Omphalocele, Varicose Vein, etc.
4. *Synonyms, eponyms, and abbreviations:* Anderson Tibial Lengthening, CBC, Clagett Procedure, EKG, Patterson Test, etc.

Instructions for Using the CPT

From a historical perspective, CPT coding has always placed procedures in general sections according to where physicians will most conveniently find them. For example, the code for a diagnostic colonoscopy, while not involving an incision, is located in the Digestive System Surgery section. Keeping the endoscopies involving a biopsy, tumor removal, or other operative interventions in proximity to the diagnostic procedure was an important consideration. Similarly, cast applications are listed in the Musculoskeletal Surgery section, in proximity to the fracture and dislocation treatments, but

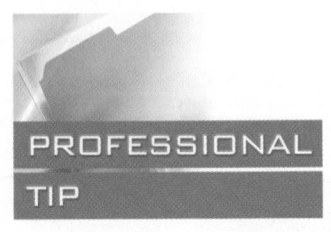

PROFESSIONAL TIP

In the CPT index, the CPT topics and subtopics are listed as the heading and a range of codes follows. The code(s) direct the coder to the code(s) where additional information on the topic(s) may be located. All topics referring to CPT code sections or chapter headings are listed in **BOLD UPPERCASE.**

clearly, cast application is not a "surgical procedure."

Code Range

A range of codes is shown when more than one code applies to an entry. Two codes, either sequential or not, are separated by a comma:

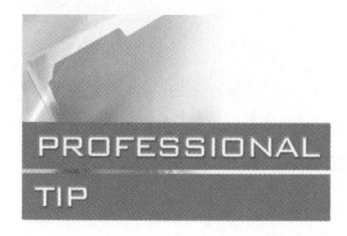

The CPT index provides a pointer to the correct code range in the main text. Using the CPT index makes the process of selecting procedural codes more efficient.

PROFESSIONAL
TIP

Biopsy

Colon...44025, 44100

More than two sequential codes are separated by a hyphen:

Biopsy

Elbow...24065–24066

Formatting and Cross-References

All CPT codes are five digits (no decimal point) followed by a **descriptor**, which is a brief description of the procedure.

Example

85002 Bleeding Time

Formatting

After searching the index for the procedure, service, or condition according to the main term and any subterms, the coder searches the section in which the code or code range is located and reads all descriptors.

A main procedure descriptor may be followed by a series of up to three indented terms that modify the main descriptor. These modifying terms should be reviewed, because these subterms have an effect on appropriate code selection. Note that the common descriptor begins with a capital letter, but the unique descriptors after the semicolon do not. The format of the terminology was originally developed as stand-alone descriptions of medical procedures.

However, to conserve space and avoid having to repeat common terminology, some of the procedure descriptors in CPT coding are not printed in their entirety, but rather refer back to a common portion of the procedure descriptor listed in a preceding entry. Within any indented series of codes, you must refer back to the first left-justified code (the *parent code*) within that series to determine the full procedure descriptor of the indented code(s). Figure 6.1 illustrates this formatting convention.

The common part of the parent code 97010, that is, the descriptor before the semicolon (in Figure 6.1, the common part descriptor reads "Application of a modality to one or more areas"), should be considered part of each of the following

Figure 6.1	97010	Application of a modality to one or more areas; hot or cold packs
	97012	traction, mechanical
Determining the full procedure descriptor.	97014	electrical stimulation (unattended)
	97016	vasopneumatic devices
	97018	paraffin bath

CPT only copyright 2007 American Medical Association. All rights reserved.

Figure 6.2	64400	Injection, anesthetic agent; trigeminal nerve, any division or branch
	64402	facial nerve
Range of procedures independently reported.	64405	greater occipital nerve
	64408	vagus nerve

CPT only copyright 2007 American Medical Association. All rights reserved.

indented codes in that series. For example, the full procedure descriptor represented by code 97012 is as follows:

> 97012 Application of a modality to one or more areas; traction, mechanical

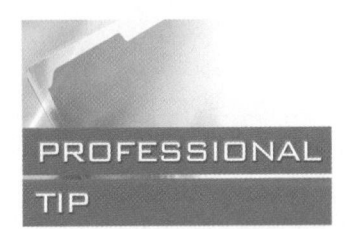

PROFESSIONAL TIP

To find the parent code, or common part of the descriptor, stop at the semicolon.

Simply because a code is indented within a series does not mean that one code from a series cannot be reported with another code within the same indented series. If two distinct procedures are performed then both procedures can be coded.

The range of procedures in Figure 6.2 can be coded independently if reported as such.

Example

The following procedures would be reported as separate codes:
64402—Injection, anesthetic agent; facial nerve
64408—Injection, anesthetic agent; vagus nerve

Cross-references

Cross-references provide additional instructions to the user. Two types of cross-references are used in the main sections.

> **See** or **Use:** These types of entries in parentheses point to another code; also used primarily for synonyms, eponyms, and abbreviations. (As an added reference in the American Medical Association's (AMA's) CPT® 2007 Standard Edition, a list of common abbreviations can be found on the back cover of the edition.)

CPT is a registered trademark of the American Medical Association.

See Also: These entries direct the coder to look under another main term if the procedure is not listed under the first main index entry.

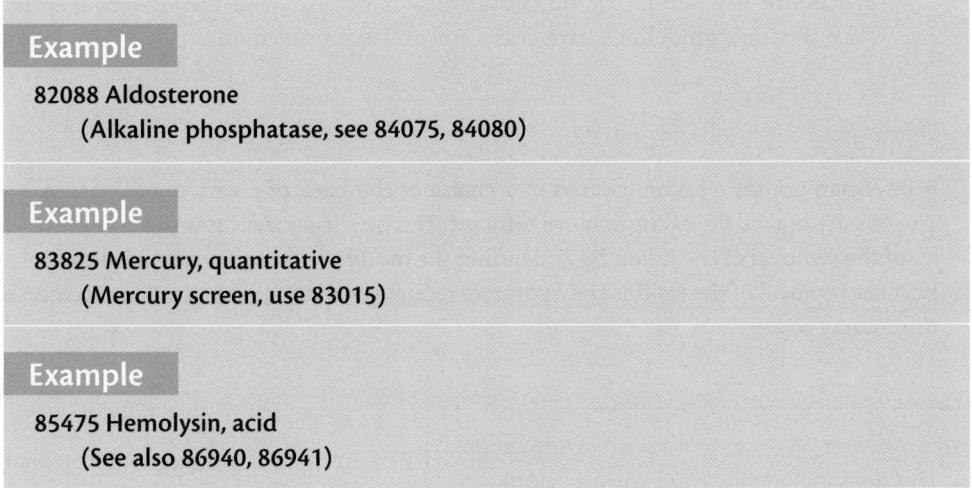

Example

82088 Aldosterone
    (Alkaline phosphatase, see 84075, 84080)

Example

83825 Mercury, quantitative
    (Mercury screen, use 83015)

Example

85475 Hemolysin, acid
    (See also 86940, 86941)

Section Guidelines

The beginning of every section has guidelines specific to that section. The guidelines provide information that is necessary to appropriately interpret and report the procedures and services found in that section. There also may be a list of modifiers, which are specific to the section. All of the guidelines and notes are there to assist the user in appropriate interpretation and application of the codes throughout the book. These guidelines are critical to using CPT coding correctly.

Modifiers

Modifiers are used with the CPT coding system to report a service or procedure that has been modified by some specific circumstance without altering or modifying the basic definition or CPT code.

The proper use of modifiers can speed up claims processing and increase reimbursement, whereas the improper use of CPT modifiers may result in claim delays or denials. The modifiers can be readily found in the CPT book in Appendix A with their full definitions. Modifiers may be used in many instances for these reasons:

- To report only the professional component of a procedure or service
- To report a service mandated by a third-party payer
- To indicate that a procedure was performed bilaterally
- To report multiple procedures performed at the same session by the same provider
- To report a portion of a service or procedure that was reduced or eliminated at the physician's discretion
- To report assistant surgeon services.

The most commonly used modifiers are discussed next.

   22 Unusual Procedural Service: This modifier is used when the service provided is higher than that usually required for the listed procedure. A special report

should be submitted with the claim. A **special report** is a report that details the reasons for a new, variable, or unlisted procedure or service; it explains the patient's condition and justifies the procedure's medical necessity. An **unlisted procedure** is a service or procedure that is not listed in the CPT codebook. Each section's guidelines have codes for unlisted procedures.

Example

A physician excises a lesion located in a crease of the back of a very obese person. The obesity makes the excision more difficult. The physician indicates the complexity of the removal of the lesion by appending the modifier 22 to the code used to report the removal of the lesion. The operative report is included with the claim to the third-party payer.

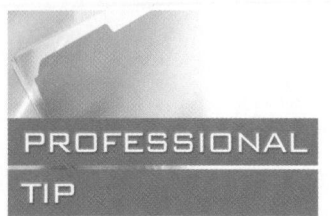

PROFESSIONAL TIP

This does include local anesthesia. Modifier 47 would not be used as a modifier for the anesthesia procedure.

47 Anesthesia by Surgeon: Regional or general anesthesia provided by the surgeon may be reported by adding modifier 47 to the basic service. This does not include local anesthesia.

Example

A surgeon performs a regional nerve block prior to performing surgery to decompress the nerve at the carpal tunnel. To report this, the physician uses code 64721, Neuroplasty and/or transposition; median nerve at carpal tunnel. Code 64415, Injection, anesthetic agent; brachial plexus, single would also be reported to describe the regional nerve block performed. The modifier "-47" is appended to the procedural code, 64721, to obtain 64721-47. The modifier alerts the third-party payer that the surgeon personally performed the anesthesia. Listing the code for the anesthesia informs the third-party payer about which nerve was blocked.

50 Bilateral Procedure: Bilateral means pertaining to two sides. Unless otherwise identified in the descriptor, bilateral procedures that are performed at the same operative session should be identified by appending modifier 50 to the procedure.

Example

A physician repairs a bilateral reducible inguinal hernia on a 2-year-old. The physician reports code 49500-50, Repair initial inguinal hernia, age 6 months to younger than 5 years, with or without hydrocelectomy; reducible. The modifier "-50" is appended to the procedure code since it was performed bilaterally.

51 Multiple Procedures: When multiple procedures are performed, other than evaluation and management (E/M) services, at the same session by the same

provider, the primary procedure may be reported as listed. The additional procedures may be identified by appending modifier 51 to the additional procedure.

Modifier 51 has four applications, namely, to identify:

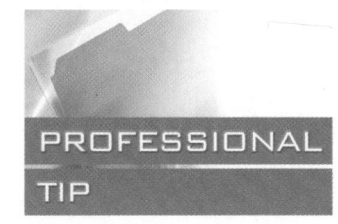

Modifier 51 should not be appended to designate add-on codes. Appendix E of the AMA's CPT summarizes the CPT codes exempt from modifier 51. Codes listed are identified in CPT® with the symbol Ø.

- Multiple medical procedures performed at the same session by the same provider
- Multiple, related operative procedures performed at the same session by the same provider
- Operative procedures performed in combination, at the same operative session, by the same provider, whether through the same or another incision or involving the same or different anatomy
- A combination of medical and operative procedures performed at the same session by the same provider.

Example

A surgeon reports code 28200, Repair tendon, flexor, foot; primary or secondary, without free graft, each tendon. The second procedure performed during the same operative session by the same provider is code 28001, Incision and drainage of the bursa, foot. The modifier "-51" is appended to the secondary procedure, 28001, resulting in a code of 28001-51.

53 Discontinued Procedure: Under certain circumstances, the physician may elect to terminate a surgical or diagnostic procedure. Due to extenuating circumstances or those that threaten the well-being of the patient, it may be necessary to indicate that a surgical or diagnostic procedure was started but discontinued. This circumstance may be reported by adding the modifier 53 to the code reported by the physician for the discontinued procedure.

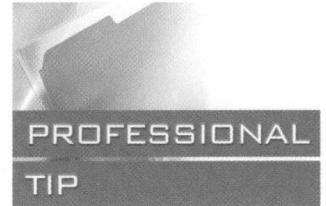

A **secondary procedure** is a procedure performed in addition to the primary procedure.

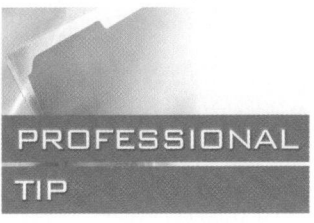

For hospital outpatient reporting of a previously scheduled procedure that is partially reduced or canceled as a result of extenuating circumstance or those that threaten the well-being of the patient prior to or after administration of anesthesia, see modifiers 73 and 74.

CPT is a registered trademark of the American Medical Association.

Example

Following anesthesia induction, the patient experiences an arrhythmia that causes the procedure to be terminated. The physician reports the code for the planned procedure with modifier 53 appended.

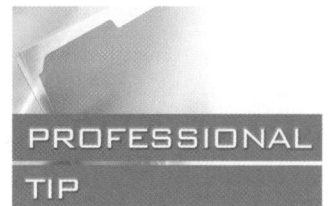

PROFESSIONAL TIP

Modifier 53 is not used to report the elective cancelation of a procedure prior to the patient's anesthesia induction or surgical preparation in the operating suite.

54 Surgical Care Only: When one physician performs a surgical procedure and another provides preoperative and/or postoperative management, surgical services may be identified by adding modifier 54 to the usual procedure number.

55 Postoperative Management Only: When one physician performed the postoperative management and another performed the surgical procedure, modifier 55 is appended to the usual procedure number.

56 Preoperative Management Only: When one physician performed the preoperative care and evaluation and another physician performed the surgical procedure, the preoperative component may be identified by adding modifier 56 to the usual procedure number.

Example

Example for Modifiers 54, 55, and 56: A physician may intend to perform all three components of a global service (preoperative management, surgical care, and postoperative management); however, after providing the preoperative management and performing the surgical procedure, he is unexpectedly called out of town. The surgeon in this case reports the surgical procedure with the modifiers 54 and 56 appended.

The physician who performed the postoperative management reports the operative procedure code with modifier 55 appended. Reporting the postoperative management indicates that the physician performed all of the postoperative care.

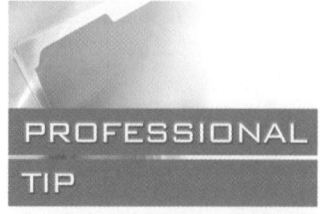

PROFESSIONAL TIP

This modifier is not used to report the treatment of a problem that requires a return to the operating room; see modifier 78 instead.

58 Staged or Related Procedure by the Same Physician During the Postoperative Period: The physician may need to indicate that the performance of a procedure or service during the postoperative period was:

1. Planned prospectively at the time of the original procedure (staged)
2. More extensive than the original procedure
3. For therapy following a diagnostic surgical procedure.

This circumstance may be reported by appending modifier 58 to the staged or related procedure.

Example

A surgeon performs a mastectomy on a patient. During the postoperative global period he inserts a permanent prosthesis. The surgeon reports the code with the 58 modifier to indicate that the service was related to the mastectomy (staged to occur at a time after the initial surgery. If the physician did not append modifier 58, a third-party payer could reject the claim because the surgery occurred during the postoperative period associated with the mastectomy.

59 Distinct Procedural Service: Under certain circumstances, the physician may need to indicate that a procedure or service was distinct or independent from other services performed on the same day. Modifier 59 is used to identify procedures that are not normally reported together, but are appropriate under the circumstances.

62 Two Surgeons: When two surgeons work together as primary surgeons performing a distinct part of a procedure, each surgeon should report his distinct operative work by adding modifier 62 to the procedure and any associated add-on codes for that procedure as long as both surgeons continue to work together as primary surgeons.

63 Procedure Performed on Infants less than 4 kg: Procedures performed on neonates and infants up to a present body weight of 4 kg may involve significantly increased complexity and physician work commonly associated with these patients. Appendix F in CPT® 2007 Standard Edition has a list of codes which are exempt from this modifier.

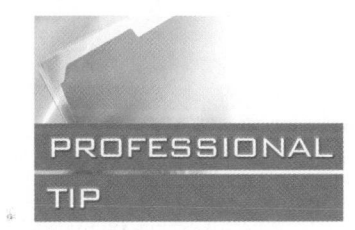

> Modifier 63 should not be appended to any CPT codes listed in the E/M Services, Anesthesia, Radiology, Pathology/Laboratory, or Medicine sections.

PROFESSIONAL TIP

66 Surgical Team: Under some circumstances, highly complex procedures (requiring the concomitant services of several physicians, often of different specialties, plus other highly skilled, specially trained personnel, and various types of complex equipment) are carried out under the "surgical team" concept.

Example

During a heart transplant, one surgeon opens the chest and inserts the chest tubes, while another surgeon prepares the great vessels for anastomosis to the donor heart. Each surgeon reports the same code with the same modifier. In this case 33945-66.

76 Repeat Procedure by Same Physician: The physician may need to indicate that a procedure was repeated subsequent to the original procedure. Documentation should be provided to the third-party payer when reporting this modifier.

77 Repeat Procedure by Another Physician: The physician may need to indicate that a basic procedure performed by another physician had to be repeated.

CPT is a registered trademark of the American Medical Association.

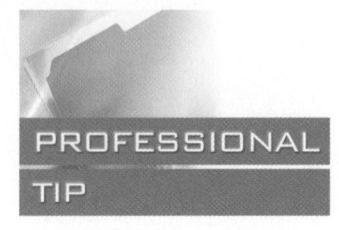

It is important that all of the physicians on the surgical team jointly write a description of each physician's general role on the heart transplant team and send the report to each third-party payer, to indicate each physician's role in the performance of surgery.

78 Return to the Operating Room for a Related Procedure During the Postoperative Period: The physician may need to indicate that another procedure was performed during the postoperative period of the initial procedure. When this subsequent procedure is related to the first and requires the use of the operating room, it may be reported by adding modifier 78 to the related procedure.

79 Unrelated Procedure or Service by the Same Physician During the Postoperative Period: The physician may need to indicate that the performance of a procedure during the postoperative period was unrelated to the original procedure.

80 Assistant Surgeon: Surgical assistant services may be identified by adding modifier 80 to the usual procedure number.

81 Minimum Assistant Surgeon: Minimum surgical assistant services are identified by adding modifier 81 to the usual procedure number.

82 Assistant Surgeon (when qualified resident surgeon not available): The unavailability of a qualified resident surgeon is a prerequisite for appending modifier 82 to the usual procedure code.

90 Outside Laboratory: When laboratory procedures are performed by a party other than the treating or reporting physician, the procedure may be identified by adding modifier 90 to the usual procedure code.

91 Repeat Clinical Diagnostic Laboratory Test: In the course of treatment of the patient, it may be necessary to repeat the same laboratory test on the same day to obtain subsequent (multiple) test results. Under these circumstances, the test's usual procedure code and the addition of modifier 91 can identify the laboratory test performed.

99 Multiple Modifiers: Under certain circumstances two or more modifiers may be necessary to completely define a service. In such situations modifier 99 should be added to the basic procedure, and other applicable modifiers may be listed as part of the description of service.

Add-on Codes (+)

Most of the procedures listed in the CPT can be reported by themselves because they represent the total procedure that was performed. These codes "stand alone" to describe the total procedure or service. Under certain circumstances, it may be necessary to report two or more "stand-alone" codes to completely describe the procedures performed. Add-on codes are used mainly with codes from the surgery section of the CPT book.

Some of the codes listed in the CPT code set describe procedures/services that must never be reported as a stand-alone code. These codes are referred to as add-on codes." **Add-on codes** describe procedures/services that are always performed in addition to the primary procedure; they are indicated by a plus sign (+) next to the code. The **primary procedure** is the most resource-intensive CPT procedure done during a patient's visit/encounter. The primary procedure code is listed first on the CMS-1500 claim form. Add-on codes can also be readily identified by specific language in the code descriptor, which includes phrases such as "each additional" or

"(List separately in addition to primary procedure)."

The multiple modifier (51) is not appended to an add-on code. These codes are exempt from the multiple procedure concept.

> Appendix E of the CPT lists the CPT codes that are exempt from the use of modifier 51; they are identified with a Ø.

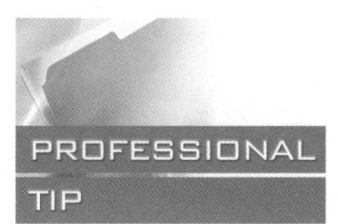

PROFESSIONAL TIP

Coding Steps

Perform the following steps:

1. **Determine the Procedures and Services to Report**   The coder chooses the name and associated code of the procedure or service that most accurately identifies and describes the services performed; then chooses names and codes for additional services or procedures. If necessary, modifiers are chosen and added to the selected service and procedure codes. Knowledge of the payers' policies is used to decide which services can be performed in the office (or which need to be referred out of office) and can be reported and billed. All services or procedures coded must also be documented in the patient's medical record.

2. **Identify the Correct Codes**   The CPT index is used to locate the main term for each procedure or service. If the term is not found, the organ or body site is looked up and then the disease or injury. Further checking can be done to locate any synonyms, eponyms, or abbreviations associated with the main term. The entries under the main term are reviewed to see if any apply, and cross-references are checked. If the main term cannot be located in the index, the coder reviews the main term selection with the physician for clarification. In some cases, there is a better or more common term that can be used.

    The main text listing, including all section guidelines and notes for particular subsections, is carefully reviewed to arrive at the final code. Items that cannot be billed separately because they are covered under another, broader code are eliminated.

    The codes to be reported for each day's service are ranked in order of highest to lowest rate of reimbursement (see Figure 6.3). The actual order in which they were performed on a particular day is not important.

3. **Determine the Need for Modifiers**   The circumstances involved with the procedure or service may require the use of modifiers. The patient's diagnosis may affect this determination.

Coding for Anesthesia

Anesthesia codes have their own section, which is located before the Surgery section. Basic anesthesia administration services are those services provided by or under the

Date	Charge	Procedure
11/22/2008	$350.00	25500
11/22/2008	$200.00	99203
11/22/2008	$85.00	73099

Figure 6.3

The codes to be reported for each day's service are ranked in order of highest to lowest rate of reimbursement.

responsible supervision of a physician. These services include general and regional anesthesia, as well as supplementation of local anesthesia. Anesthesia is reimbursed according to time. The main anesthesia codes are bundled codes. A **bundled code** is a group of related procedures covered by a single code. These bundled codes include the usual services of an anesthesiologist, which are as follows:

- Routine preoperative and postoperative visits to evaluate the patient for the planned anesthesia and monitor the patient's postsurgery recovery from anesthesia
- Administration of fluids and/or blood during the period of anesthesia care
- Interpretation of noninvasive monitoring such as electrocardiography (ECG), body temperature, blood pressure, oximetry (blood oxygen concentration), capnography (blood carbon dioxide concentration), and mass spectrometry.

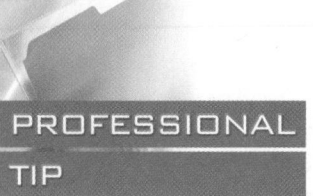

PROFESSIONAL TIP

In the CPT index, look for the code under Anesthesia. If you look first under the surgical procedure performed, the code will be for that surgical procedure and not the anesthesia given for the surgical procedure.

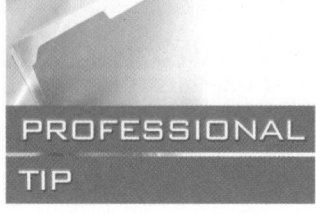

PROFESSIONAL TIP

The American Society of Anesthesiologists (ASA) provides a guide for the reporting of anesthesia services and procedures. The ASA publishes this billing and coding guide annually. It depicts and defines anesthesia services and modifiers. The guide assigns a relative value unit to anesthesia services, physical status modifiers, and qualifying circumstances that are added together to calculate anesthesia charges.

59 Distinct Procedural Service: Under certain circumstances, the physician may need to indicate that a procedure or service was distinct or independent from other services performed on the same day. Modifier 59 is used to identify procedures that are not normally reported together, but are appropriate under the circumstances.

The index is researched for the procedure under the Anesthesia section. The section's subsections are organized by body site. Under each subsection the codes are arranged by procedures. For example, under the heading "Neck," codes for procedures performed on various parts of the neck, the esophagus, thyroid, larynx, trachea; lymphatic system; and the major vessels are listed.

The **physical status modifier** is used only in the Anesthesia section with procedure codes to indicate the patient's health status. These modifiers, which are shown in Figure 6.4, range from P1 to P6.

Time spent providing the anesthesia service is reported separately when anesthesia services are coded. Anesthesia time begins when the anesthesia provider starts preparing the patient for anesthesia in the operating room or a similar location. Time ends when the patient is safely placed under postoperative supervision.

In the case of difficult and/or extraordinary circumstances such as extreme youth or age (under 1 year of age or over seventy years) or other unusual risk factors, it may be appropriate to report one or more of the qualifying circumstances by using an add-on code listed in Figure 6.5 in addition to the anesthesia services.

- P1—A normal healthy patient
- P2—A patient with mild systemic disease
- P3—A patient with severe systemic disease
- P4—A patient with severe systemic disease that is a constant threat to life
- P5—A moribund patient who is not expected to survive without the operation
- P6—A declared brain-dead patient whose organs are being removed for donor purposes

Figure 6.4

Physical status modifiers.

+99100	Anesthesia for patient of extreme age; younger than 1 one year and older than 70
+99116	Anesthesia complicated by utilization of total body hypothermia
+99135	Anesthesia complicated by utilization of controlled hypotension
+99140	Anesthesia complicated by emergency conditions (specify) (list separately in addition to code for primary anesthesia procedure)

Figure 6.5

Qualifying circumstances for anesthesia.

Answer the following questions:

1. What code is used to report the administration of anesthesia for a procedure on the esophagus? _____

2. Regional or general anesthesia provided by the surgeon also performing the procedure is reported with what CPT modifier? _____

3. What code is used to report repair of a ruptured Achilles tendon? _____ _____

4. Which physical status modifier is used to designate a patient with mild systemic disease? _____

5. What code is used to report anesthesia for a 72-year-old female for lens surgery of the right eye? _____

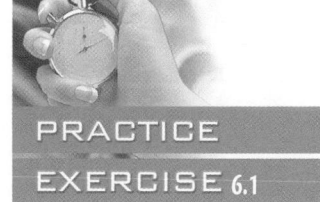

PRACTICE EXERCISE 6.1

On completion of this exercise, refer to Appendix J to check the accuracy of your work.

Surgical Coding

The Surgery section is the largest section in CPT. The subsections found in the Surgery section and how they are broken down into the body systems is shown in Figure 6.6.

Be sure you read the section guidelines!

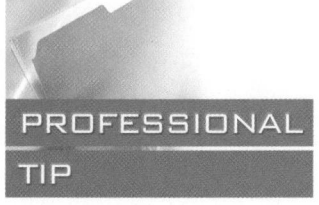

PROFESSIONAL TIP

The subsections found in the Surgery section and how they are broken down into the body systems.

Integumentary System	10021–19499
Musculoskeletal System	20000–29999
Respiratory System	30000–32999
Cardiovascular System	33010–39599
Digestive System	40490–49999
Urinary System	50010–53899
Male Genital System	54000–55980
Female Genital System	56405–58999
Maternity Care and Delivery	59000–59899
Endocrine System	60000–60699
Nervous System	61000–64999
Eye and Ocular Adnexa	65091–68899
Auditory System	69000–69979
Operating Microscope	69990

The anatomic arrangement of each subsection is as follows:

■ Head
■ Neck (Soft Tissue) and Thorax
■ Back and Flank
■ Spine (Vertebral Column)
■ Abdomen
■ Shoulder
■ Humerus (Upper Arm) and Elbow
■ Forearm and Wrist
■ Hand and Fingers
■ Pelvis and Hip Joint
■ Femur (Thigh Region) and Knee Joint
■ Leg (Tibia and Fibula) and Ankle Joint
■ Foot and Toes
■ Application of Casts and Strapping
■ Endoscopy/Arthroscopy.

Within each heading there is also a consistent theme of procedures described such as:

■ Incision
■ Excision
■ Introduction or Removal
■ Repair, Revision, and/or Reconstruction
■ Fracture and/or Dislocation
■ Arthrodesis/Amputation.

Using your CPT index, look up the following and outline how you got there:

PRACTICE
EXERCISE 6.2

1. Anesthetic injection of the facial nerve _____

_____

_____

2. Closed treatment of the clavicle _____

_____

_____

_____

3. Excision of the gallbladder _____

_____

_____

_____

On completion of this exercise, refer to Appendix J to check the accuracy of your work.

As previously discussed in this chapter, following is an example of the use of an add-on code.

Example

Additional Lesion(s)

11100 Biopsy of skin, subcutaneous tissue and/or mucous membrane (including simple closure). Unless otherwise listed (separate procedure); single lesion

+11101 each separate/additional lesion (List separately in addition to code for primary procedure)

Code 11100 is the primary procedure and code 11101 is the add-on code. Code 11101 would never be reported without first reporting code 11100. As the code descriptor indicates, code 11101 is reported for each separate/additional lesion. The parenthetical note following code 11101 instructs the user regarding the code that is considered the primary procedure for that particular add-on code.

If biopsies are performed on three separate lesions of the skin, subcutaneous tissue, and/or mucous membrane, then code 11100 would be reported for the first lesion and code 11101 would be reported twice, once for the second lesion biopsy, and again for the third lesion biopsy.

Other CPT codes are also exempt from modifier 51. These codes are identified throughout the CPT book with the Ø symbol placed before the code. The "null" symbol is a circle with a blackslash bisecting it. These codes cannot be modified with modifier

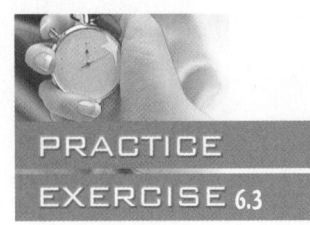

Use your CPT book to code the following:

1. Neurorrhaphy of two digital nerves _____
    _____

2. Xenograft, to trunk, arms and legs; 200 sq. cm _____
    _____

3. Arthrodesis, interphalangeal joint (3) _____
    _____

On completion of this exercise, refer to Appendix J to check the accuracy of your work.

fier 51 multiple procedures because the add-on code is used to add increments to a primary procedure, so the need for multiple procedures is represented by procedures that are added on.

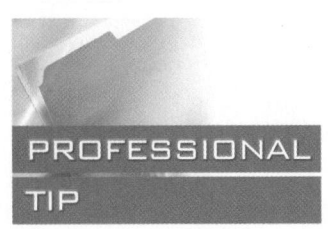

⊙ This symbol refers to the procedure that includes moderate (conscious) sedation, which is a drug induced depression of consciousness during which the patient responds purposefully to verbal commands. The provider cannot report this as a separate procedure.

Separate Procedure

A **separate procedure** is a descriptor used in the CPT for a procedure that is usually part of a surgical package but may also be performed separately or for a different purpose, in which case it may be reported separately.

Some of the codes listed in the CPT nomenclature have been identified by inclusion of the term "separate procedure" in the code descriptor. The "separate procedure" designation indicates that a certain procedure or service may be:

1. Considered an integral component of another procedure/service
2. Performed independently
3. Unrelated
4. Distinct from other procedures provided at that time.

Example

58720	Salpingo-oophorectomy, complete or partial, unilateral or bilateral (separate procedure)
58150	Total abdominal hysterectomy (corpus and cervix), with or without removal of tube(s), with or without removal of ovary(s)

When reporting a total abdominal hysterectomy with removal of the tube(s) and ovary(s), it would not be appropriate to separately report code 58720 in conjunction with code 58150. The procedure described by code 58720 is considered an integral component of the procedures described by code 58150.

However, codes designated as separate procedures should be additionally reported when performed independently, unrelated to, or distinct from other procedure(s)/service(s) provided.

Example

58720 Salpingo-oophorectomy, complete or partial, unilateral or bilateral (separate procedure)

   If removal of the fallopian tubes and ovaries is the only procedure performed, then it would be appropriate to report code 58720 to describe the procedure performed.

When a procedure or service that is designated as a separate procedure is carried out independently or considered to be unrelated to or distinct from other procedures/services provided at that time, the procedure or service designated as a separate procedure may be reported by itself, or in addition to other procedures/services by appending modifier 59 to the specific "separate procedure" code reported. This indicates that the procedure is not considered a component of another procedure, but is a distinct, independent procedure.

Surgical Package or Global Surgery Concept

A surgical CPT code is a bundled code. As mentioned earlier, a *bundled code* is a single CPT code used to report a group of related procedures as in the surgical package. **Unbundling** or **fragmented billing** occurs when separate procedures are reported that should have been included under a bundled code. This practice will result in denial of a claim.

A **surgical package** includes specific services in addition to the operation, including these:

- One related E/M encounter on the date immediately prior to or on the date of procedure, subsequent to the decision for surgery
- Preparing the patient for surgery including local infiltration, topical anesthesia
- Performing the operation, including normal additional procedures, such as debridement
- Immediate postoperative care, including dictating operative notes, talking with the family and other physicians
- Writing orders
- Evaluating the patient in the postanesthesia recovery area
- Typical postoperative follow-up.

The typical postoperative care includes follow up visits for normal uncomplicated care. Each third-party payer determines the number of days in which this follow-up care may take place. Therefore, it is important when certifying for surgery to ask the global period of the third-party payer. The **global period** refers to the number of days surrounding a surgical procedure during which all services relating to that procedure—preoperative, during the surgery, and postoperative—are considered part of the surgical package. This is also referred to as the **global surgical concept**. To determine global days, information from the insurance carrier or other payers may need to be obtained. Many publications and software packages on the market address global days for most carriers and unbundling.

Third-party payers have varying definitions of what constitutes a surgical package and varying policies about what is to be included in the surgical package. Because surgical package rules define what is or is not included in addition to the surgical procedure, the surgery also defines the services for which additional charges can or cannot be submitted.

The CPT code for a normal postoperative follow-up visit included in global service is 99024. This code is useful to the reporting physician for tracking the number of postoperative visits provided that are included in the "package" for the procedure performed.

Two types of services are not included in surgical package codes. These services are reported separately and reimbursed in addition to the surgical package fee:

- Complications, exacerbations, recurrence, or the presence of other diseases or injuries requiring additional services should be separately reported.
- Care for the condition for which a diagnostic surgical procedure was performed or of other coexisting conditions is not included and may be reported separately.

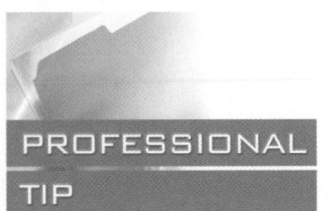

PROFESSIONAL TIP

Some examples of diagnostic procedures include endoscopy, arthroscopy, and injection procedures for radiography.

Example

A patient undergoes a diagnostic upper gastrointestinal endoscopy for suspected gastric ulcer disease. The findings of the endoscopy are positive for an acute gastric ulcer. At that time, the physician prescribes medication for treatment of the ulcer disease. The patient is instructed to return to the physician's office in 1 week for follow-up care related to the effectiveness of the medication prescribed.

In the preceding example, the follow-up visit is reported separately with the appropriate level of E/M code based on key components that have been met during the encounter. Care of the condition for which the diagnostic procedure was performed is not included and may be reported separately.

The following are some examples of what is included in a surgical procedure and cannot be billed separately:

- Positioning the patient
- Insertion of intravenous access for medication (IV)
- Administration of sedative by the physician performing the procedure
- Local infiltration of medication—topica, or regional anesthetic administered by the physician performing the procedure
- Surgical approach, including identification of landmarks, incision, and evaluation of the surgical field
- Exploration of operative area
- Fulguration of bleeding points
- Simple debridement of traumatized tissue
- Lysis of a moderate amount of adhesions

- Isolation of neurovascular tissue or muscular, bony, or other structures limiting access to the surgical field
- Surgical cultures
- Wound irrigation
- Insertion and removal of drains, suction devices, dressings, pumps into or out of same site
- Surgical closure
- Application and removal of postoperative dressings including analgesic devices
- Application of splints with musculoskeletal procedures
- Institution of patient-controlled analgesia
- Photographs, drawings, dictation, transcription to document the services provided
- Surgical supplies.

An area of great concern in medical billing is inaccurately billing separately for procedures considered incidental to the major procedure. Many CPT surgical narratives in the CPT book include "with or without" or other language to include or exclude incidental services. Numerous procedures are done in conjunction with other procedures, and often the CPT code subsection notes and guidelines will indicate that a particular code includes a variety of the supporting procedures.

The CPT book further states that follow-up care for complications, exacerbations, recurrence, and the presence of other diseases that require additional services is not included in the surgery package. General anesthesia for surgical procedures is not part of the surgical package, and the anesthesiologist bills general anesthesia services separately.

Supplies and Services

Supplies and materials provided by the physician (e.g., sterile trays/drugs) over and above those usually included with procedures rendered are listed separately. The guideline indicates that you should list the drugs, trays, supplies, and materials provided, and identify them as code 99070 or use the specific supply code, which can be found in HCPCS. According to the CPT nomenclature, supplies and materials provided by the physician are reported only if they are "over and above" those usually included with the office visit or other services rendered.

CPT code 99070 is used to report supplies provided by the physician "over and above" those usually included with the services rendered. This code could be used to report, for example, a drug, special dressings used to pack a wound, wound irrigation equipment, or a pair of crutches.

Radiology Codes

The codes in the Radiology section are used to report radiological services performed by or supervised by a physician. Radiology codes may have two parts:

1. *Results are the technical component of a service. Testing leads to results.* The **technical component** is the part of the relative value associated with the procedure that reflects the test, technologist, the equipment, and processing including preinjection and postinjection services such as local anesthesia, placement of a needle or catheter, and injection of contrast material. The technical component of taking the x-ray would be reported with the procedure code and the modifier "-TC" attached to the procedure.

2. *Results lead to interpretation. Reports are the work product of the interpretation of numerous test results.* The **professional component** is the part of the relative value associated with a procedure that represents a physician's skill, time, and expertise used in performing it, as opposed to the technical component. The reading, interpretation, and the written report of the radiological examination by the physician would be the professional component and the modifier "-26" would be attached to the procedure.

These modifiers are to be used only when the physician's office states that only part of the radiological procedure was done; otherwise, the descriptor remains as stated with no modifier.

Note that the supervision and interpretation (S&I) descriptor means that the radiology code is only for the professional component. Modifier 26 does not need to be attached. When the words "supervision and interpretation" or the acronym "S&I" appears, the code for the technical component is selected from another section.

Example

19290	**Preoperative placement of needle localization wire, breast; (For radiological supervision and interpretation, see 76942, 77031, 77032)**

The radiology code does not need any modifiers if the provider does the technical and professional component.

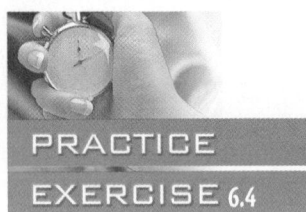

PRACTICE
EXERCISE 6.4

Code the following situation:

An orthopedic surgeon sends his patient to the radiologist for an x-ray of the leg (73592), but asks that the patient return with the x-ray for his interpretation (professional component).

1.   The radiologist would code 73592 with modifier _____

2.   The orthopedist would code 73592 with modifier _____

3.   How would it be coded if the orthopedist sent the patient to the radiologist to take the x-ray and send the report? _____

4.   Complete study, cardiac MRI for function (professional component only)

     _____

5.   Computed tomography, lumbar spine; with contrast material (technical component only) _____

On completion of this exercise, refer to Appendix J to check the accuracy of your work.

Radiology codes follow the same type of guidelines noted in the Surgery section. For example, some radiology codes are identified as separate procedure codes. These codes are usually part of a larger, more complex procedure and should not be reported as separate codes unless the procedure was done independently. Also, some codes are add-on codes, such as those covering additional vessels that are studied after the basic examination. These codes are used with the primary codes and do not stand alone.

Contrast material is commonly used for imaging enhancement. Contrast material improves visualization and evaluation of the body structure or organ studied. Some of the procedures listed in the Radiology section of the CPT book may be performed with or without the use of contrast material for imaging enhancement. The phrase "with contrast" used in the codes for procedures using contrast for imaging enhancement represents contrast material administered intravascularly, intra-articularly, or intrathecally. When contrast materials are only administered orally and/or rectally, the study does not qualify as "with contrast" and should be coded "without contrast."

Pathology and Laboratory Codes

The codes in the Pathology/Laboratory section cover services provided by physicians or by technicians under the supervision of a physician. A complete procedure includes:

- Ordering the test
- Taking and handling the sample
- Performing the actual test
- Analyzing and reporting on the test results.

The 8000 series codes are used to report the performance of specific laboratory tests only and do not include the collection of the specimen via venipuncture (or finger/heel/ear stick), arterial puncture, or other collection methodology (e.g., lumbar puncture). The collection of the specimen by venipuncture or by arterial puncture is not considered an integral part of the laboratory procedure(s) performed. Codes in the 36400–36425 series are used to report venipuncture for obtaining blood samples.

Organ or disease-oriented panels are reported with the codes from the 80048–80076 series. These panels were developed for coding purposes and should not be interpreted as clinical standards for testing. A **panel** is a group of tests ordered together to detect particular diseases or malfunctioning organs. When a panel is reported, all of the listed tests must have been performed with no substitution. If fewer tests are performed than those listed in the panel code (unbundling), then the individual code number(s) for each test should be listed rather than the panel code.

Example

80051 Electrolyte Panel
   This panel must include the following:

Carbon dioxide	(82374)
Chloride	(82435)
Potassium	(84132)
Sodium	(84295)

PRACTICE
EXERCISE 6.5

Code the following:

1. Macroscopic examination parasite _____

2. Digoxin quantitative _____

3. Drug screen, qualitative; single drug class method, each drug class _____
_____

4. Urinalysis, by dip stick or table reagent automated with microscopy _____
_____

5. TRH stimulation panel; 1 hour _____

On completion of this exercise, refer to Appendix J to check the accuracy of your work.

Procedures and services are listed in the index under the following types of main terms:

- Name of the test, such as urinalysis, drug test
- Procedure such as hormone assay
- Abbreviations such as CBC, RBS, TLC
- Panel of tests, under Blood Tests.

Some medical practices have laboratory equipment and perform their own testing. In-office labs must be certified by the **Clinical Laboratory Improvement Amendment (CLIA)** of 1988, which awards three levels of certification. The lowest level for an in-office certified lab can perform dipstick urinalysis and urine pregnancy. If the medical practice does not have a lab but obtains the specimen for the lab, the venipuncture code 36415 may be billed for obtaining the blood sample. As in every medical setting, the Occupational and Safety and Health Administration (OSHA) regulates safety.

Although Medicare does not allow physicians to bill for lab work they did not perform, other third-party payers do. When a medical practice has a contract with a lab (pays the lab for the work), it may bill for the tests reported. The modifier 90 is attached to the code for the lab test. On the CMS-1500, form locator 20 must say "yes" and the fee the medical practice pays the lab must be entered under "Charges." Also, form locator 32 must report the name and address of the lab.

Medicine Codes

The Medicine section of the CPT book contains a variety of listings for reporting procedures and services provided by many different types of healthcare providers. In addition, many services and procedures provided by nonphysician practitioners can be found in the Medicine section. For example, codes in the physical medicine and rehabilitation subsection are often used to report the services and procedures provided by physical and occupational therapists. Audiologists and speech therapists find listings in the special otorhinolaryngologic services subsection that describes some of the technical procedures and services they provide.

Codes from the Medicine section may be used with codes from any other section. Add-on codes and separate procedure codes are included in the Medicine section.

| 90471 | Immunization administration |
| 90710 | Measles, mumps, rubella, and varicella vaccine (MMRV), live, for subcutaneous use |

Figure 6.7

Immunizations require two codes.

Immunizations require two codes, one for administering the immunization and the other for the particular vaccine or toxoid that is given (see Figure 6.7).

The descriptors for injections require two codes, one for administering the immunization and the other for the particular vaccine or toxoid that is given.

Cardiac catheterizations are the most commonly performed surgical procedure, with more than 1 million performed each year. Complete coding of cardiac catheterization requires at least three codes: a code for the catheterization procedure itself, a code for the injection procedure, and a code for the imaging supervision and interpretation. Each of these has a professional and a technical component. Unless the physician owns the laboratory, those codes are billed using modifier 26.

Immunoglobulins use a different administration code. Always read the notes provided in the section before choosing the correct codes.

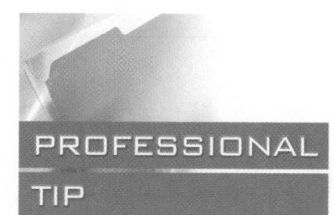

PROFESSIONAL TIP

Chapter Summary

- Reimbursement is the key to a medical practice's success. Medical office specialists should be aware of the importance of correct procedure coding.
- When using the CPT index, it is important to understand how entries to the index have been made. It cannot be stressed enough that the CPT index is not a substitute for the main text of the CPT nomenclature.
- Specific "guidelines" can be found at the beginning of each of the six sections of the CPT book. The guidelines provide information that is necessary to appropriately interpret and report procedures and services found in that section.
- Modifiers more fully describe procedures that were changed in some way, and they affect the reimbursement by increasing or decreasing the amount.
- Add-on codes describe procedures/services that are always performed in addition to the primary procedure; they are indicated by a plus sign (+) next to the code.
- A bundled code is used to report a group of related procedures as in the surgical package. Each surgical package has included in its reimbursement a certain number of days during which procedures association with a surgery are reimbursed, as determined by third-party payers.
- Anesthesia coding requires physical status modifier. The reimbursement is based on measurement of time.
- The surgery section is the largest CPT section and has fourteen subsections.
- Radiology codes have two components, technical and professional.
- A panel is a group of tests found in the laboratory section.
- The medicine section contains a variety of listings for reporting procedures and services provided by many different types of healthcare providers.

Chapter Review

True/False

Identify the statement as true (T) or false (F).

_____ **1.** CPT add-on codes are never used as primary procedure codes.

_____ **2.** In the CPT, a bundled code is used to report a group of related procedures.

_____ **3.** If a CPT code is not bilateral, a modifier is used with the code to report a bilateral service.

_____ **4.** The terms *unbundling* and *fragmented billing* in procedural coding have the same meaning.

_____ **5.** A CPT modifier is used to show that only part of a procedure has been done.

_____ **6.** An incomplete CPT code does not have a modifier attached.

_____ **7.** When a physician treats complications or recurrences that arise after surgery, these services are reported separately.

_____ **8.** All third-party payers have the same definitions for surgical package codes.

_____ **9.** A global surgical concept for a diagnostic procedure includes follow-up care related only to recovery from the procedure itself, not for care of the patient's underlying condition.

_____ **10.** Add-on codes that describe qualifying circumstances are available for use with codes from the Anesthesia section of the CPT.

_____ **11.** Codes from the Surgery section of the CPT cover only the operation itself, not postoperative care.

_____ **12.** To report a bilateral procedure, the 50 modifier (Bilateral Procedure) is attached to the CPT code for the unilateral procedure.

_____ **13.** S&I is the abbreviation for supervision and interpretation.

_____ **14.** The injection of a local or topical anesthesia by the surgeon can be billed in addition to the operation itself.

Multiple Choice

Identify the letter of the choice that best completes the statement or answers the question.

_____ 1. In the CPT, what procedure is bundled with the arthroscopy in the following entry? 23515 Open treatment of clavicular fracture, with or without internal or external fixation
   a. open treatment
   b. clavicular fracture
   c. with or without internal or external fixation
   d. none of the above

_____ 2. The divisions of the CPT, such as Anesthesia and Radiology, are referred to as
   a. parts.   c. sections.
   b. chapters.   d. components.

_____ 3. If fewer tests are performed than those listed in the panel code (unbundling), then the individual code number(s) for each test should be listed rather than the panel code as:
   a. unbundled.
   b. bundled.
   c. listed separately.
   d. none of the above.

_____ 4. The primary CPT code that is listed first for an CMS-1500 claim form is the procedure that:
   a. is performed first.
   b. is the most resource intensive.
   c. appears first in the CPT-4.
   d. none of the above.

_____ 5. Which is the correct process for selecting CPT codes?
   a. Locate the probable code, determine the procedures and services it covers, and determine the need for modifiers.
   b. Determine the procedures and services to report, identify the correct codes, and determine the need for modifiers.
   c. Determine the correct codes and modifiers, and then place them in the proper order from primary to secondary procedures.
   d. None of the above.

_____ 6. An unlisted procedure is a service or procedure that:
   a. needs a special report not listed in the index.
   b. needs a special report listed in the index.
   c. needs a special report with a modifier.
   d. needs a special report without a modifier.

_____ 7. The bundle codes in CPT's Anesthesia section generally cover:
   a. preoperative evaluation and planning.
   b. care during the procedure.

c. routine postoperative care.

d. all of the above.

_____ 8. What is required of the physician in order to report the professional component of a CPT code from the Radiology section?

a. reading the radiological examination

b. writing a report of interpretation

c. both a and b

d. neither a nor b

_____ 9. How many CPT codes are required to report an immunization?

a. one   c. three

b. two   d. four

_____ 10. A patient has an office encounter for removal of five skin tags on her hand. During the visit, she asks the physician to evaluate swelling and heat in her left knee. The physician performs an expanded history and examination with low medical decision making. What codes should be reported?

a. 11200, 99214   c. 11100, 99213-25

b. 11200, 99213-25   d. 11200, 99213-51

_____ 11. A patient had a previous surgery 15 days ago to treat a dislocated ankle. Today, the same surgeon repairs the patient's flexor tendon muscle on the other foot. What code should be reported for today's service?

a. 28200-79   c. 28200-58

b. 28200   d. 28200-51

_____ 12. Radiology codes may have two parts:

a. unlisted or guided.

b. supervision or interpretation.

c. professional or technical.

d. complete or partial.

_____ 13. Under CPT guidelines, all services related to a surgical procedure are not additionally reimbursed:

a. before the global period.   c. during the global period.

b. after the global period.   d. during the E/M period.

_____ 14. CPT codes from the Anesthesia section may use:

a. standard CPT modifiers and physical status modifiers.

b. physical status modifiers and duration modifiers.

c. either a or b.

d. neither a nor b.

_____ 15. How many subsections are in the surgery section?

a. eleven   c. fourteen

b. nine   d. fifteen

_____ 16. In CPT, a plus sign (+) next to a code indicates a(n):

a. add-on code.   c. revised code.

b. new code.   d. new/revised text.

Completion

Complete each sentence or statement.

1. In CPT, some codes have both a technical component and a(n) _____ component that represents the physician's skill, time, and expertise.

2. A(n) _____ procedure can be performed in addition to the primary procedure.

3. Codes in the Anesthesia section of the CPT are reimbursed according to _____.

4. Codes for many procedures and services provided by family practice physicians, such as immunizations, are located in the CPT's _____ section.

For Additional Practice

Provide the correct modifier for each of the following descriptions.

1. Distinct procedural service _____

2. Mandated service _____

3. Multiple modifiers _____

4. Discontinued procedure _____

5. Radiologist provides a report on a lateral chest x-ray _____

6. Multiple procedures _____

7. Bilateral procedure _____

8. Referenced outside laboratory _____

9. Postoperative management only _____

10. Unrelated procedure by the same physician during the postoperative period _____

Code the following using your CPT code book:

1. Debridement of 10 nails by any method _____

2. Chemical peel, facial; dermal _____

3. Preoperative placement of needle localization wire, breast _____

4. Mastectomy, subcutaneous _____

5. Incision and drainage (I&D of hematoma, soft tissue of neck _____

6. Manipulation, elbow, under anesthesia _____

7. Endoscopy, surgical; operative tissue ablation and reconstruction of atria, without cardiopulmonary bypass _____

8. Repair atrial septal defect, secundum, with cardiopulmonary bypass, with or without patch _____

9. Laparoscopy, surgical, appendectomy _____

10. Nephrolithotomy; secondary surgical operation for calculus _____

11. Vaginal delivery only including postpartum care _____

12. Removal of lens material; intracapsular, for dislocated lens _____

13. Radiological supervision and interpretation, percutaneous vertebroplasty or vertebral augmentation including cavity creation, per vertebral body under CT guidance _____

14. Mammary ductogram, single duct, radiological supervision and interpretation _____

15. Mammography; bilateral _____

16. Therapeutic radiology treatment, intermediate _____

17. Lipase _____

18. General health panel _____

19. Triglycerides _____

20. PSA total _____

21. Tissue culture for non-neoplastic disorders; lymphocyte _____

22. Pathology consultation during surgery _____

23. Intravenous infusion, hydration 2 hours _____

24. End-stage renal disease (ESRD) related services per full month; for patient 58 years old _____

25. Spirometry, including graphic record, total and timed vital capacity, expiratory flow rate measurement with or without maximal voluntary ventilation _____

26. Application of a modality to one or more areas; diathermy _____

27. Hospital-mandated on-call service; in-hospital (1 hour) _____

28. Ventilation assist and management, initiation of pressure or volume preset ventilators for assisted or control breathing; hospital inpatient, initial day _____

29. Tobacco use assessed (CAD, CAP, COPD, PV) _____

30. Dyspnea assessed, present (COPD) _____

Resources

American Society of Anesthesiologists website: ***www.asahq.org***
The 2007 CPT Standard Edition, published by the American Medical Association: ***www.cptnetwork.com***

Chapter 7 | HCPCS and Coding Compliance

Chapter Objectives

After reading this chapter, the student should be able to:

1. Understand the three levels of HCPCS.
2. Recognize the need for HCPCS coding and when to report HCPCS codes.
3. Learn how to use HCPCS modifiers.
4. Interpret and identify correct code linkages.
5. Review the coding for accuracy.
6. Understand federal laws, regulations, and penalties that pertain to coding compliance.
7. Understand the responsibilities of coding and coding compliance.
8. Explain the National Correct Coding Initiative.
9. Understand medical ethics for the medical coder.

Key Terms

abuse
advanced beneficiary
    notice (ABN)
advisory opinion
assumption coding
code linkage

durable medical
    equipment (DME)
fraud
HCPCS
Level I HCPCS
Level II HCPCS

Level III HCPCS
National Correct Coding
    Initiative (NCCI)
OIG fraud alerts
OIG Work Plan

Case Study
Coding Procedures and Services

The physician ordered a blood test to be completed for Mrs. Cleets who has Medicare. The medical assistant performed the venipuncture and marked the patient encounter form with the HCPCS code G0001. The billing specialist that was to post the charges, noticed that a HCPCS code was used instead of the CPT code 36415. She knew that the G0001 code was deleted in 2005 and the CPT code was to be used in its place. She corrected the error and sent out an email memo reminding staff of the change.

Questions

1. Why is it important to use only current codes and coding books?
2. How could this error have been prevented?
3. Would this claim have been denied? What are some of the effects of a denied claim?

Introduction

HCPCS (pronounced "hick-picks") is the acronym for the Health Care Procedure Coding System. This system is a uniform method used by healthcare providers and medical suppliers to report professional services, procedures, and supplies. Prior to its development in 1983 by the Health Care Financing Administration (which as of 2001 is called Centers for Medicare and Medicaid Services), there was no uniform system for coding a procedure, service, or supply for reimbursement. Competent coding is part of the overall effort being made by medical practices to comply with regulations in many areas. For instance, the diagnosis code chosen must match the procedure performed. In addition, medical office specialists who work with patient records as they code must be knowledgeable about patient privacy regulations and how to keep patient data secure.

History of HCPCS

Early in the history of medical coding, Blue Cross Blue Shield created and required the use of its own coding system; many other insurance companies also created their own method of coding physician services and procedures. Despite the addition and subtraction of codes over the nearly 30-year history, the Centers for Medicare and Medicaid Services (CMS) has maintained the essence of HCPCS, which is to:

- Meet the operational needs of Medicare/Medicaid
- Coordinate government programs by uniform application of CMS policies
- Allow providers and suppliers to communicate their services in a consistent manner
- Ensure the validity of profiles and fee schedules through standardized coding
- Enhance medical education and research by providing a vehicle for local, regional, and national utilization comparisons.

The permanent national codes serve the important function of providing a standardized coding system that is managed jointly by private and public insurers. It supplies a predictable set of uniform codes that provide a stable environment for claims submission and processing.

HCPCS Level of Codes

HCPCS has three levels of coding, each of which is a unique coding system, as discussed in the following subsections. The HCPCS codes used must be valid at the time the service is rendered.

Level I: CPT® Codes

Level I HCPCS The terms Level I and CPT codes are synonymous. An insurance carrier may require HCPCS Level I coding for medical procedures. The coder will know that this refers to the CPT book.

CPT is a registered trademark of the American Medical Association.

Level II: HCPCS National Codes

The CPT book does not contain all of the codes a medical coder might need to report certain medical services, ambulance services, or the use of durable medical equipment and supplies. **Durable medical equipment (DME)** is an appliance, apparatus, or product intended for use in assisting or treatment of a patient. The CMS developed the second level of HCPCS codes. In contrast to the five-digit codes found in Level I, **Level II HCPCS** national codes consist of one alphabetic character (a letter between A and V), followed by four digits. The codes are grouped by the type of service or supply they represent and are updated annually by the CMS with input from private insurance companies.

Example

A HCPCS code from injections that may be covered by Medicare is reported from the J series of the Level II codes used for material (drug) that is injected, rather than a CPT code.

   Ampicillin up to 500 mg; IM or IV   J0290

Level II codes are required for reporting most medical services and supplies provided to Medicare and Medicaid patients and by most private payers.

There are 22 sections, each covering a related group of items. Review Table 7.1 to become familiar with the different types of procedures covered. Codes are provided for a wide

Table 7.1	Level II HCPCS Codes	
	Transportation services	A0000–A0999
	Medical and surgical supplies	A4000–A7509
	Miscellaneous and experimental	A9000–A9999
	Enteral and parenteral therapy	B0000–B9999
	Temporary hospital outpatient PPS	C0000–C9999
	Dental procedures	D0000–D9999
	Durable medical equipment (DME)	E0000–E9000
	Procedures and services, temporary	G0000–G9999
	Rehabilitative services	H0000–H9999
	Drugs administered other than oral method	J0000–J8999
	Chemotherapy drugs	J9000–J9999
	Temporary codes for DMERCS	K0000–K9999
	Orthotic procedures	L0000–L4999
	Prosthetic procedures	L5000–L9999
	Medical services	M0000–M9999
	Pathology and laboratory	P0000–P9999
	Temporary codes	Q0000–Q9999
	Diagnostic radiology services	R0000–R9999
	Private payer codes	S0000–S9999
	State Medicaid agency codes	T0000–T9999
	Vision	V0000–V2999
	Hearing services	V5000–V5999

range of medical services, dental services, rehabilitative services, drugs, intravenous and chemotherapy treatments, and supplies. For proper reimbursement this book must be used for the specific supplies used.

National permanent HCPCS Level II codes are maintained by the HCPCS National Panel. The panel is comprised of representatives from the Blue Cross/Blue Shield Association (BCBSA), the Health Insurance Association of America (HIAA), and the CMS. The panel is responsible for making decisions about additions, revisions, and deletions to the permanent national alphanumeric codes. These codes are for the use of all private and public health insurers.

Level III: Local Codes

The **Level III HCPCS** codes are assigned and maintained by individual state Medicare carriers. Like Level II codes, these codes begin with a letter (W through Z) followed by four numeric digits, but the most notable difference is that these codes are not common to all carriers. Individual carriers assign these codes to describe new procedures that are not yet available in Level I or II. These codes can be introduced on an as-needed basis throughout the year, but carriers must send written notification to the physicians and suppliers in their area when these local codes are required. Reading and implementing the information received from these carriers will keep you up to date.

HCPCS Modifiers

HCPCS modifiers are two-digit codes, which may be either alpha (all letters) or alphanumeric (letters plus numbers). They range from AA to VP. National modifiers can be used with all levels of HCPCS codes.

Level III (local) modifiers are assigned by individual Medicare carriers and are distributed to physicians and suppliers through carrier newsletters. The carrier may change, add, or delete these local modifiers as needed.

HCPCS modifiers are used to modify procedures and services on health insurance forms filed for Medicare patients. The list of modifiers is shown in Table 7.2.

Use of the GA Modifier

An **advanced beneficiary notice (ABN)**, according to the CMS, is a written notification that must be signed by the patient or guardian prior to the provider rendering a service to a Medicare beneficiary that could potentially be denied/deemed "not medically necessary." When an ABN is on file, an HCPCS GA modifier must be appended to the code for the service in question on the CMS-1500 form. Once a Medicare beneficiary signs the ABN, he or she is legally responsible for the charges if Medicare denies payment for the service as "not medically necessary."

HCPCS Index

Because the HCPCS is organized by code number rather than by service or supply name, the index allows you to locate any code without looking through the individual range of codes. To find a code, look up in the index the medical or surgical supply, service, orthotic, prosthetic, or generic drug you need, and you will be directed to the appropriate codes. This index also references many of the brand names by which these items are known.

Table 7.2	HCPCS Modifiers
LT	Left side (used to identify procedures performed on the left side of the body)
RT	Right side (used to determine procedures performed on the right side of the body)
CA	Procedure payable only in the inpatient setting when performed emergently on an outpatient who expires prior to admission
E1	Upper left, eyelid
E2	Lower left, eyelid
E3	Upper right, eyelid
E4	Lower right, eyelid
FA	Left hand, thumb
F1	Left hand, second digit
F2	Left hand, third digit
F3	Left hand, fourth digit
F4	Left hand, fifth digit
F5	Right hand, thumb
F6	Right hand, second digit
F7	Right hand, third digit
F8	Right hand, fourth digit
F9	Right hand, fifth digit
GA	Waiver of liability statement on file
GG	Performance and payment of a screening mammogram and diagnostic mammogram on the same patient, same day
GH	Diagnostic mammogram converted from screening mammogram on same day
LC	Left circumflex, coronary artery (Hospitals use with codes 92980–92984, 92985, 92986)
LD	Left anterior descending coronary artery (Hospitals use with codes 92980–92984, 92995, 92996)
RC	Right coronary artery (Hospitals use with codes 92980–92984, 92995, 92996)
QM	Ambulance service provided under arrangement by a provider of services
QN	Ambulance service furnished directly by a provider of services
TA	Left foot, great toe
T1	Left foot, second digit
T2	Left foot, third digit
T3	Left foot, fourth digit
T4	Left foot, fifth digit
T5	Right foot, great toe
T6	Right foot, second digit
T7	Right foot, third digit
T8	Right foot, fourth digit
T9	Right foot, fifth digit

Coding Compliance

One of the most important documents in the medical record is the progress note, which updates the patient's clinical course of treatment and summarizes the assessment and plan of care. If a patient's condition, examination, and treatment plan is not documented in the chart, "it did not happen."

Providers have the ultimate responsibility for proper documentation and correct coding, as well as for compliance with regulations. Medical office specialists help to ensure that maximum reimbursement is received promptly for reported services by submitting correct claims.

Coding compliance is part of the overall effort of medical practices to comply with regulations in many areas, such as patient privacy and the security of patient data. In this sense, compliant claims are an indication of a compliant medical practice. On the other hand, claims that contain errors raise the question of whether the practice is generally acting in a fraudulent manner. To reduce the chances of being targeted for an investigation or an audit, and to reduce the risk of liability if there is an audit, medical practice staff as well as physicians must be aware of, understand, and comply with all applicable regulations and laws.

These claims, as well as the process used to create them, must comply with the rules imposed by federal and state law and by government and private payer healthcare program requirements. Correct claims reduce the chance of an investigation and the risk of liability if an audit occurs. Consequences of inaccurate coding and incorrect billing include the following:

- Denied claims
- Delays in processing claims and receiving payments
- Reduced payments
- Fines and other sanctions
- Exclusion from payers' programs
- Prison sentences
- Loss of the provider's license to practice medicine.

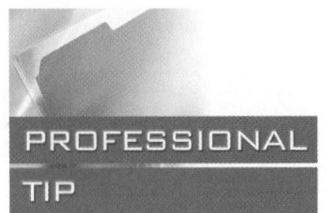

Medicare has placed a cap on the number of physical therapy treatments that Medicare patients are allowed. If a provider exceeds that amount and cannot prove that additional therapy was medically necessary, the treatment will be denied. The medical office specialist must be aware of the rules and regulations issued by Medicare and have the patient sign an ABN in advance of treatment received if treatment has exceeded the allowed amount and reimbursement may be denied. Also the GA modifier needs to be attached to the CPT code for the provider to be able to bill the patient for the denial.

Code Linkage

On a "clean claim," each reported service is connected to a diagnosis that supports the procedure as necessary to investigate or treat the patient's condition. Payers analyze this connection between the diagnostic and the procedural information, called **code linkage**, to evaluate the medical necessity of the reported charges. Correct claims also comply with many other requirements issued by government and private payers. Some regulations involve the place, frequency, or level of services. Some services are always denied as not reasonable or medically necessary or as experimental. Payers also often deny claims because of certain frequency limitation on services.

The ultimate goal of submitting claims is to be paid and not be audited after payment. If a provider is audited, it takes up time and disrupts the practice of everyday "work."

To increase the chances of submitting a "clean claim" and having it accepted without an audit, a medical office specialist should ask himself these questions before submitting the claim:

> Medicare allows one physical examination for a beneficiary within 6 months of becoming a Medicare Part B subscriber. If a provider does an annual physical after the 6 months have passed, reimbursement will be denied. Again, the patient would need to sign an ABN and a GA modifier would need to be attached to the procedure.

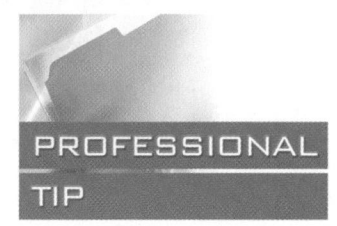

PROFESSIONAL TIP

1. Is the coded service billable?
2. Are the codes appropriate to the patient's profile (age, gender, condition)?
3. Is there a clear and correct link between each diagnosis and procedure?
4. Is the documentation in the patient's medical record adequate to support the reported services?
5. Do the reported services comply with all regulations?

Billing CPT Codes

When entering CPT codes on a CMS-1500 claim form, the most resource-intensive procedure or service should be listed first. The third-party payer or Medicare may pay the first listed code at the approved rate but reduce any following procedures by 50% or deny it as being part of the primary procedure.

Federal Law

The Federal Civil False Claims Act prohibits submitting a fraudulent claim or making a false statement or representation in connection with a claim. The False Claims Act, 31 U.S.C. §3729 False Claims, includes liability for certain acts. Any person who engages in an action listed in Figure 7.1 is submitting fraudulent claims.

The federal government encourages reporting of suspected fraud and abuse against the government by protecting and rewarding people involved in qui tam, or whistle-blower, cases.

Any person who engages in one of the following actions is submitting fraudulent claims:

- knowingly presents, or causes to be presented to an officer or employee of the U.S. Government a false or fraudulent claim for payment or approval;
- knowingly makes, uses, or causes to be made or used, a false record or statement to get a false or fraudulent claim paid or approved by the Government;
- conspires to defraud the Government by getting a false or fraudulent claim allowed or paid;
- has possession, custody, or control of property or money used, or to be used, by the Government and intending to defraud the Government or willfully to conceal the property,
- knowingly makes, uses, or causes to be made or used, a false record or statement to conceal, avoid, or decrease an obligation to pay or transmit money or property to the Government.

Figure 7.1

A list of fraudulent actions from Civil False Claims Act.

The Health Insurance Portability and Accountability Act of 1996 (HIPAA) created the Healthcare Fraud and Abuse Control Program to uncover fraud and abuse in the Medicare and Medicaid programs. The Office of Inspector General (OIG) works with the U.S. Department of Justice (DOJ), which includes the Federal Bureau of Investigation (FBI), under the direction of the U.S. Attorney General to investigate and prosecute those suspected of medical fraud and abuse. Figure 7.2 is a 2005 news release that refers to prosecution.

Figure 7.3 provides settlement amounts recovered by the Department of Health and Human Services (DHHS) and the OIG. Note that some of these recoveries were made because the professional provider did not actually administer the service and the modalities given were not one-on-one with the patient as indicated. Although this would be the responsibility of the provider of the service, the coder must be aware of the differences in the procedures when coding.

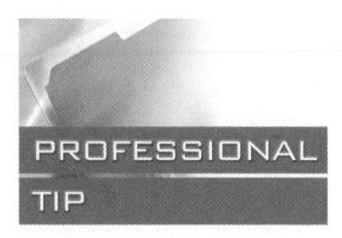

PROFESSIONAL TIP

Knowing the difference between a supervised modality and a constant attendance modality for physical therapy is required for proper coding. In the case of HealthSouth (see Figure 7.3), if the physical therapist was not in constant attendance with the patient the claim would be fraudulent. Supervised attendance does not require direct (one-on-one) contact by the provider.

Physician Self-Referral

Physician self-referral is the practice of a physician referring a patient to a medical facility in which he has a financial interest, be it ownership, investment, or a structured compensation arrangement. Critics of the practice allege an inherent conflict of interest, given the physician's position to benefit from the referral. They suggest that such arrangements may encourage overutilization of services, in turn

Figure 7.2

News Release that refers to prosecution.

WASHINGTON, Nov. 7–U.S. Newswire—The United States obtained over $1.4 billion in settlements and judgments in the fiscal year ending September 30, 2005, pursuing allegations of fraud against the federal government, the Justice Department announced today. This brings total recoveries since 1986, when Congress substantially strengthened the civil False Claims Act, to $15 billion.

Of the $1.4 billion, $1.1 billion is associated with suits initiated by whistle-blowers under the False Claims Act's *qui tam* provisions. These provisions authorize individuals, known as relators, to file suit on behalf of the United States against those who have falsely or fraudulently claimed federal funds. Such cases run the gamut of federally funded programs from Medicare and Medicaid to defense contracts, disaster assistance loans, and agricultural subsidies. Persons who claim federal funds they know they aren't entitled to are liable for three times the government's loss plus a civil penalty of $5,500 to $11,000 for each false claim. If the government intervenes in a *qui tam* action, the person who filed the suit can recover from 15 to 25 percent of any settlement or judgment attributable to the fraud identified by the whistle-blower. The relator's share increases up to 30 percent if the United States declines to intervene and the whistle-blower pursues the action alone. In fiscal year 2005, whistle-blowers were awarded $166 million.

Fraudulent claims actions, as listed in a release from the U.S. Department of Justice, Washington, D.C., November 7, 2005, U.S. Newswire.

As in the last several years, health care accounted for the lion's share of fraud settlements and judgments: **$1.1 billion**. The Department of Health and Human Services reaped the biggest recoveries, largely attributable to its Medicare and Medicaid Programs. Substantial recoveries were also made by the Office of Personnel Management, which administers the Federal Employees Health Benefits Program, the Department of Defense for its TRICARE insurance program, the Department of Veterans Affairs and the Railroad Retirement Board.

Among the most significant recoveries in fiscal year 2005 were:

$327 million from HealthSouth Corporation to settle allegations of fraud against Medicare and other federally insured health care programs. The United States alleged that HealthSouth, the nation's largest provider of rehabilitative medicine services, engaged in three major schemes to defraud the government. The first, comprising $170 million of the settlement amount, resolved Health South's alleged false claims for outpatient physical therapy services that were not properly supported by certified plans of care, administered by licensed physical therapists or for one-on-one therapy as represented. Another $65 million resolved claims that HealthSouth engaged in accounting fraud which resulted in overbilling Medicare on hospital cost reports and home office cost statements. The remaining $92 million resolved allegations of billing Medicare for a range of unallowable costs, such as lavish entertainment and travel expenses incurred for HealthSouth's annual administrators' meeting at Disney World, and other claims. Government-initiated claims accounted for $251 million of the settlement amount, with the remaining $76 million attributable to four *qui tam* lawsuits.

Five relators received $12.6 million for their contributions to the litigation. HealthSouth also entered into a corporate integrity agreement with the Inspector General of Human Health Services to prevent future misconduct.

$310 million from Gambro Healthcare for false claims for Medicare and Medicaid in connection with dialysis services. Allegations against Gambro included providing home dialysis patients with equipment and supplies through a sham durable medical equipment company to increase Medicare reimbursement, billing for phantom supplies, billing for ancillary medications and services that were not medically necessary—a requirement for Medicare reimbursement, and paying kickbacks to physicians for referring patients to Gambro clinics in violation of the Medicare Anti-Kickback Act. The company also paid $15 million to resolve state Medicaid liabilities and paid a $25 million criminal fine.

$138.5 million from AdvancePCS, a subsidiary of Caremark, Inc., in the pharmacy benefit management business, to resolve allegations that AdvancePCS exacted kickbacks, disguised as administrative fees and sales and service agreements, from drug manufacturers in exchange for marketing their drugs to providers reimbursed by federally insured health programs; and paid kickbacks to providers reimbursed by federally insured health programs to ensure that AdvancePCS was selected or retained as the pharmacy benefit manager for the health plans in the form of cash payments and rebates from drug manufacturers in exchange for marketing their drugs to providers reimbursed by federally insured health programs.

Fraudulent claims actions, as listed in a release from the U.S. Department of Justice, Washington, D.C., November 7, 2005, U.S. Newswire.

Figure 7.3

Settlement amounts recovered by the DHHS and the OIG.

driving up healthcare costs. In addition, they believe that it would create a captive referral system, which limits competition from other providers. An example of federal legislation of this situation is the Stark law, which governs physician self-referral for Medicare and Medicaid patients. The law is named for U.S. Congressman Pete Stark, who sponsored the initial bill.

Government Investigations and Advice

Civil Law

Under civil law the maximum penalty for medical fraud is $10,000 for each item or service for which fraudulent payment has been received. An amount up to three times the amount of the claim can also be fined.

Criminal Law

Because medical fraud can have criminal aspects, those found guilty can receive jail sentences of up to 10 years as well as fines. If a patient is seriously injured or dies, longer jail sentences—up to life imprisonment—are probable.

Administrative Law

Physicians can also be subject to administrative remedies, such as exclusion from participation as providers in all government health programs.

Most billing-related accusations are based on the Civil False Claims Act and on Section 231 of HIPAA, which broadened the definition of fraud to state that providers who knew or should have known that a claim for service was false can be held liable.

Fraud is an act of deception used to take advantage of another person or entity. If a person pretends to be a physician and treats patients without a valid medical license, these actions constitute fraud. Fraudulent acts are intentional because the person knows that the act is illegal and is trying to obtain a profit. In federal law, **abuse** means an action that misuses the money that the government has allocated such as Medicare funds. Abuse is illegal because the taxpayers' dollars are misspent. A health claim fraud occurs when healthcare providers or others falsely represent their services or charges to payers. A provider may bill for services that were not performed, code at a higher level to increase payment, or fail to provide complete services under a contract. The key difference between fraud and abuse is as follows: To bill when the procedure was not done is fraud; to bill when it was not necessary is abuse.

Each year the OIG announces the **OIG Work Plan**. This plan lists the year's planned projects for sampling types of billing to see if there are any problems. Each year a specific area of billing will be audited; for example, in 2006, outpatient physical therapy services billings were audited. In 2007, the place of service continues to be an issue. The OIG chooses a specific region of the country in which to conduct this audit. If the OIG finds problems with billing these codes, then it will expand their investigation nationally.

OIG fraud alerts are issued periodically by the Office of Inspector General and are posted on the CMS website to advise providers of problematic actions that have come to the OIG's attention. The OIG also issues CMS advisory bulletins that alert providers and government-sponsored program beneficiaries of potential problems. Providers are responsible for knowing the contents of the advisories and can be prosecuted for "not knowing." The medical office specialist must read the bulletins to be knowledgeable of any changes or updates in billing and coding procedures.

Errors Relating to Code Linkage and Medical Necessity

Three common types of errors are associated with the code linkage process and the question of medical necessity:

1. The CPT procedure codes must match the International Classification of Diseases, Ninth Revision, Clinical Modification (ICD-9-CM) diagnosis codes. For example, billing for drainage of a pilonidal cyst would need a diagnosis of pilonidal cyst with or without mention of abscess.
2. The procedures must not be elective, experimental, or nonessential. For example, billing for a cosmetic surgery for an eyelift when the procedure was done for appearance only and not medically necessary is not allowed. If, however, the patient had blepharoptosis, then the eyelift would be medically necessary and would not be considered an elective surgery.
3. The procedures must be furnished at an appropriate level. Coding of the E/M codes must be done at the appropriate level that meets the reason for the encounter, history, examination, and the medical decision making.

Errors Relating to the Coding Process

Other common errors include those that arise during the coding process:

1. **Assumption coding**: Reporting items or services that are not actually documented, but the coder assumes they were performed.
2. Altering documentation after the services are reported.
3. Coding without proper documentation.
4. Reporting services provided by unlicensed or unqualified clinical personnel.
5. Failure to have all necessary documentation available at the time of coding.

Errors Relating to the Billing Process

Yet other errors surround the billing process itself:

1. Reporting services that are not covered or have limited coverage.
2. Using modifiers incorrectly.
3. *Upcoding*: Using a procedure code that provides a higher reimbursement rate than the code that actually reflects the services provided.
4. *Unbundling*: Billing the parts of a bundled procedure as separate procedures.

National Correct Coding Initiative (NCCI)

Medicare's national policy on correct coding is called the Medicare **National Correct Coding Initiative (NCCI)**. The NCCI is an ongoing process to standardize bundled codes and control improper coding that could lead to inappropriate payment for Medicare claims for physician services. The NCCI list contains more than 200,000 CPT code combinations. These code combinations, called NCCI *edits*, make up the computerized screening process used by Medicare to examine claims.

The NCCI edits determine what procedures and services cannot be billed together for the same patient on the same day of service. In the Medicare environment, these are coding errors, even though in the commercial environment they may be correctly coded.

There are three types of edits for NCCI errors:

■ *Comprehensive versus component edits:* In this group, the first column of codes contains the comprehensive code, and the second column shows the component code. According to the NCCI, the comprehensive code includes all the services that are described by the component code, so the component code cannot be billed together with the comprehensive code for the same patient on the same day of service.

Example	
Comprehensive	**Component**
27370	20610, 76000, 76003

■ *Mutually exclusive edits:* This group also lists codes in two columns. According to CMS regulations, the services represented by these codes could not have reasonably been done during a single patient encounter, so they cannot be billed together. If the provider reports codes from both column 1 and column 2 for a patient on the same day, Medicare pays only the lower payout code.

Example	
Column 1	**Column 2**
50021	49061, 50020

■ *Modifier indicators:* This type of NCCI modifier is a number appearing alongside the comprehensive and component code list and the mutually exclusive code list. A provider may include an NCCI modifier to allow payment for both services within the code pair under certain circumstances. Figure 7.4 is an example taken from the Musculoskeletal System for Correct Coding for Physician Services.

Fraudulent Actions

Healthcare payers base their decision to pay or deny claims only on the diagnosis and procedure codes. The integrity of the request for payment rests on the accuracy and the honesty of the coding. Incorrect coding may be simply an error or it may represent deliberate efforts to obtain fraudulent payment. Actions that might be viewed as occasional slips or errors could also be interpreted as establishing a pattern and practice of violations, which constitutes the knowledge meant by "providers knew or should have known."

If a provider has a question as to the legality of an action, the OIG and CMS offer an advisory opinion. An **advisory opinion** is legal advice on any question regarding healthcare business. The requesting party, such as a physician, nursing home, or hospital, formally presents a situation and asks whether the way they intend to handle it is acceptable. The answer is written to the requesting parties and then becomes public so that anyone who needs to know the answer to specific questions can study the opinions. They are published without revealing the requesting parties' name. If the requesting party does not follow the OIG's advice, then they could be prosecuted. If they were in error prior to the opinion and change their practice as to the opinion, then they are immune from investigation. An advisory opinion is the best way to be sure that an intended action will not be subject to investigation.

Figure 7.4

Musculoskeletal System					
Column1/Column 2 Edits		* = In existence prior to 1996	Effective Date	Deletion Date* = no data	Modifier 0 = not allowed 1 = allowed 9 = not applicable
Column 1	Column 2				
20000	20500		19970101	*	1
20000	29580		19990101	*	1
20000	36000		20021001	*	1
20000	36410		20021001	*	1
20000	37202		20021001	*	1
20000	62318		20021001	*	1
20000	62319		20021001	*	1
20000	64415		20021001	*	1
20000	64416		20030101	*	1
20000	64417		20021001	*	1
20000	64450		20021001	*	1
20000	64470		20021001	*	1
20000	64475		20021001	*	1
20000	69990		20000605	*	0

Example from the NCCI's Musculoskeletal System for Correct Coding for Physician Services.

Source: CPT codes and descriptions only are copyright 2007 American Medical Association. All rights reserved.

Federal Compliance

The *Federal Register*, publishes the *Compliance Program Guidance for Individual and Small Group Physician Practices* developed by the OIG. The creation of compliance program guidelines is a major initiative of the OIG in its effort to engage the private healthcare community in preventing the submission of erroneous claims and in combating fraudulent conduct. Also available online is the *Medicare Carrier's Manual*, which interprets the guidelines of the Medicare program. If a physician would like to purchase a printed copy from Medicare, the cost is approximately $100. The medical office specialist must be familiar with the Medicare website, which provides information on all rules and guidelines for billing.

We should emphasize again that the excuse that a billing action was made in error because the provider "didn't know" is not acceptable when billing a government entity. Such actions will be interpreted as violations and may result in penalties and fines for fraud and abuse.

How to Be Compliant

To be compliant, a physician's practice should have a compliance plan in place. The seven components included in the OIG's *Compliance Program Guidance* provide a solid basis on which a physician's practice can create a voluntary compliance program:

- Conduct internal monitoring and auditing.
- Implement compliance and practice standards.
- Designate a compliance officer or contact.

■ Conduct appropriate training and education.
■ Respond appropriately to detected offenses and develop corrective actions.
■ Develop open lines of communication.
■ Enforce disciplinary standards through well-publicized guidelines.

This guidance for physicians' practices does not suggest that physicians' practices implement all seven components of a full-scale compliance program. Instead, the guidance emphasizes a step-by-step approach to follow in developing and implementing a voluntary compliance program. The OIG believes that the great majority of physicians are honest and share the goal of protecting the integrity of Medicare and other federal healthcare programs. To that end, all healthcare providers have a duty to ensure that the claims submitted to federal healthcare programs are true and accurate. The best way to ensure that an office is honest is to have a compliance plan in place.

Benefits of a Voluntary Compliance Program

The following are benefits of a voluntary compliance program:

■ Optimizes the speed of processing and the proper payment of claims.
■ Minimizes billing mistakes.
■ Reduces the chances that an audit will be conducted by CMS or the OIG.
■ Avoids conflicts with the self-referral and anti-kickback statutes.

A voluntary compliance plan also shows that the physician's practice is making good-faith efforts to submit claims appropriately. Practices that embrace the active application of compliance principles in their practice culture and make efforts at compliance on a continued basis can help to prevent problems from occurring in the future. A compliance program also sends an important message to a physician's practice's employees that, although the practice recognizes that mistakes will occur, employees have an affirmative, ethical duty to come forward and report erroneous or fraudulent conduct so that it may be corrected.

Ethics for the Medical Coder

The professional medical office specialist who is responsible for medical coding has a duty to code medical services and procedures to the best of his ability. The guidelines and the codes combined with the regulatory errata change on an almost daily basis. It is important that the coder know his limitations and ask for help from the provider or a more experienced coder when doubts exist as to appropriate coding for a medical situation. The AMA, national specialty medical societies, and local carriers can provide important information regarding coding, governmental regulations, and other payers' policies concerning compliance, coding, and reimbursement.

Accessing patient records is usually a necessary part of the coder's tasks. Patient confidentiality is a patient's right and should never be violated. It is never appropriate to speak of a patient's medical condition with anyone but the medical provider. All such discussions should take place in private areas far from the public ear.

The role of the professional medical office specialist will often be that of emissary and educator to providers and other members of the office staff. The coder's job is to teach and implement strategies for correct coding. When a coder's ability to code services, procedures, and diagnoses is compromised on the job by coding policies deemed fraudulent, then she should try to resolve the problem through the organization's compliance program. Only when all avenues have failed should a coder consider reporting a provider to the authorities. It is the professional coder's job to be a part of a solution, not part of a problem.

A coder should never change billing information marked on an encounter form by a provider without informing the provider of the issue. Good communication skills will serve as an invaluable tool to the professional medical specialist coder. Open dialogue with the provider is the key to success!

Chapter Summary

- HCPCS is the acronym for the Health Care Procedure Coding System.
- Each of the three HCPCS levels represents a unique coding system. Level I is CPT coding.
- Level II is HCPCS national codes, which consist of one alphabetic character (a letter between A and V), followed by four digits.
- Level III contains codes assigned and maintained by individual state Medicare carriers.
- The GA modifiers must be used when an ABN is given.
- The HCPCS is organized by code number rather than by service or supply name, so the HCPCS index is invaluable for finding a particular service and its code.
- Payers analyze the connection between the diagnostic and the procedural information, called code linkage, to evaluate the medical necessity of the reported charges.
- When entering CPT codes on a CMS-1500 claim form, the most resource-intensive procedure or service should be listed first.
- The Federal Civil False Claims Act prohibits submitting a fraudulent claim.
- The Health Insurance Portability and Accountability Act of 1996 (HIPAA) created the Healthcare Fraud and Abuse Control Program to uncover fraud and abuse in the Medicare and Medicaid programs.
- Medicare's national policy on correct coding is called the Medicare National Correct Coding Initiative.
- To be compliant a physician's practice should have a Compliance Plan in place.
- The coder's job is to teach and implement strategies for correct coding. Problems should be resolved through the facility's compliance program.

Chapter Review

True/False

Identify the statement as true (T) or false (F).

_____ **1.** NCCI is the abbreviation for National Current Coding Initiative.

_____ **2.** Fraud alerts are issued once a year by the Office of Inspector General.

_____ **3.** Work Plans are issued periodically as needed by the Office of Inspector General.

_____ **4.** OIG fraud alerts explain potentially fraudulent or noncompliant billing and reporting practices to providers.

_____ **5.** Overpayments to providers from the Medicare program are always the result of fraud and abuse.

_____ **6.** The OIG Work Plan lists the types of medical billing and reporting practices that the Office of Inspector General intends to investigate in the coming year.

_____ **7.** Coding and billing errors may be considered fraudulent when they are part of a repeated pattern found by an external auditor.

_____ **8.** Having a compliance plan helps a medical practice prevent fraud and abuse relating to reimbursement for services and procedures.

_____ **9.** A medical practice that has a compliance plan demonstrates its desire to be in compliance with rules and regulations.

_____ **10.** Reporting more than one diagnosis code indicates that the procedures are medically necessary.

_____ **11.** A provider who is found guilty of fraud and abuse against the Medicare program can be excluded from further participation as a provider in all government-sponsored healthcare programs.

_____ **12.** Under civil law, large financial penalties and fines can be levied against those guilty of fraud and abuse.

Multiple Choice

Identify the letter of the choice that best completes the statement or answers the question.

_____ **1.** Durable medical equipment (DME) such as wheelchairs covered by the Medicare program are reported using:
a. ICD-9-CM codes.　　　　c. HCPCS Level II codes.
b. CPT codes.　　　　d. local Medicare carrier codes.

_____ **2.** In Medicare's National Correct Coding Initiative, which type of code cannot be billed together with its comprehensive code for the same patient on the same day of service?
a. edit　　　　c. diagnostic
b. exclusive　　　　d. component

_____ **3.** Proposed and final rules from the CMS about the Medicare program are published in:
a. OIG advisory opinions.
b. local newspapers.
c. the _Federal Register_.
d. the National Correct Coding Initiative.

_____ **4.** Some possible consequences of inaccurate coding and incorrect billing in a medical practice are:
  a. denied claims and reduced payments.
  b. prison sentences.
  c. fines.
  d. all of the above.

Completion

Complete each sentence or statement.

1. Medicare's National Correct Coding Initiative lists procedures that cannot be billed together for the same _____ on the same _____ of service.

2. To establish compliance plans and follow up on implementation, most medical practices appoint a(n) _____.

3. Healthcare payers base their decision to pay or deny claims only on the _____ and _____ codes.

4. Providers have the ultimate _____ for _____ and _____.

5. Medical practice staff as well as physicians must be aware of, understand, and _____ with all applicable _____ and _____.

6. Each reported service connected to a diagnosis that supports the procedure results in _____.

7. Level I HCPCS codes are found in the _____ book.

8. _____ prohibits submitting a fraudulent claim or making a false statement or representation in connection with a claim.

9. _____ created the Healthcare Fraud and Abuse Control Program to uncover fraud and abuse in the Medicare and Medicaid programs.

10. NCCI means _____.

11. A(n) _____ is legal advice on any question regarding healthcare business.

12. The _____, sets forth the _Compliance Program Guidance for Individual and Small Group Physician Practices_ developed by the Office of Inspector General.

For Additional Practice

Code the following:

1. Ampicillin sodium 500 mg injection _____

2. Penicillin G benzathine and penicillin procaine 1,000,000 units _____

3. Speech screening _____

4. Ambulatory surgical boot _____

5. Oxygen tent _____

6. Roll-about chair with 6-inch casters _____

7. Hemi-wheelchair with detachable arm desk and swing-away detachable leg rests _____

Resources

Compliance Training Manual: *www.usc.edu/health/uscp/compliance/tm1.html#1*

Chapter 8   Auditing

Key Terms

audit	external audit	retrospective audit
code edits	internal audit	upcode
downcode	prospective audit	

Case Study
Auditing

Dr. Terrance is a family practice physician. He has been practicing for 30 years and his manner of documentation has been the same for all of those 30 years. With the changes in the documentation regulations, he has had to update the way he dictates. The billing supervisor still has to remind him of the need to document the connection between the level of history and examination and the level of service he wants to bill. This sometimes leads to a difference of opinion.

Questions

1. Why is it important that the MA and/or doctor document precisely and completely for every visit?

2. How can the billing supervisor make the transition easier on Dr. Terrance?

3. Could the use of EMR improve the quality of the medical documentation?

Introduction

An **audit** is a formal examination or review. An audit, whether it is performed in the office or by an external auditor, examines the documentation to determine whether it adequately substantiates the service billed and shows medical necessity. In addition to facilitating high-quality patient care, an appropriately documented medical record serves as a legal document to verify services provided.

Purpose of an Audit

Three of the most important reasons why an office should audit its charts are:

1. To assess the completeness of the medical record
2. To determine the accuracy of the physician's documentation
3. To discover lost revenue.

If audits are not performed on a regular basis, the medical office specialist will not know for a fact that the documentation was correct and appropriate for the level of service performed. If an audit is performed, any errors found can be brought to the attention of the provider and corrected for future billing. Remember that a practice should agree to regularly monitor its records to be in compliance with federal guidelines (see Chapter 7). Audits help facilitate the maintenance of accurate and complete coding and reimbursement practices. An independent medical record review (i.e., an audit) should be performed a minimum of twice a year to identify coding and documentation errors. Top coding and documentation errors include the following:

- The service is upcoded one level; documentation in the chart does not support the level of service, therefore a lower level code should have been selected. The term **upcode** means that the procedure code stated is for a procedure that is more involved than the one actually documented in the chart.
- The service is downcoded one level; documentation in the chart supports a higher level of service, however the coder has chosen a lower level code to avoid government investigation. The term **downcode** means that the procedure code stated is for a procedure that is less involved than the one actually documented in the chart.
- The chief complaint (the reason for the encounter) is missing.
- Assessment is not clearly documented; the coder cannot use "rule out," "suspected," or "probable."
- No diagnosis is given; the coder must code only signs and symptoms.
- The documentation is not initialed or signed.
- Tests ordered are not stated in the chart, but are billed on the encounter form.
- Documentation of medication is not clear.
- The diagnosis is not always referenced correctly.
- Documentation is missing.
- Dictation is lost.
- The encounter form is not available.
- The encounter form is incomplete or incorrect.

- Documentation not complete, so the code has no record that an action was taken.
- Documentation is difficult to read; the auditor will disallow the visit when she cannot read the documentation.

Types of Audits

There are three types of audits: external audit, internal audit, and accreditation audit.

External Audit

An **external audit** is a private payer's or government investigator's review of selected records of a practice for compliance. Code linkage, completeness of documentation, and adherence to documentation standards, such as signing and dating of entries by the responsible healthcare professional, may all be studied. The account records are often reviewed as well.

Third-party payers conduct a prepayment audit by their software computer edits. These edits are reviewed to verify documentation such as the date of the service provided and the insured's insurance ID number. The documentation regarding the extent of the visit is investigated after payment. A postpayment audit is conducted after payment to ensure that the providers have billed accurately as to the visit or procedure billed. Postpayment audits also investigate the complete documentation regarding the visit including progress reports, x-rays, laboratory results, appointment book and sign-in sheet, and billing records.

Internal Audit

An **internal audit** is an audit done within the practice to be sure that the practice is coding claims correctly and is compliant. This will reduce the chance of an investigation or of an employee needing to become a whistle-blower. A practice employee or a consultant may be hired to perform this audit. The internal audits should be done routinely and performed without any reason to be suspicious of fraudulent behavior.

Because of their importance and the widespread use of the evaluation and management (E/M) codes, they are always an ongoing focus of audits. It is reasonable to see why. The documentation can be used to verify the correct usage of the proper E/M code. To verify the correct E/M code, the use of an internal audit should be used by the physician's practice in their compliance plan.

A **retrospective audit** is performed retrospectively, that is, after payment. A **prospective audit** is done before the claim is submitted for payment. A prospective audit would be difficult to do in a physician's office for many reasons. The person conducting the audit would have to wait for the documentation if it had been dictated. The majority of claims are sent electronically and it would affect the accounts receivable if payment or submission of claims were delayed. A prospective audit could be performed on claims that need attachments, such as a workers' compensation claim. This type of claim is submitted on a CMS-1500 form with a progress report attached. An internal audit could be easily performed for this type of claim.

An internal audit is used for these reasons:

- To determine that procedures have been coded correctly based on the documentation.
- To analyze the coders' skill and knowledge.

- To review any need for further training or review of the practice's compliance plan and policies.
- To review the involvement of the billing staff, medical coders, and the office insurance specialist with the physician.

Many audit tools are available to the medical office staff for performing an internal audit. The documentation for the date of service with the explanation of benefits (EOB) is reviewed and checked with the audit tool. The auditor checks the documentation by the physician to determine the correct level of E/M code.

Accreditation Audits

Providers who have contracts with managed care organizations are accredited once a year. A representative from the managed care organization for example, a registered nurse, will visit the facility. The provider is informed ahead of time of the upcoming visit. Upon arrival, the nurse will request at least 20 charts of the insured patients in their plan. An audit will be conducted on each chart as to the appearance of the chart, patient's information, and any signed authorizations. Medical auditing will then be assessed as to the proper documentation of the provider for the patient's visits, ordering of tests, prescription drugs, and any follow up care.

If there seems to be a problem with inadequate documentation, the provider will be given a warning and asked to be in compliance within a certain amount of time. If the charts do not meet the requirements set forth, the provider may lose his privileges to participate in this plan.

Private Payer Regulations

Private payers require use of the American Medical Association's (AMA's) Current Procedural Terminology (CPT®) codes and the International Classification of Diseases, Ninth Revision, Clinical Modification (ICD-9-CM) codes for reimbursement. They have, however, also developed their own **code edits**, which screen for improperly or incorrectly reported procedure codes. Most states require third-party payers to give a reason for denial of a claim. The software to determine if a clean claim has been submitted may also be different and in error. The medical office specialist must be prepared to appeal a claim if there is no explanation of the reason for denial.

Third-party payers may also have their own rules and policies about submitting a clean claim. One must be familiar with the payers' policies to submit the claim. For example, Blue Cross Blue Shield may want the documentation to include the name of the serum, the dosage, and the route of administration for a hepatitis A immunization. Any third-party payer from which the provider is accepting assignments must follow the third-party payer's policies and procedures as part of their contract agreement. Documentation must also be audited internally to show that the physician's practice is in compliance with all payer regulations.

Medical Necessity for E/M Services

Compliance plans focus on the training of physicians to use the AMA's *Documentation Guidelines for Evaluation and Management Services* and to know the current codes, in order to code correctly. The key components for selecting E/M codes are the extent of the his-

CPT is a registered trademark of the American Medical Association.

tory documented, the extent of the examination documented, and the complexity of the medical decision making. These guidelines reduce the amount of subjectivity involved in making judgments about E/M codes, such as one person's opinion of an extended examination versus another's definition. They do this by describing the specific items that may be documented for each of the three key components. They also explain how many of these items are needed to place the item on the appropriate scale.

The documentation guidelines have precise number counts of these items; these counts can be used to audit as well as to initially code the service. The audit double-checks the selected code based on the documentation in the patient's medical record. The auditor looks at the medical record and with an auditing tool (see later section) that independently analyzes by number count the services documented. The auditor then compares the code reported to the code selected through the audit. When the results are not the same, the auditor has uncovered a possible problem in interpreting the documentation guidelines.

Federal law requires that all expenses paid by Medicare including expenses for E/M services be "medically reasonable and necessary":

- Medical necessity of E/M services is generally expressed in two ways: frequency of services and intensity of service (the CPT level).
- Medicare's determination of medical necessity is separate from its determination that the E/M service was rendered as billed.
- Medicare determines medical necessity largely through the experience and judgment of clinician coders along with the limited tools provided in the CPT book and by the Centers for Medicare and Medicaid Services (CMS).
- At audit, Medicare will deny or downcode E/M services that, in its judgment, exceed the patient's documented needs.

Information used by Medicare is contained within the medical record documentation of history, examination, and medical decision making. Medical necessity of E/M services is based on the following:

- Number, acuity, and severity/duration of problems addressed through history, physical, and medical decision making
- The context of the encounter among all other services previously rendered for the same problem
- The complexity of documented comorbidities that clearly influenced the physician's work
- Physical scope encompassed by the problems (number of physical systems affected by the problems).

Audit Tool

Because the E/M codes are the most widely used codes, they are also the ones that may trigger an audit. As stated in Chapter 7, the Office of Inspector General (OIG) will announce which codes will be audited and if they find a problem in a certain area, the audit will then be expanded to all regions.

To prevent errors being found after payment, an internal audit, as discussed earlier, should be performed periodically to determine if the practice is coding properly. This is an objective evaluation, which should be conducted by the office staff. Preparing for the audit should include selecting 10 to 15 charts at random, including new patient visits, established patient visits, consultations, encounter forms, and insurance information.

The EOBs should be pulled with the charts to determine if the codes billed and paid for were coded to the correct level of an E/M.

Many practices use an audit tool to conduct their internal audits. When an audit is performed either retrospectively or prospectively an audit tool such as that shown in Figure 8.1 should be utilized to determine the exact E/M code selected by the

Figure 8.1

E/M audit tool.

E/M Audit Tool

Patient Information

Patient:	Visit Date:	History Level
Examined By:		Exam Level
Patient Status:	DOB:	Decision Making
Service Type:	Sex:	Insurance Carrier

CPT® Code(s) Billed	DOCUMENTED	DIAGNOSIS CODE(S) BILLED	DOCUMENTED

History

History of Present Illness
- ❑ location
- ❑ quality
- ❑ severity
- ❑ duration
- ❑ timing
- ❑ context
- ❑ modifying factors
- ❑ associated signs and symptoms
- ❑ No. of chronic diseases

History _____

Review of Systems
- ❑ Constitutional symptoms
- ❑ Eyes
- ❑ Ears, nose, mouth, throat
- ❑ Cardiovascular
- ❑ Respiratory
- ❑ Gastrointestinal
- ❑ Genitourinary
- ❑ Integumentary
- ❑ Musculoskeletal
- ❑ Neurologic
- ❑ Psychiatric
- ❑ Endocrine
- ❑ Hematologic/lymphatic
- ❑ Allergic/immunologic

Past, Family & Social History

PAST
- ❑ current medication
- ❑ prior illnesses and injuries
- ❑ operations and hospitalizations
- ❑ age-appropriate immunizations
- ❑ allergies   ❑ dietary status

FAMILY
- ❑ health status or cause of death of parents, siblings, and children
- ❑ hereditary or high-risk diseases
- ❑ diseases related to CC, HPI, ROS

SOCIAL
- ❑ living arrangements
- ❑ marital status   ❑ sexual history
- ❑ occupational history
- ❑ use of drugs, alcohol, or tobacco
- ❑ extent of education
- ❑ current employment   ❑ other

❑ PFSH form reviewed, no change   ❑ PFSH form reviewed, updated   ❑ PFSH form new

General Multi-System Examination

Constitutional
- ❑ 3 of 7 (2 BP, pulse, respir, tmp, hgt, wgt)
- ❑ General Appearance

Eyes
- ❑ Conjunctivac, Lids
- ❑ Eyes: Pupils, Irises
- ❑ Opthal exam—Optic discs, Pos Seg

ENT
- ❑ Ears, Nose
- ❑ Oto exam—Aud canals, Tymp membr
- ❑ Hearing
- ❑ Nasal mucosa, Septum, Turbinates
- ❑ ENTM: Lips, Teeth, Gums
- ❑ Oropharynx—oral mucosa, palates

Neck
- ❑ Neck
- ❑ Thyroid

Respiratory
- ❑ Respiratory effort
- ❑ Percussion of chest
- ❑ Palpation of chest
- ❑ Auscultation of lungs

Cardiovascular
- ❑ Palpation of heart
- ❑ Auscultation of heart (& sounds)
- ❑ Carotid arteries Abdominal aorta
- ❑ Femoral arteries
- ❑ Pedal pulses
- ❑ Extrem for periph edema/varicosities

Chest
- ❑ Inspect Breasts
- ❑ Palpation of Breasts & Axillae

Gastrointestinal
- ❑ Abd (+/− masses or tenderness)
- ❑ Liver, Spleen
- ❑ Hernia (+/−)
- ❑ Anus, Perineum, Rectum
- ❑ Stool for occult blood

GU/Female
- ❑ Female: Genitalia, Vagina
- ❑ Female Urethra
- ❑ Bladder
- ❑ Cervix
- ❑ Uterus
- ❑ Adnexa/parametria

GU/Male
- ❑ Scrotal Contents
- ❑ Penis
- ❑ Digital Rectal of Prostate

Lymphatic
- ❑ Lymph: Neck
- ❑ Lymph: Axillae
- ❑ Lymph: Groin
- ❑ Lymph: Other

Musculoskeletal
- ❑ Gait (. . . ability to exercise)
- ❑ Palpation Digits, Nails
- ❑ Head/Neck: Inspect, Percuss, Palp
- ❑ Head/Neck: Motion (+/− pain, crepit)
- ❑ Head/Neck: Stability (+/− lux, sublux)
- ❑ Head/Neck: Muscle strength & tone
- ❑ Spine/Rib/Pelv: Inspect, Percuss, Palp
- ❑ Spine/Rib/Pelv: Motion
- ❑ Spine/Rib/Pelv: Stability
- ❑ Spine/Rib/Pelv: Strength and tone

- ❑ R. Up Extrem: Inspect, Percuss, Palp
- ❑ R. Up Extrem: Motion (+/− pain, crepit)
- ❑ R. Up Extrem: Stability (+/− lux, sublux)
- ❑ R. Up Extrem: Muscle strength & tone
- ❑ L. Up Extrem: Inspect, Percuss, Palp
- ❑ L. Up Extrem: Motion (+/− pain, crepit)
- ❑ L. Up Extrem: Muscle strength & tone
- ❑ R. Low Extrem: Inspect, Percuss, Palp
- ❑ R. Low Extrem: Motion (+/− pain, crepit)
- ❑ R. Low Extrem: Stability (+/− lux, laxity)
- ❑ R. Low Extrem: Muscle strength & tone
- ❑ L. Low Extrem: Inspect, Percuss, Palp
- ❑ L. Low Extrem: Motion (+/− pain, crepit)
- ❑ L. Low Extrem: Sability (+/− lux, sublux)
- ❑ L. Low Extrem: Muscle strength & tone

Skin
- ❑ Skin: Inspect Skin & Subcut tissues
- ❑ Skin: Palpation Skin & Subcut tissues

Neuro
- ❑ Neuro: Cranial nerves (+/− deficits)
- ❑ Neuro: DTRs (+/− pathological reflexes)
- ❑ Neuro: Sensations

Psychiatry
- ❑ Psych: Judgment, Insight
- ❑ Psych: Mood, Affect (depression, anxiety)

Exam Documented _____

CPT is a registered trademark of the American Medical Association.

Figure 8.1

E/M audit tool. (continued)

Number of Diagnoses/ Management Options	Points
Self-limited or minor (Stable, improved, or worsened)—Maximum 2 points in this category.	1
Established problem (to examining MD); stable or improved	1
Established problem (to examining MD); worsening	2
New problem (to examining MD); no additional workup planned—Maximum 1 point in this category.	3
New problem (to examining MD); additional workup (eg., admit/ transfer)	4
Total	

Table of Risk

Level of Risk	Presenting Problem(s)	Diagnostic Procedure(s) Ordered	Management Options Selected
Minimal	• One self-limited or minor problem, e.g., cold, insect bite, tinea corporis	• Laboratory tests requiring venipuncture • Chest x-rays • EKG/EEG • Urinalysis • Ultrasound, eg, echocardiography • KOH prep	• Rest • Gargles • Elastic bandages • Superficial dressings
Low	• Two or more self-limited or minor problem • One stable chronic illness, e.g., well-controlled hypertension, non-insulin-dependent diabetes, cataract, BPH • Acute uncomplicated illness or injury, e.g., cystitis allergic rhinitis, simple sprain	• Physiologic tests not under stress, e.g., pulmonary functions tests • Noncardiovascular imaging studies with contrast, e.g., barium enema • Superficial needle biopsies • Clinical laboratory tests requiring arterial puncture • Skin biopsies	• Over-the-counter drugs • Minor surgery with no identified risk factors • Physical therapy • Occupational therapy • IV fluids without additives
Moderate	• One or more chronic illnesses with mild exacerbation, progression, or side effects of treatment • Two or more stable chronic illness • Undiagnosed new problem with uncertain prognosis, e.g., lump in breast • Acute illness with systemic symptoms, e.g., pyelonephritis, pneumonitis, colitis • Acute complicated injury, e.g., head injury with brief loss of consciousness	• Physiologic tests under stress, e.g., cardiac stress tests, fetal contraction stress test • Diagnostic endoscopies with no identified risk factors • Deep needle or incisional biopsy • Cardiovascular imaging studies with contrast and no identified risk factors, eg, arteriogram, cardiac catheterization • Obtain fluid from body cavity, e.g., lumbar puncture, thoracentesis, culdocentesis	• Minor surgery with identified risk factors • Elective major surgery (open, percutaneous, or endoscopic) with no identified risk factors • Prescription drug management • Therapeutic nuclear medicine • IV fluids with additives • Closed treatment of fracture or dislocation without manipulation
High	• One or more chronic illnesses with severe exacerbation, progression, or side effects of treatment • Acute or chronic illnesses or injuries that pose a threat to life or bodily function, eg, multiple trauma, acute MI, pulmonary embolus, severe respiratory distress, progressive severe rheumatoid arthritis, psychiatric illness with potential threat to self or others, peritonitis, acute renal failure • An abrupt change in neurologic status, e.g., seizure, TIA, weakness, sensory loss	• Cardiovascular imaging studies with contrast with identified risk factors • Cardiac electrophysiological tests • Diagnostic endoscopies with identified risk factors • Discography	• Elective major surgery (open, percutaneous, or endoscopic) with identified risk factors • Emergency major surgery (open, percutaneous, or endoscopic) • Parenteral controlled substances • Drug therapy requiring intensive monitoring for toxicity • Decision not to resuscitate or to deescalate care because of poor prognosis

Amount and/or complexity of Data Reviewed	Points
Lab ordered and/or reviewed (regardless of # ordered)	1
X-ray ordered and/or reviewed (regardless of # ordered)	1
Medicine section (90701-99199) ordered and/or reviewed	1
Discussion of test results with performing physician	1
Decision to obtain old record and/or obtain hx from someone other than patient	1
Review and summary of old records and/or obtaining hx from someone other than patient and/or discussion with other health provider	2
Independent visualization of image, tracing, of specimen (not simply review of report)	2
Total	

Medical Decision Making	SF	LOW	MOD	HIGH
Number of Diagnoses or Treatment Options	1	2	3	4
Amount and/or Complexity of Data to be Reviewed	1	2	3	4
Risk of Complications, Morbidity, Mortality	Minimal	Low	Moderate	High
E/M Level=2 out of 3				

MDM_____

Chart Note
❑ Dictated   ❑ Handwritten
❑ Form   ❑ Illegible
❑ Note signed
❑ Signature missing

Other Services or Modalities:

Auditor:

number count. Trailblazer has published a tool for auditing for physicians' practices billing Medicare Part B. It is called the *Evaluation and Management: Coding and Documentation Pocket Reference.*

When conducting an audit with the E/M Audit Tool in Figure 8.1 the following information is analyzed.

Key Elements of Service

To code a claim correctly, the coder must determine the appropriate level of service for a patient's visit. In doing so, it is first necessary to determine whether the patient is new or already established. The physician then uses the presenting illness as a guiding factor and his or her clinical judgment about the patient's condition to determine the extent of key elements of service to be performed. The key elements of service are:

- History
- Examination
- Medical decision making.

The key elements of service and documentation of an encounter dominated by counseling and/or coordination of care are discussed below.

History

The elements required for each type of history are depicted in Table 8.1. Note that each history type requires more information as you read down the left-hand column. For example, a problem-focused history requires the documentation of the chief complaint (CC) and a brief history of present illness (HPI), whereas a detailed history requires the documentation of a CC, extended HPI, extended review of systems (ROS), and pertinent past, family, and/or social history (PFSH).

The extent of information gathered for the history is dependent on clinical judgment and the nature of the presenting problem. Documentation of patient history includes some or all of the following elements.

Table 8.1	Elements Required for Each Type of History			
Type of History	**Chief Complaint**	**History of Present Illness**	**Review of Systems**	**Past, Family, and/or Social History**
Problem Focused	Required	Brief	N/A	N/A
Expanded Problem Focused	Required	Brief	Problem	N/A
Detailed	Required	Extended	Pertinent Extended	Pertinent
Comprehensive	Required	Extended	Complete	Complete

Source: The International Classification of Diseases, Ninth Revision, published by the World Health Organization is the foundation of the ICD-9-CM. The CPT codes, descriptions, and other data only are copyright 2007 American Medical Association. All rights reserved.

Chief Complaint

A chief complaint is a concise statement that describes the symptom, problem, condition, diagnosis, or reason for the patient encounter. The CC is usually stated in the patient's own words. For example, patient complains of upset stomach, aching joints, and fatigue.

History of Present Illness

The history of present illness is a chronological description of the development of the patient's present illness from the first sign and/or symptom or from the previous encounter to the present. HPI elements include the following:

- *Location:* For example, pain in left leg.
- *Quality:* For example, aching, burning, radiating.
- *Severity:* For example, 10 on a scale of 1 to 10.
- *Duration:* For example, it started three days ago.
- *Timing:* For example, it is constant or it comes and goes.
- *Context:* For example, lifted large object at work.
- *Modifying factors:* For example, it is better when heat is applied.
- *Associated signs and symptoms:* For example, numbness.

There are two types of HPIs:

1. Brief, which includes documentation of one to three HPI elements. In the following example, three HPI elements—location, severity, and duration—are documented:
   - CC: A patient seen in the office complains of left ear pain.
   - *Brief HPI:* Patient complains of dull ache in left ear over the past 24 hours.
2. Extended, which includes documentation of at least four HPI elements or the status of at least three chronic or inactive conditions. In the following example, five HPI elements—location, severity, duration, context, and modifying factors—are documented:
   - *Extended HPI:* Patient complains of dull ache in left ear over the past 24 hours. Patient states he went swimming two days ago. Symptoms somewhat relieved by warm compress and ibuprofen.

Review of Systems

A review of systems is an inventory of body systems obtained by asking a series of questions in order to identify signs and/or symptoms that the patient may be experiencing or has experienced. There are three types of ROS:

1. Problem pertinent, which inquires about the system directly related to the problem identified in the HPI. In the following example, one system—the ear—is reviewed:

Example

CC: Earache.
ROS: Positive for left ear pain. Denies dizziness, tinnitus, fullness, or headache.

2. Extended, which inquires about the system directly related to the problem(s) identified in the HPI and a limited number (two to nine) of additional systems.

In the following example, two systems—cardiovascular and respiratory—are reviewed:

Example

CC: Follow-up visit in office after cardiac catheterization. Patient states, "I feel great."
ROS: Patient states he feels great and denies chest pain, syncope, palpitations, and shortness of breath. Relates occasional unilateral, asymptomatic edema of left leg.

---

3. Complete, which inquires about the system(s) directly related to the problem(s) identified in the HPI plus all additional (minimum of 10) body systems. In the following example, 10 signs and symptoms are reviewed:

Example

CC: Patient complains of "fainting spell."
ROS
- Constitutional: weight stable; + fatigue.
- Eyes: + loss of peripheral vision.
- Ear, nose, mouth, throat: no complaints.
- Cardiovascular: + palpitations; denies chest pain; denies calf pain, pressure, or edema.
- Respiratory: + shortness of breath on exertion.
- Gastrointestinal: appetite good, denies heartburn and indigestion; + episodes of nausea. Bowel movement daily; denies constipation or loose stools.
- Urinary: denies incontinence, frequency, urgency, nocturia, pain, or discomfort.
- Skin: + clammy, moist skin.
- Neurological: + fainting; denies numbness, tingling, and tremors.
- Psychiatric: denies memory loss or depression. Mood pleasant.

A sample of chart notes is shown in Figure 8.2.

Past, Family, and/or Social History

The past, family, and/or social history consists of a review of the patient's:

- Past history including experiences with illnesses, operations, injuries, and treatments
- Family history including a review of medical events, diseases, and hereditary conditions that may place him at risk
- Social history including an age-appropriate review of past and current activities.

There are two types of PFSH:

1. Pertinent, which is a review of the history areas directly related to the problem(s) identified in the HPI. In the following example, the patient's past surgical history is reviewed as it relates to the current HPI:
   - Patient returns to office for follow-up of coronary artery bypass graft in 2007. Recent cardiac catheterization demonstrates 50% occlusion of vein graft to obtuse marginal artery.

Patient: Summers, Lillian   DOB: 05-23-1945

DOS: 4-15-2008

ROS

+ weight gain—started 2-1-2007, 90 lbs since steroid
+ insomnia due to shortness of breath (SOB)/choking
+ pt complains of (c/o) heat intolerance, alternating with cold spells
+ chronic headache: posterior occipital
+ decreased vision: blurring > 6 months + photophobia, c/o dry eyes
- epistaxis
+ nausea, - vomiting, + constipation with occasional diarrhea
+ polydipsia, + polyuria, + nocturnal uria
+ most recent urinary tract infection (UTI) ~ 1 month ago
+ occasional dysuria
+ lower extremity edema—right ankle swelling
+ skin—dry/itching
+ poor appetite

Figure 8.2

Sample chart notes.

2. Complete, which is a review of two or all three of the areas, depending on the category of E/M service. A complete PFSH requires a review of all three history areas for services that, by their nature, include a comprehensive assessment or reassessment of the patient. A review of two history areas is sufficient for other services. At least one specific item from each of the three history areas must be documented for the following categories of E/M services:
   - Office or other outpatient services, established patient
   - Emergency department
   - Domiciliary care, established patient
   - Home care, established patient.

At least one specific item from each of the history areas must be documented for the following categories of E/M services:

   - Office or other outpatient services, new patient
   - Hospital observation services
   - Hospital inpatient services, initial care
   - Consultations
   - Comprehensive nursing facility assessments
   - Domiciliary care, new patient
   - Home care, new patient.

In the following example, the patient's genetic history is reviewed as it relates to the current HPI:

Example

Family history reveals the following:

   - **Maternal grandparents: both + for coronary artery disease; grandfather deceased at age 69; grandmother still living.**

- Paternal grandparents: grandmother, + diabetes, hypertension; grandfather, + heart attack at age 55.
- Parents: mother, + obesity, diabetes; father, + heart attack age 51, deceased age 57 of heart attack.
- Siblings: sister, + diabetes, obesity, hypertension, age 39; brother, + heart attack at age 45, living.

Sample chart notes for past medical history are shown in Figure 8.3.

Examination

An examination may involve several organ systems or a single organ system. The extent of the examination performed is based on clinical judgment, the patient's history, and nature of the presenting problem.

Table 8.2 depicts the body areas and organ systems that are recognized according to the CPT book.

There are two types of examinations that can be performed during a patient's visit:

1. A general multisystem examination, which involves the examination of one or more organ systems or body areas.
2. A single organ system examination, which involves a more extensive examination of a specific organ system.

Any physician, regardless of specialty, may perform both types of examinations. Table 8.3 compares the elements of the cardiovascular system/body area for both a general multi-system and single organ system examination. The elements required for general multi-system examinations are depicted in Table 8.4.

According to the 1997 *Documentation Guidelines for Evaluation and Management Services*, the 10 single organ system examinations are:

- Cardiovascular;
- Ear, Nose, and Throat;
- Eye;
- Genitourinary;

Figure 8.3

Sample chart notes for past medical history.

Patient: Summers, Lillian   DOB: 05-23-1945

DOS: 4-15-2008

PMH

Status post thyroid resection—1982
Status post splenectomy—1982
    DM/HTN/sickle cell anemia
    Esophagitis status post EGD/OGI

Habits

Smoker 1 pack every 4 days > 29 yrs

No allergies

SHX—disabled

Table 8.2	Body Areas and Organ Systems Recognized According to the CPT Book	
Body Areas		**Organ Systems**
Head, including face		Eyes
Neck		Ears, Nose, Mouth, and Throat
Chest, including breast and axilla		Cardiovascular
Abdomen		Respiratory
Genitalia, groin, buttocks		Gastrointestinal
Back		Genitourinary
Each extremity		Musculoskeletal
		Skin
		Neurologic
		Hematologic/Lymphatic/Immunologic
		Psychiatric

Table 8.3	Comparison of the Elements of the Cardiovascular System/Body Area for Both a General Multi-System and Single Organ System Examination	
System/Body Area	**General Multi-System Examination**	**Single Organ System Examination**
Cardiovascular	Palpation of heart (e.g., location, size, thrills).	Palpation of heart (e.g., location, size, and forcefulness of the point of maximal impact; thrills; lifts; palpable S3 or S4).
	Auscultation of heart with notation of abnormal sounds and murmurs.	Auscultation of heart including sounds, abnormal sounds, and murmurs.
	Examination of:	Measurement of blood pressure in two or more extremities when indicated (e.g., aortic dissection, coarctation).
	■ Carotid arteries (e.g., pulse amplitude, bruits);	Examination of:
	■ Abdominal aorta (e.g., size, bruits);	■ Carotid arteries (e.g., waveform, pulse amplitude, bruits, apical-carotid delay);
	■ Femoral arteries (e.g., pulse amplitude, bruits);	■ Abdominal aorta (e.g., size, bruits);
	■ Pedal pulses (e.g., pulse amplitude); and	■ Femoral arteries (e.g., pulse amplitude, bruits);
	■ Extremities for edema and/or varicosities.	■ Pedal pulses (e.g., pulse amplitude); and
		■ Extremities for peripheral edema and/or varicosities.

Table 8.4

Comparison of the Elements Required for Both General Multi-System and Single Organ System Examinations

Type of Examination	Multi-System Examinations	Single Organ System Examinations
Problem Focused	1–5 elements identified by a bullet in 1 or more organ system(s) or body area(s).	1–5 elements identified by a bullet, whether in a box with a shaded or unshaded border.
Expanded Problem Focused	At least 6 elements identified by a bullet in one or more organ system(s) or body area(s).	At least 6 elements identified by a bullet, whether in a box with a shaded or unshaded border.
Detailed	At least 6 organ systems or body areas. For each system/area selected, performance and documentation of at least 2 elements identified by a bullet is expected. **OR** At least 12 elements identified by a bullet in 2 or more organ systems or body areas.	At least 12 elements identified by a bullet, whether in a box with a shaded or unshaded border. Eye and psychiatric: At least 9 elements identified by a bullet, whether in a box with a shaded or unshaded border.
Comprehensive	Include at least 9 organ systems or body areas. For each system/area selected, all elements of the examination identified by a bullet should be performed, unless specific directions limit the content of the examination. For each area/system, documentation of at least 2 elements identified by bullet is expected.	Perform all elements identified by a bullet, whether in a shaded or unshaded box. Document every element in each box with a shaded border and at least 1 element in a box with an unshaded border.

Source: CPT copyright 2007 American Medical Association. All rights reserved.

- Hematologic/Lymphatic/Immunologic;
- Musculoskeletal;
- Neurological;
- Psychiatric;
- Respiratory; and
- Skin.

Table 8.4 compares the elements that are required for both general multi-system and single organ system examinations.

Some important points that should be kept in mind when documenting general multi-system and single organ system examinations include these:

- Specific abnormal and relevant negative findings of the examination of the affected or symptomatic body area(s) or organ system(s) should be documented. A notation of "abnormal" without elaboration is not sufficient.
- Abnormal or unexpected findings of the examination of any asymptomatic body area(s) or organ system(s) should be described.
- A brief statement or notation indicating "negative" or "normal" is sufficient to document normal findings related to unaffected area(s) or asymptomatic organ system(s). (However, an entire organ system should not be documented with a statement such as "negative.")

Patient: Summers, Lillian   DOB: 05-23-1945

DOS: 4-15-2008

PE

Obese BF
Neck—right side mass without bruit
Oropharynx clear
Lung clear
Right extremity edema
Skin—wrinkling in skin of her neck—lateral side

Sample chart notes for a physical examination.

Figure 8.4 provides a sample of chart notes for a physical examination.

Medical Decision Making

Medical decision making refers to the complexity of establishing a diagnosis and/or selecting a management option, which is determined by considering the following factors:

- The number of possible diagnoses and/or the number of management options that must be considered
- The amount and/or complexity of medical records, diagnostic tests, and/or other information that must be obtained, reviewed and analyzed
- The risk of significant complications, morbidity, and/or mortality as well as comorbidities associated with the patient's presenting problem(s), the diagnostic procedure(s), and/or the possible management options.

Table 8.5 depicts the elements for each level of medical decision making. Note that to qualify for a given type of medical decision making, **two of the three elements must either be met or exceeded.**

Table 8.5	Elements for Each Level of Medical Decision Making		
Type of Decision Making	**Number of Diagnoses or Management Option**	**Amount and/or Complexity of Data to Be Reviewed**	**Risk of Significant Complications, Morbidity, and/or Mortality**
Straightforward	Minimal	Minimal or None	Minimal
Low Complexity	Limited	Limited	Low
Moderate Complexity	Multiple	Moderate	Moderate
High Complexity	Extensive	Extensive	High

Source: CPT copyright 2007 American Medical Association. All rights reserved.

Number of Diagnoses or Management Options

The number of possible diagnoses and/or the number of management options that must be considered is based on the following:

■ The number and types of problems addressed during the encounter
■ The complexity of establishing a diagnosis
■ The management decisions that are made by the physician.

In general, decision making with respect to a diagnosed problem is easier than that for an identified but undiagnosed problem. The number and type of diagnosed tests performed may be an indicator of the number of possible diagnoses. Problems that are improving or resolving are less complex than problems that are worsening or failing to change as expected. Another indicator of the complexity of diagnostic or management problems is the need to seek advice from other healthcare professionals.

Keep these important points in mind when documenting the number of diagnoses or management options:

■ For each encounter, an assessment, clinical impression, or diagnosis should be documented, which may be explicitly stated or implied in documented decisions regarding management plans and/or further evaluation.
  ● For a presenting problem with an established diagnosis, the record should reflect whether the problem is (1) improved, well controlled, resolving, or resolved or (2) inadequately controlled, worsening, or failing to change as expected.
  ● For a presenting problem without an established diagnosis, the assessment or clinical impression may be stated in the form of differential diagnoses or as a "possible," "probable," or "rule out" diagnosis.
■ The initiation of, or changes in, treatment should be documented. Treatment includes a wide range of management options including patient instructions, nursing instructions, therapies, and medications.
■ If referrals are made, consultations requested, or advice sought, the record should indicate to whom or where the referral or consultation was made or from whom advice was requested.

Amount and/or Complexity of Data to Be Reviewed

The amount and/or complexity of data to be reviewed is based on the types of diagnostic testing ordered or reviewed. Indications of the amount and/or complexity of data being reviewed include the following:

■ A decision to obtain and review old medical records and/or obtain history from sources other than the patient (increases the amount and complexity of data to be reviewed)
■ Discussion of contradictory or unexpected test results with the physician who performed or interpreted the test (indicates the complexity of data to be reviewed)
■ The physician who ordered a test personally reviews the image, tracing, or specimen to supplement information from the physician who prepared the test report or interpretation (indicates the complexity of data to be reviewed).

Here are some important points that should be kept in mind when documenting amount and/or complexity of data to be reviewed:

- If a diagnostic service is ordered, planned, scheduled, or performed at the time of the E/M encounter, the type of service should be documented.
- The review of laboratory, radiology, and/or other diagnostic tests should be documented. A simple notation such as "White blood count elevated" or "Chest x-ray unremarkable" is acceptable. Alternatively, the review may be documented by initialing and dating the report that contains the test results.
- A decision to obtain old records or obtain additional history from the family, caretaker, or other source to supplement information obtained from the patient should be documented.
- Relevant findings from the review of old records and/or the receipt of additional history from the family, caretaker, or other source to supplement information obtained from the patient should be documented. If there is no relevant information beyond that already obtained, this fact should be documented. A notation of "Old records reviewed" or "Additional history obtained from family" without elaboration is not sufficient.
- Discussion about results of laboratory, radiology, or other diagnostic tests with the physician who performed or interpreted the study should be documented.
- The direct visualization and independent interpretation of an image, tracing, or specimen previously or subsequently interpreted by another physician should be documented.

Risk of Significant Complications, Morbidity, and/or Mortality

The risk of significant complications, morbidity, and/or mortality is based on the risks associated with the following categories:

- Presenting problem(s)
- Diagnostic procedure(s)
- Possible management options.

The assessment of risk of the presenting problem(s) is based on the risk related to the disease process anticipated between the present encounter and the next encounter. The assessment of risk of selecting diagnostic procedures and management options is based on the risk during and immediately following any procedures or treatment. The highest level of risk in any one category determines the overall risk.

The level of risk of significant complications, morbidity, and/or mortality can be:

- Minimal
- Low
- Moderate
- High.

Some important points that should be kept in mind when documenting level of risk are as follows:

- Comorbidities/underlying diseases or other factors that increase the complexity of medical decision making by increasing the risk of complications, morbidity, and/or mortality should be documented.

■ If a surgical or invasive diagnostic procedure is ordered, planned, or scheduled at the time of the E/M encounter, the type of procedure should be documented.
■ If a surgical or invasive diagnostic procedure is performed at the time of the E/M encounter, the specific procedure should be documented.
■ The referral for or decision to perform a surgical or invasive diagnostic procedure on an urgent basis should be documented.

Table 8.6 can be used to assist in determining whether the level of risk of significant complications, morbidity, and/or mortality is minimal, low, moderate, or high. Because determination of risk is complex and not readily quantifiable, the table includes common clinical examples rather than absolute measures of risk.

Documentation of an Encounter Dominated by Counseling and/or Coordination of Care

When counseling and/or coordination of care dominates (i.e., is more than 50% of) the physician/patient and/or family encounter (face-to-face time in the office or other outpatient setting, floor/unit time in the hospital or nursing facility), time is considered the key or controlling factor to qualify for a particular level of E/M services. If the level of service is reported based on counseling and/or coordination of care, the total length of time of the encounter should be documented and the record should describe the counseling and/or activities to coordinate care. For example, if 25 minutes was spent face to face with an established patient in the office and more than half of that time was spent counseling the patient or coordinating his or her care, CPT code 99214 should be selected. Figure 8.5 can be used as a reference to determine the correct code.

Use the following tips to correctly code E/M Services based on medical necessity:

1. Identify all of the presenting complaints and or reasons for the visit for which physician work occurred.
   ● Demonstrate clearly the history, physician, and extent of medical decision making associated with each problem.
   ● Demonstrate clearly how physician work (expressed in terms of mental effort, physical effort, time spent, and risk to the patient) was affected by comorbidities or chronic problems listed.
2. Ensure that the nature of the patient's presentation corresponds to the CPT book's contributory factors of nature of the presenting problem and/or patient status descriptions for the code reported. For instance:
   ● 99231—Usually the patient is stable, recovering or improving.
   ● 99232—Usually the patient is responding inadequately to therapy or has developed a minor complication.
   ● 99233—Usually the patient is unstable or has developed a significant complication or a significant new problem.
3. Utilize clinical examples in Appendix C of the CPT book. The Appendix C, located in the back of the CPT book, gives the coder or provider clinical examples for evaluation and management coding properly.
   ● The clinical examples are believed by the CPT coding to represent the physician work that is reasonable and necessary in order to provide appropriate patient care in the specified clinical circumstance of the example.
   ● Understand that Medicare expects actual documentation of services similar to the ones in the examples to also satisfy CMS documentation requirements to demonstrate that the service billed was provided.

Table 8.6	**Table of Risk**

Level of Risk	Presenting Problem(s)	Diagnostic Procedure(s) Ordered	Management Options Selected
Minimal	One self-limited or minor problem, e.g., cold, insect bite, tinea corporis.	Laboratory tests requiring venipunture. Chest x-rays. Electrocardiogram/ electroencephalogram. Urinalysis. Ultrasound e.g., echocardiography. Potassium Hydroxide prep.	Rest. Gargles. Elastic bandages. Superficial dressings.
Low	Two or more self-limited or minor problems. One stable chronic illness, e.g., well controlled hypertension, non-insulin-dependent diabetes, cataract, benign prostatic hyperplasia. Acute uncomplicated illness or injury, e.g., cystitis, allergic rhinitis, simple sprain.	Physiologic tests not under stress, e.g., pulmonary functions tests. Non-cardiovascular imaging studies with contrast, e.g., barium enema. Superficial needle biopsies. Clinical laboratory tests requiring arterial puncture.	Over-the-counter drugs. Minor surgery with no identified risk factors. Physical therapy. Occupational therapy. Intravenous fluids without additives.
Moderate	One or more chronic illnesses with mild exacerbation, progression, or side effects of treatment. Two or more stable chronic illnesses. Undiagnosed new problem with uncertain prognosis, e.g., lump in breast. Acute illness with systemic symptoms, e.g., pyelonephritis, pneumonitis, colitis. Acute complicated injury, e.g., head injury with brief loss of consciousness.	Physiologic tests under stress, e.g., cardiac stress test, fetal contraction stress test. Diagnostic endoscopies with no identified risk factors. Deep needle or incisional biopsy. Cardiovascular imaging studies with contrast and no identified risk factors, eg., arteriogram, cardiac catheterization. Obtain fluid from body cavity, e.g., lumbar puncture, thoracentesis, culdocentesis.	Minor surgery with identified risk factors. Elective major surgery (open, percutaneous or endoscopic) with no identified risk factors. Prescription drug management. Therapeutic nuclear medicine. Intravenous fluids with additives. Closed treatment of fracture or dislocation without manipulation.
High	One or more chronic illnesses with severe exacerbation, progression, or side effects of treatment. Acute or chronic illnesses or injuries that pose a threat to life or bodily function, e.g., multiple trauma, acute MI, pulmonary embolus, severe respiratory distress, progressive severe rheumatoid arthritis, psychiatric illness with potential threat to self or others, peritonitis, acute renal failure. An abrupt change in neurologic status, e.g., seizure, translent ischemic attact, weakness, sensory loss.	Cardiovascular imaging studies with contrast with identified risk factors. Cardiac electrophysiological tests. Diagnostic endoscopies with identified risk factors. Discography.	Elective major surgery (open, percutaneous, or endoscopic) with identified risk factors. Emergency major surgery (open, percutaneous, or endoscopic). Parenteral controlled substances. Drug therapy requiring intensive monitoring for toxicity. Decision not to resuscitate or to de-escalate care because of poor prognosis.

1 HISTORY

HPI (History of Present Illness): Characterize HPI by considering either the Status of chronic conditions or the number of elements recorded.

☐ 1 condition ☐ 2 conditions ☐ 3 conditions

OR

☐ Location ☐ Severity ☐ Timing ☐ Modifying factors
☐ Quality ☐ Duration ☐ Context ☐ Associated signs and symptoms

☐ Status of 1-2 chronic conditions	☐ Status of 1-2 chronic conditions	☐ Status of 3 chronic conditions	☐ Status of 3 chronic conditions
☐ Brief (1-3)	☐ Brief (1-3)	☐ Extended (4 or more)	☐ Extended (4 or more)

ROS (Review of Systems):

☐ Constitutional (wt loss, etc.) ☐ Ears, nose, mouth, throat ☐ GI ☐ Integumentary (skin, breast) ☐ Endo
☐ Eyes ☐ Card/vasc ☐ GU ☐ Neuro ☐ Hem/lymph
☐ Musculo ☐ Psych ☐ Resp ☐ All/immuno

N/A	☐ Pertinent to problem (1 system)	☐ Extended (Pert and others) (2-9 systems)	☐ Complete (Pert and all others) (10 systems)

PFSH (Past medical, Family, Social History) areas:

☐ Past history (the patient's past experiences with illnesses, operation, injuries and treatments)
☐ Family history (a review of medical events in the patient's family, including diseases that may be hereditary or place the patient at risk)
☐ Social history (an age-appropriate review of past and current activities)

N/A	N/A	☐ Pertinent (1 history area)	☐ *Complete (2 or 3 history areas)

*Complete PFSH: 2 history areas: a) established patients - office (outpatient) care, domiciliary care, home care; b) emergency department; c) subsequent nursing facility care; d) subsequent hospital care; and, e) follow-up consultations.

3 history areas: a) new patients - office (outpatient) care, domiciliary care, home care; b) initial consultations; c) initial hospital care; d) hospital observation; and, e) comprehensive nursing facility assessments.

PROBLEM-FOCUSED	EXP. PROBLEM-FOCUSED	DETAILED	COMPREHENSIVE

Final History requires all 3 components above met or exceeded

2 EXAMINATION

CPT Exam Description	95 Guideline Requirements	97 Guideline Requirements	CPT Type of Exam
Limited to affected body area or organ system	One body area or organ system	1-5 bulleted elements	PROBLEM-FOCUSED EXAM
Affected body area or organ system and other symptomatic or related organ systems	2-7 body areas and/or organ systems	6-11 bulleted elements	EXPANDED PROBLEM-FOCUSED EXAM
Extended exam of affected body area or organ system and other symptomatic or related organ systems	2-7 body areas and/or organ systems	12-17 bulleted elements for 2 or more systems	DETAILED EXAM
General multi-system	8 or more body areas and/or organ systems	18 or more bulleted elements for 9 or more systems	COMPREHENSIVE EXAM
Complete single organ system exam	Not defined	See requirements for individual single system exams	

3 MEDICAL DECISION-MAKING

Final Result of Complexity for Medical Decision-Making Level				
A. Number of diagnoses and/or management options	≤ 2 Minimal	3-4 Limited	5-6 Multiple	≥ 7 Extensive
B. Amount and complexity of data reviewed/ordered	≤ 1 None/Minimal	2 Limited	3 Multiple	≥ 4 Extensive
C. Risk	Minimal	Low	Moderate	High
Type of medical decision-making	Straightforward	Low Complexity	Moderate Complexity	High Complexity

Final Medical Decision-Making requires 2 of 3 components above met or exceeded

A. Number of Diagnoses and/or Management Options (see Table A.1)	#DX	#TX	#DX + #TX
New or est problem(s), no evaluation/management mentioned and problem **is not** clearly co-morbid condition.	0	0	0
New or est problem(s), no evaluation/management mentioned and problem **is** a co-morbid condition.		0	
New or established problem(s), evaluation/management mentioned.			
		TOTAL	

Figure 8.5 Tool to determine the correct CPT code.

3 MEDICAL DECISION-MAKING (continued)

A.1 Treatments and Therapeutic Options	
DO NOT COUNT AS TREATMENT OPTIONS NOTATIONS SUCH AS Continue "same" therapy or "no change" in therapy (including drug management) without further description (record does not document what the current therapy plan is nor that the physician reviewed it)	0
Continue "same" therapy or "no change" in therapy without further description (record clearly documents what the current therapy plan is and that the physician reviewed it); or scheduled monitoring without specific therapy	1
Drug management, new prescriptions, or changes in dosing for current medications	1
Complex drug management (more than 3 medications/prescriptions and/or over-the-counter) new prescriptions or changes in dosing for current medications	2
Open or percutaneous therapeutic cardiac, surgical or radiological procedure – minor or major	1
Physical, occupational or speech therapy or other manipulation	1
Closed treatment for fracture or dislocation	1
IV fluids	1
Complex insulin prescription (SC or combo of SC/IV), hyperalimentation, insulin drip or other complex IV admix prescription	2
Conservative measures such as rest, ice, bandages, dietary	1
Radiation therapy	1
IM injection/aspiration or other pain management procedure	1
Patient educated on self or home care topics/techniques	1
Hospital admit	1
Hospital admit – other physician(s) contacted	2
Referral to another physician, consultation	1
Other – specify	
TOTAL	

B. Amount and/or Complexity of Data Reviewed or Ordered	
Order and/or review results of clinical lab tests	1
Order and/or review results of tests in Radiology section of CPT	1
Order and/or review results of tests in Medical section of CPT	1
Discuss case with consultant or order consultation or discuss case with other physician also managing the patient	1
Discuss test results with performing physician	1
Order (identify specific source of records ordered) and/or summarize old or other health care records (simple statements to the effect that other or old outside records were reviewed is insufficient to count)	1
Physiologic monitoring	1
Independently visualize and report findings from images, tracings, pathological specimens themselves (not the reports) for procedures and tests for which interpretation not separately billed by the provider	1
TOTAL	

C. Risk of Complication and/or Mortality (see Table C.1)

	Minimal	Low	Moderate	High
Nature of the presenting illness	Minimal	Low	Moderate	High
Risk conferred by diagnostic options	Minimal	Low	Moderate	High
Risk conferred by therapeutic options	Minimal	Low	Moderate	High

Final Risk determined by highest of 3 components above

C.1 Risk of Complications and/or Morbidity or Mortality

LEVEL OF RISK	PRESENTING PROBLEM(S)	DIAGNOSTIC PROCEDURE(S) ORDERED	MANAGEMENT OPTIONS SELECTED
Minimal	• One self-limited or minor problem, e.g., cold, insect bite, tinea corporis	• Laboratory tests requiring venipuncture • Chest x-rays • EKG/EEG • Urinalysis • Ultrasound, e.g., echo • KOH prep	• Rest • Gargles • Elastic bandages • Superficial dressings
Low	• Two or more self-limited or minor problems • One stable chronic illness, e.g., well-controlled hypertension or non-insulin dependent diabetes, cataract, BPH • Acute uncomplicated illness or injury, e.g., cystitis, allergic rhinitis, simple sprain	• Physiologic tests not under stress, e.g., pulmonary function tests • Non-cardiovascular imaging studies with contrast, e.g., barium enema • Superficial needle biopsies • Clinical laboratory tests requiring arterial puncture • Skin biopsies	• Over-the-counter drugs • Minor surgery with no identified risk factors • Physical therapy • Occupational therapy • IV fluids without additives

C.1 Risk of Complications and/or Morbidity or Mortality

LEVEL OF RISK	PRESENTING PROBLEM(S)	DIAGNOSTIC PROCEDURE(S) ORDERED	MANAGEMENT OPTIONS SELECTED
Moderate	• One or more chronic illnesses with mild exacerbation, progression, or side effects of treatment • Two or more stable chronic illnesses • Undiagnosed new problem with uncertain prognosis, e.g., lump in breast • Acute illness with systemic symptoms, e.g., pyelonephritis, pneumonitis, colitis • Acute complicated injury, e.g., head injury with brief loss of consciousness	• Physiologic tests under stress, e.g., cardiac stress test, fetal contraction stress test • Diagnostic endoscopies with no identified risk factors • Deep needle or incisional biopsy • Cardiovascular imaging studies with contrast and no identified risk factors, e.g., arteriogram cardiac cath • Obtain fluid from body cavity, e.g., lumbar procedure, thoracentesis, culdocentesis	• Minor surgery with identified risk factors • Elective major surgery (open, percutaneous or endoscopic) with no identified risk factors • Prescription drug management • Therapeutic nuclear medicine • IV fluids with additives • Closed treatment of fracture or dislocation without manipulation
High	• One or more chronic illnesses with severe exacerbation, progression, or side effects of treatment • Acute or chronic illnesses or injuries that may pose a threat to life or bodily function, e.g., multiple trauma, acute MI, pulmonary embolus, severe respiratory distress, progressive severe rheumatoid arthritis, psychiatric illness with potential threat to self or others, peritonitis, acute renal failure • An abrupt change in neurologic status, e.g., seizure, TIA, weakness or sensory loss	• Cardiovascular imaging studies with contrast with identified risk factors • Cardiac electrophysiological tests • Diagnostic endoscopies with identified risk factors • Discography	• Elective major surgery (open, percutaneous or endoscopic with identified risk factors) • Emergency major surgery (open, percutaneous or endoscopic) • Parenteral controlled substances • Drug therapy requiring intensive monitoring for toxicity • Decision not to resuscitate or to de-escalate care because of poor prognosis

Figure 8.5   (continued)

(4) LEVEL OF SERVICE

OUTPATIENT, CONSULTS (OUTPATIENT AND INPATIENT) AND ER

	New Office/Consults/ER						Established Office			
	Requires 3 components within shaded area						Requires 2 components within shaded area			
History	PF / ER: PF	EPF / ER: EPF	D / ER: EPF	C / ER: D	C / ER: C	Minimal problem that may not require presence of physician	PF	EPF	D	C
Examination	PF / ER: PF	EPF / ER: EPF	D / ER: EPF	C / ER: D	C / ER: C		PF	EPF	D	C
Complexity of Medical Decision	SF / ER: SF	SF / ER: L	L / ER: M	M / ER: M	H / ER: H		SF	L	M	H
Average Time (minutes) (ER have no average time)	10 New (99201) 15 Outpt cons (99241) 20 Inpat cons (99251) ER (99281)	20 New (99202) 30 Outpt cons (99242) 40 Inpat cons (99252) ER (99282)	30 New (99203) 40 Outpt cons (99243) 55 Inpat cons (99253) ER (99283)	45 New (99204) 60 Outpt cons (99244) 80 Inpat cons (99254) ER (99284)	60 New (99205) 80 Outpt cons (99245) 100 Inpat cons (99255) ER (99285)	5 (99211)	10 (99212)	15 (99213)	25 (99214)	40 (99215)
Level	I	II	III	IV	V	I	II	III	IV	V

INPATIENT

	Initial Hospital/Observation			Subsequent Inpatient/Follow-up		
	Requires 3 components within shaded area			Requires 2 components within shaded area		
History	D or C	C	C	PF interval	EPF interval	D interval
Examination	D or C	C	C	PF	EPF	D
Complexity of Medical Decision	SF/L	M	H	SF/L	M	H
Average Time (minutes) (Observation care has no average time)	30 Init hosp (99221) Observ care (99218)	50 Init hosp (99222) Observ care (99219)	70 Init hosp (99223) Observ care (99220)	15 Subsequent (99231)	25 Subsequent (99232)	35 Subsequent (99233)
Level	I	II	III	I	II	III

NURSING FACILITY

	Annual Assessment/Admission			Subsequent Nursing Facility			
	Old Plan Review	New Plan	Admission				
	Requires 3 components within shaded area			Requires 2 components within shaded area			
History	D/C	C	C	PF interval	EPF interval	D interval	C interval
Examination	D/C	C	C	PF	EPF	D	C
Complexity of Medical Decision	SF	M	M	SF	L	M	H
No Average Time Established (Confirmatory consults and ER have no average time)	(99304)	(99305)	(99306)	(99307)	(99308)	(99309)	(99310)
Level	I	II	III	I	II	III	IV

DOMICILIARY (REST HOME, CUSTODIAL CARE) AND HOME CARE

	New					Established			
	Requires 3 components within shaded area					Requires 2 components within shaded area			
History	PF	EPF	D	C	C	PF interval	EPF interval	D interval	C
Examination	PF	EPF	D	C	C	PF	EPF	D	C
Complexity of Medical Decision	SF	L	M	M	H	SF	L	M	H
Average Time (minutes)	20 Domiciliary (99324) 20 Home care (99341)	30 Domiciliary (99325) 30 Home care (99342)	45 Domiciliary (99326) 45 Home care (99343)	60 Domiciliary (99327) 60 Home care (99344)	75 Domiciliary (99328) 75 Home care (99345)	15 Domiciliary (99334) 15 Home care (99347)	25 Domiciliary (99335) 25 Home care (99348)	40 Domiciliary (99336) 40 Home care (99349)	60 Domiciliary (99337) 60 Home care (99350)
Level	I	II	III	IV	V	I	II	III	IV

PF = Problem focused   EPF = Expanded problem focused   D = Detailed   C = Comprehensive   SF = Straightforward   L = Low   M = Moderate   H = High

Figure 8.5   Tool to determine the correct CPT code. (continued)

Tips for Preventing Coding Errors with Specific E/M Codes

The medical coder needs to realize that coding mistakes happen. If you are unsure about which code to use or have not been given enough information in the patient medical record, ask for help. Some common coding errors and how to help prevent them are listed here.

1. *High-level services and the "comprehensive" codes:* Understand the CPT code requirements.
   - All codes in the following code sets require three of the three key components to be documented according to the CMS guidelines to meet published CPT definitions:

     New patient office services
     Initial hospital services
     Initial consultations (inpatient and outpatient)
     Emergency department services
     Comprehensive nursing facility assessments.
   - All of the following codes require not just three of the three key components to be documented, but also require comprehensive history and comprehensive examination:

     99204 and 99205 (New patient office services)
     99222 and 99223 (Initial hospital services)
     99244 and 99245 (Office consultations)
     99254 and 99255 (Initial in-patient consultations)

2. *Emergency department services:* Pay attention to the unique record kept in most emergency departments (EDs). Multiple individuals, including hospital staff, contribute to the ED service and the ED record, but Part B must not pay the physician for services rendered by hospital staff. Physician coding should be based on the physician's E/M work (or work shared by a physician and non-physician practitioner in the same group). All history obtained and recorded by triage and other hospital nursing staff must be specifically repeated by the physician and either re-recorded or annotated with specific comments, additions, and/or corrections and notation of the element of work personally performed by the physician.

3. *Subsequent hospital services:* Pay attention to medical necessity. When coding, strongly consider the CPT book's "nature of the presenting problem" contributory factors and/or other patient status descriptions.

     99231—Usually the patient is stable, recovering or improving
     99232—Usually the patient is responding inadequately to therapy or has developed a minor complication
     99233—Usually the patient is unstable or has developed a significant complication or a significant new problem.

4. *Consultations:* Before coding a consultation, ask and answer questions about the service. If the answer is "no" to any of the following questions, do not report the service as a consultation:
   - Did you receive a request for an opinion from another physician?
   - Does the documentation of the service clearly demonstrate who made the request and the nature of the opinion requested?
   - Has the provider provided a written report of his or her opinion/advice to the referring physician?

- Though the referring physician may have asked for a "consultation," should the E/M service truly be reported as a consultation?
- Will the provider's opinion be used by, and in some manner affect, the requesting physician's own management of the patient?
- Will the referring physician be involved in subsequent decision making about the problem for which the referral has been made?
- For preoperative "consultations" is the service requested specifically for preoperative clearance that is medically necessary considering the patient's condition and the procedure planned?

5. *Critical care:* Before coding critical care, ask and answer the following questions about the service. If the answer is "no" to any of these questions, do not report the service as critical care:
- Does the record demonstrate work performed during the encounter that is more intense than the work of other E/M codes of the same time duration?
- Does the physician's documentation demonstrate all of the following?:

  Direct personal management

  Frequent personal assessment and manipulation (not generally a once-daily visit).

  High-complexity decision making to assess, manipulate, and support vital system function(s) to treat single or multiple organ system failure and/or to prevent further life-threatening deterioration.

  Intervention of a nature such that failure to initiate these interventions on an urgent basis would likely result in sudden clinically significant or life-threatening deterioration in the patient's condition.
- What about the time spent providing critical care?

  Is it specifically recorded?

  Is it reasonable considering the documented work provided?

  Does it exclude time spent performing procedures for which separate payment is made?

  If it includes time spent with family, was the family member operating as a surrogate decision maker because the patient was unable to make decisions?

Chapter Summary

- If audits are not performed on a regular basis, the medical office specialist will not know for a fact that the documentation was correct and appropriate for the level of service performed. If an audit is performed, any errors found can be brought to the attention of the provider and corrected for future billing.
- There are three types of audits: internal, external, and accreditation.
- The auditor looks at the medical record and with an auditing tool independently analyzes by number count the services documented. The auditor then compares the code reported to the code selected through the audit.
- The three key elements of service are the history documented, the examination documented, and the medical decision making.

Chapter Review

True/False

Identify the statement as true (T) or false (F).

_____   1. There are four types of audits.

_____   2. An accreditation audit is performed by the facility prior to claims submission.

_____   3. Code edits are conducted by the medical coder.

_____   4. When conducting an internal audit the three key elements reviewed are history, examination, and medical decision making.

_____   5. Code edits screen for improperly or incorrectly reported procedure codes.

_____   6. Compliance plans focus on training of physicians to use the AMA documentation guidelines for E/M services.

_____   7. *Downcoding* refers to a coding method in which lower level codes are selected to avoid government investigation.

_____   8. The term *external audit* may refer to an audit conducted by a consultant that the medical practice has hired.

_____   9. Both insurance carriers and agencies of the federal government may conduct external audits of medical practices' claims.

_____ 10. An internal audit is conducted to verify that a medical practice is in compliance with reporting regulations.

_____ 11. A prospective audit is also called an external audit.

_____ 12. To comply with regulations, all codes that are reported must be current, correct, and complete.

_____ 13. Retrospective internal audits permit the auditor to see which codes have been rejected or downcoded by the payer and set up ways to avoid making the same errors in the future.

_____ 14. Evaluation and management (E/M) codes are an ongoing focus of external audits because they are reported by so many medical practices.

_____ 15. Auditors may use an audit tool based on E/M documentation guidelines to determine whether a practice's selection of E/M codes complies with regulations.

Multiple Choice

Identify the letter of the choice that best completes the statement or answers the question.

_____ 1. What type of audit is performed internally after claims are submitted?
a. accreditation audit
b. routine payer audit
c. retrospective audit
d. prospective audit

_____ 2. What type of external audit is performed by payers before claims are processed?
a. retrospective
b. prospective
c. prepayment
d. postpayment

_____ 3. The term _downcode_ means that the procedure code stated is for a procedure that is _____.
a. more involved
b. in the hospital
c. less involved
d. less than per diem

_____ 4. The AMA documentation guidelines set up the rules for the correct selection of:
a. evaluation and management codes.
b. anesthesia codes.
c. surgery codes.
d. none of the above.

Completion

Complete each sentence or statement.

1. Correct code linkage establishes the medical _____ for a service or procedure.

2. A retrospective is performed _____.

3. Assigning a higher level of CPT code than is warranted by the documented service is called _____.

4. Coding _____ is part of a medical practice's overall effort to follow regulations in many areas.

5. In addition to facilitating high-quality patient care, an appropriately _____ medical record serves as a legal document to verify services provided.

6. An _____ is performed to judge whether a medical practice complies with applicable regulations for correct coding and billing.

Resources

American Academy of Neurology: **_www.aan.com_**

Medical Claims

The medical office specialist must have the knowledge and skills to submit a claim with no errors so that full reimbursement will be received. In the physician's office, as much as 80% of the physician's income can be generated by the submission of insurance claims and the reimbursement received from the insurance carrier. Chapter 9, Physician Medical Billing, will walk the student through the steps necessary to document all services provided accurately and in detail.

In the hospital setting, physicians' bills for inpatient care are much larger than the bills for services rendered in a physician's office. The majority of hospital reimbursement is from insurance companies; however, it is becoming more difficult for patients with insurance coverage to pay their share of the bill. As a result, accurate and timely billing with good follow-up and collection techniques is essential. Chapter 10, Hospital Medical Billing, presents detailed information on the inpatient billing process, coding and reimbursement methods, and presents the skills required to accurately bill for hospital services.

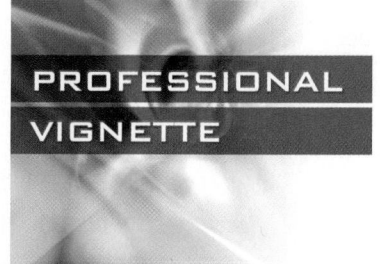

PROFESSIONAL VIGNETTE

My name is Lorraine Papazian-Boyce and for over 25 years I've worked with several specialties of physicians, as well as hospitals, cancer centers, community mental health, long term care, and alternative care providers. I even owned a medical billing business for 7 years. I thrive on the challenge of learning something new on a daily basis!

In my first job as the insurance biller for a group of psychologists, all of our claims were handwritten or typed on a typewriter. We didn't even use CMS-1500 forms. Many other changes have occurred over the years, and more are yet to come. Each experience I've had better prepares me for future changes.

Chapter 9 Physician Medical Billing

Chapter Objectives

After reading this chapter, the student should be able to:

1 Differentiate and complete medical claim forms accurately, both manually and electronically.

2 Define claim form parts, sections, and required information.

3 Exhibit the ability to complete claim forms without omitting information.

4 Understand the common reasons why claim forms are delayed or rejected and submit a claim without payer rejection.

5 File a secondary claim.

Key Terms

assignment of benefits form
audit/edit report
billing services
birthday rule
claim attachment
clean claims
clearinghouse
CMS-1500 claim form
dirty claim
electronic claims, electronic media claims (EMCs)
employer identification number (EIN)

facility provider number (FPN)
form locators
group provider number (GPN)
guarantor
National Provider Identifier number (NPI)
optical character recognition (OCR)
patient information form
provider identification number (PIN)
release of information form

secondary insurance
state license number
superbills
supplemental insurance
tax identification number (TIN)
UB-04 claim form
Unique Physician Identification Number (UPIN)
verification of benefits (VOB) form

Case Study
Physician
Medical
Billing

William arrived at Dr. Spence's office and gave the medical office specialist his insurance cards. Recently, William's wife had gone back to work and they now have two insurance plans. The front desk assistant asked William which insurance was primary. William did not understand the question. It was explained that it meant which insurance was to be billed first. William asked that his wife's be billed first because it had better coverage. The medical office specialist explained that this is not possible unless it is specifically set up as primary. His insurance would have to be billed first and his wife's secondary.

Questions

1. Why can't the office bill the wife's insurance first?

2. What would be the result of billing the wife's insurance as primary?

3. Will there be cases when the spouse's insurance may be primary?

Introduction

Services that are provided by a physician are generally covered by the patient's health insurance. As much as 80% of a physician's income can be generated by the submission of insurance claims and the reimbursement received from the insurance carrier. A medical office specialist must have the knowledge and skills to submit a claim with no errors so that full reimbursement will be received. The physician and her office staff, both clinical and clerical, must document all services provided accurately and in detail.

Patient Information

Billing insurance carriers for medical services provided in a medical office setting requires information from many different departments and people. Because insurance billing provides the majority of a physician's income, it is extremely important to gather accurate information so that claims can be processed without delay.

When a new patient registers at a medical office, he is asked to complete a **patient information form** (Figure 9.1). This form contains demographic, employment, and insurance information. The form varies from one practice or facility to another. Some facilities may have a multipage form requesting allergy or personal/family medical history. Although the patient (or parent/guardian) is asked to write his insurance information on the patient information form, it is necessary to obtain a copy (front and back) of the patient's insurance card as well. Some practices also request a copy of the driver's license to confirm the patient/parent identity.

The patient, if an adult, or the guardian (often referred to as the **guarantor**, the person who is ultimately responsible for paying for the services) is also asked to sign an **assignment of benefits form** (Figure 9.2) and a **release of information form** (Figure 9.3)

Assignment of benefits means that the patient/guarantor is asking the insurance carrier to send the money for the services rendered and billed directly to the provider who performed the services instead of to the patient/guarantor. If an assignment of benefits form is not signed and the office submits the claim to the insurance carrier, the money will be sent directly to the patient. An assignment of benefits form is usually signed once a year.

The release of information form specifies which healthcare information from the medical chart may be released and to whom it may be released. If there is no signed release of information form on file, you cannot submit the claim to the carrier. A signed release of information form is referred to as the "signature on file" form in most medical offices. This form must be signed once a year, however, some facilities require the patient to sign the release of information every six months.

The phrase *healthcare information* refers to information recorded in any form or medium that identifies the patient and relates to the patient's history, diagnosis, treatment, or prognosis. It is commonly know as the patient's *medical record*.

Generally there is a designated person or persons in the office/clinic who will verify patients' insurance benefits. One cannot assume that just because a patient has an insurance card, it is valid. Verifying the insurance benefits is accomplished by contacting the insurance carrier listed on the patient's insurance card. This can be done by telephone, fax, and sometimes over the Internet. Some insurance carriers have a service on their website to verify a patient's coverage and basic benefits.

Before you verify the patient's insurance benefits, you will need to gather some basic information about the patient and the policyholder (the person who took out the

Capital City Medical—123 Unknown BLVD, Capital City,
NY 12345-2222 (555)555-1234

Phil Wells, MD, Mannie Mends, MD, Bette R. Soone, MD

Patient Information Form

Tax ID: 75-0246810

Group NPI: 1513171216

Patient Information:

Name: (Last, First) _____ ❑ Male ❑ Female Birth Date: _____

Address: _____ Phone: ( ) _____

Social Security Number: _____ Full-Time Student: ❑ Yes ❑ No

Marital Status: ❑ Single ❑ Married ❑ Divorced ❑ Other

Employment:

Employer: _____ Phone: ( ) _____

Address: _____

Condition Related to: ❑ Auto Accident ❑ Employment ❑ Other Accident

Date of Accident: _____ State _____

Emergency Contact: _____ **Phone: ( )** _____

Primary Insurance: _____ Phone: ( ) _____

Address: _____

Insurance Policyholder's Name: _____ ❑ M ❑ F DOB: _____

Address: _____

Phone: _____ Relationship to Insured: ❑ Self ❑ Spouse ❑ Child ❑ Other

Employer: _____ Phone: ( ) _____

Employer's Address: _____

Policy/ID No: _____ Group No: _____ Percent Covered: ___%, Copay Amt: $____

Secondary Insurance: _____ Phone: ( ) _____

Address: _____

Insurance Policyholder's Name: _____ ❑ M ❑ F DOB: _____

Address: _____

Phone: _____ Relationship to Insured: ❑ Self ❑ Spouse ❑ Child ❑ Other

Employer: _____ Phone: ( ) _____

Employer's Address: _____

Policy/ID No: _____ Group No: _____ Percent Covered: ___%, Copay Amt: $____

Reason for Visit: _____

Known Allergies: _____

Were you referred here? If so, by whom?: _____

Figure 9.1

Sample patient information form.

Figure 9.2

Sample assignment of benefits form.

I authorize payment of medical benefits to Allied Medical Center or the specified physician below.

Alison R. Smith, M.D.   Samson Westheimer, M.D.

_____   _____
Patient/Guarantor's Signature   **Date**

Figure 9.3

Sample release of information form.

I, _____ **ACTING ON**
BEHALF OF: (Print Name of Patient or Legally Authorized Representative)

_____ **HEREBY AUTHORIZE THE RELEASE**
(Print Name of Patient) _____
OF INFORMATION AS INDICATED:

My Healthcare Information

_____ I authorize disclosure of healthcare information (related to my medical history, diagnosis, treatment, or prognosis) to all inquiries or only to the following people or entities (for example, family friends, employer, insurance companies, clergy, etc.):

List Names:

_____
_____

Limited Healthcare Information

_____ I wish to limit disclosure of only certain kinds of healthcare information (related to my medical history, diagnosis, treatment, or prognosis) to the following people or entities:

List Names   **List information that may be released**

_____   _____
_____   _____

No Information

_____ I do not authorize release of any information.

_____   _____
(Signature of Patient or Legally Authorized representative)   **(Date)**

insurance policy). You will need the patient's name (as it appears on the insurance card) and date of birth, the insured's/policyholder's name, insurance identification number (also referred to as certificate number or policy number), insurance group number, date of service, patient's reason for the visit (routine or problem-specific), name of attending physician (the physician with whom the patient has scheduled an appointment), the attending physician's tax identification number and the specific

Patient's Name: _____ Chart #: _____ Appt. Date: _____

D.O.B._____ Policy ID # _____ Gr# _____

Policyholder: _____ DOB: _____

Insurance Co. Name: _____ Referral# Required: ❑ No ❑ Yes

Telephone #_____ Referral #: _____

Mailing Address: _____

Employer's Name: _____

Employer's Phone #: _____

Effective Date: _____ Lifetime maximum: _____

Pre-Cert Required: ❑ Yes ❑ No

Deductible Met:

Copay_____ Deductible_____ ❑ No ❑ Yes

Pays @_____%

Exclusion/Preexisting: _____

Chief Complaint/Diagnosis: _____

Insurance Rep's Name: _____ Ext# _____

Voice Tracking #: _____ Date: _____ Time: _____

Verified by_____Date: _____

Figure 9.4

Insurance verification of benefits worksheet.

identification number assigned to the physicians' by the insurance carrier. Different facilities will ask different questions, but there are some basic answers every facility wants to know:

- What is the effective date for this insurance coverage/policy?
- Is this patient subject to any preexisting clauses (a clause in the contract that may exclude coverage for a condition the patient had prior to the effective date of the insurance policy)?
- Is this patient and/or type of service subject to a deductible amount and, if so, how much is the deductible amount and has any of it been met?
- Is this type of service subject to a copayment amount and, if so, what is the amount?
- Is this (office visit, test, etc.) a covered benefit?
- Does this plan require a referral or prior authorization?
- What is the claims mailing address?
- What is your first and last name (of the insurance carrier representative on the phone)?

Most facilities have a **verification of benefits (VOB) form** (Figure 9.4) on which to write the answers to these questions. It is important to document everything. A VOB form may come in handy if the insurance carrier pays the claim incorrectly or denies the claim after giving you information to the contrary when you verified benefits.

Superbills

Superbills, also referred to as encounter forms, charge slips, or routing slips, contain International Classification of Diseases (ICD-9-CM; diagnostic) and Current Procedural

Figure 9.5

A sample superbill.

Patient Name _____

Capital City Medical
123 Unknown Boulevard, Capital City, NY 12345-2222

Date of Service
_____

New Patient			Other Invasive/Noninvasive			Laboratory	
Problem Focused	99201		Arthrocentesis/Aspiration/Injection			Amylase	82150
Expanded Problem, Focused	99202		Small Joint	20600		B12	82607
Detailed	99203		Interm Joint	20605		CBC & Diff	85025
Comprehensive	99204		Major Joint	20610		Comp Metabolic Panel	80053
Comprehensive/High Complex	99205		**Other Invasive/Noninvasive**			Chlamydia Screen	87110
Well Exam Infant (up to 12 mos.)	99381		Audiometry	92552		Cholesterol	82465
Well Exam 1–4 yrs.	99382		Cast Application			Digoxin	80162
Well Exam 5–11 yrs.	99383		Location Long Short			Electrolytes	80051
Well Exam 12–17 yrs.	99384		Catheterization	51701		Ferritin	82728
Well Exam 18–39 yrs.	99385		Circumcision	54150		Folate	82746
Well Exam 40–64 yrs.	99386		Colposcopy	57452		GC Screen	87070
			Colposcopy w/Biopsy	57454		Glucose	82947
			Cryosurgery Premalignant Lesion			Glucose 1 HR	82950
			Location (s):			Glycosylated HGB A1C	83036
			Cryosurgery Warts			HCT	85014
Established Patient			Location (s):			HDL	83718
Post-Op Follow Up Visit	99024		Curettement Lesion			Hep BSAG	87340
Minimum	99211		Single	11055		Hepatitis panel, acute	80074
Problem Focused	99212		2–4	11056		HGB	85018
Expanded Problem Focused	99213		>4	11057		HIV	86703
Detailed	99214		Diaphragm Fitting	57170		Iron & TIBC	83550
Comprehensive/High Complex	99215		Ear Irrigation	69210		Kidney Profile	80069
Well Exam Infant (up to 12 mos.)	99391		ECG	93000		Lead	83655
Well exam 1–4 yrs.	99392		Endometrial Biopsy	58100		Liver Profile	80076
Well Exam 5–11 yrs.	99393		Exc. Lesion Malignant			Mono Test	86308
Well Exam 12–17 yrs.	99394		Benign			Pap Smear	88155
Well Exam 18–39 yrs.	99395		Location			Pregnancy Test	84703
Well Exam 40–64 yrs.	99396		Exc. Skin Tags (1–15)	11200		Obstetric Panel	80055
Obstetrics			Each Additional 10	11201		Pro Time	85610
Total OB Care	59400		Fracture Treatment			PSA	84153
Injections			Loc			RPR	86592
Administration Sub. / IM	90772		w/Reduc w/o Reduc			Sed. Rate	85651
Drug			I & D Abscess Single/Simple	10060		Stool Culture	87045
Dosage			Multiple or Comp	10061		Stool O & P	87177
Allergy	95115		I & D Pilonidal Cyst Simple	10080		Strep Screen	87880
Cocci Skin Test	86490		Pilonidal Cyst Complex	10081		Theophylline	80198
DPT	90701		IV Therapy—To One Hour	90760		Thyroid Uptake	84479
Hemophilus	90646		Each Additional Hour	90761		TSH	84443
Influenza	90658		Laceration Repair			Urinalysis	81000
MMR	90707		Location Size Simp/Comp			Urine Culture	87088
OPV	90712		Laryngoscopy	31505		Drawing Fee	36415
Pneumovax	90732		Oximetry	94760		Specimen Collection	99000
TB Skin Test	86580		Punch Biopsy			**Other:**	
TD	90718		Rhythm Strip	93040			
Unlisted Immun	90749		Treadmill	93015			
Tetanus Toxoid	90703		Trigger Point or Tendon Sheath Inj.	20550			
Vaccine/Toxoid Admin <8 Yr Old w/ Counseling	90465		Tympanometry	92567			
Vaccine/Toxoid Administration for Adult	90471						

Diagnosis/ICD-9: _____

I acknowledge receipt of medical services and authorize the release of any medical information necessary to process this claim for healthcare payment only. I do authorize payment to the provider.

Patient Signature _____

Total Estimated Charges: _____

Payment Amount: _____

Next Appointment: _____

Terminology (CPT®; procedure) codes for the services that the office routinely provides (Figure 9.5). Superbills vary in appearance because medical practices design their own to meet the specific needs of the practice. As an example, a superbill for a specialty practice will contain ICD-9-CM and CPT codes relating only to that specialty, whereas a family practice will have a superbill with a myriad of ICD and CPT codes dealing with different body systems.

In preparation for a day's activities, the medical office specialist prints a superbill (either from the medical billing software or from preprinted forms inserted into the computer printer) for each scheduled appointment and attaches it to the patient's chart, if a paper chart is used. The superbill follows the patient throughout the visit. The professional staff (physician, nurse, physician's assistant, etc.) mark on the superbill the procedures and treatments performed during the visit, as well as the diagnosis and return it to the business office staff to use as the source document for entering data into a computerized accounting system. Because this document contains most of the critical information for the billing process, it serves as a link between the professional staff and the business office staff, which files the insurance claims and bills the patient.

When a patient or physician returns the superbill to the front office or cashier, the medical office specialist opens the patient's account in the computer and keys ("posts") the charge and diagnosis data from the superbill.

Once the patient demographics, insurance information, diagnosis, and charges are posted to the patient account, it is time to send a claim form to the patient's insurance carrier for the services that were provided. Without the information provided on the patient information form, superbill, insurance card, and verification of benefits form, billing the patient's insurance carrier would be impossible. Physicians bill insurance carriers using the **CMS-1500 claim form**. Hospitals bill carriers using the **UB-04 claim form**. Both the CMS-1500 and UB-04 form are universal claim forms for filing all medical claims.

Types of Insurance Claims: Paper vs. Electronic

Insurance claims are sent to insurance carriers either on paper or electronically. The term *encounter record* is a buzz term for a claim. A *paper claim* is one that is submitted on paper, including optically scanned claims that are converted to electronic form by insurance companies. Paper claims may be typed or generated by computer and sent through the U.S. Postal Service. Some claims require additional information for processing. In this instance, the claim is printed to paper and the additional information is sent as a **claim attachment** to the insurance carrier. Claim attachments are forms of documentation that support the medical necessity of a claim, such as an x-ray report or an operative report.

Electronic claims, also called **electronic media claims** or **EMCs**, are submitted to the insurance carrier via a central processing unit (CPU), tape diskette, direct data entry, direct wire, telephone line via modem, or personal computer. Electronic claims are never printed on paper. When claims are sent electronically to the insurance carriers for processing, an electronic signature is used to verify that the information received is true and correct.

Electronic claims have a number of advantages:

■ Administrative costs are lower because fewer personnel hours are needed to prepare forms, and supply and postage costs are lower.

CPT is a registered trademark of the American Medical Association.

■ Fewer claims are rejected because technical errors are detected and corrected before the claim arrives at the payer.

■ Payment is faster. An electronic claim is received by the payer in minutes, and payment can be transferred electronically to the provider's bank, eliminating delays in cash flow. These payments are referred to as *electronic remittances*.

Electronic claims also have disadvantages:

■ Claims transmission can be disrupted occasionally due to power failures, or computer hardware or software problems that might require claims to be re-submitted.

■ Many patient billing programs cannot create an electronic attachment, so when a claim attachment is required, the electronic claim must be sent separately from mailed attachments, which sometimes causes problems for the payer in matching up the two. In some cases, the claim must instead be submitted on paper when it must be accompanied by a claim attachment.

Electronic claims, which are the leading method of claims submission by providers, are submitted through a clearinghouse, a billing service, or directly to the carrier. A physician who plans to use electronic billing must contact all major insurers and carriers for a list of the vendors approved to handle electronic claims, and must have a signed agreement with each. Each carrier has special electronic billing requirements and is knowledgeable in which systems meet their criteria and which are compatible in format. The field data that is requested by the carriers is almost identical to the information on the CMS-1500 claim form. Insurance carriers also provide information about how to submit an electronic bill for patients who have secondary coverage. Medicare provides the software and training for electronic submissions. Medicare, Medicaid, TRICARE, and many private insurance carriers allow providers to submit insurance claims directly to them with no "middle man." In this type of system, the medical practice must have special software or the physician must lease a terminal from the carrier to key in claims data. The data is transmitted via modem (dedicated telephone line) directly to the carrier's computer for processing.

If the physician is not sending the data directly to the carrier, a clearinghouse may be used. A **clearinghouse** is a company that receives claims from providers, puts them through a series of audits to check for errors, and then forwards them to the appropriate insurance carrier in the carrier's required data format. Clearinghouses may charge a flat fee per claim or charge a percentage of the claim's dollar value. It is very important for the physicians' practices to negotiate the best possible fee for using a clearinghouse's services.

The clearinghouse conducts an audit to determine if any data on the claim is incorrect or missing; such a claim is referred to as a **dirty claim**. The results of the audit are sent back to the provider from the clearinghouse in the form of an **audit/edit report**. The audit/edit report shows which claims need corrections and which claims have been forwarded on to the appropriate carrier. Figures 9.6 through 9.9 show the various types of reports generated by a clearinghouse. The medical office specialist will need to correct any claims with incorrect data (as indicated on the audit/edit report) and resubmit them to the clearinghouse.

Dirty claims will not be transmitted to the carriers. When the claims are corrected and resubmitted to the clearinghouse, they are considered **clean claims**, which are then formatted and forwarded to the carrier. Each time the claim is returned there is an additional charge, so the medical office specialist should ensure that clean claims are transmitted initially.

Title: Acknowledgment Report

Purpose: To let the submitter know that claims were received and how they were handled (E, D R)

Comment: None

ACKNOWLEDGMENT REPORT for NAME OF DOCTOR MD - 03-01-2008

E = Submitted Electronically; D = Duplicate; R = Rejected

File: PPSZ-ECS.116

1 WATSON, BRENDA 922253 SOUTHWEST ADMIN /LA 02-06-08 $42.90 E
2 RIVERA, ESAU 922318 LAWRENCE HEALTH CAR 02-09-08 $43.80 E
3 MARTIN, DAN 922582 UNITED HEALTHCARE / 02-10-08 $73.20 E
4 LEGGETT, NEDRA 922621 BLUE CROSS /BLUE CA 02-10-08 $259.80 E
5 THORERNER, ROBERT 922649 BLUE CROSS /P.B. OX 02-09-08 $43.80 E
6 DOBALIAN, IVY 922651 BLUE CROSS /OXNARD- 02-09-08 $70.20 E
7 LEGGETT, NEDRA 922684 BLUE CROSS /BLUE CA 02-06-08 $111.60 E
8 LEGGETT, NEDRA 922689 BLUE CROSS /BLUE CA 02-06-08 $33.00 E
9 WATKINS, CHARLES 925031 FIRST HEALTH /KENT 02-16-08 $43.80 E
10 THOMPSON, ANNA 925052 METRAHEALTH /RR-MED 02-18-08 $43.80 E
11 RAMIREZ, VERA 925064 MAXICARE /LA-861059 02-18-08 $43.80 E

TOTAL ELECTRONIC CLAIMS 11 $809.70

TOTAL CLAIMS RECEIVED AND PROCESSED 11 $809.70

Figure 9.6

Sample acknowledgment report.

Title: Accepted Claims Report

Purpose: From Envoy. To let the submitter know that claims for the named people were accepted into the system and sent on to the insurance company.

Comment:

03/02/08 --

ACCEPTED CLAIMS for NAME OF DOCTOR MD-03/02/08

1. TABB, DONNA   2. ALVAREZ, ELIA   3. REED, ALDOLPHUS
4. JUDD, GEORGE   5. NABER, MIRIAM   6. REED, ALDOLPHUS
7. REED, PATRICIA   8. JUDD, LINDI   9. RAHAL, RIMA
10. RAHAL, RIMA   11. NAMDARKHAN, JAFAR   12. BARRETT, CLEMENTINA
13. BARRETT, CLEMENTINA   14. WATERS, MADALAINE   15. WATERS, MADALAINE
16. BIRD, STACIE   17. SHAO, SEN   18. MANJARREZ, ESTEBAN   19. JR, DARRELL B
20. REYES, MARIO   21. REYES, MARIO   22. AKHAVAN, MOHSEN   23. EHRENPREIS, JACQUELI   24. JOE, BOBBY   25. JOE, BOBBY   26. MONTOYA, ANTONIO
27. OBERG, CAROL   28. RAUCH, URSULA   29. RAUCH, URSULA   30. CHANDRA, VINOD   31. CHANDRA, VINOD   32. RAHAL, AHMAD   33. RAHAL, AHMAD
34. PHAM, NHUTHUY   35. PHAM, NHUTHUY

Figure 9.7

Sample accepted claims report.

Figure 9.8

**Sample rejected claims
report.**

Title: Rejected Claims Report

Purpose: To let the submitter know which claims were rejected and the reason
(sometimes, very cryptic) for the rejection.

Comment: None

03/02/08 ....

REJECTED CLAIMS for NAME OF DOCTOR MD-03/02/08

PATIENT	DATA in ERROR	DESCRIPTION
922387	97118	PROCEDURE INVALID FOR PAYER USE HCPC

Figure 9.9

**Sample claims settlement
report.**

Title: Claims Settlement Report

Purpose: To let the submitter know which claims were settled (not necessarily paid) by
the insurance company.

Comment: Some insurance companies will return this report, not all.

03/02/09 ....

CLAIM SETTLEMENT for NAME OF DOCTOR MD - 03/02/09

COMPLETED: EXPENSES INCURRED PRIOR TO COVERAGE

PATIENT	STATEMENT DATES		PAYER	TOTAL AMOUNT	
	FROM	THRU		CHARGES	PAID
911851	06/25/08	07/02/08	METROPOLITAN LIFE	599.00	0.00
911879	08/13/08	08/18/08	METROPOLITAN LIFE	560.00	0.00

COMPLETED: PAYMENT MADE ACCORDING TO PLAN PROVISIONS

PATIENT	STATEMENT DATES		PAYER	TOTAL AMOUNT	
	FROM	THRU		CHARGE	PAID
917914	10/27/08	10/27/08	CIGNA	274.00	0.00
917914	10/27/08	10/27/08	CIGNA	274.00	0.00
917922	10/29/08	10/31/08	CIGNA	560.00	0.00
917922	10/29/08	10/31/08	CIGNA	560.00	0.00
917922	10/29/08	10/31/08	CIGNA	560.00	0.00
917922	10/29/08	10/31/08	CIGNA	560.00	0.00
917922	10/29/08	10/31/08	CIGNA	560.00	0.00
917922	10/29/08	10/31/08	CIGNA	560.00	0.00
917922	10/29/08	10/31/08	CIGNA	560.00	0.00
917894	09/29/08	09/29/08	CIGNA	274.00	0.00
917894	09/29/08	09/29/08	CIGNA	274.00	0.00
917922	11/04/08	11/06/08	CIGNA	553.00	0.00
917922	11/04/08	11/06/08	CIGNA	553.00	0.00
917922	11/04/08	11/06/08	CIGNA	553.00	0.00
917922	11/04/08	11/06/08	CIGNA	553.00	0.00

COMPLETED: NO PAYMENT WILL BE MADE FOR THIS CLAIM

Figure 9.9

(continued)

| PATIENT STATEMENT DATES | | | TOTAL AMOUNT | |
	FROM THRU	PAYER	CHARGES	PAID
911851	06/25/08-07/02/08	METROPOLITAN LIFE	599.00	0.00
911851	07/02/08-07/02/08	METROPOLITAN LIFE	371.00	0.00
911879	08/13/08-08/18/08	METROPOLITAN LIFE	560.00	0.00

Billing services are companies that provide data processing and claims processing services to physicians' offices for a fee. The office staff supplies the billing service company with copies of the necessary information for them to create the claims that go to the carriers. This information includes personal information, copies of the insurance card, and the patient superbills. The billing company then enters all of the data into their computer system, creates the claims, and forwards them to the specific carriers. Billing companies might also use the services of a clearinghouse to check the claims that they send out for the physicians. When the carriers adjudicate the claims, reimbursement is sent to the billing service, which then posts the checks to the doctor's accounts.

A digital fax claim is sent to the insurance carrier as a paper claim via fax, but it is never printed to paper at the receiving end. Instead, the fax is encrypted by an optical code reader and transmitted to a computer screen, where it can be unencrypted. Encryption is the process of scrambling information during transmission so that it cannot be intercepted and read by anyone except the intended recipient.

Optical Character Recognition

Optical character recognition (OCR) devices (scanners) are being used frequently across the nation for processing paper insurance claims because of their speed and efficiency. A scanner can transfer printed or typed text and bar codes to the insurance company's computer memory. Scanners read at such a fast speed that they reduce the cost of data entry and decrease the processing time. More control is gained over data input by using OCR. It improves accuracy, thus reducing coding errors because the claim is entered exactly as coded by the medical office specialist.

The CMS-1500 form, discussed next, was developed so insurance carriers could process claims efficiently by OCR. Keying a form for OCR scanning requires different techniques than preparing one for standard claims submission. Because the majority of insurance carriers accept the OCR format, it is suggested that it be routinely used.

Successful OCR begins with the proper submission of claims data. Printed characters must conform to the preprogrammed specifications relative to character size and alignment on the CMS-1500 form. Only the current CMS-1500 form with red dropout ink is acceptable for OCR. These characteristics cannot be copied; therefore, original forms are necessary. You can obtain CMS-1500 forms through various vendors including the American Medical Association (AMA) or the U.S. Government Printing Office.

CMS-1500 Provider Billing Claim Form

The CMS-1500 form was developed by the Centers for Medicare and Medicaid Services (CMS) to facilitate the process of billing by easily arranging diagnoses and services provided that were necessary to treat patients. This information is attached to a claim form that is submitted to insurance carriers—private or government—and used to process claims for billing. The boxes to be completed on the form are referred to as **form locators**.

The CMS-1500 form is divided into two major sections:

Patient and Insured Information (Form locators 1–13)
Physician or Supplier Information (Form locators 14–33)

The CMS-1500 is printed in red ink so that it is recognizable by OCR scanners. Because it was developed by CMS for Medicare claims, Medicare has made it mandatory for all claims submissions. Private insurance carriers have also accepted the claim form for submission of their claims, although its use is not mandatory.

The upper portion of the CMS-1500 form consists of 13 form locators that contain 11 data elements and two signature form locators. The lower portion of the form consists of 20 form locators numbered 14 through 33, which contain 19 data elements, and one signature form locator

Specific guidelines exist for completing a CMS-1500 claim form. TRICARE, CHAMPVA, Medicare, Medicaid, and workers' compensation carriers have their own rules. Because guidelines vary at the state and local levels for completing the CMS-1500, the medical office specialist should check with his local intermediaries or private carriers. For Blue Cross Blue Shield claims, the medial office specialist should refer to the provider manual for their state's Blue Cross Blue Shield plans for guidelines for completing the CMS-1500 claim form. Blue Cross Blue Shield plans are similar to other insurance carriers and they do not have their own set of recognized rules for completing the CMS-1500 insurance claim form; therefore, form locators specific to Blue Cross Blue Shield are not listed separately in the text.

 For electronic billing, the Health Insurance Portability and Accountability Act of 1996 (HIPAA) developed standards and regulations that the health industry must follow in order to standardize patient care. The law that regulates electronic billing is known as the Administrative Simplification Subsection of HIPAA, which covers entities such as health plans, clearinghouses, and healthcare providers. HIPAA refers to these entities as *covered entities*, which encompasses the medical practice or health plan and all of its employees. These regulations govern your job and behavior. When people working with billing in the medical field refer to HIPAA, they are generally referring to this subsection. The Administrative Simplification Subsection has four distinct components:

1. Transaction and Code Sets
2. Uniform Identifiers
3. Privacy
4. Security.

When information is exchanged electronically, both parties to the transaction must agree to use the same format in order to make the information intelligible to the receiver. Before HIPAA, transactions for every insurance plan used a format that contained variations that made it different from another plan's format. This meant that the plans could not easily exchange or forward claims. Providers were limited when sending electronic claims. HIPAA standardized these formats by requiring specific transaction standards as follows:

- Claims or Equivalent Encounters and Coordination of Benefits
- Remittance and Payment Advice
- Claims Status

- Eligibility and Benefit Inquiry and Response
- Referral Certification and Preauthorization
- Premium Payment
- Enrollment and Un-enrollment in a Health Plan
- Health Claims Attachment
- First Report of Injury
- Retail Drug Claims, Coordination of Drug Benefits and Eligibility Inquiry.

In an electronic transaction, certain portions of the information are sent as codes. For the receiving entity to understand the content of the transaction, both the sender and the receiver must use the same codes. CPT, HCPCS, and ICD-9-CM are examples of the codes required for electronic transmission. Standards have also been set for codes for sex, race, type of provider, relation of the policyholder to the patient, and hundreds of others.

General guidelines for filling out each form locator on the CMS-1500 are discussed next. Before learning about the form locators, however, review the abbreviations given in Table 9.1 and the CMS-1500 form itself, shown in Figure 9.10.

Table 9.1	CMS-1500 Abbreviations

AMA—American Medical Association	HMO—Health maintenance organization
BLK Lung—Black lung	ICD-9-CM—Internal Classification of Disease, Ninth Revision, Clinical Modification
CCYY—Year, indicates entry of four digits for the century (CC) and year (YY)	ID—Identification
CHAMPUS—Civilian Health and Medical Program of the Uniformed Services	ID #—Identification number
	INFO—Information
CHAMPVA—Civilian Health and Medical Program of the Department of Veterans Affairs	LMP—Last menstrual period
	M—Male
CLIA—Clinical Laboratory Improvement Amendments	MM—Month, indicates entry of two digits for the month
CMS—Centers for Medicare and Medicaid Services, formerly HCFA	NDC—National Drug Code
COB—Coordination of benefits	No.—Number
CPT—Current Procedural Terminology, 4th Edition	NPI—National Provider Identifier
DD—Day, indicates entry of two digits for the day	NUCC—National Uniform Claim Committee
DME—Durable medical equipment	NUCC-DS—National Uniform Claim Committee Data Set
EIN—Employer identification number	PH #—Phone number
EMG—Emergency	QUAL.—Qualifier
EPSDT—Early and Periodic Screening, Diagnosis, and Treatment (Medicaid program)	REF.—Reference
	SOF—Signature on file
F—Female	SSN—Social Security number
FECA—Federal Employees' Compensation Act	UPC—Universal Product Code
GTIN—Global trade item number	UPIN—Unique physician identification number
HCFA—Health Care Financing Administration, currently CMS	USIN—Unique supplier identification number
	VP—Vendor product number
HCPCS—Health Care Procedure Coding System	
HIBCC—Health Industry Business Communications Council	YY—Year, indicates entry of two digits for the year; may also be noted as CCYY, which allows for entry of four digits for the century (CC) and year (YY)
HIPAA—Health Insurance Portability and Accountability Act of 1996	

Figure 9.10   **CMS-1500 claim form.**

Instructions for Completing the CMS-1500 Claim Form

The areas to be completed on the CMS-1500 claim form are referred to as Form Locators in this textbook. Additional names for these areas that may be used by other entities are Item Number, Item, Block, and Field.

We now take a detailed look at how to complete a CMS-1500 claim form by reviewing how to fill out the information required for each form locator.

Form Locators for the CMS-1500 Form

Form Locator 1: Type of Insurance
Form locator 1 identifies what type of insurance the patient carries. The form lists five government plans: Medicare, Medicaid, TRICARE/CHAMPUS, CHAMPVA, and FECA Black Lung. There are two other options: Group Health Plan and Other. These are utilized based on what type of plan the insured is enrolled in.

Form Locator 1a: Insured's ID Number
Form locator 1a asks for the insured's insurance ID number as reflected on the insurance card. The insured could be the patient or it could be someone else such as spouse, mother, or father.

Form Locator 2: Patient's Name
In form locator 2, enter the name of the patient who received services. This information is input last name, first name, and middle name or initial. The spelling should match the insurance card exactly. If the name on the card is misspelled, then the name in the computer should be misspelled until the patient provides a new card with the correct spelling.

Form Locator 3: Patient's Date of Birth/Sex
In form locator 3, enter the patient's date of birth and sex/gender. The date of birth is entered using the eight-digit format: MMDDCCYY. The patient's sex/gender is identified as either male or female.

Form Locator 4: Insured's Name
Form locator 4 asks for the name of the person who is the insured. This may or may not be the patient. If the patient is the insured, the word "Same" should be entered. The insured's name should be entered last name, first name, middle name or initial.

Form Locator 5: Patient's Address
Enter the patient's home address and telephone number in form locator 5. This information is taken from the patient information form when the patient registers in the office. The address should include the street name and number, city, state (two-letter abbreviation), and zip code. Do not use commas, periods, or other punctuation in the address. When entering a nine-digit zip code, include the hyphen. Do not use a hyphen or space as a separator within the telephone number.

Form Locator 6: Patient's Relationship to the Insured
Once form locator 4 has been completed, in form locator 6 enter an X in the correct box to indicate the patient's relationship to the insured. Options include Self, Spouse, Child, or Other. If the patient is the insured person, the "Self" entry is marked here. Only one box can be marked.

Form Locator 7: Insured's Address

In form locator 7, enter the insured's address. If the insured person is not the patient (see form locator 4), then this field should be completed. This information should include the street name and number, city, state (two-letter abbreviation), zip code, and phone number. If the patient is the insured, leave this form locator blank.

Form Locator 8: Patient Status

Indicate the patient's status in form locator 8: Single, Married, or Other. It also requires the patient's employment status: Employed, Full-Time Student, or Part-Time Student. Enter an X in the box for the patient's marital status and for the employment or student status. Only one box on each line can be marked.

Full-Time Student indicates that the patient is registered as a full-time student as defined by the postsecondary school or university. This information is important for determination of liability and coordination of benefits.

Form Locator 9: Other Insured's Name

If form locator 11d is marked YES, complete form locators 9 and 9a–d; otherwise, leave them blank. Form locator 9 indicates that there is a holder of another policy that may cover the patient. When there is additional group health coverage, enter the other insured's full last name, first name, and middle initial of the enrollee in another health plan if it is different from that shown in form locator 2. If there is no secondary policy, form locator 9 is left blank.

Form Locator 9a: Other Insured's Policy or Group Number

Enter the policy number or group number of the secondary insurance policy in form locator 9a. The number should be entered exactly as it appears on the insurance card.

Form Locator 9b: Other Insured's Date of Birth/Sex

Form locator 9b requires the date of birth of the insured of the secondary policy. The date of birth should be entered in the eight-digit format: MMDDCCYY. Choose either male or female accordingly.

Form Locator 9c: Employer's Name or School Name

Enter the name of the insured's employer or school in form locator 9c.

Form Locator 9d: Insurance Plan Name or Program Name

Form locator 9d asks for the name of the secondary insurance plan. This information is taken directly from the secondary insurance card. Enter the name exactly as it appears on the card.

Form Locator 10a–c: Is Patient's Condition Related To?

Form locator 10 identifies whether the patient's visit was related to an employment accident, auto accident, or other accident. This form locator is used when filing workers' compensation claims, auto accident claims, or claims for other types of injuries. If the patient's visit does not pertain to an accident of any kind, the default answer will be NO. Enter an X in the correct box.

Form Locator 10d: Reserved for Local Use

Different insurance carriers for different reasons use form locator 10d. One example of use would be a specific insurance carrier requiring the word "Attachment" to be placed here in the event that there are paper attachments with the claim.

Form Locator 11: Insured's Policy Group or FECA Number

If form locator 4 is completed, then form locator 11 should be completed. Form locator 11 identifies the insured's policy group number listed on the insurance card. This number should be entered exactly as it appears on the insurance card. A FECA number (nine-digit alphanumeric identifier) is listed here when employees of the federal government are filing workers' compensation claims.

Form Locator 11a: Insured's Date of Birth/Sex

In form locator 11a, list the date of birth of the insured. The date of birth should be listed in the eight-digit format: MMDDCCYY. If the patient and the insured are the same person, this space can be left blank. Choose either male or female accordingly. If gender is unknown, leave blank.

Form Locator 11b: Employer's Name or School Name

In form locator 11b, list the insured's place of employment or school that is attended. If the patient/insured is unemployed, leave blank.

Form Locator 11c: Insurance Plan Name or Program Name

Form locator 11c identifies the insurance plan name. The information should be taken directly from the insurance card and spelled exactly as it appears on the card.

Form Locator 11d: Is There Another Health Benefit Plan?

In form locator 11d, indicate whether there is another health benefit plan. If there is another plan, YES is marked with an X and the information is entered into form locators 9a–d. If there is no additional insurance plan, NO is marked.

Form Locator 12: Patient's or Authorized Person's Signature

Form locator 12 is where the patient or guarantor signs, allowing the release of any medical information to the insurance company for billing purposes. This release is only valid for billing information. Any other request for records will require a formal release of information form to be signed by the patient or guarantor. This signature is good for 1 year from the date it is signed and should be updated annually. When submitting claims the words "Signature on File" or "SOF" may be added here in place of a signature. The actual patient signature will be on file in the patient's chart. Enter the date in the six-digit format (MM/DD/YY) or eight-digit format (MM/DD/CCYY). If there is no signature on file, leave blank or enter "No Signature on File."

Form Locator 13: Insured's or Authorized Person's Signature

Form locator 13 is where the patient or insured signs, authorizing the insurance company to reimburse the physician or supplier directly. As just stated, the words "Signature on File" or "SOF" may be added here in place of a written signature when filing claims. If there is no signature on file, leave blank or enter "No Signature on File."

Form Locator 14: Date of Current: Illness, Injury, Pregnancy

Indicate the first date of the current illness, injury, or pregnancy in form locator 14. The date should be entered in the six-digit (MM/DD/YY) or eight-digit format (MM/DD/CCYY). For a pregnancy, the first day of the woman's last menstrual period (LMP) is used. If this information is not known, leave blank.

Form Locator 15: If Patient Has Had Same or Similar Illness

In form locator 15, enter the first date of treatment for the same or similar illness in the past. The date should be entered in the six-digit (MM/DD/YY) or eight-digit format (MM/DD/CCYY). If the information is not known, leave blank.

Form Locator 16: Dates Patient Unable to Work in Current Occupation

In form locator 16, list the dates the patient is unable to work due to his illness or injury. These dates will be required when filing workers' compensation or disability claims. The dates should be entered in the six-digit (MM/DD/YY) or eight-digit format (MM/DD/CCYY). If the information is not required, leave blank.

Form Locator 17: Name of Referring Physician or Other Source

Form locator 17 requests the name of the physician referring the patient. Some insurance companies, such as health maintenance organizations (HMOs) or exclusive provider organizations (EPOs), require this information to be on a claim. The information entered should include the physician's last name, first name, and credentials. If multiple providers are involved, enter one provider using the following priority order:

1. Referring provider
2. Ordering provider
3. Supervising provider.

If there is no referring physician, leave blank.

Form Locator 17a: ID Number of Referring Physician

The ID number of the referring, ordering, or supervising provider is reported in form locator 17a in the shaded area. The qualifier indicating what the number represents is reported in the qualifier field, which is the small box to the immediate right of the "17a." The NUCC defines the following qualifiers:

0B State license number
1B Blue Shield provider number
1C Medicare provider number
1D Medicaid provider number
1G Provider UPIN number
1H TRICARE/CHAMPUS identification number
E1 Employer identification number
G2 Provider commercial number
LU Location number
N5 Provider plan network identification number
SY Social Security number (The Social Security number may not be used for Medicare.)
X5 State industrial accident provider number
ZZ Provider taxonomy.

The non-NPI number of the referring, ordering, or supervising provider refers to the payer-assigned unique identifier of the professional. This box allows for the entry of 2 characters in the qualifier box and 17 characters in the larger box to the right.

Form Locator 17b: NPI Number

Enter the NPI number of the referring, ordering, or supervising provider in form locator 17b. The NPI number refers to the HIPAA National Provider Identifier number (see earlier discussion in this section), which is a 10-digit number.

Form Locator 18: Hospitalization Dates Related to Current Services

Enter the dates the patient has been hospitalized in relation to the current services in form locator 18. If the patient has been discharged from the hospital, the dates should include the day admitted and the day discharged. If the patient is still hospitalized include only the day admitted. The dates should be entered in the six-digit or eight-digit format. If the patient has not been hospitalized, leave blank.

Form Locator 19: Reserved for Local Use

Form locator 19 is reserved for local use depending on the insurance policy. Some payers ask for certain identifiers in this field. If identifiers are reported in this field, enter the appropriate qualifiers describing the identifier. Do not enter a space, hyphen, or other separator between the qualifier code and the number. Refer to Form Locator 17a for a list of qualifiers.

Form Locator 20: Outside Lab

Form locator 20 is used to indicate if lab work was done that was performed outside the office. A YES answer indicates that an entity other than the entity billing for the service performed the purchased services. If YES is chosen, enter the purchased price under Charges. When YES is chosen, form locator 32 must be completed. When billing for multiple purchased services, each service should be submitted on a separate claim form. Only one box can be marked. A NO answer indicates that no purchased services are included on the claim. When the answer is YES, the dollar amount must be entered in the $ Charges area. There is a limit of nine characters.

Form Locator 21: Diagnosis or Nature of Illness or Injury

In form locator 21, the ICD-9 codes for the diagnoses applied to this claim are entered. At least one code must be entered and up to four codes can be used on a claim. They are placed in order of precedence, line 1 being the primary diagnoses, and so forth. No written diagnoses are used on a claim form. The ICD-9 codes should be checked for medical necessity to make sure they are used appropriately with the CPT codes used in form locator 24D.

Relate lines 1, 2, 3, and 4 to the lines of service in 24E by line number.

> Always make sure that the ICD-9 codes used are the most recent, up-to-date codes utilized to avoid denials. Codes used should be coded to the highest level of specificity (see Chapter 4).

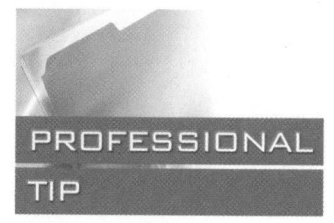
PROFESSIONAL TIP

Form Locator 22: Medicaid Resubmission Code

If required, form locator 22 is where the Medicaid resubmission code used for Medicaid claims is entered. List the original reference number and the code for resubmitted claims.

> **Example**
>
> **22. MEDICAID**   **ORIGINAL REF NO.**
> **RESUBMISSION**   **ABC1234567890**
> **CODE**
> **123**

Form Locator 23: Prior Authorization Number

Some insurance plans, such as those of HMOs, EPOs, and preferred provider organizations (PPOs), require a prior authorization number. If required, when preauthorization is obtained from an insurance company for services, the number assigned is input in form locator 23. Also, HMO required referral numbers are input in this form locator. Any of the following can be entered here: prior authorization number, referral number, mammography precertification number, or Clinical Laboratory Improvement Amendments (CLIA) number, as assigned by the payer for the current service. Do not enter hyphens or spaces within the number. If prior authorization is required and is omitted, the claim will be denied. If no prior authorization is required, leave blank.

Section 24

The six service lines in Section 24 have been divided horizontally to accommodate submission of both the NPI and another/proprietary identifier during the NPI transition and to accommodate the submission of supplemental information to support the billed service. The top area of the six service lines is shaded and is the location for reporting supplemental information. (It is not intended to allow the billing of 12 lines of service.)

The supplemental information is to be placed in the shaded section of 24A through 24G as defined in each item number. Providers must verify this supplemental information with the payer.

Form Locator 24A: Dates of Service

In form locator 24A, enter the dates of service for the services provided. Depending on the insurance carrier, these columns are filled in using different formats. Some require both the To and From dates to be listed in six-digit format (MM/DD/YY). Some require just the From date to be listed or just the To date. If the same procedure was provided multiple times on a single date, the specific date is entered once and the number of procedures is listed in form locator 24G.

Form Locator 24B: Place of Service

Place of service in form locator 24B is a mandatory field to be completed because it describes the place where the procedure or service was performed. This place could be many places, such as the physician's office, hospital, emergency department, skilled nursing facility, or even the patient's home. A code is used (see following list) to indicate the place of service.

Note that the CMS has stated that the place of service must also be fully written out in form locator 32.

Consider this example: The patient was an inpatient (hospital) and the physician saw the patient in the hospital for an evaluation and management service. Therefore, the code 21 (see following list) would be entered in form locator 24B and the following entered in form locator 32:

Allied Hospital
210 Frankford Road
Carrollton, TX 12345

Common place of service codes include the following:

11. Physician's office
12. Private residence
13. Assisted living facility
20. Urgent care facility
21. Inpatient hospital
22. Outpatient hospital
23. Hospital emergency department
24. Ambulatory surgical center
25. Birthing center
26. Military treatment facility
31. Skilled nursing facility
34. Hospice
81. Independent laboratory.

Form Locator 24C: EMG (Emergency)
Form locator 24C is used to indicate whether the service was provided on an emergency basis. This form locator should be marked with a Y for YES or left blank for NO. The definition of an emergency can be defined differently by each payer.

Form Locator 24D: Procedures, Services, or Supplies
In form locator 24D, enter the CPT or HCPCS codes used to identify the procedures, services, or supplies provided. Modifiers are also listed in form locator 24D. If more than three modifiers are used, list 99 here and enter the modifiers in form locator 19.

Form Locator 24E: Diagnosis Pointer
Form locator 24E indicates the number (1, 2, 3, and 4) of the diagnosis code listed in form locator 21 as it relates to each service or procedure. If more than one diagnosis is attached to a single procedure or service, list the primary diagnosis first.

Form Locator 24F: Charges
Form locator 24F lists the charges that are assigned to each CPT or HCPCS code listed. The amount should be entered without a decimal point or dollar sign. If multiple units are entered in form locator 24G, the charges should reflect the amount of the procedure times the number of units. Charges should be updated on a regular basis to follow appropriate billing guidelines.

Form Locator 24G: Days or Units
Enter the number of units per procedure or service provided to a patient in form locator 24G. If billing for anesthesia, the amount entered should be entered in minutes and calculated accordingly. If billing for multiple services, such as liters of oxygen, list the

actual number of liters. If multiple units are entered in 24G, the charges should reflect the amount of the procedure multiplied by the number of units.

When required by payers to provide supplemental information such as the National Drug Code (NDC) units in addition to the HCPCS units, enter the applicable NDC units' qualifier and related units in the shaded line. The following qualifiers are to be used when reporting NDC units:

F2	International Unit	ML	Milliliter
GR	Gram	UN	Unit

Form Locator 24H: EPSDT Family Plan

Form locator 24H is used to identify whether the patient is receiving her services through Medicaid's Early and Periodic Screening, Diagnosis, and Treatment (EPSDT) program. If there is no state requirement to report a reason code for EPSDT, enter "Y" for YES. Only enter "Y" for yes or "N" for NO.

If there is a requirement to report a reason code for EPSDT, enter the appropriate reason code as noted below. (A "Y" or "N" response is not entered with a code.) The two-character code is entered in the top shaded area of the field.

The following codes are for EPSDT:

AV   Available—Not used (Patient refused referral.)

S2   Under treatment (Patient is currently under treatment for referred diagnostic or corrective health problem.)

ST   New service requested (Referral to another provider for diagnostic or corrective treatment/scheduled for another appointment with screening provider for diagnostic or corrective treatment for at least one health problem identified during an initial or periodic screening service, not including dental referrals.)

NU   Not used (Used when no EPSDT patient referral was given.)

If the service is for family planning, enter "Y" for YES or "N" for NO in the bottom, unshaded area of the field.

Form Locator 24I:

Enter in the shaded area of form locator 24I the qualifier identifying whether the number is a non-NPI number. The other ID number of the rendering provider is then reported in form locator 24J in the shaded area. Refer to form locator 17a for a list of qualifiers.

The rendering provider is the person or company (laboratory or other facility) who rendered or supervised the care. In the case where a substitute provider was used, enter that provider's information here. Report the identification number in form locators 24I and 24J only when different from data recorded in form locators 33a and 33b.

Form Locator 24J: Rendering Provider

The individual rendering the service is reported in form locator 24J. Enter the non-NPI ID number in the shaded area of the field. Enter the NPI number in the unshaded area of the field.

Form Locator 25: Federal Tax I.D. Number

List in form locator 25 the physician's federal tax I.D. number or his employer identification number (EIN). Do not enter hyphens with numbers. The appropriate box (SSN or EIN) should be marked with an X.

Form Locator 26: Patient's Account Number

In form locator 26, enter the patient's account number assigned by the medical office. The computer system used in the office will generate the number and it should be entered on the claim. This in turn will allow for the account number to appear on the Explanation of Benefits (EOB) form, which makes it easier to locate the correct patient to post insurance payments.

Form Locator 27: Accept Assignment?

Form locator 27 is used to indicate whether or not the physician accepts assignment on this claim. If the physician does accept assignment and the patient has signed form locator 13, the insurance carrier will pay the physician directly for services provided. If the physician does not accept assignment, the insurance carrier will send the reimbursement to the patient.

Form Locator 28: Total Charge

Form locator 28 lists the total charges, added together from those listed in form locator 24F. The charges should be checked for accuracy to ensure proper reimbursement. Do not use decimal points or dollar signs in this entry.

Form Locator 29: Amount Paid

Form locator 29 indicates the amount paid on this claim. This amount is usually added after the primary EOB is received and payment is posted. A secondary claim is printed to be sent to the secondary insurance carrier along with a copy of the primary insurance carrier's EOB. Do not use decimal points or dollar signs in this entry.

Form Locator 30: Balance Due

Form locator 30 is used to record the difference between the amounts in form locators 28 and 29. This amount is the balance due for the claim being submitted. When a claim is submitted electronically this locator or "balance due" does not appear. Do not use decimal points or dollar signs in this entry.

Form Locator 31: Signature of Physician or Supplier Including Degrees or Credentials

Form locator 31 identifies the name of the physician or supplier who has provided the services to the patient along with his credentials (M.D., PA-C, or NP).

If a paper claim is submitted, the physician or supplier's name must be typed/printed or the signature of the physician's or supplier's representative, or enter "Signature on File" or "SOF." Enter a six-digit date (MM/DD/YY), eight-digit date (MM/DD/CCYY), or alphanumeric date. A signature stamp may be used instead of a written signature. The stamp must leave a clear, nonsmeared image on the claim.

Form Locator 32: Name and Address of Facility Where Services Were Rendered

Form locator 32 identifies the name of the facility where services were provided. Enter the name, address, zip code, and NPI number when billing for purchased diagnostic tests. When more than one supplier is used, a separate CMS-1500 form should be used for each supplier.

Form Locator 32a: NPI Number

Enter the NPI number of the service facility location in form locator 32a.

Form Locator 32b: Other ID Number

Enter the two-digit qualifier identifying the non-NPI number followed by the ID number. Do not enter a space, hyphen, or other separator between the qualifier and number. Refer to form locator 17a. for a list of qualifiers.

Form Locator 33: Billing Provider Information and Phone Number

Enter the provider's or supplier's billing name, address, zip code, and phone number in form locator 33. The phone number is to be entered in the area to the right of the field title. Enter the name and address information in the following format:

> First line: Name
> Second line: Address
> Third line: City, state, and zip code.

Form Locator 33a: NPI Number

Enter the NPI number of the billing provider in form locator 33a. The NPI number refers to the HIPAA National Provider Identifier number, which allows for the entry of 10 characters.

Form Locator 33b: Other ID Number

Enter the two-digit qualifier identifying the non-NPI number followed by the ID number. Do not enter a space, hyphen, or other separator between the qualifier and number. Refer to form locator 17a. for a list of qualifiers.

Remember that the non-NPI ID number of the billing provider refers to the payer-assigned unique identifier of the professional.

Physicians' Identification Numbers

Insurance companies and federal and state programs require certain identification numbers on health insurance claims (HIC) forms submitted from individuals and facilities who provide and bill for services to patients. Although the NPI will eventually replace all of these numbers except a few, an understanding of these numbers is imperative for the medical biller. The use of the various numbers can be confusing to the beginner, as well as to someone experienced in insurance billing procedures, so an explanation is provided here.

> **State license number**: To practice within a state, each physician must obtain a physician's **state license number**. Sometimes this number is requested on forms and used as a provider number; for example, Texas Workers' Compensation (form locator 33).
>
> **Employer identification number**: In a medical group or solo practice, each physician must have her own federal tax identification number, known as an **employer identification number (EIN)**, or **tax identification number (TIN)**. This number is issued by the Internal Revenue Service for income tax purposes (form locator 25). Each physician may have one or more TIN for financial reasons. Examples of additional TINs would be a group practice that bills from different entities, for example, an orthopedic office that provides physical therapy. An EIN would be used for the physician visits and a TIN for the physical therapy visits. Also if a group practice has satellite offices, those offices might have different TINs.

Social Security number (SSN): In addition, each physician has a SSN for other personal use. Social Security numbers are not typically used on the claim form unless the provider does not have an EIN.

Provider numbers: Claims may require three provider identification numbers: one for the referring physician (form locator 17a), one for the ordering physician (form locator 17a), and one for the performing physician (form locator 24K or form locator 33 for the billing entity). The ordering physician and the performing physician can be the same (form locators 17a and 33). On rare occasions, the number may be the same for all three, but more frequently three different numbers are required, depending on the circumstances of the case. For placement on the CMS-1500 claim form, keep in mind what role the physician(s) and their numbers represent in relationship to the provider listed in form locator 33. To assist with claims completion, a reference list of providers' numbers could be compiled for all ordering physicians and physicians who frequently refer patients. Physicians' provider numbers can be obtained by calling their offices or through the Medicare carrier.

Provider identification number: Every physician who renders services to patients may be issued a carrier-assigned **provider identification number (PIN)** by the insurance company.

Unique Physician Identification Number: The Medicare program issues each physician a **Unique Physician Identification Number (UPIN)**.

Group provider number: The **group provider number (GPN)** is used instead of the individual PIN for the performing provider who is a member of a group practice that submits claims to insurance companies under the group name (form locator 33). In this case, the PIN is reported in form locator 24J for the specific performing provider.

National Provider Identifier Number: As of May 2007, all providers have a **National Provider Identifier Number (NPI)**. This number is a lifetime 10-digit number that is recognized by the Medicaid, Medicare, TRICARE, and CHAMPVA programs and will be used by all private insurance carriers. It will replace the existing identification numbers.

Durable medical equipment number: Medicare providers who charge patients a fee for supplies and equipment, such as crutches, urinary catheters, ostomy supplies, surgical dressings, and so forth, must bill Medicare using a durable medical equipment (DME) number.

Facility provider number: Each facility (e.g., hospital, laboratory, radiology office, skilled nursing facility) is issued a **facility provider number (FPN)** to be used by the performing physician to report services done at the location.

Although most facilities send insurance claims electronically, it is necessary to be familiar with the form locators on both the CMS-1500 and the UB-04 claim forms. When submitting an insurance claim, the medical office specialist must make sure the claim has all of the needed information completed in order for the claim to be processed by the carrier. As mentioned earlier, a claim that has no mistakes/missing information is referred to as a *clean claim*. If needed information is missing from a claim (referred to as a *dirty claim*), the carrier will not process it, resulting in the added time and expense needed to correct the claim and resend it. Prior to sending claims electronically, the medical office specialist must look over the claims on the computer screen to make sure they are clean. Being familiar with the locators will assist in this process.

Practice Exercises

The following exercises will familiarize the medical office specialist with the form locators and the information required on the claim forms. By completing claims by hand, the medical office specialist can get a feel for the information that is required on claim forms.

NOTE: The following practice exercises are date sensitive to the date on which the patient presented, which for the student is today's date. Please read the case studies in the exercises and enter the applicable dates. For instance, if the patient was told to return to the office in 3 days, the student would enter a date that is 3 days from today's date, which is the initial date of service.)

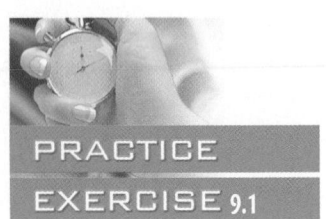

PRACTICE EXERCISE 9.1

Completion of CMS-1500 (Section I)

Fill out form locators 1 through 13 on the CMS-1500 form based on the information given here. To complete this exercise, copy the CMS-1500 form provided in Appendix D or download it from the CD-ROM that accompanies this text.

Michael Louis Putnam is a patient in the medical office where you work. This information appears on his patient information form:

Name:	Michael Louis Putnam
Gender:	Male
Birth Date:	May 23, 1945
Phone:	972-555-2233
Address:	765 South Parker
	Frisco, TX 12345
Marital Status:	Single
Employer:	Big Lots
Social Security number:	459-12-5555
Insurance carrier	C 16 NA
Insurance ID number:	459-12-5555
Group number:	FMR1235
Other Health Insurance:	None

Mr. Putnam has signed an authorization form to release medical records and an assignment of benefits on February 10, 2008. The patient's encounter form indicates diagnoses of essential hypertension (401.9). The diagnosis is not related to the patient's previous employment or an accident.

Check the accuracy of your work by comparing your claim form to the completed claim form shown in Figure 9.11.

Your Practice Exercise 9.1 claim form should look like the one shown in Figure 9.11.

AREA

HEALTH INSURANCE CLAIM FORM

PICA		PICA

1. MEDICARE MEDICAID TRICARE CHAMPVA GROUP FECA OTHER	1a. INSURED'S I.D. NUMBER (For Program in Item 1)

1. MEDICARE   MEDICAID   TRICARE   CHAMPVA   GROUP HEALTH PLAN   FECA BLK LUNG   OTHER
☐(Medicare #)   ☐(Medicaid #)   ☐(Sponsor's SSN)   ☐(Member ID#)   ☒(SSN or ID)   ☐(SSN)   ☐(ID)

1a. INSURED'S I.D. NUMBER   (For Program in Item 1)
459-12-5555

2. PATIENT'S NAME (Last Name, First Name, Middle Initial)
PUTNAM MICHAEL L

3. PATIENT'S BIRTH DATE   SEX
MM | DD | YY
05 | 23 | 1945   M ☒   F ☐

4. INSURED'S NAME (Last Name, First Name, Middle Initial)
SAME

5. PATIENT'S ADDRESS (No, Street)
765 SOUTH PARKER

6. PATIENT RELATIONSHIP TO INSURED
Self ☒   Spouse ☐   Child ☐   Other ☐

7. INSURED'S ADDRESS (No, Street)

CITY   **FRISCO**   STATE   **TX**

8. PATIENT STATUS
Single ☒   Married ☐   Other ☐

Full-Time   Part-Time
Employed ☒   Student ☐   Student ☐

CITY   STATE

ZIP CODE   **12345**   TELEPHONE (Include Area Code)   **(082) 555-2233**

ZIP CODE   TELEPHONE (Include Area Code)   ( )

9. OTHER INSURED'S NAME (Last Name First, Name, Middle Initial)

10. IS PATIENT'S CONDITION RELATED TO:

11. INSURED'S POLICY GROUP OR FECA NUMBER
FMR1235

a. OTHER INSURED'S POLICY OR GROUP NUMBER

a. EMPLOYMENT? (Current or Previous)
☐YES   ☒NO

a. INSURED'S DATE OF BIRTH   SEX
MM | DD | YY   M ☐   F ☐

b. OTHER INSURED'S DATE OF BIRTH   SEX
MM | DD | YY   M ☐   F ☐

b. AUTO ACCIDENT?   PLACE (State)
☐YES   ☒NO

b. EMPLOYER'S NAME OR SCHOOL NAME
BIG LOTS

c. EMPLOYER'S NAME OR SCHOOL NAME

c. OTHER ACCIDENT?
☐YES   ☒NO

c. INSURANCE PLAN NAME OR PROGRAM NAME
CIGNA

d. INSURANCE PLAN NAME OR PROGRAM NAME

10d. RESERVED FOR LOCAL USE

d. IS THERE ANOTHER HEALTH BENEFIT PLAN?
☐YES   ☒NO   *If yes*, return to and complete item 9 a-d

READ BACK OF FORM BEFORE COMPLETING & SIGNING THIS FORM.

12. PATIENT'S OR AUTHORIZED PERSON'S SIGNATURE I authorize the release of any medical or other information necessary to process this claim. I also request payment of government benefits either to myself or to the party who accepts assignment below.

SIGNED   **SIGNATURE ON FILE**   DATE   **02102006**

13. INSURED'S OR AUTHORIZED PERSON'S SIGNATURE I authorize payment of medical benefits to the undersigned physician or supplier for services described below.

SIGNED   **SIGNATURE ON FILE**

Figure 9.11   **Practice Exercise 9.1 CMS-1500 form.**

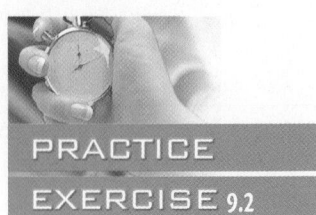

Completion of CMS-1500 (Section I)

Fill out form locators 1 through 13 on the CMS-1500 form based on the information given here. To complete this exercise, copy the CMS-1500 form provided in Appendix D or download it from the CD-ROM that accompanies this text.

Liz Mary Smith is a patient in the medical office where you work. This information appears on her patient information form:

Name:	Liz Mary Smith
Gender:	Female
Birth Date:	July 1, 1996
Marital Status:	Single
Phone:	214-555-2984
Address:	4591 Explorer Drive
	Plano, TX 12345
Responsible Person:	Harry L. Smith (father)
Insured's DOB:	August 5, 1950
Insured's Gender:	Male
Insured's Home Address:	5419 W. 8th Street, Apt. 306
	Norman, OK 12345
Insured's Employer Address:	Vines Lumber Co.
	6840 Judy Street
	Norman, OK 12345
Social Security number:	425-68-3030
Insurance Carrier:	BMA
	P.O. Box 7459
	Memphis, TN 12345
Insurance Certificate Number:	78815-080-07-000
Insurance Group Number:	G123456

Treatment and progress notes in the patient medical record indicate diagnosis of left acute otitis media (382.9), on January 13, 20XX. The medical office collects only the coinsurance and waits for payment directly from the insurance carrier. Guarantor's signature on file for charges to be paid directly to provider, FORM SIGNED January 13, 20XX.

Authorization to release medical information on file.

Check the accuracy of your work by comparing your claim form to the completed claim form in Appendix J.

Completion of CMS-1500 (Section II)

Fill out form locators 14 through 33 on the CMS-1500 form based on the information given here. To complete this exercise, copy the CMS-1500 form provided in Appendix D or download it from the CD-ROM that accompanies this text.

Physician Information:

Name:	Forrest M. Sherwood, M.D.
	325 Nichols Road, Suite 20B
	Brookfield, Wisconsin 12345
Phone:	414-555-6790
Federal Tax ID Number:	52-9753211
UPIN:	S985621
NPI:	1226449762

Patient's Encounter Form:

Name:	Daniel M. Williams
Date:	Today's date
	T-101 P-90 R-18 BP-132/76 WT-175
CC:	Swollen neck glands, fever, headache, general malaise since yesterday
DX:	Peritonsillitis (475)
RX:	Rest, fluids, Tylenol for headaches prn. Return in 5 days for recheck
Date:	Today's date (5 days after initial visit)
	T-98 P-88 R-18 BP-130/60
CC:	Fever, pain, and swelling of tonsils and adenoids
DX:	Hypertrophy of tonsils and adenoids (474.10)
RX:	Ampicillin 500 mg. #16 Ampicillin 500 mg IM. Return in 2 days
Date:	Today's date (2 days after last visit)
	T-98.8 P-80 R-16 BP-132/74
RX:	Recheck, improvement, continue meds, recheck in 2 weeks

List of Fees for Services:

Date:	Today's date
DX:	Peritonsillitis DIAGNOSIS CODE: 475
Services and Charges:	Office visit, expanded problem focused history & exam, medical decision making of low complexity. $60.00, CPT CODE: 99213

(continued)

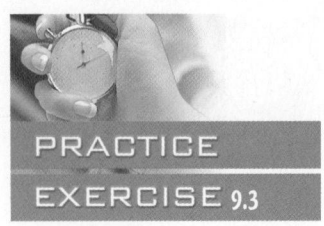

PRACTICE
EXERCISE 9.3

(continued)

Date:	Today's date (5 days after initial visit)
DX:	Hypertrophy of Tonsils and Adenoids, DIAGNOSIS CODE: 474.10
Services and Charges:	Office visit, problem focused history and exam, straightforward decision making. $35.00, CPT CODE: 99212 IM Ampicillin 500 mg $20.00, CPT CODE: 90788
Date:	Today's date (2 days after previous visit)
DX:	Hypertrophy of Tonsils and Adenoids DIAGNOSIS CODE: 474.10
Services and Charges:	Office visit, problem focused history and exam, straightforward decision making $35.00, CPT CODE: 99212

Patient Ledger:

Insurance Carrier:	United Health Care
Filing Date:	Today's date
	Provider accepts assignment.

Check the accuracy of your work by comparing your claim form to the completed claim form in Appendix J.

Completion of CMS-1500 (Section II)

Fill out form locators 14 through 33 on the CMS-1500 form based on the information given here. To complete this exercise, copy the CMS-1500 form provided in Appendix D or download it from the CD-ROM that accompanies this text.

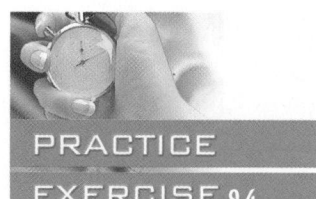

PRACTICE EXERCISE 9.4

Physician Information:

Name:	Forrest M. Sherwood, M.D.
Address:	325 Nichols Road, Suite 20B
	Brookfield, WI 12345
Phone:	414-555-6790
Federal Tax ID Number:	52-9753211
UPIN:	S985621
NPI:	1226449762

Patient Encounter Form:

Name:	Martha M. Butler
Date:	Today's date
	T-98.8 P-68 R-15 BP-178/98 WT 155
CC:	This a.m. while going to get mail pt fell on sidewalk; a neighbor brought her in c/o pain and disability in left hip area, SOB, chest pain
EXAM:	Pt in distress, x-ray L hip two views—negative, ECG T-wave inversion
LAB:	Cardiac enzymes, electrolytes
DX:	Sprained L hip, essential hypertension, R/O angina pectoris
RX:	Injection 2.0 mL Norflex IM, moist heat, Norflex tablets #12, Inderal capsules 80 mg #30 Return in 3 days for lab results and recheck
Date:	Today's date (3 days after initial visit)
	T-98.6 P-68 R-15 BP-150/88
LAB:	Within normal limits
EXAM:	Hip improving, ECG negative
DX:	Essential hypertension, angina pectoris
RX:	Continued prescribed meds. Nitrostat tablets, one tab dissolved under tongue at first sign of angina attack

(continued)

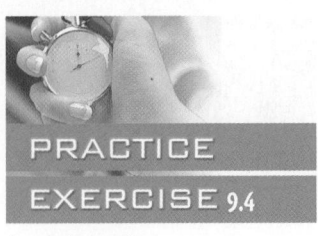

PRACTICE EXERCISE 9.4

(continued)

List of Fees for Services:

Date:	Today's date
DX:	Sprained L hip (843.9), essential hypertension (401.9)
Services and Charges:	Office visit, detailed history and detailed exam, moderate complexity decision making $80.00 (**99214**), DX: 843.9, 401.9
	Venipuncture for collections $18.00 (**36415**). DX: 401.9
	Lab (sent to Nottingham Laboratory Services, 1435 N. 12th St., Milwaukee, WI 53002).
	X Ray L hip two views $90.00 (**73510**), DX: 843.9
	Injection 2.0 mL Norflex IM $12.00 (**90782**), DX: 843.9
	ECG routine, 12 leads interpretation & report $55.00 (**93000**) DX: 401.9
Date:	Today's date (3 days after initial visit)
DX:	Essential hypertension (401.9), angina pectoris (413.9)
Services and Charges:	Office visit, problem focused history & exam, straightforward decision making $35.00 (**99212**)

Patient Ledger:

Patient's Account number:	BUTMA0 (Date: Today's Date $55.00)
Insurance Carrier:	US Life
Filing Date:	Today's date

Check the accuracy of your work by comparing your claim form to the completed claim form in Appendix J.

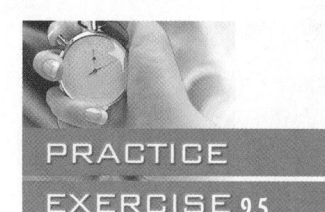

PRACTICE EXERCISE 9.5

Completion of CMS-1500 (Section II)

Fill out form locators 14 through 33 on the CMS-1500 form based on the information given here. To complete this exercise, copy the CMS-1500 form provided in Appendix D or download it from the CD-ROM that accompanies this text.

Physician Information:

Name:	Forrest M. Sherwood, M.D.
Address:	325 Nichols Road, Suite 20B
	Brookfield, WI 12345
Phone:	414-555-6790
EIN:	52-9753211
Insurance Carrier:	Cigna
Cigna PIN:	17FMs53
UPIN:	5569821
NPI:	1226449762

Patient's Encounter Form:

Name:	Audrey Janell Smith
Account Number:	SMIAU
DOB:	2/8/1961
Date:	Today's date
	T-98 P-85 R-15 BP-150/96 WT-164 HT-73
CC:	Patient came in for CPX (complete physical exam) (V70.0)
HEENT:	Within normal limits
Chest:	Normal
Back:	Normal
Breast:	Normal
Heart:	Normal
Abdomen:	Normal
Pelvic:	Normal
Chest:	X-ray: 2 views—normal
ECG:	Normal
UA complete-dip:	Normal
UA-micro:	Normal
DX:	High Blood Pressure (796.2)
RX:	Return tomorrow for recheck on BP
Date:	Today's date (1 day after initial visit)
BP check:	148/94
Date:	Today's date (1 week after initial visit)
BP:	152/96, reviewed with patient results of exam.
DX:	Essential Hypertension (401.9)
RX:	Maxzide 25 mg one tablet daily, return for recheck in one week

(continued)

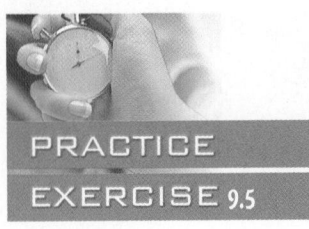

PRACTICE

EXERCISE 9.5

(continued)

List of Fees for Services:

Date: Today's date

DX: Annual Physical Exam (V70.0), High Blood
                                         Pressure (796.2)

Service and Charges: Initial preventive medicine, new patient:
                                         $125.00 CPT: (**99386**) DX: (V70.0)

                                         X-ray chest, 2 views: $45.00 CPT: (**71020**) DX:
                                         (V70.0) (796.2)

                                         ECG routine, 12 lead: $55.00 CPT: (**93000**) DX:
                                         (V70.0) (796.2)

                                         Complete UA: $15.00 CPT: (**81000**) DX:
                                         (V70.0)

Date: Today's date (1 day after initial visit) DX:
                                         High Blood Pressure (796.2)

Service and Charges: Follow-up office visit—problem focused his-
                                         tory and exam, straightforward decision
                                         making. $35.00 CPT: (**99212**) DX: (796.2)

Date: Today's date (1 week after initial visit)

DX: Essential Hypertension (401.9)

Services and Charges: Expanded problem focused history and exam-
                                         ination (reviewed results of physical exami-
                                         nation), medical decision making of low
                                         complexity $60.00 CPT: (**99213**) DX:
                                         (401.9)

Patient Ledger:

Insurance Carrier: Cigna

Date: Today's date $240.00

Date: 1 day after initial visit $35.00

Date: 1 week after initial visit $60.00

Filing Date: 1 week after initial visit

Check the accuracy of your work by comparing your claim form to the completed claim form in
Appendix J.

Completion of CMS-1500 (Sections I and II)

Fill out the form locators on the CMS-1500 form based on the information given here. To complete this exercise, copy the CMS-1500 form provided in Appendix D or download it from the CD-ROM that accompanies this text.

PRACTICE EXERCISE 9.6

Physician Information:
Name:	Len M. Handelsman, M.D.
Address:	325 Nepperhan Avenue
	Yonkers, NY 12345
Phone:	914-555-6790
Federal Tax ID Number:	52-9683211
UPIN:	H658743
Insurance Carrier:	Aetna
Aetna Pin Number:	56991
NPI:	3335224814

Patient Information Form:
Name:	Gloria Poyner-Chin
Sex:	Female
DOB:	July 1, 1945
Marital Status:	Single
Account Number:	POYNEGL0
Address:	1221 Avenue of the Bronx
	Bronx, NY 12345
Phone Number:	(914) 555-2166
Social Security number:	814-51-0303
Insured's Employer	Country Club Bingo Hall
Insurance Carrier:	Aetna
Insurance Carrier Address:	1900 Seventh Avenue
	New York, NY 12100
Insurance Certificate number:	445-80-0701
Insurance Group Number:	G020456

Patient's Encounter Form:
Date:	Today's date
	T-99 P-90 R-18 BP-132/76 WT-125
CC:	Pain in elbow and forearms following tennis game, 11-12-02
DX:	Elbow sprain (841.9)
RX:	Rest

List of Fees for Service:
Date:	Today's date
DX:	Elbow sprain (841.9)
Services and Charges:	Office visit, problem focused history and exam, straightforward decision making $35.00 CPT: (**99212**) DX: 841.9
Signature on file:	Signed Today's date

Check the accuracy of your work by comparing your claim form to the completed claim form in Appendix J.

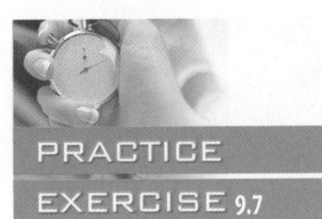

Completion of CMS-1500 (Sections I and II)

Fill out the form locators on the CMS-1500 form based on the information given here. To complete this exercise, copy the CMS-1500 form provided in Appendix D or download it from the CD-ROM that accompanies this text.

Physician Information:

Name:	William F. Bonner, M.D.
Corporation Name:	Youngblood and Associates
Address:	2128 East 144th Street, Suite 15
	Chicago, IL 12345
Phone:	312-555-7690
EIN:	56-3342560
UPIN:	5248120
NPI:	5524998733
CIGNA Physician ID Number:	3266113
Cigna Group Number:	0655872
Group NPI:	6625897130

Patient's Information Form:

Name:	Randall Jay Tillman
DOB:	February 19, 1989
Sex:	Male
Marital Status:	Single
Patient Address:	1212 Fry Street
	Des Plaines, IL 12345
	312-555-4993
Account Number:	TILLRA
Responsible Party:	Theresa Mae Tillman (mother)
Insured's DOB:	January 3, 1958
Insured's Sex:	Female
Address:	4225 Benton Avenue, Apt. 6
	Des Plaines, IL 12345
Phone:	312-555-4993
Insured's Employer:	Des Plaines Chevrolet
Social Security number:	421-80-6060
Insurance Carrier:	Cigna
Insurance Carrier Address:	P.O. Box 3490
	Chicago, IL 60671
Insurance ID Number:	753-00865
Insurance Group Number:	DP 139
Signature on File:	Yes, form signed

(continued)

Patient's Encounter Form:

Date: Today's date
Date of first symptom: 3 days ago
                               WT-45 HT-50 T-100.4 P-94 R-20 BP- 90/60
CC: Wheezing, coughing, dyspnea, fever 3 d
DX: Bronchitis with influenza (487.1)
RX: EryPed 200 1 tsp Q.I.D., Tussi-Organidan 1 tsp
                                  in AM and 1 tsp at night
                               Return 3 days for recheck

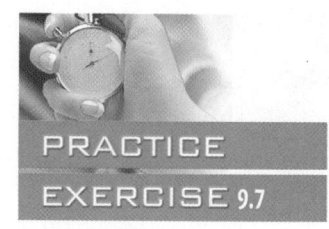

PRACTICE EXERCISE 9.7

(continued)

List of Fees for Service:

Date: Today's date
DX: Bronchitis with influenza (487.1)
Services and Charges: Office visit, problem focused history and
                                  exam, straightforward decision making
                                  $50.00 CPT: (**99202**) DX: (487.1)
Filing Date: Today's date

Check the accuracy of your work by comparing your claim form to the completed claim form in Appendix J.

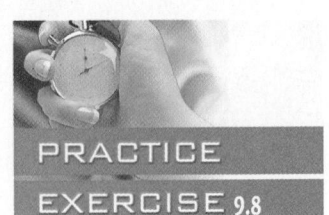

Completion of CMS-1500 (Sections I and II)

Fill out the form locators on the CMS-1500 form based on the information given here. To complete this exercise, copy the CMS-1500 form provided in Appendix D or download it from the CD-ROM that accompanies this text.

Physician Information:

Name:	Mary Ann Brock, M.D.
Corporation Name:	PCL Medical Associates
Address:	1720 Front Street
	Philadelphia, PA 12345
Phone:	215-555-3000
Employer ID Number:	51-4290642
UPIN:	5569882
BS Pin Number:	49-5529-78
Group Number:	BS 0862
NPI:	9998755667
Group NPI:	6666455522

Patient Information Form:

Name:	Amy Louise Lynch
Address:	893 Bay Street
	Philadelphia, PA 12345
Phone:	215-555-0081
DOB:	January 9, 1999
Student Status:	Full-Time Student
Sex:	Female
Marital Status:	Single
Account Number:	LYNAM
Responsible Party:	Fred K. Lynch (father)
Insured's DOB:	June 15, 1947
Insured's Sex:	Male
Insured's Address:	1776 Liberty Road
	Philadelphia, PA 12345
Insured's Phone:	215-555-0704
Insured's Employer:	WDAF Radio
Insured's SS Number:	512-53-9751
Insurance Carrier:	Blue Cross Blue Shield of Pennsylvania
Insurance Carrier Address:	P.O. Box 7476
	Philadelphia, PA 19174
Insurance ID Number:	512-53-9751
Insurance Group Number:	W45980
Signature on File:	Yes, Today's date
Additional Insurance:	Metropolitan Family
Insured:	Jessie M. Lynch (mother)
DOB:	August 5, 1950
Sex:	Female

(continued)

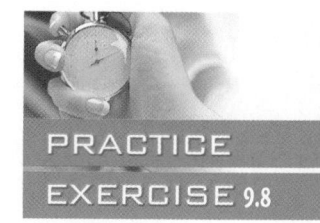

Employer: Southerland Lumber
Insurance Carrier Address: 414 East Franklin Road
Philadelphia, PA 12345
Insurance ID Number: 491-51-0003A
Insurance Group Number: 7989

Patient's Encounter Form:

Date: Today's date
T-104 P-115 R-25
CC: Fever, pain in left ear, sensitive to touch, L ear
red, tympanic membrane retracted
DX: Acute Otitis Media, left ear (382.00)
RX: Amoxil pediatric suspension 30 mL bottle,
2.5 mL q 8 hrs
Return 3 days for recheck

List of Fees for Service:

Date: Today's date
DX: Acute Otitis Media (382.00)
Services and Charges: Office visit, problem focused history and
exam, straightforward decision making
$40.00 CPT: (**99212**) DX: (382.00)
Physician Accepts
Assignment—Filing Date: Tomorrow's Date

Check the accuracy of your work by comparing your claim form to the completed claim form in Appendix J.

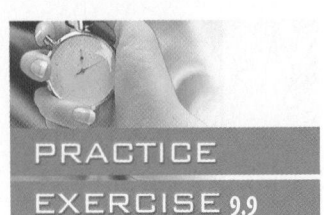

Completion of CMS-1500 (Sections I and II)

Fill out the form locators on the CMS-1500 form based on the information given here. To complete this exercise, copy the CMS-1500 form provided in Appendix D or download it from the CD-ROM that accompanies this text.

Physician Information:

Name:	Paul Erickson, M.D.
Corporation Name:	Family Medicine, P.C.
Address:	2500 East Avenue, Olathe, KS 12345
Phone:	913-555-2700
Employer ID Number:	53-1919011
Primary Health ID Number:	90-ERICKSO-993
Medicare UPIN:	CBR923 (Participating)
Cigna PPO ID Number:	04-5657
Cigna Group Number:	567203
NPI:	4531118907
Group NPI:	7221160934

Laboratory Information:

Name:	Johnson County Lab Services
Address:	15107 South Locust Olathe, KS 12345
Provider ID Number:	528761
NPI:	0325644443
Independent Laboratory:	Johnson County Laboratory Services

Patient Information Form:

Name:	Veronica Lee Bowman
DOB:	June 7, 1961
Sex:	Female
Marital Status:	Single
Account Number:	BOWVE1
Responsible Party:	Self
Address:	25 Elm Street Gardner, KS 12345
Phone:	913-555-7779
Employer:	Frito Lay
Social Security number:	312-23-4489
Insurance Carrier:	Cigna
Insurance Carrier Address:	P.O. Box 16139 Topeka, KS 12345
Insurance ID Number:	26-30254
Insurance Group Number:	FR 2856
Signature on file:	Yes

Patient Encounter Form:

Date:	Today's date T-99 P-80 R-16 BP-132/78
CC:	Fever, cough, rhinorrhea X 2 days
DX:	Upper respiratory infection (487.1)

(continued)

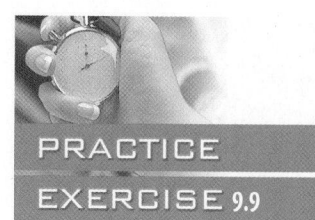

RX:	Actifed with codeine, Amoxil capsule 500 mg #16 one cap q 8 hrs
	Return in 2 days for recheck
Date:	Today's date (2 days after initial visit)
	T-99 P-86 R-18 BP-130/80
CC:	Pt still complains of fever, coughing with sputum, chills, chest pain
	Auscultation revealed rales
	Chest x-ray, two views, frontal and lateral, revealed consolidation
	Sputum culture STAT, WBC 13,000 (Sent to Johnson County Laboratory Services)
DX:	Pneumonia (487.0)
RX:	Continue meds, bed rest, fluids, return next day
Date:	Today's date (3 days after initial visit)
	Sputum culture revealed mycoplasma pneumonia
DX:	Mycoplasma Pneumonia (483.0)
RX:	Discontinue previous meds; erythromycin capsules #24 mg one cap, one hr before meals q 6 hrs
	Return 2 days

List of Fees for Services:

Date:	Today's date
DX	Upper respiratory infection (487.1)
Services and Charges:	Office visit, problem focused history and examination, straightforward decision making $60.00 CPT: (**99212**) DX: (487.1)
Date:	Today's date (2 days after initial visit)
DX:	Pneumonia (487.0)
Services and Charges:	Office visit, detailed history and examination, moderately complex decision making $100.00 CPT: (**99214**) DX: (487.0)
	X-ray, chest single view, 2 views $45.00 each CPT: (**71010**) DX: (487.0)
	Sputum culture $18.00 lab fee charge $12.00 CPT: (**87015**) DX: (487.0)
	WBC test $17.00 lab fee charge $10.00 CPT: (**85025**) DX: (487.0)
Date:	Today's date (3 days after initial visit)
DX	Mycoplasma Pneumonia (483.0)
Services and Charges:	Office visit, expanded problem focused history and examination, low complexity medical decision making. $75.00 CPT: (**99213**) DX: (483.0)

Physician Accepts Assignment

Check the accuracy of your work by comparing your claim form to the completed claim form in Appendix J.

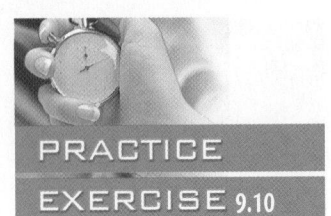

Completion of CMS-1500 (Sections I and II)

Fill out the form locators on the CMS-1500 form based on the information given here. To complete this exercise, copy the CMS-1500 form provided in Appendix D or download it from the CD-ROM that accompanies this text.

Physician Information:

Name:	Tina Harris, M.D.
Address:	16670 West 95 Terrace
	Overland Park, KS 12345
Phone:	913-555-9706
Employer ID Number:	55-1530016
NPI:	8954433148
Referring Physician:	Charles Henderson, M.D.
Referring Doctor UPIN:	08623
Referring Doctor NPI:	0815094410

Patient Information Form:

Name:	Kathy Ann Black
Sex:	Female
DOB:	January 20, 1949
Marital Status:	Married
Account Number:	BLAKA
Social Security number:	476-91-3852
Address:	79 North West Terrace
	Kansas City, KS 12345
Phone:	913-555-1560
Responsible Party:	Jason Darnell Black (husband)
Insured's SS Number:	512-19-2583
Insured's DOB:	April 1, 1945
Insured's Address:	Same
Insured's Employer:	EDS
Insurance Carrier:	Fortis Insurance Company
Pre Certification Number:	52521212
ID Number:	60923
Group Number:	2222
Signature on File:	Yes, form signed 09/15/20XX.

Patient's Encounter Form:

Date:	Today's date
Date of Current Illness:	3 days ago
	T-98.6 P-70 R-16 BP-180/92
CC:	Patient has felt lumps in both breasts
Breasts:	Masses felt in both R and L breast, breast biopsy bilateral STAT
DX:	Breast mass bilateral, high blood pressure
RX:	Aldomet tablets 250 mg #100, one tab T.I.D. for first 48 hours
	Return tomorrow for BP check and results of biopsy

(continued)

Date: Today's date (1 day after initial visit)
BP-176/92
Biopsy reveals breast carcinoma

(NOTE: 3 days Pt. admitted to Metropolitan Medical Center, NPI 0066677889 153 Slater Road, Leawood, KS 66206 for mastectomy bilateral.)

Date: Today's date (3 days after previous visit)
Initial Hospital Admission

Date: Today's date (1 day after admission)
Bilateral Radical Mastectomy performed no complication.

Date: Today's date (3 days after mastectomy)
Hospital discharge exam. Pt. is to return to office in 1 week for follow-up exam and BP check

List of Fees for Service:

Date: Today's date
DX: Breast mass, elevated blood pressure (611.72)
Services and Charges: New patient office visit, expanded history and examination, straightforward decision making $150.00 CPT: (**99204**) DX: (611.72)
Breast biopsy (bilateral) $350.00 CPT: (**19100-50**) DX: (611.72)

Date: Today's date (1 day after initial visit)
DX: Breast carcinoma, Essential hypertension, (174.9)
Services and Charges: Office visit, problem focused $40.00 CPT: (**99214**) DX: (174.9)

Date: Today's date (3 days after previous visit)
DX: Breast carcinoma, essential hypertension (174.9)
Services and Charges: Initial Hospital Care $150.00 CPT: (**99221**) DX: (174.9)

Date: Today's date (1 day after admission)
DX: Breast carcinoma, essential hypertension (174.9)
Services and Charges: Bilateral Mastectomy Radical including pectoral muscles, axillary lymph nodes. $3,700.00 CPT: (**19200-50**) DX: (174.9)

Date: Today's date (3 days after mastectomy)
DX: Breast carcinoma, essential hypertension (174.9)
Services and Charges: Hospital discharge, day management $50.00 CPT: (**99238**) DX: (174.9)

Claim Filed: 3 days after discharge with operative report

PRACTICE EXERCISE 9.10

(continued)

Check the accuracy of your work by comparing your claim form to the completed claim form in Appendix J.

Common Reasons for Delayed or Rejected CMS-1500 Claim Forms

The medical office specialist should be aware of common billing errors and how to correct them for quicker claims settlements and to reduce the number of appeals. This may help avoid additional administrative burdens, such as making telephone calls, re-submitting claims, and writing appeal letters. Figure 9.12 is a list of some reasons why claims are rejected or delayed and suggested solutions when completing the CMS-1500 insurance claim form locators.

Figure 9.12

Suggested solutions to problems that may arise when completing the CMS-1500 form.

Problem: Form locator 1. Claim submitted to the secondary insurer instead of the primary insurer.

Solution: Verify with the patient the two carriers and determine which is the primary carrier, either by using the birthday rule, the effective date of coverage, or depending on the illness, injury, or accident during the initial office visit. The **birthday rule** states that the parent whose day of birth is earlier in the calendar year will be considered the primary insurer. Submit the claim to the primary carrier and then after being paid or denied by the primary carrier submit a claim with the EOB form to the secondary carrier.

Problem: Form locators 1–13. Information missing on patient portion of the claim form.

Solution: Obtain a complete registration form from which information can be extracted. Educate patients on data requirements at the time of the first visit to the physician's office as patients fill out their portion of the form. Review the patient's information form before having the patient seen by the physician. If information is missing, highlight it with a color marker and ask the patient to complete.

Problem: Form locator 1a. Patient's insurance number is incorrect or transposed (especially in Medicare and Medicaid cases).

Solution: Proofread numbers carefully from source documents. Always photocopy front and back of insurance identification card.

Problem: Form locator 2. Patient's name and insured's name are entered as the same when the patient is a dependent.

Solution: Verify the insured party and check for Sr., Jr., and correct birth date.

Problem: Form locator 3. Incorrect gender identification, resulting in a diagnosis or procedure code that is inconsistent with patient's gender.

Solution: Proofread claim before mailing and review patient's medical record to locate gender, especially if the patient's first name could be male or female.

Problem: Form locators 9a–d. Incomplete entry for other insurance coverage.

Solution: Accurately abstract data from the patient's registration form. Telephone the patient if information is incomplete.

Problem: Form locator 10. Failure to indicate whether patient's condition is related to employment or an "other" type of accident.

Solution: Review patient's medical history to find details of injury or illness and proofread claim before mailing. Telephone the employer and verify the injury has been reported as a workers' compensation injury and the employer has workers' compensation insurance (Texas only).

Figure 9.12

(continued)

Problem: Form locator 12 and 13. Patient's signature is missing.
Solution: Always make sure the signature form locators are completed with "Signature on File" or "SOF" except in government (participating physician) or workers' compensation claims. Verify that the signature is on file in the medical record.

Problem: Form locator 14. Date of injury, date of last menstrual period (LMP), or dates of onset of illness are missing. This information is important for determining whether accident benefits apply, patient is eligible for maternity benefits, or there was a preexisting condition.
Solution: Do not list unless dates are clearly documented in the patient's medical record. Read the patient's medical history and call the patient to obtain the date of accident or LMP. Compose an addendum to the record, if necessary. Always proofread the claim before mailing.

Problem: Form locators 17, 17a, and 17b. Incorrect or missing name and/or PIN/NPI numbers of referring physician on claim for consultation or other services requiring this information. The referring physician may also be the ordering physician.
Solution: Check the patient registration form and the chart note for reference to the referring physician. Obtain a list of PIN/NPI numbers for all physicians in the area. Enter the provider's (ordering) name and NPI if there is no referring physician.

Problem: Form locator 19. Refer to the most current instructions from the applicable public or private payer regarding the use of this field.
Solution: Contact the carrier and inquire what information they require. Locator 19 is generally left blank, however, some carriers do require information inserted.

Problem: Form locator 21. The diagnostic code is missing, incomplete, invalid, not coded to the highest level of specificity, certainty (e.g., fourth or fifth digit is missing), or the diagnosis code does not match the CPT code.
Solution: Update encounter forms annually when the addendum comes out in October of each year. Conduct a chart audit every 6 months. Check with physician to verify the diagnosis code that belongs with the CPT code.

Problem: Form locator 22: The Medicaid resubmission number is missing.
Solution: List the original reference number for resubmitted claims and the resubmission code for Medicaid.

Problem: Form locator 23: Prior authorization number missing.
Solution: Enter any of the following: prior authorization number, referral number, mammography precertification number, or CLIA number as assigned by the payer.

Problem: Form locator 24A. Omitted, incorrect, overlapping, or duplicate dates of service.
Solution: Verify against the encounter form or medical record that all dates of services are listed and accurate and appear on individual lines. Date spans for multiple services must be adequate for the number and types of services provided.

Problem: Form locator 24B. Missing or incorrect place of service.
Solution: Verify the place of service from the encounter form or medical record and list the correct code for place of service and submitted procedure.

Problem: Form locator 24C: EMG: Was visit an emergency?—Yes or no.
Solution: NEW: Enter "Y" for YES if emergency; leave blank if not.

Problem: Form locator 24D. Procedure codes are incorrect, invalid, or missing.
Solution: Verify the coding system used by the insurance company and submit correct procedure code(s) by referring to a current CPT book. For Medicare patients and certain private payers, check the HCPCS manual for CMS national and local procedure codes.

(continued)

Figure 9.12

(continued)

Problem: Form locator 24D. Missing or incorrect modifiers.
Solution: Verify the need for modifiers. Submit correct modifiers using a current CPT book or HCPCS.

Problem: Form locator 24E: Diagnosis pointer does not match the CPT.
Solution: Check that the diagnosis pointer refers to the line number in form locator 21 and relates to the reason the service was performed.

Problem: Form locator 24F. Omitted or incorrect amount billed.
Solution: Be certain the fee column is filled in. Check the amounts charged as the UCR, MFS, or workers' compensation fee.

Problem: Form locator 24G. Days do not match dates of service (From and To; e.g., hospital visits); units of time are incorrectly billed (e.g., 1 unit may equal 15 minutes).
Solution: Depending on the error, check the documentation from the encounter form or chart and correct. Check to make sure the third-party payer accepts the units of time, etc.

Problem: Form locator 24I. Provider's NPI is missing.
Solution: Verify the physician's NPI and insert the number in this block if it is different from form locators 33a and 33b.

Problem: Form locator 24J. The number of the individual rendering the service is missing.
Solution: Enter the non-NPI number in the shaded area of the field. Enter the NPI number in the unshaded area of the field.

Problem: Form locator 25. The federal tax ID number is missing.
Solution: Enter the physician's EIN number. Do not use the Social Security number.

Problem: Form locator 27. Accept Assignment not checked.
Solution: Make sure that this box is checked YES. If not, the money will go to the patient.

Problem: Form locator 28. Total amounts do not equal itemized charges.
Solution: Total the charges for each claim and verify amounts with the patients' account. If the number of units in 24G is more than 1, multiply the units by the fee listed in 24F and add to all other charges listed.

Problem: Form locator 31. Physician's signature is missing.
Solution: Have the physician or physician's representative sign the claim form or use an ink stamp with the physician's signature on it.

Problem: Form locator 32. No place of service is recorded.
Solution: Enter the place of service where the procedure was performed, for example, office, hospital, or laboratory.

Problem: Form locator 32a. Missing NPI number.
Solution: Enter the NPI number of the service facility location listed in form locator 32a.

Problem: Form locator 32b. Missing other ID number.
Solution: Enter the two-digit qualifier identifying the non-NPI number followed by the ID number.

Problem: Form locator 33. Provider's billing name, address, or phone number is missing.
Solution: Enter the provider's or supplier's billing name, address, zip code, and phone number. The phone number is to be entered in the area to the right of the field title.

Problem: Form locator 33a. Missing NPI number.
Solution: Enter the NPI number of the billing provider in 33a.

HIPAA Compliance Alert

With the advent of HIPAA, a number of federal laws now apply to insurance claims submissions. HIPAA security standard rules were adopted to safeguard and protect the confidentiality, integrity, and availability of electronic health information. The rules were needed because no standard measures existed in the healthcare industry that addressed all aspects of the security of electronic health information while it is in use, being stored, or during the exchange of that information between entities. HIPAA mandated security standards to protect an individual's health information, while permitting the appropriate access and use of that information by healthcare providers, clearinghouses, and health plans without evidence of fraud or abuse issues.

To authorize the release of information, a patient must sign either form locator 12 on the CMS-1500 form or a consent document with similar wording to be retained in the office files. Often the release of information is incorporated into the new patient's information form.

Filing Secondary Claims

A patient may have coverage under more than one group insurance plan; additional insurance policies are referred to as **secondary insurance**. For example, a person may have primary insurance through his employer and also be covered under his spouse's insurance, making that his secondary insurance.

Supplemental insurance is an insurance plan that covers part of a patient's expenses, such as coinsurance, that the policyholder is otherwise responsible for. Supplemental insurance is exactly what it sounds like—it supplements the primary insurance. If the primary policy does not cover a service, supplemental does not cover it either. Supplemental insurance is generally limited to Medigap policies. Medigap policies are insurance policies that supplement Medicare payments.

Finding out which policy will be the primary one is important because insurance policies contain a provision called *coordination of benefits* (COB). The concept of coordination of benefits was originally developed by Blue Cross Blue Shield to prevent overpayment on a claim. If the secondary plan did not know what the primary plan had paid, the amount

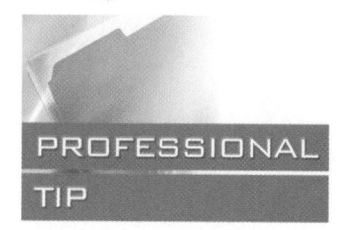

The difference between supplemental insurance and secondary insurance is that the secondary insurance policy may cover items that the primary insurance does not cover.

PROFESSIONAL TIP

paid by the two plans could exceed the provider's charge. The COB rule states that when a patient is covered by more than one policy, benefits paid by all policies are limited to 100 percent of the charge. This clause prevents people from having a number of plans and making a profit by collecting from each one. With coordination of benefits, insurance carriers exchange information with each other regarding payments and payment denials.

Determining Primary Coverage

Various standards are available for determining primary coverage:

- If the patient only has one policy, it is the primary one.
- If the patient has coverage under two plans under which she is the primary policyholder, the plan that has been in effect for the patient for the longest

period of time is the primary one. However, if the patient is an active employee of a company and has a plan with her present employer but is still covered by a former employer's plan (as would be the case with, say, a retiree or laid-off employee), the current employer's plan is the primary plan.

■ If the patient is covered as a dependent under another insurance policy, such as a spouse's policy, the patient's plan is the primary plan.

■ If an employed patient has coverage under the employer's plan and additional coverage under a government-sponsored plan, the employer's plan is the primary one. For example, if the patient is enrolled in a PPO through employment and is also on Medicare, the PPO is primary.

■ If a retired patient is covered by a spouse's employer's plan, and the spouse is still employed, the spouse's plan is the primary, even if the retired person has Medicare. Medicare is the primary for individuals and family members who are retired and receiving coverage under a group policy from a previous employer.

■ If the patient is a dependent child covered by both parents' plans, and the parents are not separated or divorced (or if they have joint custody of the child), the primary plan is determined by which parent's date of birth is earlier in the calendar year (the birthday rule).

■ If two of more plans cover dependent children of separated or divorced parents who do not have joint custody of their children, the children's primary plan is determined in this order:

  ● The plan of the custodial parent
  ● The plan of the spouse of the custodial parent (if the parent has remarried)
  ● The plan of the parent without custody.

When two insurance policies are involved, one is considered primary and the other is secondary. The patient's signature should always be acquired for release of information and assignment of benefits for both insurance companies. The initial CMS-1500 is submitted with primary and secondary insurance information in form locators 9a–d. Form locator 11d would be answered "yes." After payment is received from the primary payer, a claim form with a copy of the primary carrier's EOB is submitted to the secondary carrier.

Some physician practices and hospitals will automatically file for secondary insurance benefits, while others require the patient to do so. When submitting a secondary claim, you must attach a copy of the primary carrier's EOB to the completed CMS-1500 or CMS-1450/UB-04. Most secondary claims are not submitted electronically.

It is important to remember that a referral or prior authorization number may still be required even if that insurance carrier provides secondary coverage for the patient. Without the authorization number and primary carrier EOB, the claim will be denied.

Practice Exercises

Practice Exercises 9.11 through 9.15 are designed to help the reader learn how to complete claim forms when the patient has secondary insurance. For Practice Exercises 9.11 through 9.15, complete the primary CMS-1500 form manually. Then complete the EOB. Complete the secondary CMS-1500 manually adding the payment from the primary EOB. Hand in the secondary claim and EOB to your instructor.

To complete these exercises, copy the CMS-1500 form provided in Appendix D or download it from the CD-ROM that accompanies this text.

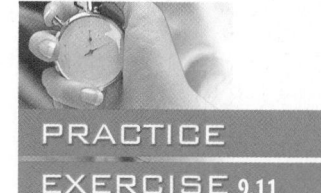

Secondary Claim

Patient Information:

Name:	Barbara Ward
Address:	214 Band Road
	Frisco, TX 12345
Phone:	972-555-8943
Sex:	F
DOB:	08/02/56
Social Security number:	214-68-9852
Marital Status:	M
Employment Status:	Full-time
Employer:	Allied Career Center
Address:	1933 E Frankford Road #110
	Carrollton, TX 12345
	972-555-3982
Insurance Plan:	Oxford Health
	12030 Plano Parkway
	Plano, VA 43098
	555-800-0302
Insurance ID/Policy Number:	214689852
Insurance Group Number:	54790012

Other Insured:

Name:	Charles Ward
DOB:	10/09/53
Address:	Same
Relationship:	Spouse
Telephone:	Same
Social Security number:	622-64-8701
Employer:	Dalmeth Enterprises
Address:	100023 Main Street
	Dallas, TX 12345
	214-555-9984
Insurance Plan:	Aetna Health
Address:	PO Box 855
	Irving, TX 75062
	222-889-9751
Insurance ID/Policy Number:	622648701
Insurance Group Number:	2223389
Provider Information:	James Brown, M.D.
	Phone 555-345-7654
NPI:	5598565422
	1400 Last Street
	Dallas, TX 12345
EIN:	16-8749532
UPIN:	865431
Oxford Health Pin:	B0228 Aetna Pin #: AET06
Visit Information:	Barbara Ward

(continued)

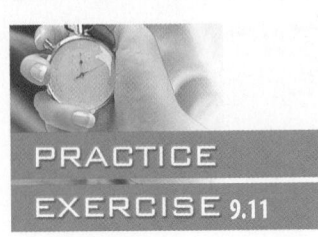

PRACTICE EXERCISE 9.11
(continued)

List of fees for services:

DOS:
DX:
99203:

Today's date
401.1 Benign Hypertension
New Patient Expanded Problem Focused:
$150.00

Assignment of benefits on file
Release of information form on file

Check the accuracy of your work by comparing your claim form to the completed claim form in Appendix J.

For Student Use Only

Payer's Name and Address

Oxford Health
12030 Plano Parkway
Plano, Virginia 43098

Today's Date:
CHECK #287613

Provider's Name and Address

Dr. James Brown
1400 Last Street
Dallas, TX 12345

This statement covers payments for the following patient(s):

Claim Detail Section

Patient Name: Ward, Barbara	**Patient Account #:** 0654	
Patient ID#: 214689852	**Insured's Name:** Same	**Group #:** 54790012
Provider Name: Dr. Brown	**Inventory #:** 33782	**Claim Control #:** 55502

Service Date(s)	Procedure	Total Billed	Allowed Charges	Contract Adjust	Deduct	Coins	Paid Amt.	Total Paid	
Claim Date	99203	150.00	125.00		00.00		80%		
TOTALS									

BALANCE DUE FROM PATIENT: PT'S DED/NOT COV $_____

PT'S COINSURANCE $_____

PAYMENT SUMMARY SECTION (Totals)

Charges	Adjustment	Allowed	Copay	Deduct/Not Covered	Coins	Total Paid

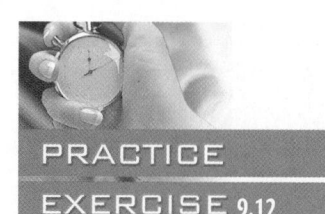

Secondary Claim

Physician Information:

Name:	Francis J. Boyer, M.D.
	916 E. Frisco Rd.
	Ithaca, NY 12345
	555-888-2233
Employer ID Number:	56-3342560
Cigna PIN:	123266
NPI:	5562811442

Patient Information Form:

Name:	Jay Wagner (NP)
Date of Birth:	February 19, 1989
Social Security number:	889-27-6623
Address:	265 First Street
	Ithaca, NY 12345
Phone:	312-555-4993
Gender:	Male
Marital Status:	Single
Responsible Party:	Theresa Wagner (mother)
Address:	Same
Insured's Date of Birth:	January 3, 1958
Insured's Sex:	Female
Phone:	312-555-4993
Insured's Employer:	The Famous Gourmet
	2241 Eatery Avenue
	Ithaca, NY 12345
Social Security number:	421-80-6060
Insurance Carrier:	Cigna
Insurance Carrier Address:	243 Harrison Avenue
	Hartford, CT 06897
Ins. Phone:	800-678-1212
Insurance ID/Policy Number:	753-00865
Insurance Group Number:	DP 139
Signature on File:	Yes

Secondary Insurance Information: Father

Name:	Howard Wagner
DOB:	September 21, 1958
Address:	Same as spouse
Phone:	Same as spouse
Social Security number:	455-59-8692
Employer:	The Print Shop
Address:	6654 Waverly Avenue
	Syracuse, NY 12345
Phone:	555-894-5521

(continued)

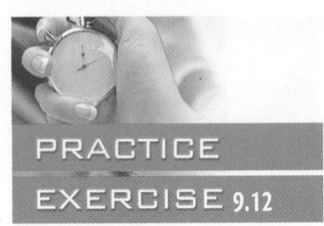

Insurance Carrier:	Allmerica Insurance
	P.O. Box 123658
	Erie, PA 12345
Phone:	215-555-7621
Insurance ID/Policy Number:	ASD56987
Insurance Group Number:	1256893
Signature on File:	Yes

Patient's Encounter Form:

Date:	Today's date
Date of first symptom:	Three days ago
	WT 45 HT 50 T 100.4 P 94 R 20 BP 90/60
CC:	Wheezing, coughing, dyspnea, fever 3 d. Auscultation of lung: Rales and congestion.
Dx:	Bronchitis.(490.0)
Rx:	EryPed 200 1 tsp Q.I.D., Tussi-Organidan 1 tsp in AM and 1 tsp at night, return 3 days for recheck.

List of Fees for Service:

Date:	Today's date
Dx:	Bronchitis. (490.0)
Services and Charges:	New Patient Office visit–99203: $150.00

Assignment of benefits on file

Release of information form on file

Check the accuracy of your work by comparing your claim form to the completed claim form in Appendix J.

For Student Use Only

Payer's Name and Address

| Cigna Health Insurance Company |
| 243 Harrison Avenue |
| Hartford, CT 06808 |

Today's Date:

CHECK #8822469

Provider's Name and Address

| Francis J. Boyer, M.D. |
| 916 E. Frisco Road |
| Ithaca, NY 12345 |

Patient Name: Jay Wagner   **Patient Account #:** WAGJ00
Patient ID#: 753-00865   **Insured's Name:** Theresa Wagner   **Group #:** DP139
Provider: Francis J. Boyer, M.D.   **Inventory Control #:** 3987540

Service Date(s)	Procedure	Total Charges	Contract Amount	Copay	Deduct/Not Covered	Coins	Paid Amt.	Total Paid	Remarks
Claim Date	99203	150.00	125.00	10.00	0.00	0.00	100%		
TOTALS									

BALANCE DUE FROM PATIENT: PT'S DED/NOT COV $_____

PT'S COINSURANCE $_____

PAYMENT SUMMARY SECTION (Totals)

Charges	Adjustment	Allowed	Copay	Deduct/Not Covered	Coins	Total Paid

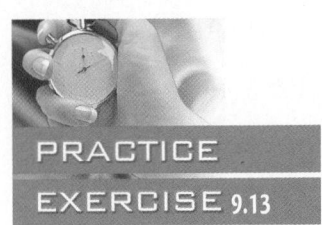

Secondary Claim

Physician Information: David Rosenberg, M.D.
                                     1400 West Center Street
                                     Toledo, Ohio 12345
                                     999-555-2121
Tax ID Number: 16-1246791
UPIN: 1001239
BCBS Number: B002
NPI: 5556214735

Patient Information Form:

Name: Stephanie Gross
                                     310 Farm Road
                                     Toledo, Ohio 12345
                                     Phone #: 789-555-3641
                                     SS#: 258-65-8902
Insurance Plan: Blue Cross Blue Shield
                                     P.O. Box 810
                                     Columbus, Ohio 44321
Phone: 800-789-1722
ID Number: 78235606
Gr Number: ED856
Sex: F
                                     Patient's copay is $15.00
Birth Date: 08/02/56
Marital Status: M
Employer: EDS Company
Employment Address: 2225 Logan Drive
                                     Toledo, OH 12345
Phone: 800-555-9293
Employment Status: Full time

Secondary Insurance Information: (Spouse)

Employer: Stewart's Tuxedos
Address: 1795 Mall Ave
                                     Toledo, OH. 12345
Phone: 800-555-1234
Husband: John J. Gross
Social Security number: 323-54-2234
DOB: 9/4/1953
Phone: Same
Address: Same
Insurance Plan: Cigna
                                     PO Box 952
                                     Plano, TX 75022
Phone: 972-380-0880
Policy/ID Number: 323542234
Gr Number: JC7843

(continued)

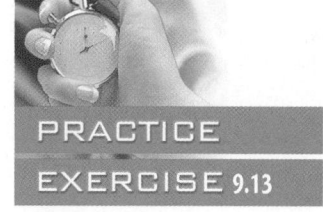

Patient's Encounter Form:

Date:	Today's Date
DX:	465.9 Upper Respiratory Infection
Service:	99213: $75.00

Assignment of benefits on file

Release of information form on file

Check the accuracy of your work by comparing your claim form to the completed claim form in Appendix J.

For Student Use Only

Payer's Name and Address

Blue Cross Blue Shield
P.O. Box 810
Columbus, Ohio 44321

Today's Date:

CHECK #19562

Provider's Name and Address

David Rosenberg, M.D.
1400 West Center Street
Toledo, Ohio 12345

This statement covers payments for the following patient(s):

Claim Detail Section

Patient Name: Gross, Stephanie   **Patient Account #:** GROST

Patient ID#: 78235606

Provider Name: David Rosenberg, M.D.   **Claim Control #** 002456

Service Date(s)	Procedure	Charges	Adjustment	Allowed	Copay	Deduct/Not Covered	Coins	Paid Amt.	Total Paid
Claim Date	99213	75.00	8.75		15.00	0.00	0.00	100%	
TOTALS									

BALANCE DUE FROM PATIENT: PT'S DED/NOT COV $_____

PT'S COINSURANCE $_____

PAYMENT SUMMARY SECTION (Totals)

Charges	Adjustment	Allowed	Copay	Deduct/Not Covered	Coins	Total Paid

PRACTICE
EXERCISE 9.14

Secondary Claim

Physician Information:	Christopher M. Brown, M.D.
	234 Haverford Road
	Haverford, Ohio 12345
	999-555-3111
Federal Tax ID:	34-086541
Physician's Choice	
Services Provider ID:	B4321
NPI:	8903789447
Patient Information:	Sandra Henderson
	15 Main Street
	Wadsworth, Ohio 12345
Phone Number:	703-555-6969
Gender:	F
Marital Status:	M
DOB:	06/05/1966
Social Security number:	331779183
Insurance:	U.S. Life
	2788 Broadway
	New York, NY, 00006
	703-877-0874
Group Number:	931
Policy/ID Number:	3317891
Employer:	Compaq Computers
Address:	10 Compaq Way
	Haverford, OH 12345
Phone:	999-555-6543
Employment Status:	Full Time

Secondary Insurance Information (Spouse):

Insured:	Charles Henderson
Gender:	M
Marital Status:	M
Social Security number:	177-36-2854
Employment:	Full Time
DOB:	08/22/1960
Employer:	Dell Computer
Address:	25 Dell Blvd.
	Haverford, OH 12345
Phone:	999-555-2599
Insurance:	Physicians Choice Services
	900 Blue Rock Turnpike
	Clarkville, Ohio 60817
Group Number:	K 2565
ID/Policy Number:	5076 241
Phone:	800-793-1257

Patient's Encounter Form:

DOS:	Today's Date

(continued)

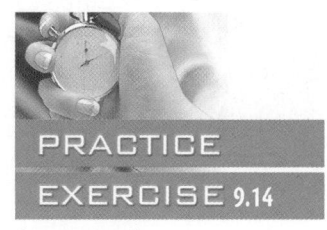

PRACTICE
EXERCISE 9.14

(continued)

CPT:	99203	150.00 New Patient
	73070	50.00 Radiological view elbow (2 views)
	73090	50.00 Radiological view forearm (2 views)

Assignment of benefits on file

Release of information form on file

Check the accuracy of your work by comparing your claim form to the completed claim form in Appendix J.

For Students Use Only

Payer's Name and Address

U.S. Life
2788 Broadway
New York, NY 25783

Today's Date:

CHECK #21763

Provider's Name and Address

Christopher M. Brown, M.D.
234 Haverford Road
Haverford, Ohio 12345

This statement covers payments for the following patient(s):

Claim Detail Section (If there are numbers in the SEE REMARKS column, see the Remarks Section for explanation.)

Patient Name: Henderson, Sandra   **Patient Account #:** Hen03

Patient ID#: 331779183   **Insured's Name:** Sandra Henderson

Provider Name: Christopher M. Brown, M.D.   **Inventory #:** 25133   **Claim Control #** 55614

Service Date(s)	Procedure	Charges	Adjustment	Allowed	Copay	Deduct/Not Covered	Coins	Paid Amt.	Remarks
Claim Date	99203	150.00	0.00		0.00	100.00		80%	01
Claim Date	73070	50.00	0.00		0.00	0.00		80%	
Claim Date	73070	50.00	0.00		0.00	0.00		80%	
TOTALS									

BALANCE DUE FROM PATIENT: PT'S DED/NOT COV $_____

PT'S COINSURANCE $_____

PAYMENT SUMMARY SECTION (Totals)

Charges	Adjustment	Allowed	Copay	Deduct/Not Covered	Coins	Total Paid

REMARKS SECTION: 01 Deductible

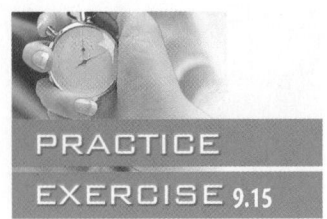

Secondary Claim

Physician Information:

Name:	Mary Ann Brock, M.D.
Address:	1547 Sampson Street
	Philadelphia, PA 12345
Phone:	215-555-3000
Tax Identification Number:	51-4290642
UPIN:	8869075
Blue Cross Blue Shield	
Provider ID Number:	495529
NPI:	6632588874

Patient Information:

Name:	Amy Louise Lynch
Address:	1776 Liberty Road
	Philadelphia, PA 12345
Phone:	215-555-9632
Social Security number:	123-45-6789
Date of Birth:	January 9, 1998
Sex:	Female
Marital Status:	Single
Employer:	Full-time student

Responsible Party (Both parents are insured):

Name:	Fred K. Lynch (father)
Insured's Address:	1776 Liberty Road
	Philadelphia, PA 12345
Phone:	215-555-9632
Insured's DOB:	July 15, 1967
Insured's Sex:	Male
Insured's Social Security number:	512-53-9751
Insured's Employer:	WDAF Radio
	200 Ester Lane
	Philadelphia, PA 12345
Phone:	215-555-9321
Insurance Carrier:	Blue Cross Blue Shield of Pennsylvania
	P.O. Box 354
	Philadelphia, PA 19174
Phone:	215-668-2334
Insured's ID/Policy Number:	512-53-9751
Insured's Group Number:	W45980

(continued)

Additional Insurance:

Name:	Jessie M. Lynch (mother)
Insured's Address	1776 Liberty Road
	Philadelphia, PA 12345
	215-555-9632
Date of Birth:	May 6, 1969
Sex:	Female
Social Security number:	491-51-0003
Employer:	Southerland Lumber
	5145 Frontier Lane
	Philadelphia, PA 12345
Phone:	215-555-1722
Insurance Carrier:	Metropolitan Family Insurance Company
	414 East Franklin Road
	Philadelphia, PA 19111
Phone:	800-555-4141
Insured's ID/Policy Number:	491-51-0003
Insured's Group Number:	7989

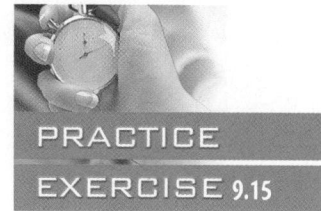

PRACTICE EXERCISE 9.15

(continued)

Patient's Encounter Form/List of Fees for Service:

Date of Service:	Today's date
Diagnosis:	V70.0 Annual Physical Examination
Services:	99385 Physical Examination Preventive Medicine Visit: $85.00

Assignment of benefits on file

Release of information form on file

Check the accuracy of your work by comparing your claim form to the completed claim form in Appendix J.

For Student Use Only

The charges are being paid at 80%.

Payer's Name and Address

| |
| |
| |
| |

Today's Date:

CHECK #24466

Provider's Name and Address

| Mary Ann Brock, M.D. |
| 1547 Sampson Street |
| Philadelphia, PA 12345 |

This statement covers payments for the following patient(s): Lynch, Amy
Claim Detail Section (If there are numbers in the SEE REMARKS column, see the
Remarks Section for explanation.)

Patient Name: Lynch, Amy	**Patient Account #:** Lyncham1
Patient ID#:	**Insured's Name:**
Group #:	
Provider Name: Mary Ann Brock, M.D.	**Inventory #:** 44562 **Claim Control #:** 28081

Service Date(s)	Procedure	Charges	Adjustment	Allowed	Copay	Deduct/Not Covered	Coins	Paid Amt.	Remarks
Claim Date	99385	85.00	0.00		0.00	0.00		80%	
TOTALS									

BALANCE DUE FROM PATIENT: PT'S DED/NOT COV $_____

PT'S COINSURANCE $_____

PAYMENT SUMMARY SECTION (Totals)

Charges	Adjustment	Allowed	Copay	Deduct/Not Covered	Coins	Total Paid

Chapter Summary

■ Insurance claims are sent to insurance carriers either on paper or electronically. Electronic claims have a number of advantages such as low administrative costs, reduced claim rejection, and faster payment.

■ The CMS-1500 form was developed so insurance carriers could process claims efficiently by OCR. Keying a form for OCR scanning requires different techniques than preparing one for standard claims submission. Because the majority of insurance carriers accept the OCR format, it is suggested that it be routinely used.

■ Specific guidelines are available for completing a CMS-1500 form. Because guidelines vary at the state and local levels for completing the CMS-1500, the medical insurance specialist should check with his local intermediaries or private carriers.

■ Insurance companies and federal and state programs require certain identification numbers on health insurance claim forms submitted from individuals and facilities who provide and bill for services to patients.

■ The medical office specialist should be aware of common billing errors and how to correct them for quicker claims settlements and to reduce the number of appeals.

■ A patient may have coverage under more than one group insurance plan; additional insurance policies are referred to as secondary insurance. For example, a person may have primary insurance through his employer and also be covered under his spouse's insurance, making that his secondary insurance.

Chapter Review

True/False

Identify the statement as true (T) or false (F).

_____ 1. If the patient is the insured person, the "Self" entry is marked under Patient Relationship to Insured on the CMS-1500 claim form.

_____ 2. If the patient has additional insurance through a spouse, this information must be provided on the CMS-1500 claim form.

_____ 3. Form locator 15 on the CMS-1500 is where the physician's unique identification number is entered.

_____ 4. An audit of an electronic CMS-1500 claim by a clearinghouse tells the submitter if required data is missing.

_____ 5. The birthday rule states that the parent whose day of birth is earlier in the calendar year will be considered the primary insurer.

_____ 6. Assignment of benefits refers to the minor giving the guarantor authority to see her medical records.

_____ 7. The CMS-1500 is a universal claim form for filing all medical claims.

Multiple Choice

Identify the letter of the choice that best completes the statement or answers the question.

_____ 1. The first 13 form locators on the CMS-1500 form refer to the:
   a. patient.
   b. provider.
   c. authorization to release information.
   d. medical practice.

_____ 2. Form locators 14 through 33 on the CMS-1500 form refer to the:
   a. patient.   c. third-party payer.
   b. physician or supplier.   d. secondary insurance plan.

_____ 3. The patient's birth date on the CMS-1500 form is entered in which of the following formats?
   a. MM/DD/YY   c. MM/DD/CCYY
   b. DD/MM/YY   d. DD/MM/CCYY

_____ 4. HIPAA developed standards and regulations to be used by all providers, carriers, billing services, and clearinghouses in order to:
   a. standardize patient care.   c. expedite claims processing.
   b. protect patient confidentiality.   d. eliminate errors.

_____ 5. Where is the facility information located on the CMS-1500 form?
   a. form locator 32   c. forms locator 20–25
   b. form locator 14   d. forms locator 1 and 5

_____ 6. Locator 24B requires a place of service to be identified. Which of the following is a common place of service code?
   a. urgent care facility   c. birthing center
   b. hospice   d. all of the above

Matching

Match the acronym with the correct definition.

   a. FPN   f. TIN
   b. EIN   g. NPI
   c. GPN   h. HIC
   d. UPIN   i. PIN
   e. SOF   j. LMP

_____ 1. Also known as federal tax identification number

_____ 2. Provider identification number, issued by the carrier

_____ 3. National Provider Identifier issued by the CMS

_____ 4. Member of a group practice who submits claims under the group's name

_____ **5.** Denotes signature on file

_____ **6.** Unique Physician Identification Number issued by Medicare

_____ **7.** Health insurance claim

_____ **8.** Last menstrual period

_____ **9.** Number issued by the Internal Revenue Service for income tax purposes

_____ **10.** A facility provider number used by the performing physician to report services done at that location

For Additional Practice

Complete the CMS-1500 form based on the information given here copy the CMS-1500 form provided in Appendix D or download it from the CD-ROM that accompanies this text.

Physician Information:

Physician Name:	Ralph Wiggum, M.D.
Address:	333 Forrest Lane
	Dallas, TX 75225
Phone:	214-388-5050
EIN:	72-5786322
NPI	2222233333
Aetna PIN:	CNC041

Patient Information Form:

Name:	Charlotte Watson
	124 Dallas Dr.
	Dallas, TX 75201
Phone:	214-388-5072
Social Security number:	555-88-8888
DOB:	07/08/44
SEX:	Female, Single
Patient Account Number:	WATCH001
Employer:	GPX Incorporated
Insurance Carrier:	Aetna (HMO)
Insurance Address:	5555 Walkway Ave
	New York, NY. 10000
Insurance ID Number:	555-88-8888
Insurance Group Number:	56885

Patient's Encounter Form:

Date:	Today's date
	T-98 P-85 R-15 BP-150/96 WT-164 HT -73
CC:	No complaints, physical examination

List of Fees for Services:

Date: Today's date
DX: Physical exam (V70.0)

Initial preventive medicine, new patient $80.00 (99386) (DX: V70.0)
X-ray, chest, 2 views $45.00 each (71020) (DX: V70.0)
ECG routine, 12 leads $55.00 (93000) (DX: V70.0)
Complete UA $15.00 (81000) (DX: V70.0)

Assignment of benefits and release of information on file, form signed Today's date, claim submitted to carrier on Today's date.

Resources

Healthcare Financial Management Association: *www.hfma.org* (type in under search box, patient friendly billing)

Chapter 10   Hospital Medical Billing

Chapter Objectives

After reading this chapter, the student should be able to:

1   Understand the inpatient billing process used by hospitals.

2   Submit accurate and timely hospital claims and practice good follow-up and collection techniques.

3   Identify the different types of facilities and differentiate between inpatient and outpatient services.

4   Understand that hospital billing and coding are based on revenue.

5   Recognize that hospital reimbursement is not a fee for service but a fixed fee payment based on the diagnosis, rather than on time or services rendered.

6   Complete the UB-04 hospital billing claim form.

Key Terms

admitting physician
Ambulatory Payment
   Classification (APC)
   system
ambulatory surgical center
   (ASC)
ambulatory surgical unit
   (ASU)
attending physician
charge description master
   (CDM)

comorbidity
cost outlier
Diagnosis Related Group
   (DRG)
emergency care
grouper
hospice
inpatient care
master patient index
operating physician
outpatient care

Outpatient Prospective
   Payment System (OPPS)
patient control number
   (PCN)
principal diagnosis
prospective payment
   system
registration
rendering physician
skilled nursing facility (SNF)
urgent care

Case Study
Hospital Medical Billing

Stacy has recently suffered from appendicitis. The morning it began she contacted her physician's office, and was sent directly to the emergency room. After several procedures, including CAT scans and examinations, she was scheduled for an appendectomy. She stayed in the hospital for several days due to the severity of her case. After everything was complete, she began to receive several bills. She was confused as to why she received so many bills from so many different places, some that she had never even heard of. She contacted the hospital and spoke with a billing manager who explained everything.

Questions

1. What types of bills might Stacy have received?
2. Why would she not recognize all of the offices the bills originated from?
3. In general, what types of codes may have been used to bill the hospital visit?

Introduction

A hospital bill for inpatient care is much larger than the usual bill for services rendered in a physician's office. Patients are admitted to hospitals for severe health problems and many require major surgery, resulting in considerable expense to the patient. The majority of most hospitals' reimbursement comes from insurance companies. However, it is becoming more difficult for patients with insurance coverage to pay their share of the bill. Consequently, accurate and timely hospital billing and good follow-up and collection techniques are in demand.

Inpatient Billing Process

The insurance billing division is often part of the hospital's business office or patient account service (PAS) department and used to be placed near the admission department, hospital cashier, or main lobby (entry and exit) of the hospital. In today's environment, however, it is more common for the PAS to be located off-site. To centralize the claims process, the off-site facility may handle not only the claims for the state in which it is located, but also for surrounding states.

The inpatient billing process involves many people and departments in and outside the hospital. Each hospital has a **master patient index**, which is the main database of all of the hospital's patients. As a patient arrives and goes through the registration or admission process, the patient is assigned a **patient control number (PCN)**, which is a unique number provided for each hospital admission. All charges and payments are posted to this number. **Registration** or admission is the process of collecting a patient's personal information, including insurance information, and entering it into the hospital's computer system. Copies of the admitting face sheet, which is similar to the patient information form, are sent to the primary care physician or surgeon's office. Registration information, copies of all authorization and signature documents, a copy of the insurance card(s), and a copy of the emergency department's report, if the patient was admitted through the emergency department, are scanned in paperless facilities or assembled in a financial folder using a traditional system.

Hospitals bill for services only after the discharge summary is completed and signed by the physician. Ideally, hospital charts should be completed within 3 to 4 days and no more than 14 days after the patient is discharged, otherwise a cash flow problem could result. A discharge analyst checks the completeness of each patient's medical record for dictated reports and signatures. She completes a deficiency sheet that is put on the medical record indicating any documentation deficiencies. The medical office specialist can help by scheduling adequate time for the physician to complete the medical records.

Charge Description Master

All services and items provided to the patient are keyed into a computer system to assist with a high volume of billing for services received by hospital patients. This may occur in one of two ways: In the first way, a designated person in each hospital department keys in all services and procedures using an internal code. This is referred to as *order entry*. In the second way, a charge sheet that has services and procedures checked

Department Number	Service Code	HCPCS Code	Description	Revenue Code	Charge
0100	001	99281	ER Visit Level 1	450	$100.00
100	002	99282	ER Visit Level II	450	$125.00
100	003	99283	ER Visit Level III	450	$150.00
100	004	99284	ER Visit Level IV	450	$200.00
100	005	99285	ER Visit Level V	450	$250.00
100	006	71010	Room/Board/Pvt	110	$500.00
100	007	71020	Intensive Care	190	$750.00
200	001	76705	Chest x-ray, AP	324	$100.00
200	002	Q0081	Chest x-ray, AP & Lat	324	$125.00
200	006	93005	Abdominal Ultrasound	320	$275.00
300	001		IV Therapy	260	$350.00
400	001		EKG	730	$250.00

Figure 10.1

A sample charge master.

off is sent to the data processing department where a data processor keys in the information using internal codes. These services, coded with the internal codes, link up in a computer system called a **charge description master (CDM)**, also commonly referred to as a *charge master* (Figure 10.1). The CDM includes the following information:

1. *Procedure code:* CPT® and HCPCS codes appear on a detail bill, outpatient bill, or outpatient uniform bill claim form UB-04, but not usually on the inpatient form.
2. *Procedure description:* This is a detailed narrative of each procedure (surgery, laboratory test, and radiological test).
3. *Service description:* This is a detailed narrative of each service (evaluation and management, observation, emergency department visits, and clinical visits).
4. *Charge:* The dollar amount for each service or procedure is recorded. This is the standard fee for the item and not the actual amount paid by the third-party payer.
5. *Revenue code:* This is a three-digit code number representing a specific accommodation, ancillary service, or billing calculation related to the service.

Each patient's data, consisting of revenue codes, procedure codes, descriptions, charges, and medical record data, are organized by the CDM and printed onto a hospital Uniform Bill claim form, commonly known as a UB-04 form or sometimes a CMS-1450 form. The charge master database must be kept current and accurate to obtain proper reimbursement. It must be regularly audited; otherwise, negative impacts such as overpayment, underpayment, undercharging for services, claim rejections, fines, and/or penalties may result. There is usually a lag time, for example, 4 days after patient discharge, to be sure that all charges have been entered prior to claim submission. A sample charge master is shown in Figure 10.1.

Types of Payers

Hospitals negotiate their fees through different types of payers, including health maintenance organizations (HMOs), preferred provider organizations (PPOs), exclusive

CPT is a registered trademark of the American Medical Association.

provider organizations (EPOs), point-of-service (POS) plans, commercial and indemnity plans, Medicare, Medicaid, TRICARE Prime (HMO), TRICARE Extra (PPO), TRICARE Standard, CHAMPUS, CHAMPVA, and workers' compensation.

Coding and Reimbursement Methods

Three basic reimbursement methods are used for inpatient hospital services:

1. Prospective payment system
2. Fee for service
3. Per diem.

The **prospective payment system** is the most recognized, but a number of carriers utilize other methods. The prospective payment system was initiated by Medicare, which established payment rates to hospitals prospectively, which means before services are rendered.

Fee for services is the oldest method for which actual charges rendered to the patient are paid if found to be medically necessary. This is based on the diagnosis as related to the treatment rendered the patient.

The third type of reimbursement is the per diem type, which pays a fixed rate per day for all services performed or provided by the hospital facility. This is based on a daily rate for the type of admission and level of service provided to the patient. This method is used by rehabilitation centers and other facilities for negotiating reimbursement by third-party carriers.

An outpatient classification system developed by Health Systems International and used by the Centers for Medicare and Medicaid Services (CMS) is **Ambulatory Payment Classification (APC) System**. This system is based on procedures rather than diagnoses. Services associated with a specific procedure or visits are bundled into the APC reimbursement. More than one APC may be billed if more than one procedure is performed, but discounts may be applied to any additional APCs. APCs are applied to:

- Ambulatory surgical procedures
- Chemotherapy
- Clinic visits
- Diagnostic services and diagnostic tests
- Emergency department visits
- Implants
- Outpatient services furnished to nursing facility patients not packaged into a nursing facility consolidated billing. (These are services commonly furnished by hospital outpatient departments that nursing facilities are not able to provide, e.g., computed tomography, magnetic resonance imaging, or ambulatory surgery.)
- Partial hospitalization services for community mental health centers
- Preventive services (colorectal cancer screening)
- Radiology, including radiation therapy
- Services for patients who have exhausted Medicare Part A benefits
- Services to hospice patients for treatment of a nonterminal illness
- Surgical pathology.

CMS provides a list of reimbursement rates for the APC system. CMS refers to it as **Outpatient Prospective Payment System (OPPS)**. When a patient undergoes multiple processes and services, multiple APCs are generated and the payments are added together. APC software automatically discounts multiple APCs when appropriate.

Diagnosis Related Group System

Another form of the prospective payment system is the **Diagnosis Related Group (DRG)** system, which categorizes diagnoses and treatments into groups.

The DRG reimbursement system is a patient classification method that categorizes patients who are medically related with respect to diagnosis and treatment and who are statistically similar in terms of their length of hospital stay. The DRG system is used to both classify past cases to measure the relative resources hospitals have expanded to treat patients with similar illness and to classify current cases to determine payment. The classifications were formed from more than 10,000 International Classification of Diseases, Ninth Revision, Clinical Modification (ICD-9-CM) codes that were divided into 25 major diagnostic categories (MDCs). These diagnoses were assigned a specific DRG number from 001 to 511 and specific values commensurate with geographic area, type of hospital, depreciation value, teaching status, and other specific criteria. TRICARE and other private insurance companies that utilize DRGs use DRG numbers 600 to 900. Most MDCs are based on a particular organ system of the body. Payments for each DRG are based on a "relative weight" assigned to each case and on the hospital's individual rate. The relative weight represents the average resources necessary to provide services for a specific diagnosis. Within MDCs, DRGs are either medical or surgical. Seven variables are responsible for DRG classifications:

- Principal diagnosis
- Secondary diagnosis (up to eight)
- Surgical procedures (up to six)
- Comorbidity and complications
- Age and sex
- Discharge status
- Trim points (number of hospital days for a specific diagnosis).

When a patient is admitted to the hospital, the admission process can be done by either the attending physician or the admitting physician. The **admitting physician** only admits the patient to the hospital. An example of this would be an emergency department physician who admits a patient. An **attending physician** is primarily responsible for the patient's care. A **rendering physician** is a provider who renders a service, for example, a radiologist. If the patient requires an operation, the physician who conducts the operation is referred to as the **operating physician.** Throughout the patient's stay, diagnoses are established and coded from the **principal diagnosis** to the secondary. The UB-04 form allows up to ten diagnoses, including the principal and admitting diagnoses. The assignment of the DRG is not performed by the facility. It is assigned by the carrier at the time the claim is processed, much like the billing of the APC. The facility has the ability to determine the DRG that should be assigned and the expected reimbursement based on the seven variables of the DRG classification given in the preceding list.

The facility may determine their charges for DRGs by using a case mix index (CMI). Each facility has a standardized dollar amount assigned to it by Medicare, determined by factors such as the CMI, local wage index, type of facility, the number of low income patients, type of institution, and so forth. A case mix is simply an average of all the DRG weights. Other factors that contribute to the facility's case mix are:

- Severity of illness
- Prognosis
- Treatment difficulty
- Need for intervention
- Resource intensity.

Although the DRG is assigned by the carrier at the time the claim is processed, the facility can determine their reimbursement by working with the DRGs. This is done by an individual in the health information management (HIM) department, which is also known as the medical records department. This individual obtains the pertinent patient case history information and codes the principal and secondary diagnoses and operative procedures. Using a computer software program called a **grouper**, this information is keyed in and the program calculates and assigns the DRG payment group. The grouper is not able to consider any differences between chronic and acute conditions. Looping is the grouper process of searching all listed diagnoses for the presence of any comorbid conditions or complications or searching all procedures for operating room procedures or more specific procedures. If any factors that affect the DRG assignment change or are added, the new information is entered and the case is assigned the new DRG.

Let's look at an example of a patient with chronic bronchitis who is admitted to the hospital with pneumonia. His medical record shows that he has had emphysema for many years, and it lists chronic obstructive pulmonary disease (COPD) as the principal diagnosis with pneumonia as a secondary diagnosis—this DRG assignment, however, is inaccurate. As stated, the assignment entitles the hospital to receive $2723.66. However, if the pneumonia diagnostic code were listed as the principal diagnosis with two secondary diagnoses, emphysema and chronic bronchitis, then the hospital would be entitled to $3294.17—an additional $570.00 when the DRGs are assigned correctly.

Cost Outliers

A case that cannot be assigned an appropriate DRG because of an atypical situation is called a **cost outlier**. These atypical situations are as follows:

- Unique combinations of diagnoses and surgeries causing high costs
- Very rare conditions
- Long length of stay (referred to as a *day outlier*)
- Low-volume DRGs
- Inliers (in which the hospital case falls below the mean average or expected length of stay)
- Death
- Leaving against medical advice
- Admitted and discharged on the same day.

The current federal reimbursement plan for outliers is to pay the full DRG rate plus an additional payment for services provided. An unethical practice, *DRG creep*, is to code a patient's DRG category for a more severe diagnosis than indicated by the patient's condition. This is also called upcoding. The amount of payment may be increased by documenting in the patient's medical record any comorbid conditions or complications. When referring to DRGs, the abbreviation "CC" is used to indicate such complications comorbidities. **Comorbidity** is defined as a preexisting condition that, because of its

Alcoholism	Diabetes mellitus, insulin-dependent
Anemia, due to blood loss, acute/chronic	Furuncles
Angina pectoris	Hematemesis
Atelectasis	Hematuria
Atrial fibrillation	Hypertensive heart disease
Cachexia	Malnutrition
Cardiomyopathy	Pneumothorax
Cellulitis	Renal failure; acute/chronic
Chronic obstructive pulmonary disease	Respiratory failure
Decubitus ulcer	Urinary retention
Dehydration	Urinary tract infection

Figure 10.2

Examples of comorbidities that could change the amount of a reimbursement.

effect on the specific principal diagnosis, will require intensive therapy or cause an increase in length of stay by at least 1 day in approximately 75% of cases (Figure 10.2).

If a patient is admitted because of two or more conditions and the physician fails to indicate the "most resource-intensive" or "most specific" diagnosis as the principal diagnosis, which is the diagnosis established after study or testing, the DRG assessment will be incorrect, resulting in decreased reimbursement to the healthcare facility. It is the responsibility of the attending physician to decide on a principal diagnosis based on her best judgment.

ICD-9-CM Procedural Coding

The principal diagnosis and principal procedure are the reason for the hospital stay. Volumes 1 and 2 of ICD-9-CM are utilized to determine the proper diagnosis. Volume 3 of ICD-9-CM is used only for hospital procedures and should be utilized when the following conditions exist:

- The procedure is surgical in nature.
- The procedure carries a procedural risk.
- The procedure carries an anesthetic risk.
- The procedure requires specialized training.

Table 10.1 shows the major categories listed in the ICD-9-CM Volume 3 procedure index.

UB-04 Hospital Billing Claim Form

In 1982 the UB-82 claim form was developed for hospital claims and was printed in green ink. A revision was issued in 1992 because it was determined that an update was needed. The 1992 Uniform Billing (UB-92) claim form, also known as the CMS-1450, was the result of this update. With the passage of the Health Insurance Portability and Accountability Act of 1996, the UB-92 was revised and is now referred to as the UB-04.

The new form freed up space on the paper form and improved alignment of the paper claim to the electronic claim. The UB-04 form is divided into four sections and includes 81 different form locators. The four sections are:

1. Patient information (form locators 1–41)
2. Billing information (form locators 42–49 and claim line 23)

Table 10.1	ICD-9-CM Volume 3 Index

Operations on the Nervous System (01–05)

Operations on the Endocrine System (06–07)

Operations on the Eye (08–16)

Operations on the Ear (18–20)

Operations on the Nose, Mouth, and Pharynx (21–29)

Operations on the Respiratory System (30–34)

Operations on the Cardiovascular System (35–39)

Operations on the Hemic and Lymphatic System (40–41)

Operations on the Digestive System (42–54)

Operations on the Urinary System (55–59)

Operations on the Male Genital Organs (60–64)

Operations on the Female Genital Organs (65–71)

Obstetrical Procedures (72–75)

Operations on the Musculoskeletal System (76–84)

Operations on the Integumentary System (85–86)

Miscellaneous, Diagnostic and Therapeutic Procedures (87–99)

3. Payer information (form locators 50–65)
4. Diagnosis information (form locators 66–81)

The numbering system begins with 1 at the top of the form and moves from left to right and top to bottom to form locator 81. Each form locator name describes the type of information that is to be input into the field. The form is printed in red ink on white paper for processing with optical scanning equipment. Figure 10.3 is an example of a blank UB-04.

The UB-04 is considered a summary document supported by an itemized or detailed bill. The UB-04 is required by CMS and is accepted by private payers. It is used by institutional facilities to submit claims for inpatient and outpatient services. Let's take a look at the types of facilities that use the UB-04 form.

Inpatient care refers to a hospital confinement of more than 24 hours. Hospice facilities, which care for patients with terminal illnesses such as cancer and liver disease, also use the UB-04 for billing. **Hospice** is a type of coordinated care that can be delivered to either outpatients or inpatients to provide palliative services for terminally ill patients and their families.

Skilled nursing facilities (SNF) are another type of inpatient care. SNF units care for patients who have been in the hospital and do not require a hospital stay any longer but are still unable to take care of themselves at home. The services provided to patients in a SNF unit are given by licensed nurses under the direction of a physician. A SNF may be in the hospital or in an independent facility. A rehabilitation center is an independent facility that also cares for patients who have been in the hospital. An example would be a patient who was treated for a cerebrovascular accident (CVA) or stroke in the hospital and is recovering well. The patient may not have complete use of her limbs yet so, instead of being discharged home, the physician refers the patient to a rehabilitation center.

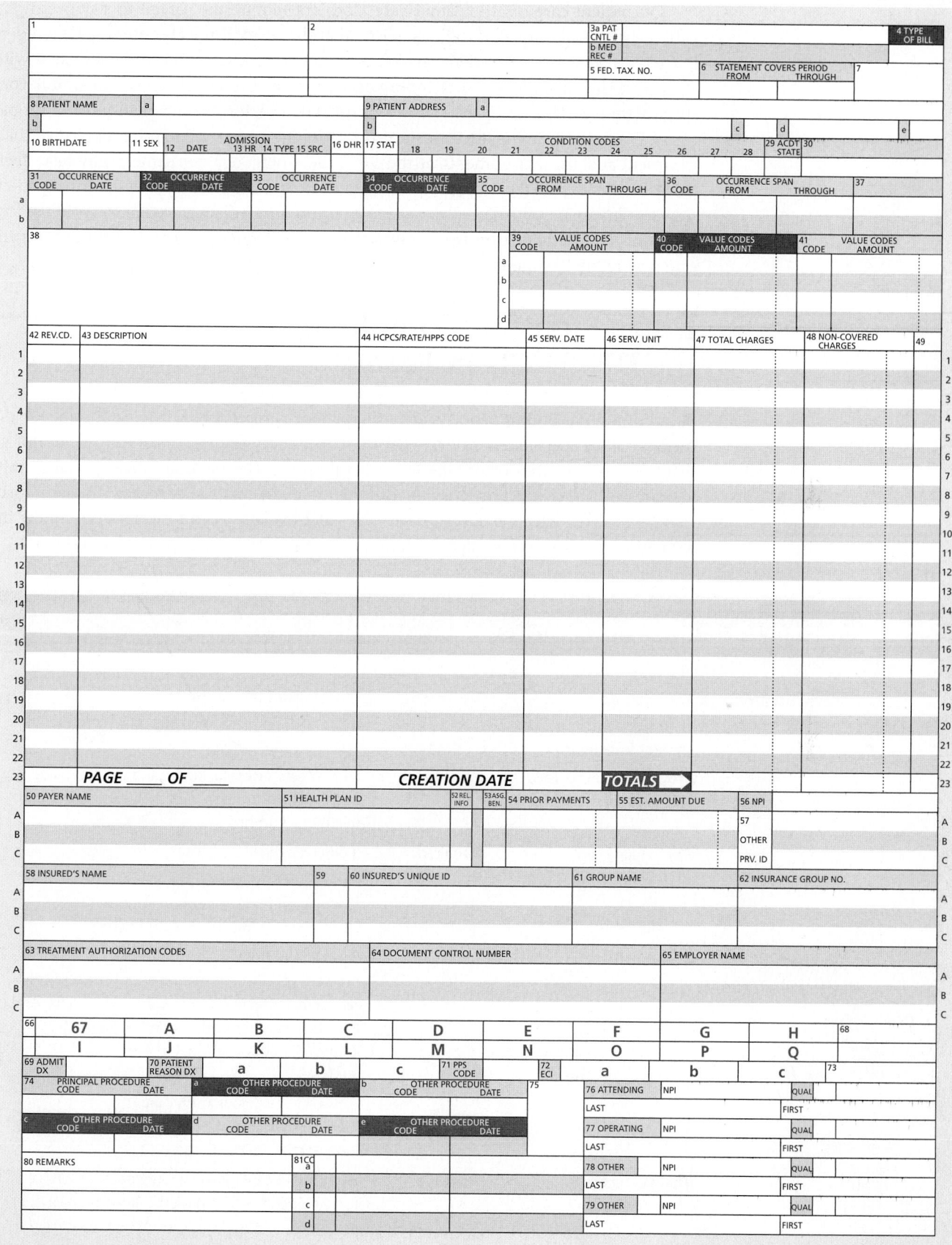

Figure 10.3   Sample UB-04 form.

Outpatient care or ambulatory care, does not require the patient to stay overnight. Different types of outpatient centers exist. An **ambulatory surgical center (ASC)** is a designated center where outpatient services are offered to patients. It may be affiliated with a particular hospital but is a freestanding building away from the hospital. An **ambulatory surgical unit (ASU)** is a department in a hospital that performs outpatient services for patients. **Emergency care** is also considered outpatient care because patients receive their treatment and are sent home. If, at the time, the emergency department physician feels the patient needs further care, the patient will be admitted to the hospital for inpatient services. Emergency situations are ones that require immediate attention to avoid the loss of life or limb. **Urgent care** is slightly different from emergency care. Although urgent care may require immediate attention, there is no risk of losing life or limb.

Instructions for Completing the UB-04 Claim Form

Because hospital billing happens after the patient is discharged, it is important for the medical office specialist to know what information is required in each form locator so that it can be gathered before the claim is submitted. The medical office specialist must choose the correct selection from the different types of codes in order for the claim form to be completed with the correct data. Table 10.2 explains each form locator and the information required to complete each of them. (*Note:* "N/A" means not applicable.)

Table 10.2   Explanation of Form Locators and Required Information

Form Locator	Description	Required?	Completion Instructions
	Patient Information		
1	Provider name, address, and telephone number	Required	Enter the name of the facility and the complete address of the location with a 9 digit zip code and telephone number.
2	Pay to name	Required	If different than FL 1.
3a–b	Patient control number	Optional	**Not required by Medicare.** *Line a:* Enter patient account number. *Line b:* Enter medical record number.
4	Type of bill	Required	Enter a valid three-digit "type of bill" code, which provides specific information about the services rendered. **Note:** Medicare requires four digits. Add 0 to the beginning of the code. See Table 10.3 for Type of Bill Codes.
5	Federal tax number	Required	A sub-ID can be reported if the facility has different wings, e.g., a rehabilitation wing. Provider indicated in box 1 assigned by the Internal Revenue Service (IRS).
6	Dates of service (from/through)	Required	Enter the beginning and ending dates of service for the period reflected on the claim in MMDDYY format.
7	Untitled	N/A	

| Table 10.2 | Explanation of Form Locators and Required Information (continued) |

Form Locator	Description	Required?	Completion Instructions
8a–b	Patient ID Patient name	Required	a. Patient ID **(not required by Medicare)** b. Last, first, and middle initial
9	Patient address	Required	a. Street address or P.O. box b. City c. State d. Zip code e. Country code (if applicable)
10	Birth date	Required	MMDDCCYY
11	Sex	Required	Refer to Table 10.4 for sex codes
12	Admission date	Required	MMDDYY
13	Admission hour	Optional	**Not required by Medicare. See Table 10.5 for codes**
14	Admission type	Required	See Table 10.6 for codes.
15	Admission source	Required	See Table 10.7 for codes
16	Discharge hour	Optional	**Not required by Medicare. See Table 10.5 for codes.**
17	Discharge status	Required	See Table 10.8
18–28	Condition code	Required	Enter the appropriate two-digit code. See Table 10.9
29	Accident state	Optional	Enter state in which accident occurred, if applicable.
30	Untitled	N/A	
31a–34b	Occurrence codes (31a–34a, 31b–34b)	Required	The two-digit code and the date must be entered. Begin with 31a and continue through the "a" entries before completing the "b" entries. See Table 10.10. Eight occurrence codes can be used.
35–36	Occurrence span code	Required	Enter the code and the dates from/through MMDDYY. See Table 10.11
37	Untitled	N/A	
38	Responsible party	Required	Enter responsible party's name, street address, city, state, and zip code.
39–41	Value codes	Required	Enter the value codes and related dollar amounts; covered days, noncovered days, coinsurance, etc. See Table 10.12
	Billing Information		
42	Revenue codes (A maximum of 22 services can be billed on one claim form with total charges and page number of claim entered on line 23.)	Required	Enter the standard three-digit uniform billing revenue codes to describe each type of accommodation and ancillary service billed. **Note:** Medicare requires four digits. Add 0 to the beginning of the code. "001" must be the final entry on all bills to identify total claim charges billed. See Table 10.13
43	Description (revenue code description)	Optional	**Not required by Medicare.** Enter the descriptor or standard abbreviation for each revenue code in FL 42.

(continued)

Table 10.2   Explanation of Form Locators and Required Information (continued)

Form Locator	Description	Required?	Completion Instructions
44	HCPCS/CPT-4, inpatient room rates, rehab rates	Required	If billing for an inpatient in a hospital, enter only the room rate. For outpatient billing, list all applicable HCPCS/CPT-4 codes.
45	Line item service dates for outpatient claims	Required	Enter the service date in MMDDYY format.
46	Service units	Required	*Inpatients:* Enter number of days. *Ancillary services:* Enter number of units. *Outpatient services:* Enter number of units when HCPCS/CPT-4 codes used.
47	Total charges	Required	Enter the charge amount for each line item reported.
48	Noncovered charges	Required	Include telephone, gift store, television.
49	Untitled	N/A	Data entered will be ignored.
23	Claim line 23	Required	End of revenue codes Page X of X Creation date: MMDDYY TOTALS: $$$.$$
	Payer Information		
50A–C	Payer name	Required	*Line A:* Primary Insurance *Line B:* Secondary Insurance *Line C:* Tertiary Insurance
51A	Health plan ID	Required	Enter the health plan provider number.
51B 51C	Secondary health plan Tertiary health plan	Required	If available, list the NPI.
52A–C	Release of information certification indicator	Required by HIPAA, state and federal laws	A "Y" indicates that a signed statement is on file permitting release of information to other organizations in order to adjudicate the claim. An "I" code indicates that informed consent has been given when a signature has not been obtained.
53A–C	Assignment of benefits	Required	**Not required by Medicare.** Data entered will be ignored. For each insurance carrier enter Y if an assignment of benefits form is on file, or N if no assignment of benefits form is on file.
54A	Prior payments	Required	**Other than inpatients should be reported in this field.** (For example, an outpatient who pays his deductible before a procedure.) **May not request prior payment from a Medicare patient unless it is the policy of the facility to request payment from all patients.** Report all prior payments for the claim. Attach an EOB from other carrier when applicable.
55	Estimated amount due	Optional	
56	National provider identifier	Required	This is the 10-digit NPI. Enter the valid NPI number of the servicing provider.
57A–C	Other provider's ID	Optional	Legacy provider numbers for other carriers (A–C).

Table 10.2	Explanation of Form Locators and Required Information (continued)		
Form Locator	**Description**	**Required?**	**Completion Instructions**
58 A–C	Insured's name	Required	Enter the name of the policyholder who is the subscriber/insured for each insurance indicated in FL 50A–C. **For Medicare enter the beneficiary's name (last, first, middle initial).**
59 A–C	Patient's relationship to insured	Required	Enter the applicable code that indicates the relationship of the patient to the insured noted in FL 58. See Table 10.14
60A–C	Health insurance claim identification number, Medicare ID, Medicaid ID, and/or subscriber's ID	Required	Enter the insured's identification number assigned by the payer organization, Medicare, Medicaid number, or the subscriber's number.
61A–C	Group name	Required	Enter the group name of the plan for the primary, secondary, and tertiary payer through which coverage is provided to the insured. **If Medicare is primary insurer, not required.**
62A–C	Insurance group number	Required	Enter the insurance group number if known.
63A–C	Treatment authorization codes	Required	When an authorization or referral is assigned by the payer, enter the authorization codes.
64A–C	Document control number	Required	Enter the control number assigned to the original bill by the health plan.
65A–C	Employer name	Required	Enter the name of the employer that provides health coverage for the individual identified on the same line in FL 58.
	Diagnosis Information		
66	Diagnosis qualifier	Required	Enter "9," which refers to the edition of the ICD that was used. ICD-9 is the only currently accepted version.
67	Principal diagnosis code	Required	The hospital enters the ICD code for the principal diagnosis.
67A–67Q	Other diagnosis codes— inpatient	Required	The hospital enters the full ICD codes for up to eight additional conditions if they coexist at the time of admission or developed subsequently and had an effect on the treatment or the length of stay. **Medicare will ignore date submitted in 67I–67Q.**
68	Untitled	N/A	
69	Admitting diagnosis	Required	For inpatient hospital claims the admitting dx is required.
70A–C	Patient's reason for visit	Required	Patient's reason for visit is required for all unscheduled outpatient visits for outpatient bills.
71	PPS code	Optional	Enter the prospective payment system code.
72	ECI codes	Optional	Enter external cause of injury (ECI) codes when applicable. **Not required by Medicare.** Data entered will be ignored.

(continued)

Table 10.2	Explanation of Form Locators and Required Information (continued)

Form Locator	Description	Required?	Completion Instructions
73	Untitled	N/A	
74	Principal procedure code and date	Required	Required on inpatient claims when a procedure was performed. Required for outpatient surgeries. **Medicare does not require for outpatient claims.**
74A–E	Other procedures and dates	Conditional	Required on inpatient claims when additional procedures are performed. Not used on outpatient claims.
75	Not used	N/A	
76	Attending provider name, NPI, and other identifiers	Required	Enter attending provider's last name, first name, and NPI. The secondary identifier qualifiers are: OB—state license number 1G—provider UPIN number G2—provider commercial number
77	Operating provider, name, NPI, and other identifiers	Required	Required when a surgical procedure code is listed on this claim. Enter provider's last, first name, and NPI. The secondary identifier qualifiers are: OB—state license number 1G—provider UPIN number E1—employer's identification number SY—Social Security number
78–79	Other provider type qualifier codes	Required	Enter the name and ID number of the individual corresponding to the qualifier category indicated in this section of the claim. The provider type qualifier codes are: DN—*Referring provider* is the provider who sends the patient to another provider for services. Required on an outpatient claim when the referring provider is different than the attending provider. ZZ—*Other operating provider* is the healthcare professional performing a secondary surgical procedure or assisting the operating physician. 82—*Rendering provider* is the healthcare professional who delivers or completes a particular medical or nonsurgical procedures. Refer to the secondary qualifiers as listed in FL 76-77.
80	Remarks	Conditional	Add any additional information pertaining to the claim. For durable medical equipment, show the rental rate, cost, and anticipated months of usage.
81	Code list qualifiers	Optional	A1—condition codes (FL 18–28) A2—occurrence codes (FL 31–34) A3—occurrence span codes (FL 35–36) A4—value codes (FL 39–41) B3—healthcare provider taxonomy codes (HPTC)

Codes for Use on the UB-04 Claim Form

The UB-04 requires different codes to be used to specify for the fiscal intermediary the type of bill, patient condition and cause, responsible party, rooms, occurrences, dates, time of admission and discharge, and other pertinent details. Revenue codes identify the department in which the services were rendered or from which supplies came. Value codes identify services and benefit days for Medicare patients. The following figures refer to specific form locators and provide examples of the information the code represents.

Revenue codes were originally three-digit codes. The need for additional codes mandated that the revenue codes become four-digit codes. The first digit should be a 0 followed by the three-digit code. The first two digits indicate which department rendered the service or supply.

Type of Bill Codes (Form Locator 4)

The type of bill code is a three-digit code that provides information about the type of bill, type of care, and the episode of care. Table 10.3 lists the acceptable type of bill codes.

All positions must be fully coded.

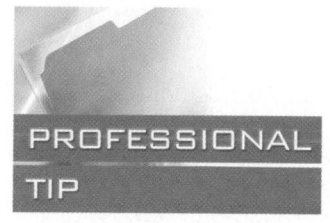

PROFESSIONAL TIP

Table 10.3	Examples of Types of Bill Codes for Use with Form Locator 4	
First Digit	**Type of Facility**	
1XX	Hospital	
11X	Inpatient (including Medicare Part A)	
12X	Inpatient (Medicare Part B only)	
13X	Outpatient	
14X	Other	
18X	Swingbed	
2XX	Skilled Nursing Facility	
21X	Inpatient (Medicare Part A)	
22X	Inpatient (Medicare Part B)	
23X	Outpatient	
3XX	Home Health Facility	
32X	Inpatient (Medicare Part B only)	
33X	Outpatient	
34X	Other	
4XX	Hospital—Christian Science	

(continued)

Table 10.3   Examples of Types of Bill Codes for Use with Form Locator 4 (continued)

First Digit	Type of Facility	
41X	Christian Science (Hospital)	
5XX	Extended Care—Christian Science (Medicare Part A)	
7XX	Clinic	
71X	Rural Health	
72X	Hospital-Based or Independent Renal Dialysis Center	
73X	Freestanding Provider-Based Federally Qualified Health Care Centers (FQHC)	
74X	Outpatient Rehabilitation Facility (ORF)	
75X	Comprehensive Outpatient Rehabilitation Facility (CORF)	
76X	Community Mental Health Center (CMHC)	
79X	Other	
8XX	Special Facilities Only	
81X	Hospice (Non-Hospital-Based)	
82X	Hospice (Hospital-Based)	
83X	Ambulatory Surgical Center Services to Hospital	
84X	Freestanding Birthing Center	
85X	Critical Access Hospital	
89X	Other	

Second Digit	Bill Classification	
X1X	Inpatient (Medicare Part A)	
X2X	Inpatient (Medicare Part B only)	
X3X	Outpatient	
X4X	Other (Part B), includes diagnostic clinical laboratory services to "nonpatients," and referred diagnostic services	
X5X	Intermediate Care Level I	
X6X	Intermediate Care Level II	
X8X	Swingbed	
X9X	Other	

Third Digit	Frequency	
XX1	Admit through Discharge Claim	Use this code for a bill encompassing an entire inpatient confinement or course of outpatient treatment for which the provider expects payment from the payer.
XX2	Interim—First Claim	Used for the first of an expected series of bills for which utilization is chargeable or which will update inpatient deductible for the same confinement or course of treatment.
XX4	Interim—Last Claim	Use this code for a bill for which utilization is chargeable and which is the last of a series for this confinement or course of treatment.

Table 10.3	Examples of Types of Bill Codes for Use with Form Locator 4 (continued)

Third Digit	Frequency	
XX7	Replacement of Prior Claim	Use to correct a previously submitted bill. Apply this code to the corrected or new bill.
XX8	Void/Cancel of Prior Claim	Use this code to indicate this bill is an exact duplicate of an incorrect bill previously submitted. A code "7" (replacement of prior claim) is being submitted showing corrected information.

NOTE: This three-digit code requires one digit of each, in the following sequence:

For Medicare use a 0 before the three digits.

1. Type of facility
2. Bill classification
3. Frequency.

Sex Codes (Form Locator 11)

The type of sex code is a one-digit code that is used to complete form locator 11, which must be filled out. See Table 10.4 for a list of sex codes.

Admission/Discharge Hour Codes (Form Locators 13 and 16)

The admission/discharge hour codes are listed in military time. Table 10.5 lists the admission/discharge hour codes.

Table 10.4	Sex Codes for Use with Form Locator 11

Code	Definition
M	Male
F	Female
U	Unknown

Table 10.5	Admission/Discharge Hour Codes for Use with Form Locators 13 and 16			
Code	**Time (A.M.)**		**Code**	**Time (P.M.)**
00	12:00–12:59 Midnight		12	12:00–12:59 Noon
01	01:00–01:59		13	01:00–01:59
02	02:00–02:59		14	02:00–02:59
03	03:00–03:59		15	03:00–03:59
04	04:00–04:59		16	04:00–04:59
05	05:00–05:59		17	05:00–05:59
06	06:00–06:59		18	06:00–06:59
07	07:00–07:59		19	07:00–07:59
08	08:00–08:59		20	08:00–08:59
09	09:00–09:59		21	09:00–09:59
10	10:00–10:59		22	10:00–10:59
11	11:00–11:59		23	11:00–11:59
			99	Hour Unknown

Source: Copyright (2005) by the National Uniform Billing Committee (NUBC). All rights reserved.

Admission Type Codes (Form Locator 14)

The type of admission codes establish the level of urgency for admission. See Table 10.6.

Table 10.6	Admission Type Code Examples for Use with Form Locator 14	
Code	**Definition**	
1	Emergency	The patient requires immediate medical intervention as a result of severe, life-threatening, or potentially disabling conditions.
2	Urgent	The patient requires immediate attention for the care and treatment of a physical or mental disorder.
3	Elective	The patient's condition permits adequate time to schedule the service.
4	Newborn	Use of this code necessitates the use of special source of admission codes (Form Locator 15).
5	Trauma	Visit to a trauma center/hospital as licensed or designated by the state or local government authority authorized to do so, or as verified by the American College of Surgeons and involving trauma activation. (Use revenue code 068 to capture trauma activation charges.)
9	Information Not Available	Information not available.

Source: Copyright (2005) by the National Uniform Billing Committee. All rights reserved.

Table 10.7	Admission Source Code Examples for Use with Form Locator 15

Code	Definition
1	Physician Referral
2	Clinic Referral
3	HMO Referral
4	Transfer from a Hospital
5	Transfer from a SNF
6	Transfer from Another Facility
7	Emergency Room
8	Court/Law Enforcement
9	Information Not Available
A	Transfer from a Critical Access Hospital (CAH)
B	Transfer from Another Home Health Agency
C	Readmission to Same Home Health Agency
D	Transfer from Hospital Inpatient to Same Facility Resulting in a Separate Claim to the Payer.

Source: Copyright (2005) by the National Uniform Billing Committee. All rights reserved.

Source of Admission (Form Locator 15)

The source of admission tells the payer how the patient was admitted and from where. *For newborn admissions only*, the source would be the type of delivery.

Table 10.7 provides admission source code examples.

Discharge Status Codes (Form Locator 17)

The type of discharge status defines where the patient was discharged to. This is especially important for Medicare patients for determining a covered benefit period. Table 10.8 includes discharge status code examples.

Condition Codes (Form Locators 18–28)

If applicable, enter specific condition codes pertaining to the patient's admission. Up to 11 conditions may be entered. These codes identify conditions that may affect the payer's processing of the bill because they identify special circumstances, events, room accommodations, or conditions that surround the services provided. Condition codes should be entered in alphanumeric sequence. See Table 10.9 for a list of condition codes.

Occurrence Code Examples (Form Locators 31–34)

Form locators 31 through 34 are used to describe the accident or mishap responsible for the patient's admission to the hospital and the date. The occurrence codes are used

Table 10.8	Discharge Status Code Examples for Use with Form Locator 17

Code	Definition
01	Discharged to home or self-care (routine discharge)
02	Discharged/transferred to a short-term general hospital for inpatient care
03	Discharged/transferred to an SNF with Medicare certification in anticipation of covered skilled care
05	Discharged/transferred to another type of health care institution not defined elsewhere in this code list
06	Discharged/transferred to home under care of an organized home health service organization in anticipation of covered skilled care
07	Left against medical advice or discontinued care
08	Discharged/transferred to home under care of home IV therapy provider
09	Admitted as an inpatient to this hospital
20	Expired (or did not recover)
30	Still a patient or expected to return for outpatient services
31–39	Still a patient to be defined at state level, if necessary
40	Expired at home (for hospice care only)
41	Expired in a medical facility such as a hospital, SNF, ICF, or freestanding hospice (for hospice care only)
42	Expired, place unknown (for hospice care only)
50	Discharged to hospice-home
51	Discharged to hospice-medical facility

Source: Copyright (2005) by the National Uniform Billing Committee. All rights reserved.

Table 10.9	Condition Codes for Use with Form Locators 18 through 28

Code	Description	Definition
01	Military Service Related	Medical condition incurred during military service.
02	Employment Related	Condition is employment related.
03	Ins Coverage Not Listed	Indicates that patient/patient representative has stated that coverage may exist beyond that reflected on this bill.
04	HMO Enrollee	Indicates bill is submitted for information only and the Medicare beneficiary is enrolled in a risk-based HMO and the provider expected to receive payment from the HMO.
05	Lien Has Been Filed	Provider has filed legal claim for recovery of funds potentially due a patient as a result of legal action initiated by, or on behalf of, the patient.
06	ESRD Patient in First Entitlement Period Covered by Employer Group Health Insurance	Code indicates Medicare may be a secondary insurer if the patient is also covered by employer group health insurance during patient's first entitlement period of end-stage renal disease (ESRD) entitlement.
07	Treatment of Nonterminal Condition for Hospice Patient	Code indicates the patient is a hospice enrollee, but the provider is not treating patient's terminal condition and is, therefore, requesting regular Medicare.

Table 10.9	Condition Codes for Use with Form Locators 18 through 28 (continued)

Code	Description	Definition
08	Pt Refuses Other Payer Info	Beneficiary would not provide information concerning coverage.
09	Neither Patient nor Spouse Employed	Indicates that in response to registration questions, the patient and spouse have denied any employment.
10	Patient and/or Spouse Is Employed but No EGHP Exists	Code indicates that in response to development questions, the patient and/or spouse have indicated that one or both are employed but have no group health insurance from an employer group health plan (EGHP) or other employer-sponsored or -provided health insurance that covers the patient.
17	Patient Is over 100 Years Old	Indicates that the patient is over 100 years old at date of admission or outpatient services.
20	Beneficiary Requested Billing	
21	Billing for Denial Notice	
31	Full-Time Student	
ACCOMMODATIONS		
37	Ward Accommodation at Patient Request	Patient assigned to ward accommodations at patient's request.
38	Semi-Private Room Not Available	Indicates that either private or ward accommodations were assigned because semiprivate accommodations were not available.
39	Private Room Medically Necessary	Patient needs a private room for medical requirements.
40	Same Day Transfer	Patient transferred to another facility before midnight on the day of admission.

to determine liability, coordinate benefits, and administer subrogation clauses. Please note that the occurrence span codes listed in Table 10.11 refer to dates only and do not relate to the occurrence codes Table 10.10. The from/through dates are used for repetitive Part B services to show a period of inpatient hospital care or outpatient surgery during this billing period. These codes also determine the patient's liability period.

Value Codes (Form Locators 39–41)

Value codes are two-digit codes that give the number of services provided and the amount. These form locators are also used for Medicare patients with regard to covered days, noncovered days, coinsurance days, and the lifetime reserve days. Table 10.12 includes value code examples for use in completing form locators 39 through 41.

Revenue Codes (Form Locator 42)

Revenue codes describe the department, type of care, service, or supply rendered. A maximum of 22 services may be billed on one claim form. Table 10.13 lists revenue code examples.

Table 10.10	**Occurrence Codes for Use with Form Locators 31 through 34**

Code	Description	Definition
01	Auto Accident	Code indicating the date of an auto accident.
02	No-Fault Insurance Involved (Including Auto Accident/Other)	Code indicating the date of an accident including auto or other where state has applicable no-fault liability laws (i.e., legal basis for settlement without admission or proof of guilt).
03	Accident/Tort Liability	Code indicating the date of an accident resulting from a third party's action that may involve a civil court process in an attempt to require payment by the third party, other than no-fault liability.
04	Accident/Employment Related	Code indicating the date of an accident allegedly relating to the patient's employment.
11	Onset of Illness	Code indicating the date patient first became aware of symptoms/illness.
18	Date of retirement for patient/beneficiary	
24	Insurance denied	Date insurance was denied.

Source: Copyright (2005) by the National Uniform Billing Committee. All rights reserved.

Table 10.11	**Occurrence Span Codes**

Code	Description	Definition
74	Leave of Absence	The from/through dates of a period at a noncovered level of care in an otherwise covered stay, excluding any period reported by **occurrence span code 76 or 77 below.** These codes are also used for repetitive Part B services to show a period of inpatient hospital care or outpatient surgery during the billing period. This code is also used for home health agency or hospice services billed under Part A.
76	Patient Liability Period	The from/through dates of a period of noncovered care for which the provider is permitted to charge the Medicare beneficiary. Code should be used only where the Peer Review Organization (PRO) or intermediary has approved such charges in advance and patient has been notified in writing at least 3 days prior to the from date of this period.
77	Provider Liability	The from/through dates of a period of noncovered care for which the provider is liable. The beneficiary's record is charged with Part A days, part A or part B deductible, and/or part B coinsurance. The provider may collect the part A or part B deductible and coinsurance from the beneficiary.

Source: Copyright (2005) by the National Uniform Billing Committee. All rights reserved.

Table 10.12	Value Code Examples for Use with Form Locators 39 through 41

Code	Description
12	Working aged
37	Pints of blood furnished
50	Physical therapy visits
53	Cardiac rehabilitation visits
80	Covered days
81	Noncovered days
82	Coinsurance days
83	Lifetime reserve days

Source: Copyright (2005) by the National Uniform Billing Committee. All rights reserved.

Patient Relationship (Form Locator 59)

The patient relationship form locator determines the relationship to the insured listed in form locator 58. Table 10.14 includes patient relationship code examples.

Practice Exercises

Complete Practice Exercises 10.1 through 10.5 by filling out the form locators on the UB-04 form based on the information given in each exercise and this chapter. This form can be located in Appendix D of the text.

Table 10.13	Revenue Code Examples for Use with Form Locator 42

Code	Definition
10X	All-Inclusive Rate
11X	R&B (Private/Med/Gen)
19X	Subacute Care
20X	Intensive Care
21X	Coronary Care
32X	Radiology—Therapeutic

Source: Copyright (2005) by the National Uniform Billing Committee. All rights reserved.

Table 10.14	Patient Relationship Code Examples for Use with Form Locator 59	
Code	**Definition**	
01	Spouse	
18	Patient Is Insured	
19	Natural Child—Insured Has Financial Responsibility	
43	Natural Child—Insured Does Not Have Financial Responsibility	
22	Handicapped Dependent	
29/53	Life Partner	
32	Mother	
33	Father	

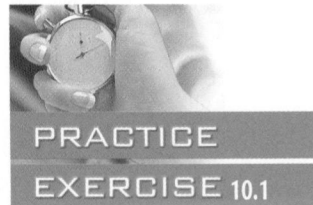

PRACTICE

EXERCISE 10.1

Fill out the form locators on the UB-04 form (located in Appendix D) based on the information given here. To complete this exercise, copy the UB-04 form provided in Appendix D or download it from the CD-ROM that accompanies this text.

Patient Information:

	Marion K. Perry
	1601 Amber Way
	Lancaster, TX 12345
	214-555-3456
DOB:	12-14-1970
Patient ID:	450-10-4320
	Single, Female
Employer:	Benefits Assistance
	1710 Firman St., #400
	Lancaster, TX 12345
	214-555-1928
	Full-time

Insurance Information:

	Great West Life Insurance Co.
	2300 Main Street
	Dallas, TX 75234
ID Number:	450104320
Group Number:	G12345

(continued)

History of Present Illness (HPI): Marion Perry was seen in the emergency room on January 3, 2009, at 1:15 p.m. She presented with severe chills for three hours. Patient has a past history of being hospitalized for pneumonia. She has had past difficulties with shortness of breath and respiratory difficulties that required steroids and antibiotics. Patient denies nausea, vomiting, diarrhea, or cough. She was admitted to the hospital for fever of unknown origin. Discharged at 3:30 p.m. on January 7, 2009.

PRACTICE
EXERCISE 10.1

(continued)

Attending Provider:	William F. Bonner, M.D.	
NPI:	2556622146	
UPIN:	654321	
Facility:	Presbyterian Hospital Dallas	
	2600 Walnut Hill Lane	
	Dallas, TX 12345	
	214-555-0001	
NPI:	5985561421	
Federal Tax Number:	75-1234567	3 Days are approved by carrier
Patient Control Number:	0100045	
Medical Record Number:	INI001PE	
Treatment Authorization Code:	2323444	
Health Plan ID Number:	5985561421	

List of Fees:

Revenue Codes			Date of Service
110	Room/Board/Semi.	$650.00	01/03/2009 to 01/07/2009
320	X-ray	$100.00	01/03/2009
324	X-ray/Chest	$275.00	01/03/2009
301	Lab Chemistry	$200.00	01/03/2009
981	ER Doctor	$300.00	01/03/2009
730	EKG	$175.00	01/03/2009
260	IV Therapy (4)	$250.00	01/03/2009 to 01/05/2009
262	IV Solutions (4)	$800.00	01/03/2009 to 01/05/2009
264	IV Supplies (4)	$400.00	01/03/2009 to 01/05/2009
001	TOTAL	$	

Principal DX: 491.21, 414.00, 272.4, 300.4
Admitting DX: 780.6
Principal Procedure Code: 99.21 (01-03-2009)

Assignment of benefits/release of information on file.

Check the accuracy of your work by comparing your claim form to the completed claim form in Appendix J.

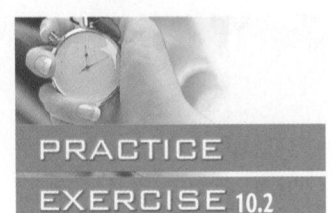

Fill out the form locators on the UB-04 form (located in Appendix D) based on the information given here. To complete this exercise, copy the UB-04 form provided in Appendix D or download it from the CD-ROM that accompanies this text.

Patient Information:

	Janet K. Stephens
	6589 Ridge Crest Lane
	Dallas, TX 12345
	214-555-9894
DOB:	3-21-55
Social Security number:	555-89-9877
	Married, female
Employer:	Homemaker

Insurance Information:

Insured's Name:	John D. Stephens (spouse)
Address:	Same
DOB:	11-14-54
Carrier:	Blue Cross Blue Shield
Carrier Address:	4899 S. Insurance Processing Blvd.
	Bluespring, MO 45898
ID Number:	658-88-3328
Group Number:	65432
Employer:	Jane's Video
	1616 Lovers Lane
	Dallas, TX 12345
	214-555-6544

History of Present Illness (HPI): Janet Stephens showed up at Trinity Medical Center emergency room on May 1, 2009, at 7:05 p.m. She was complaining of severe head pain and shortness of breath. She was admitted to the hospital for further evaluation and discharged on May 3, 2009, at 1:30 p.m.

Attending Physician:

	Francis J. Brown, M.D.
NPI:	2348810011
BCBS ID:	551012
UPIN:	208321
Facility:	Trinity Medical Center
	1234 Avenue
	Carrollton, TX 12345
	972-555-4300
NPI:	9876223551
Federal Tax Number:	75-1215977
Medical Record Number:	695247
Treatment Authorization Code:	1012559 Approved: 3 days
Health Plan ID Number:	9876223551

(continued)

List of Fees:
Revenue Codes

110	Room/Board/Semi (2)	$615.00	05/01/2009 to 05/03/2009
740	EEG	$400.00	05/01/2009
351	CT Scan	$940.00	05/02/2009
610	MRI	$1050.00	05/01/2009
250	Pharmacy	$630.00	05/01/2009
900	Respiratory Services (10)	$456.00	5/1/2009, 5/2/2009
450	Emergency Room	$770.50	05/01/2009
990	Personal Items	$25.50	05/01/2009

Principal DX:	437.3
Admitting DX:	786.05
Principal Procedure Code:	331 (05-01-2009)
Patient Control Number:	0010015

Assignment of benefits/release of information on file.

Check the accuracy of your work by comparing your claim form to the completed claim form in Appendix J.

PRACTICE EXERCISE 10.2

(continued)

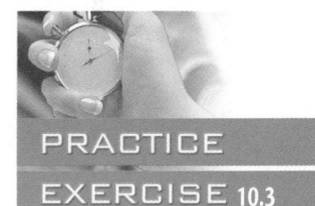

PRACTICE EXERCISE 10.3

Fill out the form locators on the UB-04 form (located in Appendix D) based on the information given here. To complete this exercise, copy the UB-04 form provided in Appendix D or download it from the CD-ROM that accompanies this text.

Patient Information:

	Michael R. James
	5489 Slow Bend Drive
	Dallas, TX 12345
	214-555-9458
DOB:	7-1-1968
Social Security number:	555-55-5544
	Married, male
Employer:	Jim's Wholesale Club
	1698 Forest Lane
	Dallas, TX 12345
	214-555-4900
	Full-time

(continued)

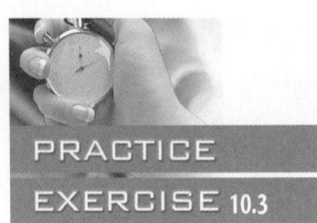

Insurance Information:

Insured's Name:	Jennifer M. James (spouse)
Address:	same
DOB:	4-11-1968
Carrier:	Cigna PPO
Carrier Address:	4899 S. Insurance Processing Blvd.
	East Insurance City, MO 45898
ID Number:	555-66-6548
Group Number:	8488
Employer:	NASTEC, Inc.
	222 Career Center
	Dallas, TX 12345
	972-555-2525

History of Present Illness (HPI): Michael James arrived at University Medical Center Emergency Room at 11:15 p.m. on January 21, 2009, patient complaining of severe lower abdominal pain. He was admitted to the hospital and released on January 23, 2009, at 10:00 a.m.

Attending Physician:	Dennis J. O'Connor, M.D.
NPI:	4589854428
Cigna Pin:	27069
Facility:	University Medical Center
	1700 Jose Lane
	Carrollton, TX 12345
	972-555-4400
NPI:	5874446521
Federal Tax Number:	75-251487
Medical Record Number:	232774
Treatment Authorization
Code:	551478 Approved: 2 days
Health Plan ID Number:	5874446251

List of Fees:

Revenue Codes (1 unit each)			Dates of Service
110	Room/Board Private	$615.00	01/21–01/23/2009
320	X-ray	$275.00	01/21/2009
305	Lab/Chemistry	$180.00	01/22/2009
260	IV Therapy	$125.00	01/22/2009
250	Pharmacy	$208.00	01/23/2009
730	EKG/ECG	$210.00	01/23/2009

Principal DX:	531.00 Acute Gastric Ulcer with hemorrhage
Admitting DX:	789.09 Abdominal Pain
Principal Procedure Code:	44.41 (01-21-2009)
Patient Control Number:	0030087

Assignment of benefits/release of information forms on file.

Check the accuracy of your work by comparing your claim form to the completed claim form in Appendix J.

Fill out the form locators on the UB-04 form (located in Appendix D) based on the information given here. To complete this exercise, copy the UB-04 form provided in Appendix D or download it from the CD-ROM that accompanies this text.

Patient Information:

	Olive Westcot
	5 Apple Lane
	West Hartford, CT 12345
	860-555-2269
DOB:	3-2-49
Social Security number:	144-40-1442
	Single, Female
Employer:	Jamison Casket
	68 West Avenue
	Hartford, CT 12345
	860-555-8956
	Full-time

Insurance Information:

	Aetna
	215 Sisson Avenue
	Hartford, CT 06106
ID Number:	005598JA
Group Number:	JAM908
Admitting Physician:	Charles W. Henderson, M.D.
PIN:	56891T
NPI:	0006667999

History of Present Illness (HPI): Ms. Westcott presented herself to the emergency room complaining of abdominal pain. She was evaluated and admitted to the hospital at 1:35 p.m. on 02/26/2009. She was discharged at 9:45 a.m. on 02/28/2009.

Facility:

	Presbyterian Hospital Dallas
	2600 Walnut Hill Lane
	Dallas, TX 12345
	214-555-0001
NPI:	5985561421
Federal Tax Number:	75-1234567 3 Days are approved by carrier
Patient Control Number:	987625941
Medical Record Number:	OLIWES0226
Treatment Authorization Code:	900ASC
Health Plan ID Number:	5985561421

(continued)

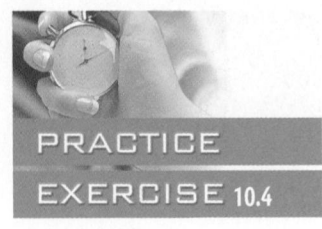

PRACTICE
EXERCISE 10.4

(continued)

List of Fees:

Revenue Codes			Date of Service
110	Semiprivate room	$340.00	02/26/2009
730	ECG	$95.00	02/27/2009
997	Admission Kit	$25.00	02/26/2009
351	CT Scan	$1,536.00	02/27/2009
300	Lab	$356.00	02/26/2009
981	ER Doctor	$300.00	02/26/2009
001	TOTAL	$2992.00	

Principal DX:	574.50	Hepatolithiasis
Admitting DX:	789.09	Abdominal Pain
Principal Procedure Code:	51.41	(02-26-2009)

Assignment of benefits/release of information forms on file.

Check the accuracy of your work by comparing your claim form to the completed claim form in Appendix J.

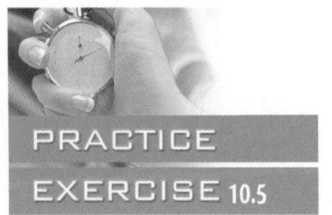

PRACTICE
EXERCISE 10.5

Fill out the form locators on the UB-04 form (located in Appendix D) based on the information given here. To complete this exercise, copy the UB-04 form provided in Appendix D or download it from the CD-ROM that accompanies this text.

Patient Information:

Alyssa M. Smith
10552 Candlewood
Las Cruces, NM 12345
505-555-0669

DOB: 4/2/1971
Social Security number: 563-88-5691
Single, Female
Employer: Olive's Garden
10305 Gateway West
Las Cruces, NM 12345
505-555-3611
Full-time

Insurance Information:

BCBS HMO
6933 Coit
Dallas, TX 75206
ID Number: ZGY563885691

(continued)

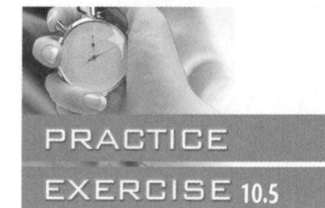

PRACTICE EXERCISE 10.5

(continued)

Group Number:	00063952
Admitting Physician:	Francis J. Bonner, M.D.
PIN:	110992F
NPI:	5555555555

History of Present Illness (HPI): Alyssa Smith was given orders from her physician to have an outpatient radiology procedure done. She came to the outpatient registration department at 8:00 a.m. on 1/10/2009 for her procedure. She was registered and sent to the radiology department for her test.

Facility:	University Medical Center
	1700 Josey Lane
	Carrollton, TX 12345
	972-555-4400
NPI:	5116523337
Federal Tax Number:	75-251487 1 Visit approved by carrier
Patient Control Number:	36249967
Medical Record Number:	SMI4291ALY
Treatment Authorization Code:	693358924
Health Plan ID Number:	5116523337

List of Fees:

Revenue Codes (1 unit each)	Date of Service
341 Radioisotope scan of the liver (78205)	01/10/2009
001 TOTAL $ 756.50	

Principal DX:	572.4 Hepatorenal Syndrome	
Principal Procedure Code:	92.02	(01/10/2009)

Assignment of benefits/release of information forms on file.

Check the accuracy of your work by comparing your claim form to the completed claim form in Appendix J.

Chapter Summary

- Each hospital has a master patient index, which is the main database of all the hospital's patients. As a patient arrives and goes through the registration or admission process, the patient is assigned a patient control number (PCN), which is a unique number given for each hospital admission.
- Each patient's data, consisting of revenue codes, procedure codes, descriptions, charges, and medical record data, are organized by the charge description master and printed onto a hospital Uniform Bill claim form, the UB-04, also known as the CMS-1450.
- Hospitals contract with managed care organizations and government health plans and negotiate fees for reimbursement.

- Three basic reimbursement methods are used for inpatient hospital services: prospective payment system, fee-for-service, and per diem.
- The DRG prospective payment system is a patient classification method that categorizes patients who are medically related with respect to diagnosis and treatment and who are statistically similar in terms of their length of hospital stay.
- ICD-9-CM Volume 3 is used for coding hospital procedures.
- The UB-04 is considered a summary document supported by an itemized or detailed bill. It is used by institutional facilities (e.g., inpatient and outpatient departments, rural health clinics, chronic dialysis services, and adult day health care) to submit claims for inpatient and outpatient services.
- The four sections of the UB-04 are patient information, billing information, payer information, and diagnosis information.

Chapter Review

True/ False

Identify the statement as true (T) or false (F).

_____ 1. The DRG indicates the medications the patient is taking while in the hospital.

_____ 2. Hospitals bill for services only after the discharge summary is completed and signed by the physician.

_____ 3. An occurrence code describes the accident or mishap responsible for the patient's admission.

_____ 4. The revenue code is a five-digit code number representing a specific accommodation, ancillary service, or billing calculation related to the service.

_____ 5. Ambulatory Payment Classification (APC) system is based on procedures rather than diagnoses.

_____ 6. An inpatient is one who has been seen in the emergency department.

_____ 7. A case that cannot be assigned an appropriate DRG because of an atypical situation is called a budget outlier.

_____ 8. The type of discharge status defines where the patient was discharged to.

_____ 9. The rendering provider is the provider who attended the patient.

_____ 10. The PCN is the unique number given to the patient at admission.

_____ 11. Patient's reason for visit is required only on scheduled outpatient visits for outpatient bills.

_____ **12.** Birth dates on the UB-04 form should be shown in the MMDDCCYY format.

_____ **13.** The UB-04 form requires information about the source of a patient's admission.

_____ **14.** A charge master contains a hospital's list of services, codes, and charges.

Multiple Choice

Identify the letter of the choice that best completes the statement or answers the question.

_____ **1.** A hospice is a facility that cares for:
   a. auto accident victims.   c. Medicare patients.
   b. patients with a terminal illness. d. individuals without insurance.

_____ **2.** A charge description master or *charge master* includes the following information:
   a. patient's demographics   c. procedure codes
   b. number of clinic visits   d. superbill

_____ **3.** Which term describes the patient's condition that is the diagnosis established after study or testing?
   a. inpatient   c. principal procedure
   b. principal diagnosis   d. admitting diagnosis

_____ **4.** Which term describes the patient's condition upon hospital admission?
   a. inpatient   c. admitting diagnosis
   b. principal diagnosis   d. principal procedure

Matching

Choose the best word or phrase that matches the description.

   a. admitting physician   h. ambulatory payment classification
   b. ASC   i. ASU
   c. attending physician   j. comorbidity
   d. DRG   k. grouper
   e. rendering physician   l. principal diagnosis
   f. prospective payment system   m. Outpatient Prospective Payment System
   g. patient control number   n. charge master

_____ **1.** Unique number given to the patient for each hospital admission.

_____ **2.** Sheet that contains the following information: procedure code, procedure, description, service description, charge and the revenue code.

_____ **3.** Outpatient payment classification system based on procedures.

_____ **4.** Established payment rates for hospitals prior to services being rendered.

_____ **5.** A form of PPS that categorizes diagnoses and treatments into groups.

_____ **6.** OPPS

_____ **7.** A program that calculates and assigns the DRG payment group.

_____ **8.** The physician who only admits the patient to the hospital.

_____ **9.** Preexisting condition that affects the principal diagnosis.

_____ **10.** Department in the hospital that performs outpatient services for patients.

_____ **11.** Designated center where outpatient services are offered to patients.

_____ **12.** A provider who is primarily responsible for the patient's care.

_____ **13.** The reason for the hospital stay.

_____ **14.** Provider who renders a service.

For Additional Practice

Complete the UB-04 form (located in Appendix D) with the following information:

Patient Information:

Name:	Charlotte Webb
	6589 Slow Curve Lane
	Dallas, TX 12345
	214-555-9874
Social Security number:	555-89-9877
DOB:	3/14/36
	Married, Female
Employer:	Bob's Crab Shack
	1629 Lovers Lane
	Dallas, TX 12345
	214-555-6786
	Employed Full Time

Primary Insurance:

Insured's Name:	Michael Webb (Husband)
Employer:	ABC Incorporated
Employer address:	2222 Stillwater Blvd Dallas, TX 12345
Blue Cross Blue Shield ID Number:	XYC555
Group Number:	551489

Case Information:

Patient arrived at the Presbyterian emergency room on January 9, 2009, at 10:45 p.m. She presented with symptoms of low abdominal pain. She has been complaining of pain to her right side. She was admitted to the hospital on January 9, 2009, @ 10:45 p.m. and discharged on January 12, 2009 @ 1:00 p.m.

Attending Physician:

	Dr. William Fredrickson
NPI:	5555005555
UPIN Number:	6654321
BCBS ID Number:	665599

Facility:

Presbyterian Hospital Dallas   3 Days are approved
2600 Walnut Hill Lane
Dallas, TX 12345
214-555-8989

NPI:	2354498762
Federal Tax ID Number:	74-1258923
Patient Control Number:	9877773 Claim filed to carrier on 01-12-2009
Medical Record Number:	CW1515633
Treatment Auth Code:	1973888
Health Plan ID Number:	2354498762

Assignment of Benefits and Release of Information on file

List of Fees:
Revenue Codes:

010	Room & Board:	$300.00 per day (3)	01-09-2009
320	X-ray: 2 views:	$250.00	01-09-2009
981	ER Doctor:	$200.00	01-09-2009
300	Lab:	$375.00	01-10-2009

Principal Dx:	540.0
Admitting Dx:	789.09
Principal Procedure:	86.0
Principal Procedure Date:	1/10/20XX

Resources

The website for the National Uniform Billing Committee (NUBC) should be visited frequently to be aware of any changes in the billing form. The reader should go to this website listed below and click on "What's New" in the menu to find any new information. *http://www.nubc.org*

Government Medical Billing

This section will provide the student with the knowledge to accurately file Medicare, Medicaid, and TRICARE claims. Medicare is a federal health insurance program established by Congress for the elderly, people with disabilities, and individuals who have end-stage renal disease. A large percentage of elderly Americans and those with disabilities are covered by the Medicare program, so it is important that the medical office specialist have a thorough understanding of Medicare claims processing. Chapter 11 discusses Medicare billing in detail.

Medicaid is a federal/state entitlement program that pays for medical assistance for certain individuals and families with low incomes and resources. Medicaid is the largest source of funding for medical and health-related services for low-income individuals, some of whom may have no medical insurance or inadequate medical insurance. Medicaid is also available for individuals who have disabilities or are blind and for pregnant women and children, though certain requirements must be met. Chapter 12 provides detailed information on Medicaid guidelines and claims filing.

TRICARE is the Department of Defense's medical entitlement program. It covers eligible uniformed services beneficiaries for medically necessary care. Chapter 13 provides an in-depth look at TRICARE and CHAMPVA, submitting claims to TRICARE on the Internet, and completing the CMS-1500 claims form for TRICARE.

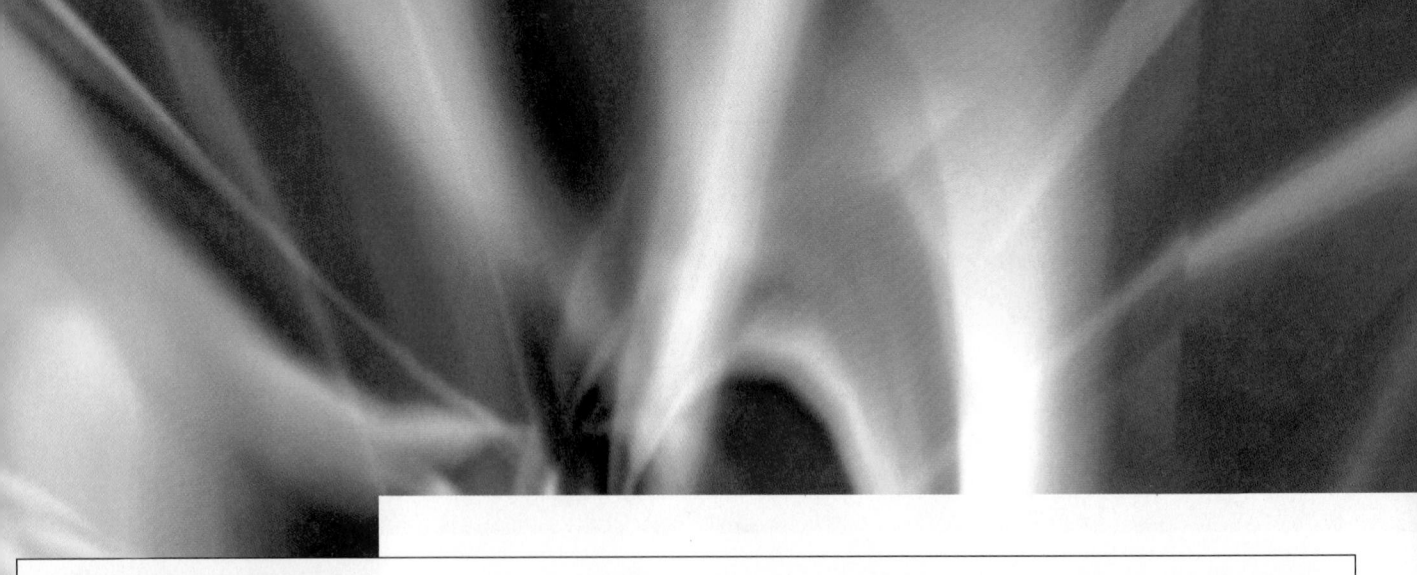

My name is Sharon Goucher-Norris. I started working at Medicare 3 months after the Medicare program came into existence in 1966. After 6 years there, I went to work for a plastic surgeon, then a community hospital. I eventually ended up at Blue Cross, first in customer service, then in training, where I spent the majority of my career. Today I am teaching the next generation of medical billers and claims processors.

I have seen the industry go from entirely paper-based, to terminals to PCs, to complete electronic claims processing. What the job insurance specialists do today is more specialized and requires more knowledge than in the past. The easy claims are processed entirely by the computer. The ones that edit out for human intervention are the more complex cases, requiring more investigation and a greater understanding of medical procedures and insurance rules. Education and training are essential in today's environment.

The keys to success in this field are openness to change and being a good communicator, with both internal and external customers. There is much opportunity for growth and advancement in the insurance side of the business, as larger companies conduct internal training and support external education as well. It really makes my day when I see one of my students get a new job.

Chapter 11 Medicare Medical Billing

Chapter Objectives

After reading this chapter, the student should be able to:

1. Discuss government billing guidelines.
2. Determine the amount due from the patient for a participating provider.
3. Understand the different Medicare Fee Schedules.
4. Examine and complete accurate Medicare claims forms.
5. Identify the types of Medicare fraud and abuse that can occur.

Key Terms

benefit period
Consolidated Omnibus
   Budget Reconciliation
   Act of 1985 (COBRA)
crossover
end-stage renal disease
   (ESRD)
intermediaries
limiting charge
Local Coverage
   Determinations (LCDs)

Medicare abuse
Medicare Advantage
   (MA)
Medicare Development
   Letter
Medicare fraud
Medicare Part A
Medicare Part B
Medicare Part D
Medicare Remittance
   Notice (MRN)

Medicare secondary payer
   (MSP)
Medicare Summary Notice
   (MSN)
Medigap
non-par MFS
Physician Quality
   Reporting Initiative
   (PQRI)
Tax Relief and Health Care
   Act (TRHCA)

Ramon has received a bill for his recent visit to the doctor's office. He is confused, because he has Medicare and American Association of Retired Persons (AARP) insurance and does not believe he should owe anything. He called AARP and they stated they never received a bill for the visit. He had been told that all claims would come directly from Medicare. He then called Medicare and asked why they had not sent the claim to AARP. Medicare stated that the physician's office had not listed AARP as a secondary insurance carrier on the claim. Ramon realized that he had not given the office his AARP card at his visit.

Questions

1. How could his physician's office have prevented this problem?
2. What is it called when Medicare forwards a claim to the secondary insurance?
3. If this claim had fallen under the Medicare deductible, would the secondary insurance pick up the change?

Introduction

Medicare is a federal health insurance program established by Congress for the elderly, people with disabilities, and individuals afflicted with **end-stage renal disease (ESRD)**. A large percentage of elderly Americans and those with disabilities are covered by the Medicare program. The network of Medicare administrators, contractors, and providers throughout the United States is kept quite busy serving the needs of Medicare beneficiaries.

Medicare History

Since the beginning of the 20th century, healthcare issues have continued to escalate in importance for our nation. There has long been broad agreement in the United States on the real need for some form of universal health insurance to alleviate the unpredictable and uneven costs associated with medical care.

In 1965, Congress acted to create a comprehensive program called Medicare that would provide medical insurance for elderly people who needed assistance with medical expenses. In 1972, Medicare benefits were also given to individuals with disabilities and those with ESRD. Today, more than 39 million Americans are enrolled in the Medicare program.

Medicare is divided into two main programs: **Medicare Part A**, which is hospital insurance, and **Medicare Part B**, which is medical insurance. In 1997 a new option was added called Medicare+Choice. This is now known as **Medicare Advantage** or **MA** for short.

Medicare Advantage offers expanded benefits for a fee through private health insurance programs such as health maintenance organizations and preferred provider organizations that have contracts with Medicare. This program is commonly referred to as Part C, although the Medicare administration does not label it as such. In 2006 **Medicare Part D** became available to participants for prescription drug coverage.

Medicare Administration

The Medicare program is administered by the Centers for Medicare and Medicaid Services (CMS), a division of the U.S. Department of Health and Human Services, located in Baltimore, Maryland. CMS (formerly called the Health Care Financing Administration) was created in 1977 by Congress to serve as a consolidated agency that would administer both Medicare and Medicaid—the two largest healthcare programs in the United States. CMS serves the Medicare program and Medicare beneficiaries in many ways. Its roles include:

- Establishing policy for the reimbursement of providers
- Conducting research into healthcare management and treatment
- Assessing the quality of healthcare facilities and services.

The agency's primary function is to ensure that its contractors and state agencies properly administer Medicare. CMS has established several regional offices throughout the nation to ensure support for all Medicare contractors.

The Social Security Administration (SSA) also assists CMS to administer Medicare by enrolling new Medicare beneficiaries into the program. The SSA also collects Medicare premiums and maintains the Medicare master beneficiary record.

Medicare is administered on the regional level by Medicare contractors. A Medicare contractor is an organization that has an agreement with CMS to administer the local Medicare program for all providers in their specified state or region. There are many contractors throughout the nation. Individual Medicare contractors may administer Medicare Part A, Medicare Part B, or both programs for their locale.

Medicare Part A contractors are called **intermediaries**, while Medicare Part B contractors are called carriers.

Medicare Part A: Intermediaries

Some of the roles and responsibilities of Medicare Part A intermediaries include:

- Determining costs and reimbursement amounts
- Maintaining records
- Establishing controls
- Safeguarding against fraud and abuse or excess use
- Conducting reviews and audits
- Making the payments to providers for services
- Assisting both providers and beneficiaries as needed.

Medicare Part B: Carriers

Some of the roles and responsibilities of Medicare Part B carriers include:

- Determining charges allowed by Medicare
- Maintaining quality of performance records
- Assisting in fraud and abuse investigations
- Making payments to physicians and suppliers for services that are covered under Part B
- Assisting both suppliers and beneficiaries as needed.

The primary responsibility of intermediaries and carriers is to process (adjudicate) and reimburse Medicare claims submitted by providers.

Medicare Part A Coverage and Eligibility Requirements

Medicare Part A coverage (also known as *hospital insurance*) includes the following:

- Inpatient hospital care
- Inpatient care in a skilled nursing facility (SNF)
- Home health care
- Hospice care.

The intermediary determines payment and processes claims for Part A facilities for covered items and services provided by the facility. Part A provides benefits for inpatient services provided at hospitals and SNFs. There is no premium if the beneficiary is eligible for Medicare.

To qualify for Medicare Part A, individuals must meet Medicare's eligibility requirements under one of it beneficiary categories:

1. *Individuals 65 or older:* Individuals age 65 or older who have paid or the beneficiary's spouse has paid FICA taxes or Railroad Retirement Board taxes for at least 40 calendar quarters.
2. *Adults with disabilities:* Individuals who have been receiving Social Security disability benefits or Railroad Retirement Board disability benefits for more than 2 years. Coverage begins 5 months after the 2 years of entitlement.
3. *Individuals who became disabled before age 18:* Individuals under the age of 18 who meet the disability criteria of the Social Security Act.
4. *Spouses of entitled individuals:* Spouses of deceased or retired individuals or individuals with disabilities who were or still are entitled to Medicare benefits.
5. *Retired federal employees enrolled in the Civil Service Retirement System (CSRS):* Retired CSRS employees and their spouses.
6. *Individuals with ESRD:* Individuals of any age who receive dialysis or a renal transplant for ESRD. Coverage typically begins on the first day of the month following the start of dialysis treatments. In the case of a transplant, entitlement begins the month the individual is hospitalized for the transplant (the transplant must be completed within 2 months). The donor is covered for services related to the donation of the organ only.

Individuals who are over age 65 who do not receive social security benefits may purchase Part A insurance by paying a premium of $410.00 a month (as of 2007).

Inpatient Hospital Care

Medicare Part A provides coverage for inpatient hospital care. A patient is eligible for 90 days of hospital care in a benefit period, as long as medical necessity for the admission and the number of days has been proven. Coverage includes semiprivate rooms, meals, general nursing, and other hospital services and supplies. This does not include private duty nursing or a television or telephone in the room. It also does not include a private room, unless medically necessary. The patient also has a lifetime reserve of 60 days that could be used once the 90 days have been exhausted. Once the reserve days have been used, they are not replenished.

Skilled Nursing Facility

Part A provides coverage for a skilled nursing facility. A patient is eligible for 100 days of care in a SNF during a benefit period, as long as medical necessity for the admission and the number of days has been proven. Semiprivate room, meals, skilled nursing and rehabilitative services, and other services and supplies (after a related 3-day inpatient hospital stay) are also covered.

Home Health Care

Part A provides coverage for home health care. Home health care is defined as part-time or intermittent skilled nursing care and home health aide services, physical therapy, occupational therapy, speech-language therapy, medical social services, durable medical equipment (such as wheelchairs, hospital beds, oxygen, and walkers), medical supplies, and other services. There is no time limit on home health care as long as medical necessity has been proven.

Hospice Care

Part A provides coverage for hospice care. Hospice care is for individuals with a terminal illness and includes drugs for symptom control and pain relief, medical and support services from a Medicare-approved hospice, and other services not otherwise covered by Medicare. Hospice care can be given in the home. However, Medicare covers short-term hospital and inpatient respite care (care given to a hospice patient so that the usual caregiver can rest).

Inpatient Benefit Days

A **benefit period** is a period of time during which medical benefits are available to an insurance beneficiary. For Medicare Part A, a benefit period:

- Starts the day a patient enters the hospital if the patient has not been an inpatient or a SNF patient in the last 60 days.
- Ends when the patient has not been an inpatient or SNF patient for 60 consecutive days.

With Medicare Part A, a patient may be allowed up to 150 days of coverage when you include the regular 90-day benefit period (60 basic days and 30 coinsurance days) and the 60 lifetime reserve days. The different types of days are discussed next.

Basic Days

Basic days are the first 60 days of acute inpatient care provided to a beneficiary during a benefit period. Medicare Part A criteria for the basic days are as follows:

- The beneficiary's financial responsibility is limited to the benefit period deductible.
- There is no coinsurance.
- If exhausted, these days are recycled once a new benefit period begins.

Table 11.1 illustrates how the deductibles for Medicare patients have been changed over the years.

Table 11.1	Changes in Deductibles for Medicare Patients for Days 1 through 60 of Each Benefit Period	
	Year	Deductible
	2004	$876.00
	2005	$912.00
	2006	$952.00
	2007	$992.00

Coinsurance Days

Medicare patients hospitalized for more than 60 days in a benefit period must pay coinsurance if they remain in the hospital.

> ### Example
>
> | Days 1–60 | Full benefits |
> |---|---|
> | Days 61–90 | Coinsurance |
> | Days 91–150 | Lifetime reserve |
>
> **Coinsurance is a daily charge of one-quarter of the current Part A deductible:**
>
> | $992.00 (2007) | $952.00 (2006) |
> |---|---|
> | × 0.25 | × 0.25 |
> | $248.00 per day | $238.00 per day |

Lifetime Reserve Days (LTR)

Once a patient with Medicare Part A has used 90 days in one benefit period (60 basic days and 30 coinsurance days), he or she becomes eligible to start using 60 lifetime reserve days for the 91st through 150th day of acute inpatient care during that same benefit period.

- Once the reserve days have been used, they cannot be renewed. That is, if the beneficiary elects to use these days, they can never be reused.
- The charge to the beneficiary for using reserve days is one-half of the current Part A deductible.

An example of the cost of using lifetime reserve days is calculated in the following example.

> ### Example
>
> **Lifetime reserve days include a daily charge (coinsurance) of one-half of the current Medicare Part A deductible:**
>
> | $992.00 (2007) | $952.00 (2006) |
> |---|---|
> | × 0.5 | × 0.5 |
> | $496.00 per day | $476.00 per day |

Skilled Nursing Facility Days

The coinsurance for stays in an SNF as of 2007 were:

- $0 for the first 20 days of each benefit period
- $124.00 per day for days 21 through 100 of each benefit period.

Medicare Part B Coverage and Eligibility Requirements

Medicare Part B insurance helps pay for physician services in both hospital and nonhospital settings, outpatient hospital services, emergency departments, diagnostic tests, clinical laboratory services, outpatient physical therapy, speech therapy services, durable medical equipment, ambulance transportation, and rural health clinic services.

To qualify for Medicare Part B, individuals must meet Medicare's eligibility requirements under one of it beneficiary categories:

> Medicare Part B also covers diagnostic and emergency department services for inpatients if the beneficiary does not have or has exhausted Part A coverage.

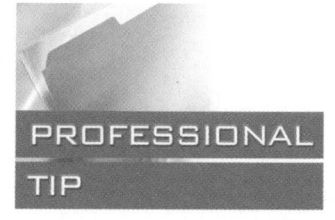
PROFESSIONAL TIP

- Must meet requirements for Medicare Part A
- Or have purchased Medicare Part A.

To purchase Medicare Part B a monthly premium is required to obtain this coverage even if the beneficiary is Medicare Part A eligible. As of 2007, the Medicare Part B premium is determined by the patient's yearly income. The minimum for 2007 is $93.50 per month. Each year the patient must meet his deductible before services are paid. The deductibles may increase annually. Review the deductibles, coinsurance requirements, and copayments for 2006 and 2007 in Table 11.2. The carrier determines payment to Part B providers for covered items and services.

Medicare Part C

In 1997, Congress created a set of healthcare options known as Medicare Part C, or Medicare+Choice now known as Medicare Advantage plans. These plans offer the same benefits as Medicare Parts A and B. In addition, many of the plans offer benefits for services not covered by the "traditional" Medicare programs, such as hearing aids, dentures, and prescription drugs (Medicare Part D). The scope of additional coverage is

Table 11.2	Medicare Deductibles, Coinsurances, and Copayments for 2006 and 2007	
	2006	**2007**
Deductible	$124.00 per year	$131.00 per year
Coinsurance	20% of approved amount	Same
Monthly premium	$88.50	$93.50
Mental health	50% of approved amount	Same
Other covered services	Copay and a coinsurance	Same
Outpatient hospital services	Coinsurance or copayment that varies by service	Same

based on the individual policy and plan; the individual has the option to choose additional coverage with Medicare Part C, which can include:

- Preventive care
- Medicare Part D
- Eyeglasses
- Dental care
- Hearing aids.

About 17 percent of all Medicare beneficiaries today choose to have their Medicare services coordinated by a managed care health program, like an HMO. Managed care plans for Medicare are prepaid healthcare plans that offer regular Part A and Part B Medicare coverage in addition to coverage for other services.

The types of Medicare Part C plans are:

- Health maintenance organization (HMO)
- Competitive medical plan (CMP)
- Point-of-service (POS) option
- Provider sponsored organization (PSO)
- Preferred provider organization (PPO)
- Medical savings account (MSA)
- Fee-for-service (FFS) plan
- A religious fraternal benefit society plan.

Medicare Part D

Medicare Part D provides prescription drug coverage. Beginning January 1, 2006, Medicare offered insurance coverage for prescription drugs. Anyone eligible for Medicare Parts A and B may enroll in Medicare Part D. The enrollee must pay a premium depending on the coverage chosen.

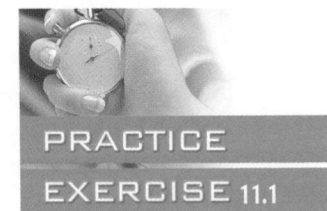

PRACTICE EXERCISE 11.1

Indicate whether the following statements about Medicare are true or false:

1. Medicare is a state health insurance program for the poor and medically indigent. _____

2. Medicare is a federal health insurance program for the elderly, people with disabilities, and ESRD patients. _____

3. Medicare is a health insurance program enacted by Congress in 1965 that today serves more than 39 million elderly Americans and those with disabilities. _____

4. Medicare is a federal health insurance program created to alleviate the unpredictable and uneven costs associated with medical care for the elderly, people with disabilities, and ESRD patients. _____

On completion of this exercise, refer to Appendix J to check the accuracy of your work.

Services Not Covered by Medicare Parts A and B

Medicare doesn't cover everything. Items and services that are not covered include, but are not limited to, the following:

- Acupuncture
- Deductibles, coinsurance, or copayments when a beneficiary receives health-care services
- Dental care and dentures (with only a few exceptions)
- Cosmetic surgery
- Custodial care (help with bathing, dressing, using the bathroom, and eating) at home or in a nursing home
- Eye refractions
- Health care received while traveling outside of the United States
- Hearing aids and hearing exams for the purpose of fitting a hearing aid
- Hearing tests (other than for fitting a hearing aid) that haven't been ordered by the doctor
- Long-term care, such as custodial care in a nursing home
- Orthopedic shoes (with only a few exceptions)
- Prescription drugs
- Routine foot care such as cutting of corns or calluses (with only a few exceptions)
- Routine eye care and most eyeglasses
- Routine or yearly physical exams
- Screening tests and screening laboratory tests
- Vaccinations
- Some diabetic supplies.

There are exceptions to the rules on Medicare Part A and Part B covered services. Items and services that are covered include:

- Services provided in Canada when the beneficiary travels between Alaska and another state while on board a ship in U.S. territorial waters
- One pair of eyeglasses with standard frames after cataract surgery that includes implanting an intraocular lens
- A one-time physical exam within the first 6 months of receiving Part B benefits
- Tests such as bone mass measurements are covered once every 24 months, or more if medically necessary; cardiovascular screenings (every 5 years to test cholesterol, lipid, and triglyceride levels); colorectal cancer screenings (screening colonoscopy once every 120 months unless patient is at high risk then every 24 months); diabetes screening (up to two screenings every year based on history and test results); Pap test and pelvic exam (every 24 months except for women at high risk then every 12 months); prostate screening (once every 12 months for the PSA); and mammograms (once every 12 months)
- Pneumococcal shot, hepatitis B shots, and flu shots. Hepatitis shots are covered for patients with high or medium risk for hepatitis B. This would be a patient with hemophilia, ESRD, or a condition that lowers his resistance to infection.
- Syringes or insulin unless the insulin is used with an insulin pump or the patient has Medicare Part D

Medigap, Medicaid, and Supplemental Insurance

A Medicare beneficiary may have additional coverage to pay for any parts of a claim not covered by Medicare. In these cases, Medicare is always primary for Medigap and Medicaid.

Medigap is a privately offered, Medicare supplemental health insurance policy designed to provide additional coverage for services that Medicare does not pay for. It also helps to satisfy deductibles or any coinsurance payments. Medigap is not available to patients enrolled in HMOs.

Be aware that not all Medicare supplemental insurance is Medigap. Only certain insurance companies are authorized to offer Medigap insurance to Medicare beneficiaries. The Medigap policies offered by these companies are regulated by Medicare law. When a Medicare beneficiary has elected to purchase a Medigap policy, Medicare must be informed that the beneficiary wishes to have his claims information sent to a Medigap insurer. The notification is made by the information provided on the claim. The reassignment of the gaps in coverage is called **crossover**, and eliminates the need for the beneficiary to file a separate claim with his Medigap insurer. To enable the crossover process, beneficiaries must sign a release of information/assignment of benefits form with each of their providers. This authorization is kept in the patient's medical file. Form locator 13 on the CMS-1500 form is signed for direct payment from the Medigap carrier.

Medicaid is a federally and state-funded program through which certain categories of the nation's poor and people with disabilities are entitled to medical and health-related benefits. The federal government provides broad guidelines for eligibility, but allows each state to:

- Dictate more defined eligibility standards
- Determine the coverage of services
- Set rates of payment
- Administer the program.

Medicaid is known as the payer of last resort. If the patient has any additional coverage, Medicaid will always be secondary. Medicaid is discussed in detail in Chapter 12.

Requirements for Medical Necessity

For a service to be considered medically necessary, the following criteria must be met:

- Procedure matches the diagnosis
- Is not an elective procedure
- Is not an experimental or investigational procedure
- Is an essential treatment; that is, not performed for the patient's convenience
- Is delivered at the most appropriate level that can be safely and effectively administered to the patient.

Medicare Coverage Plans

Medicare beneficiaries may receive benefits in two ways:

1. *Fee-for-service benefits.* Benefits that require patients to pay a deductible (if not previously met) and any applicable coinsurance each time a service is rendered. Patients

are also responsible for paying noncovered services (program exclusion), or any items for which they signed an advance beneficiary notice (ABN).

2. *Managed care plan*: A plan in which the beneficiaries prepay a set amount (usually a copayment) for items or services provided by physicians or other healthcare providers. Most managed care programs today are run by HMOs, although some are also competitive medical plans.

Fee-for-Service: The Original Medicare Plan

The type of insurance coverage offered under the original Medicare plan was a fee-for-service plan. A fee-for-service plan is a method of reimbursement that paid the provider his standard charge for each procedure. Medicare uses the *resource-based relative value scale* (RBRVS) reimbursement method to determine its fees for service.

Fee-for-service Medicare benefits allow beneficiaries to go to almost any doctor, hospital, or other healthcare provider they desire. Generally, a fee is charged to the patient each time a service is rendered by a provider (i.e., coinsurance, Medicare deductible, costs for Medicare noncovered services, or costs of services that are the result of an ABN.)

Participating Providers should have their 9 digit zip code on file with Medicare's Provider File Master Address for correct locality reimbursement!

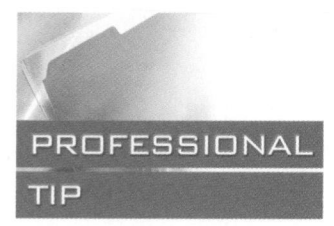

PROFESSIONAL TIP

The traditional fee-for-service Medicare program does not cover all medical expenses of Medicare patients. Beneficiaries pay for the medical services not covered by the fee-for-service plan. An ABN must be given and on file for the provider to collect from the patient. When billing the noncovered or excluded service, use the modifier GA.

Medicare beneficiaries who choose the fee-for-service benefit option are required to pay a deductible and coinsurance.

Medicare Advantage Plans or Medicare Part C

Medicare Advantage plans (Medicare Part C) are health plan options that are part of the Medicare program. Except in emergencies, beneficiaries who choose a managed care plan typically receive all of their care from the doctors, hospitals, and other healthcare providers who are a part of that plan. This coverage includes prescription drug coverage. Medicare pays a set amount of money for the care every month to these private health plans whether the services are rendered or not. Most of these plans generally provide extra benefits and have lower copayments than the original fee-for-service Medicare plan just discussed.

The types of Medicare Advantage Plans include HMOs and PPOS. In an HMO, patients must choose a primary care physician (PCP) and usually pay a copayment at each visit. A primary care physician is the medical provider chosen by an insured or subscriber to provide initial medical care prior to seeing a specialist. Patients also have the choice of receiving services from providers outside the network for an additional fee.

In a PPO patients are given a financial incentive to use doctors within a network but may choose to go outside the network. Visits outside the network incur additional costs that may include a higher copayment or coinsurance. The two types of PPOs are:

1. Local PPOs that serve individual counties
2. Regional PPOs that serve an entire region, which may be a single state or multistate area. In a regional PPO, members have added protection for Medicare Part A and Medicare Part B benefits. They have an annual limit on their out-of-pocket costs; the limit varies depending on the plan.

Medicare Providers

A healthcare person or organization that supplies beneficiaries with healthcare services and products is called a *provider*. A participating provider is a physician or an organization that agrees to provide medical service to a payer's policyholders according to the terms of a contract. All providers (regardless of participation) must file claims on behalf of Medicare patients.

Part A Providers

Part A providers are healthcare facilities such as hospitals, skilled nursing facilities, nursing homes, and others.

All Part A providers must become certified with Medicare to be able to provide services to Medicare patients. Part A provider certification occurs through formal inspections by state agencies that verify whether or not a healthcare facility has the appropriate staff, equipment, facility, and medical licensing to perform quality medical services for Medicare patients.

Part B Providers

Part B providers are physicians, nonphysician practitioners, or suppliers who have agreed with Medicare to supply services for their Medicare patients and accept the Medicare fee as payment in full. The Medicare fee includes the amount paid by the patient and the amount paid to the provider by Medicare.

Physician

A physician is considered a doctor of medicine or osteopathy, dental medicine, dental surgery, podiatric medicine, optometry, or chiropractic medicine legally authorized to practice by the state in which she performs. The **Tax Relief and Health Care Act (TRHCA)** of 2006 authorized the establishment of a physician quality reporting system by CMS. The **Physician Quality Reporting Initiative (PQRI)** establishes a financial incentive for eligible professionals to participate in a voluntary quality reporting program. No registration or enrollment is required to participate. Those who successfully report a designated set of quality measures on claims may earn a 1.5% bonus, subject to a cap.

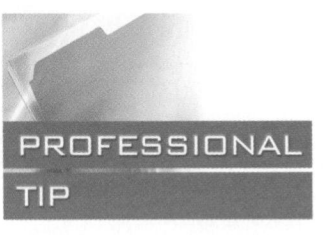

PROFESSIONAL TIP

Chiropractic services that provide acute or chronic active/corrective treatment must be billed with the AT modifier. If codes 98940-98942 are billed without the AT modifier, the treatment will be considered maintenance and will not be covered.

An ABN should be given when chiropractic manipulations are done for the sole purpose of maintenance.

Nonphysician Practitioner

A nonphysician practitioner includes, but is not limited to, an anesthesia assistant, an independent billing psychologist, an independent billing audiologist, a certified clinical nurse specialist, a family nurse practitioner, a clinical psychologist, a certified registered nurse practitioner, and a licensed clinical social worker.

Supplier

The description of a supplier includes, but is not limited to, organizations such as a screening mammography center, an ambulance service supplier, a portable x-ray supplier, an independent diagnostic testing facility, and an independent laboratory.

Participating versus Nonparticipating Medicare Part B Providers

A nonparticipating provider is a physician that chooses not to participate in a Medicare Plan. A nonparticipating provider can treat Medicare patients and choose to accept assignment or not accept assignment.

Accepting assignment refers to a provider who has agreed to accept the allowed charge of a rendered service as payment in full.

Not accepting assignment refers to a provider who will not accept the allowed charge as payment in full.

When the provider does not accept assignment, the payment will be sent directly to the patient. The medical office specialist should collect payment at the time of service.

A participating provider is a physician who contracts with Medicare to provide treatment for beneficiaries of Medicare Part B. Medicare participating providers receive benefits that nonparticipating providers do not. These benefits include:

- Reimbursement directly from Medicare rather than the patient
- Medigap insurance automatically crosses over (if the requirements for crossover are met)
- Access to beneficiary eligibility information.

If a nonparticipating provider accepts assignment, then he:

- Must still file all Medicare claims on behalf of Medicare patients
- Accepts a 5% lower fee allowances for services
- Understands that Medigap/supplemental insurance does not automatically cross over
- Does not have access to beneficiary eligibility information.

Part B providers who choose not to participate and not to accept assignment may charge a limiting charge, as discussed next.

Limiting Charge

Physicians who are not participating and not accepting assignment may charge a **limiting charge**. The limiting charge is 115% more than the nonparticipating provider's Medicare Fee Schedule (MFS). To calculate this number, take the **non-par MFS** and multiply it by 115%. The limiting charge does not apply to immunizations, supplies, or ambulance service.

The Medicare Comprehensive Limiting Charge Compliance Program was created to prevent nonparticipating physicians from collecting the balance from Medicare patients. Physicians who collect amounts in excess of the limiting charge are subject to financial penalties.

Patient's Financial Responsibility

Patients who choose the fee for service benefits can choose their providers. The amount due by the patient will depend on what type of provider they choose.

1. **Par Provider Accepting Assignment:** Patient pays 20% of the Medicare Fee Schedule
2. **Non-Par Provider Accepting Assignment:** Patient pays 20% of the Non-Par Medicare Fee Schedule
3. **Non-Par Provider, Not Accepting Assignment:** Patient is responsible for the limiting charge. The patient will only be reimbursed by Medicare at 80% of the Non-Par Medicare Fee Schedule. Patient out of pocket expense will be the difference between the limiting charge and the reimbursement of 80% of the Non-Participating Fee. The payment will be made directly to the patient.

Determining the Medicare Fee and Limiting Charge

Complete Practice Exercises 11.2 through 11.5 to determine the amount owed by the patient to a participating provider, a nonparticipating provider who accepts assignment, and a nonparticipating provider who does not accept assignment. To help you get started, the following example shows how to determine the Medicare fee and limiting charge.

Example

MFS: $200.00
Participating provider: $200.00
Nonparticipating, accepting assignment provider: $200.00 × 95% = $190.00
Nonparticipating, not accepting assignment provider's limiting charge:
    $190.00 × 115% = $218.50

1. The participating Medicare provider accepting assignment receives 100% of the MFS plus other incentives for participating; in this case, $200.00.
2. The nonparticipating, accepting assignment provider receives 5% less than the MFS, or 95% of $200.00: $190.00. This is also called the *non-par MFS*.
3. The nonparticipating provider who is not accepting assignment is allowed to charge 115% of the non-par MFS, which is 5% less than the MFS. This is called the *limiting charge*. In this example, the non-par MFS is $190.00, so $190.00 × 115% = $218.50.

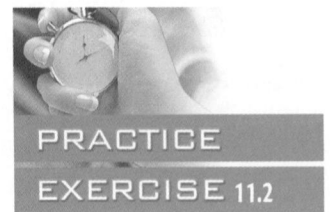

PRACTICE EXERCISE 11.2

Determine the amount owed by the patient in the following situations:

Participating Provider:

Physician's standard fee: $175.00

Medicare fee: $140.00

1. Medicare pays 80%:   _____
2. Patient or supplemental plan pays 20%:   _____
3. Provider adjustment (write-off):   _____

(continued)

Nonparticipating Provider Accepting Assignment:

Physician's standard fee: $175.00

Medicare Fee: $140.00

1. Medicare non-par fee: _____

2. Medicare pays 80%:   _____

3. Patient or supplemental plan pays 20%:   _____

4. Provider adjustment (write-off):   _____

Nonparticipating Provider Not Accepting Assignment:

Physician's standard fee: $175.00

Medicare Fee: $140.00

1. Medicare non-par fee: _____

2. Limiting charge: _____

3. Patient billed: _____

4. Medicare pays patient: _____

5. Total provider can collect: _____

6. Patient out-of-pocket expense: _____

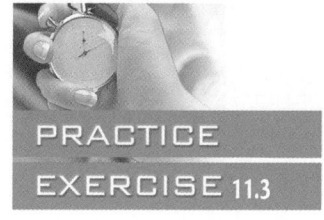

PRACTICE
EXERCISE 11.2

(continued)

On completion of this exercise, refer to Appendix J to check the accuracy of your work.

Determine the amount owed by the patient in the following situations:

Procedure Code	Physician's Fee	Medicare Fee
99212	$75.00	$38.32

Participating Provider:

1. Physician's standard fee: _____

2. Medicare fee: _____

3. Medicare pays 80%:   _____

4. Patient or supplemental plan pays 20%:   _____

5. Provider adjustment (write-off):   _____

PRACTICE
EXERCISE 11.3

(continued)

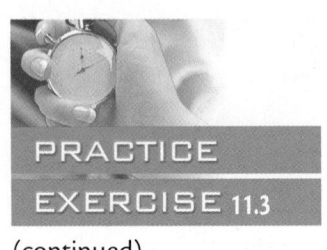

PRACTICE EXERCISE 11.3
(continued)

Nonparticipating Provider Accepting Assignment:

1. Physician's standard fee: _____

2. Medicare non-par fee: _____

3. Medicare pays 80%:   _____

4. Patient or supplemental plan pays 20%:   _____

5. Provider adjustment (write-off):   _____

Nonparticipating Provider Not Accepting Assignment:

1. Physician's standard fee: _____

2. Medicare non-par fee: _____

3. Limiting charge: _____

4. Patient billed: _____

5. Medicare pays patient: _____

6. Total provider can collect: _____

7. Patient out-of-pocket expense: _____

8. Patient out-of-pocket with Medigap: _____

9. Provider adjustment: _____

On completion of this exercise, refer to Appendix J to check the accuracy of your work.

PRACTICE EXERCISE 11.4

Determine the amount owed by the patient in the following situations:

Procedure Code	Physician's Fee	Medicare Fee
99213	$100.00	$52.12

Participating Provider:

1. Physician's standard fee: _____

2. Medicare fee: _____

3. Medicare pays 80%:   _____

4. Patient or supplemental plan pays 20%:   _____

5. Provider adjustment (write-off):   _____

Nonparticipating Provider Accepting Assignment:

1. Physician's standard fee: _____

2. Medicare non-par fee: _____

(continued)

3. Medicare pays 80%: _____

4. Patient or supplemental plan pays 20%: _____

5. Provider adjustment (write-off): _____

PRACTICE EXERCISE 11.4

(continued)

Nonparticipating Provider Not Accepting Assignment:

1. Physician's standard fee: _____

2. Medicare non-par fee: _____

3. Limiting charge: _____

4. Patient billed: _____

5. Medicare pays patient: _____

6. Total provider can collect: _____

7. Provider adjustment (write-off): _____

On completion of this exercise, refer to Appendix J to check the accuracy of your work.

Determine the amount owed by the patient in the following situations:

Procedure Code	Physician's Fee	Medicare Fee
99203	$150.00	$95.75

PRACTICE EXERCISE 11.5

Participating Provider:

1. Physician's standard fee: _____

2. Medicare fee: _____

3. Medicare pays 80%: _____

4. Patient or supplemental plan pays 20%: _____

5. Provider adjustment (write-off): _____

Nonparticipating Provider Accepting Assignment:

1. Physician's standard fee: _____

2. Medicare non-par fee: _____

3. Medicare pays 80%: _____

4. Patient or supplemental plan pays 20%: _____

5. Provider adjustment (write-off): _____

(continued)

332   Section V   Government Medical Billing

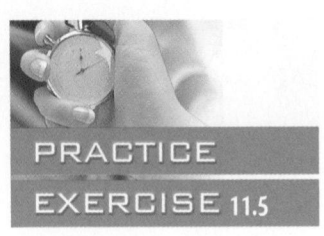

PRACTICE
EXERCISE 11.5

(continued)

Nonparticipating Provider Not Accepting Assignment:

1. Physician's standard fee: _____
2. Medicare non-par fee: _____
3. Limiting charge: _____
4. Patient billed: _____
5. Medicare pays patient: _____
6. Total provider can collect: _____
7. Provider adjustment (write-off):   _____

On completion of this exercise, refer to Appendix J to check the accuracy of your work.

Patient Registration

As a medical office specialist (MOS) who receives initial patient information, three major tasks need to be performed that are vital to the efficiency and financial welfare of the healthcare organization. These tasks are:

1. Copying the Medicare card
2. Obtaining essential patient information through the use of completed medical information/history and insurance forms
3. Determining Medicare as primary or secondary

The medical office specialist should check patients' Medicare eligibility every 6 months.

Copying the Medicare Card

The Medicare enrollee receives a health insurance card (Figure 11.1). It is very important for the MOS to obtain a copy of the beneficiary's card during a patient's first visit with the facility. Medicare also recommends that the beneficiary's insurance information be verified periodically to determine if any changes have occurred. If changes have occurred, patient records should be updated accordingly.

The pieces of information to record from the patient's card are:

- Exact name
- Claim number—include all numbers and letters
- Type of coverage
- Effective dates of coverage for Part A and Part B.

Recording the information from the Medicare card accurately is extremely important because that information will be used on many claims forms and medical documentation materials throughout the patient's history with the facility. The need for recording the information exactly as it appears on the card even extends to mis-

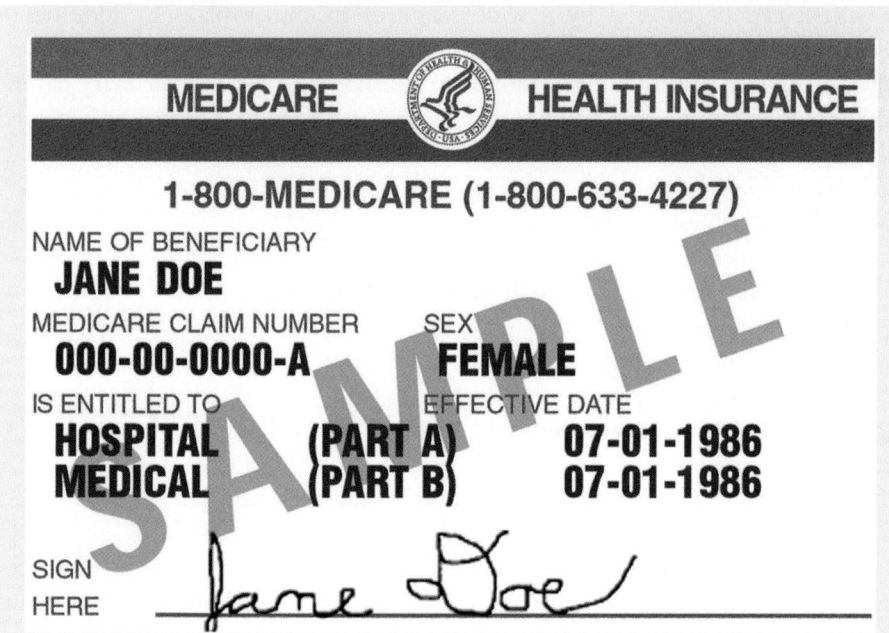

Figure 11.1

Medicare card.

spelling the patient's name in the computer if it is misspelled on the Medicare card! If there is a misspelling, it is the patient's responsibility to call Medicare and have it corrected.

If the MOS makes a mistake when recording information from the Medicare card, these mistakes can carry over to Medicare claims forms, causing claim rejections, delays in processing, and even denials. These mistakes cause more work and can be quite costly for the practice.

Obtaining Patient Signatures

Having the appropriate patient signatures on Medicare claim forms or on file is essential. Rather than have patients sign each time a claim is processed, Medicare provides a document that patients can sign which lasts a lifetime: the Lifetime Beneficiary and Claim Authorization Form. A facility may use their own form to obtain authorization for release of information and payments. When the Medicare claim is submitted the signature of the patient or SOF (signature on file) must be noted on locator 12. If the patient has Medigap the signature or SOF must be noted on locator 13 in order for the provider to receive payment instead of the patient. If the provider is non-participating the Medigap payment will always be paid directly to the patient.

The UB-04/CMS-1450 and CMS-1500 claims forms are good references to use for developing a release of information form for the office. The information on the release of information form should at least encompass the information necessary to fill out the Medicare claims forms correctly.

Determining Primary and Secondary Payers

When registering a hospital patient, the medical office specialist will be required to have the patient complete a Medicare questionnaire similar to that shown in Appendix D.

A patient can be covered by a wide range of insurance plans in addition to Medicare. In cases where a patient has additional coverage, Medicare may be considered the "secondary payer" and the additional insurance carrier the "primary payer."

You should ask patients a number of questions to make sure you have obtained complete and correct information about their insurance coverage:

1. Is your injury/illness due to:
   - A work-related accident or condition?
   - A condition covered under the federal Black Lung Program?
   - An automobile accident?
   - An accident other than an automobile accident?
   - The fault of another party?
2. Are you eligible for coverage under the Veterans Administration?
3. Are you employed?
   - Do you have coverage under an employer group health insurance?
4. Is your spouse employed?
   - Do you have coverage under your spouse's employer group health insurance?
5. Are you a dependent covered under a parent or guardian's employer group health plan?

The preceding questions will help the MOS determine if the beneficiary is:

- Covered under another policy or government program
- Potentially eligible for coverage by a different insurer due to an accident or injury that makes a third party liable for medical expenses
- Eligible for coverage of all expenses over the amount that Medicare covers.

6. Have you had outpatient or emergency department services in the last 3 days? This question is asked to determine if any outpatient charges occurred within the last 3 days prior to an inpatient admission (72 hours). This is called the *72-hour rule* (also the *3-day payment window rule*). The Medicare rule states that if a patient receives diagnostic tests and hospital outpatient services within 72 hours of admission to a hospital, then all such tests and services are combined with inpatient services. The preadmission services become part of the DRG payment to the hospital and may not be billed or paid separately.
7. Do you currently reside in a nursing home? If the patient answers yes, list the name of the nursing home.
8. Has the patient given up his Medicare and replaced it with a HMO? If yes, the HMO is primary. If no, the HMO will be secondary.

Plans Primary to Medicare

When an individual is employed and receives coverage through the employer's group health plan, Medicare is the secondary payer. Medicare is also the secondary payer when an individual age 65 or older receives coverage through a spouse's employer (the spouse does not have to be 65 or older).

On the other hand, **Medicare is the primary payer for individuals 65 or older:**

- Who are working for an employer with 20 employees or fewer
- Who are covered by another policy that is not a group policy
- Who are enrolled in Part B, but not Part A, of the Medicare program
- Who must pay premiums to receive Part A coverage

- Who are retired and receiving coverage under a group policy from a previous employer
- Who are retired and receiving coverage under a group policy from a previous employer
- Who are receiving coverage under Cobra

Consolidated Omnibus Budget Reconciliation Act of 1985

The **Consolidated Omnibus Budget Reconciliation Act of 1985 (COBRA)** requires employers to allow employees, their spouses, and their dependents to continue group health insurance coverage for a minimum of 18 months after their employment with the company ends. The employee pays premiums without any contribution from the employer. COBRA is primary to Medicare.

People with Disabilities

If an individual has a disability, is under age 65, and receives coverage through an employer's group health plan (which may be held by the individual, a spouse, or another family member), Medicare is the secondary payer. If the individual or family member is not actively employed, Medicare is the primary payer.

People with End-Stage Renal Disease

During a coordination of benefits period (currently 30 months), Medicare is the secondary payer for individuals with ESRD who receive coverage through an employer-sponsored group health plan and who fail to apply for ESRD-based Medicare coverage. The coordination of benefits period begins the first month the individual is eligible for or entitled to Part A benefits based on an ESRD diagnosis. This rule is in effect regardless of whether the individual is employed or retired.

Workers' Compensation

If an individual is receiving treatment for a work-related job injury, Medicare is not filed. The workers' compensation claim is paid in full for the allowed amount for that injury only by the employer's workers' compensation carrier.

Automobile, No-Fault, and Liability Insurance

Medicare is always the secondary payer when treatment is for an accident-related claim. Medicare is not responsible for any payment until the patient has reached his maximum allowed benefits from the primary payer. In that case, a copy of the letter of denial is sent to Medicare with the claim.

Veteran Benefits

If a veteran is entitled to Medicare benefits, he may choose whether to receive coverage through Medicare or through the Veterans Administration.

Medicare Coordination

Information on eligibility and benefits entitlement can be obtained from the Coordination of Benefits Central File Contractor. This is a service that is used to facilitate accurate

PROFESSIONAL TIP

All Medicare secondary payer (MSP) inquiries, including the reporting of potential MSP situations, changes in a beneficiary's insurance coverage, changes in employment, and general MSP questions or concerns, should be directed to the COB. The toll free number is 800-999-1118.

payment. The Coordination of Benefits Contractor is not affiliated with the local Medicare carrier or intermediary. The COB contractor will provide customer service to all callers from any source, including but not limited to beneficiaries, attorneys, or other beneficiary representatives, employers, insurers, providers, and suppliers.

When contacting the COB contractor, have the following information available:

- Patient's name
- Patient's Medicare or Social Security number
- Date of incident
- Date of illness
- Name and address of the other insurance
- Name of injured
- Policy/claim number
- Medicare provider number.

Medicare as the Secondary Payer

When Medicare is clearly the secondary payer, the provider's organization needs to follow certain steps when submitting the claim. The medical office specialist must complete the required form locator fields in the computer and the claim will be processed without any attachment. Medicare does not require the primary insurance remittance notice when submitting **Medicare Secondary Payer (MSP)** claims electronically. The medical office specialist will need to keep the remittance notice on file and make it available to Medicare on request. The fields that need to be completed are:

1. The primary insurance allowed amount (form locator 28)
2. The primary insurance paid amount (form locator 29)
3. The Obligated to Accept as Payment in Full (OTAF) amount, if any (form locator 30).

Medicare will no longer accept paper attachments.

Conditional Payment

In liability cases where the beneficiary's medical expenses may be covered by a third party's insurance, the provider has a choice of actions. These choices include:

1. *Bill the insurer:* The provider can bill the liability insurer directly. If it is determined that the primary payer will not pay promptly (within 120 days after billing the liability insurer), the provider may file a claim with Medicare for conditional primary payment. If a Medicare conditional payment is made, the provider or supplier may no longer bill the primary insurer or the beneficiary for services that were covered by the Medicare conditional payment. They may only bill the beneficiary for applicable Medicare deductibles and coinsurance.

2. *File a lien:* When the patient sues the liability insurer for damages, the provider may file a lien against the settlement proceeds of the liability case. If it is determined that the primary payer will not pay promptly (within 120 days after billing the liability insurer), the provider may file a claim with Medicare for conditional primary payment. If a Medicare conditional payment is made, the provider or supplier may no longer bill the primary insurer or the beneficiary for services that were covered by the Medicare conditional payment. They may only bill the beneficiary for applicable Medicare deductibles and coinsurance.

Medicare Documents

As we have discussed, some Medicare documents need to be signed by the insured. The documents that require the insured's signature, the advance beneficiary notice and the Lifetime Beneficiary Claim Authorization and Information Release (lifetime release form), can be copied from the Medicare website, which ensures that the documents are worded correctly.

The advance beneficiary notice (ABN) is proof that the office has given patients notice that the services about to be provided may not be covered by Medicare because they are not medically reasonable or necessary, and that the patient is responsible for the charges. If a procedure, service, or supply that the patient is receiving is questionable as to its coverage under Medicare, an ABN form should be given to the patient to sign before services are rendered. An ABN should also be given to the patient prior to receiving a noncovered or excluded service.

For Medicare to determine if the patient has been notified in advance that he will be responsible for payment, a GA modifier is used with the procedure. This demonstrates to the carrier that the provider has a notice on file. If the patient refuses to sign the ABN for a nonassigned claim, use a GZ modifier, which alerts the carrier that the form was presented and the patient refused to sign it. A GY modifier indicates that the item or service is statutorily excluded or does not meet the definition of any Medicare benefit. If no notice is given prior to service, the provider must write off the entire charge for the service.

If the provider chooses to make an ABN, rather than use the one from the Medicare website, the notice must include the following information:

- The patient's name
- Date(s)
- Description of item or service
- Reason(s) why the item or service may not be considered medically necessary.

Refer to the ABN in Appendix D. An ABN notice must be signed and dated by the patient each time an item is given or service is rendered that may not be deemed "medically necessary." In contrast, a lifetime release form is signed once by the patient and filed in his record.

Development Letter

A **Medicare Development Letter** is sent from Medicare to a provider when a claim is filed that needs additional information or documentation. These letters usually detail what information is necessary in order for Medicare to resume processing a specific claim or claims. The MOS may be responsible for gathering and sending the information

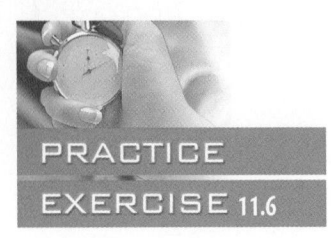

PRACTICE
EXERCISE 11.6

Indicate whether the following statements about Medicare are true or false:

1. The advance beneficiary notice is a notice from Medicare that a claim submitted by your provider organization cannot be processed without additional information and/or documentation.

2. A Medicare Development Letter is sent to a provider when a claim is filed that needs additional information or documentation. There is no time limit on responding, but a claim may be denied if the wrong information is sent.

3. The advance beneficiary notice must include the patient's name, date(s), a description of the item or service provided, and the reason(s) why the item or service may not be considered medically necessary.

On completion of this exercise, refer to Appendix J to check the accuracy of your work.

that Medicare requests. A time limit is usually placed on return of the requested information. If the additional information is not sent to Medicare within the time frame communicated in the development letter, the services at issue will be denied payment by Medicare.

Medicare Insurance Billing Requirements

The Healthcare Common Procedure Coding System (HCPCS) is used to report procedures and services for Medicare patients. This system is also used to report services for Medicaid patients. HCPCS consists of the following three levels of codes:

Level I codes, which are copyrighted by the American Medical Association's Current Procedural Terminology, Fourth Edition (CPT-4®)

Level II codes, which are five-position alphanumeric codes proved and maintained jointly by the Alpha Numeric Panel (consisting of the CMS, the Health Insurance Association of America, and the Blue Cross Blue Shield Association). The American Dental Association copyrights the D code series in Level II HCPCS.

Level III codes, which are used by regional insurance companies throughout the country.

The Health Insurance Portability and Accountability Act (HIPAA) Transaction and Code Set Rule requires providers to use the medical code set that is valid at the time that the service is provided. Providers should be aware that as of January 1, 2005, carriers, Durable Medical Equipment Regional Carriers (DMERC), and fiscal intermediaries no longer accepted discontinued HCPCS codes for dates of service January 1 through March 31 of the current year (beginning in 2005) that are submitted prior to April 1. In addition, effective January 1, 2005, CMS no longer allowed a 90-day grace period for discontinued codes resulting from any midyear HCPCS updates.

CPT is a registered trademark of the American Medical Association.

Medicare Part A providers bill insurance claims (if submitting on paper) using the UB-04/CMS-1450 claim form. Medicare Part B providers bill insurance claims (if submitting on paper) using the CMS-1500 claim form.

Completing Medicare Part B Claims

Providers are required by law to submit all Medicare claims for services performed on Medicare beneficiaries. Medicare providers can submit their claims in two ways: the claim form (CMS-1500) or electronically (EMC) through a computer, a modem, and an approved billing software (NSF/ANSI). Medicare prefers that claims be sent electronically. However, if a paper claim does need to be submitted, the medical office specialist needs to obtain the proper mailing address. All paper claims throughout the country are processed using an optical character recognition (OCR) system located in Dallas, Texas. Failure to send paper claims to the correct P.O. box in Dallas for a particular region may result in delayed reimbursement.

Once a claim is received and entered into the computer system, it is processed through an edits and audits system to verify its accuracy and completeness. The system also determines Medicare's liability for the claim and issues payment. CMS mandates contractors to process claims in a timely manner. The turnaround time for OCR claims is 29 days and 14 days for an electronic claim.

Form Locators 1 through 13 for Medicare Part B Claims

As you know from Chapter 9, form locators 1 through 13 on the CMS-1500 form are used to record patient information.

Form Locator 1: Type of Insurance   Form locator 1 identifies what type of insurance the patient carries. The form lists five government plans: Medicare, Medicaid, TRICARE, CHAMPVA, and FECA Black Lung. There are two other options: Group Health Plan and Other. These are utilized based on what type of plan the insured is enrolled in.

Form Locator 1a: Insured's ID Number   Form locator 1a asks for the insured's insurance ID number as reflected on the insurance card. The health insurance claims (HIC) number should be nine digits, followed by a valid suffix; for example: 123456789A. The following are examples of valid HIC number suffixes:

Code Type

A	Primary claimant
B	Aged wife A62 (1st claimant)
B1	Aged husband (1st claimant)
C1–C9	Child (includes child with a disability or student child)
D	Aged widow A60 (1st claimant)
D1	Aged widower (1st claimant)
E1	Surviving divorced mother
E5	Surviving divorced father
M	Uninsured beneficiary (not qualified for automatic health insurance benefits [HIB])
M1	Uninsured beneficiary (qualified for automatic HIB but requests supplemental medical insurance SMI only)
T	Uninsured beneficiary

| W | Disabled widow |
| W1 | Disabled widower |

Note: Railroad retirement beneficiaries' HIC number has the "letter" in front of the numbers versus the "letter" after the numbers.

Form Locator 2: Patient's Name   In form locator 2, enter the name of the Medicare patient. Use the name as it appears on the Medicare card. *The spelling must match the insurance card exactly.*

Form Locator 3: Patient's Date of Birth and Sex   In form locator 3, enter the patient's date of birth and sex/gender. The date of birth is entered using the eight-digit format: MMDDCCYY. The patient's sex/gender is identified as either male or female.

Form Locator 4: Insured's Name   In form locator 4, enter the name of the person who is the insured. This may or may not be the patient. If the patient is the insured, the word "Same" should be entered. The insured's name should be entered last name, first name, middle name or initial. **If Medicare is primary, leave blank.**

Form Locator 5: Patient's Address   Form locator 5 lists the patient's home address and telephone number. This information is taken from the patient information form when the patient register's in the office. The address should include the street name and number, city, state (two-letter abbreviation), and zip code. When entering the patient's telephone number do not use commas, periods, or other punctuation in the address. When entering a nine-digit zip code, include the hyphen. Do not use a hyphen or space as a separator within the telephone number.

Form Locator 6: Patient Relationship to Insured   If form locator 4 has been filled out, then enter an X in the correct box of form locator 6 to indicate the patient's relationship to the insured. Options include Self, Spouse, Child, or Other. Only one box can be marked.

Form Locator 7: Insured's Address   Form locator 7 asks for the insured's address. If form locator 4 is completed, then this field also needs to be completed. This information should include the street name and number, city, state (two-letter abbreviation), zip code, and phone number. If the patient is the insured enter the word "Same".

Form Locator 8: Patient Status   Form locator 8 indicates the patient status: single, married, or other. It also identifies the patient's employment status: Employed, Full-Time Student, or Part-Time Student. Enter an X in the box for the patient's marital status and for the employment or student status. Only one box on each line can be marked.

Form Locator 9: Other Insured's Name   If form locator 11d is marked yes, complete form locators 9 and 9a–d; otherwise leave blank.

Form Locator 9a: Other Insured's Policy or Group Number   Enter the policy and/or group number of the Medigap insured preceded by MEDIGAP, MG, or MGAP.

Form Locator 9b: Other Insured's Date of Birth and Sex   Enter the date of birth and sex of the Medigap insured. It should be entered in the eight-digit format: MMDDCCYY.

Form Locator 9c: Employer's Name or School Name   Leave blank if a Medigap payer ID is entered in item 9d. Otherwise enter the claims processing address of the Medigap insurer. Use the abbreviated street address, two-letter state abbreviation, and zip code copied from the Medigap insured's Medigap identification card.

Form Locator 9d: Insurance Plan Name or Program Name Enter the nine-digit Payer ID number of the Medigap insurer. If no Payer ID number exists, then enter the Medigap insurance program or plan name.

Form Locators 10a–c: Is Patient's Condition Related To? In form locator 10, identify whether the patient's visit was related to an employment accident, auto accident, or other accident. This form locator is used when filing workers' compensation claims, auto accident claims, or claims for other types of injuries. If the patient's visit does not pertain to an accident of any kind, the default answer will be NO. Enter an X in the correct box.

Form Locator 10d: Reserved for Local Use Use this form locator for Medicaid information. If the patient is entitled to Medicaid, enter the patient's Medicaid number preceded by MCD.

Form Locator 11: Insured's Policy Group or FECA Number (REQUIRED) This form locator must be completed. It is a required field. By completing this item, the physician/supplier acknowledges having made a good-faith effort to determine whether Medicare is the primary or secondary payer. If there is insurance primary to Medicare, enter the insured's policy or group number and proceed to items 11a–c. **Form locators 4, 6, and 7 must also be completed. If Medicare is secondary, enter the insured's policy or group number.** If there is no insurance primary to Medicare, enter the word "None" and proceed to form locator 12.

Form Locator 11a: Insured's Date of Birth and Sex In form locator 11a, list the date of birth of the insured. The date of birth should be listed in the eight-digit format: MMDDCCYY. If the patient and the insured are the same person, this space can be left blank. Choose either male or female accordingly. If gender is unknown, leave blank.

Form Locator 11b: Employer's Name or School Name If there is a change in the insured's insurance status, for example, retired, enter either a six-digit or eight-digit retirement date preceded by the word "Retired." For a Medicare patient the only change Medicare is concerned with is employment versus retired.

Form Locator 11c: Insurance Plan Name or Program Name If there is insurance primary to Medicare indicated in form locator 11, enter the nine-digit payer ID number of the primary insured. If no payer ID exists, enter the complete payer's program name or plan name.

Form Locator 11d: Is There Another Health Benefit Plan? Leave blank. Not required by Medicare.

Form Locator 12: Patient's or Authorized Person's Signature Form locator 12 is where the patient or authorized representative signs unless the signature is on file. In lieu of signing the claim, the patient may sign a release statement to be retained in the provider, physician, or supplier file. If the patient is physically or mentally unable to sign, a representative may sign on the patient's behalf. In this event, the statement's signature line must indicate the patient's name followed by "by" the representative's name, address, relationship to the patient, and the reason the patient cannot sign. The authorization is effective indefinitely unless the patient or the patient's representative revokes this arrangement.

"Signature on File" or "SOF" may be used here in place of a signature. The actual patient signature will be on file in the patient's chart. Enter the date in the six-digit format or eight-digit format. If there is no signature on file, leave blank or enter "No Signature on File."

Form Locator 13: Insured's or Authorized Person's Signature   The signature in this form locator authorizes payment of mandated Medigap benefits to the participating physician or supplier if required by Medigap information included in form locator 9 and its subdivisions. The signature must be on file as a separate Medigap authorization. The Medigap assignment on file with the participating provider of service must be insured specific. It may state that the authorization applies to all occasions of service until it is revoked.

Form Locators 14 through 33 for Medicare Part B Claims

Form locators 14 through 33 record information about the service provider.

Form Locator 14: Date of Current: Illness, Injury, or Pregnancy   Use form locator 14 to indicate the first date of the current illness, injury, or pregnancy. The date should be entered in the six-digit format: MM/DD/YY. For a pregnancy, the first day of the woman's last menstrual period (LMP) is used. If this information is not known, leave blank. For chiropractic services, enter a six-digit format for the date of the initiation of the course of treatment and enter a six-digit date in form locator 19.

Form Locator 15: If Patient Has Had Same or Similar Illness   Leave blank. Not required by Medicare.

Form Locator 16: Dates Patient Unable to Work in Current Occupation   Form locator 16 indicates the dates the patient is unable to work due to her illness or injury. These dates will be required when filing workers' compensation or disability claims. The dates should be entered in the six-digit (MM/DD/YY) or eight-digit format (MM/DD/CCYY). If the information is not required, leave blank.

Form Locator 17: Name of Referring Provider or Other Source   Form locator 17 asks for the name of the provider referring the patient. Enter the name of the referring or ordering physician if the service or item was ordered or referred by a physician. A *referring provider* is a physician who requests an item or service for the beneficiary for which payment may be made under the Medicare program. An *ordering physician* is a physician who orders nonphysician services for the patient such as diagnostic laboratory tests, clinical laboratory tests, pharmaceutical services, durable medical equipment, and services incident to that physician's or nonphysician practitioner's service.

Form Locator 17a: ID Number of Referring Physician   The ID number of the referring, ordering, or supervising provider is reported in form locator 17a in the shaded area. The qualifier indicating what the number represents is reported in the qualifier field to the immediate right of the "17a." The National Uniform Claim Committee (NUCC) defines the following qualifiers, which are the same as those used in the electronic 837 Professional 4010A1:

0B	State license number
1B	Blue Shield provider number
1C	Medicare provider number
1D	Medicaid provider number
1G	Provider UPIN number
1H	TRICARE/CHAMPUS identification number
E1	Employer identification number
G2	Provider commercial number

LU	Location number
N5	Provider plan network identification number
SY	Social Security number (*Note:* The Social Security number may not be used for Medicare.)
X5	State industrial accident provider number
ZZ	Provider taxonomy (Taxonomy codes, also known as specialty codes, identify a provider's specialty category.).

The non-National Provider Identifier (NPI) number of the referring, ordering, or supervising provider refers to the payer-assigned unique identifier of the professional. This field allows for the entry of 2 characters in the qualifier field and 17 characters in the Other ID Number field.

Form Locator 17b: NPI Number   Enter the NPI number of the referring, ordering, or supervising provider in form locator 17b. The NPI number refers to the HIPAA National Provider Identifier number, which is a 10-digit number.

Form Locator 18: Hospitalization Dates Related to Current Services   Enter the dates the patient has been hospitalized in relation to the current services in form locator 18. If the patient has been discharged from the hospital, the dates should include the day admitted and the day discharged. If the patient is still hospitalized, only include the day admitted. The dates should be entered in the six-digit (MM/DD/YY) or the eight-digit format (MM/DD/CCYY). If the patient has not been hospitalized, leave blank.

Form Locator 19: Reserved for Local Use

A. When an independent physical or occupational therapist or podiatrist providing routine foot care submits claims, enter the six-digit date the patient was last seen by their attending physician with the NPI of the attending physician. The attending physician is the individual who wrote the prescription for the treatment. For physical and occupational therapists, entering this information certifies that the required physician certification is being kept on file. Do not enter a space, hyphen, or other separator between the qualifier code and the number. The National Uniform Claim Committee (NUCC) defines qualifiers listed in form locator 17a.

B. *Chiropractic treatment:* Enter a six-digit x-ray date for chiropractor services (if an x-ray, rather than a physical examination, was the method used to demonstrate the subluxation). By entering an x-ray date and the initiation date for course of chiropractic treatment in form locator 14, the chiropractor is certifying that all the relevant information requirements along with the x-ray are available for carrier review.

C. *Not Otherwise Classified (NOC) Drugs:* Enter the drug's name and dosage when submitting a claim for NOC.

D. *Unlisted procedure code or an NOC code:* Enter a concise description of an "unlisted procedure code" or an NOC code if one can be given within the confines of this box. Otherwise, an attachment shall be submitted with the claim.

E. *Multiple modifiers per line:* Enter all applicable modifiers when −99 (multiple modifiers) is entered in form locator 24d. If modifier −99 is entered on multiple line items of a single claim form, all applicable modifiers for each line item containing a −99 modifier should be listed as follows: 1 = (mod), where the number 1 represents the line item and "mod" represents all modifiers applicable to the referenced line item.

F. Enter the statement "Homebound" when an independent laboratory renders an EKG tracing or obtains a specimen from a homebound or institutionalized patient.

G. *Beneficiary refuses to assign benefits:* Enter the statement "Patient refuses to assign benefits" when the beneficiary absolutely refuses to assign benefits to a participating provider. In this case, no payment may be made on the claim.

H. *Hearing aid:* Enter the statement "Testing for hearing aid" when billing services involving the testing of a hearing aid, which is used to obtain intentional denials when other payers are involved.

I. *Dental examination:* When dental examinations are billed, enter the specific surgery for which the exam is being performed.

Form Locator 20: Outside Lab   Complete this field when billing for diagnostic tests subject to purchase price limitations. Enter the purchase price under charges if the "Yes" block is checked. A "Yes" check indicates that an entity other than the entity billing for the service performed the diagnostic test. A "No" check indicates "no purchased tests are included on the claim." When "Yes" is marked, locator 32 shall be completed.

Form Locator 21: Diagnosis or Nature of Illness or Injury   In form locator 21, the ICD-9 codes for the diagnoses applied to this claim are entered. At least one code must be entered and up to eight codes can be used on claim for electronic billing. They are placed in order of precedence, with line 1 being the primary diagnosis, and so forth. No written diagnoses are used on a claim form. The ICD-9 codes should be checked for medical necessity to make sure they are used appropriately with the CPT codes used in form locator 24D. Relate lines 1, 2, 3, and 4 to the lines of service in form locator 24E by line number.

PROFESSIONAL TIP

Always make sure that the ICD-9 codes used are the most recent, up-to-date codes utilized to avoid denials. Codes used should be coded to the highest level of specificity.

Form Locator 22: Medicaid Resubmission Code   Leave blank. Not required by Medicare.

Form Locator 23: Prior Authorization Number   Some insurance plans, such as those of HMOs, exclusive provider organizations (EPOs), and preferred provider organizations (PPOs), require a prior authorization number. If required, when preauthorization is obtained from an insurance company for services, the number assigned is input in form locator 23. Also, HMO required referral numbers are input in this form locator. Any of the following can be entered here: prior authorization number, referral number, mammography precertification number, or Clinical Laboratory Improvement Amendments (CLIA) 10-digit number, as assigned by the payer for the current service. Do not enter hyphens or spaces within the number. If prior authorization is required and is omitted, the claim will be denied. If no prior authorization is required, leave blank.

Section 24

The six service lines in Section 24 have been divided horizontally to accommodate submission of both the NPI and another/proprietary identifier during the NPI transition and to accommodate the submission of supplemental information to support the billed service. The top area of the six service lines is shaded and is the location for reporting supplemental information. (It is not intended to allow the billing of 12 lines of service.)

The following types of supplemental information can be entered in the shaded lines of Section 24:

- Anesthesia duration in hours and/or minutes with start and end times
- Narrative description of unspecified codes
- NDCs for drugs
- Vendor product number from the Health Industry Business Communication Council (HIBCC)
- Product number from the Health Care Uniform Code Council—Global Trade Item Number (GTIN), formerly Universal Product Code (UPC) for products
- Contract rate.

The following qualifiers are used when reporting these services:

7	Anesthesia information
ZZ	Narrative description of unspecified code
N4	NDCs
VP	Vendor product number from the HIBCC labeling standard
OZ	Product number from the Health Care Uniform Code Council (GTIN)
CTR	Contract rate.

If required to report other supplemental information not listed above, follow payer instructions for the use of a qualifier that pertains to the information being reported. When reporting a service that does not have a qualifier, enter two blank spaces before entering the information. To enter supplemental information, begin at 24A by entering the qualifier and then the information. Do not enter a space between the qualifier and the number/code/information. Do not enter hyphens or spaces within the number/code.

Form Locator 24A: Dates of Service   Enter the dates of service for the services provided in form locator 24A. Depending on the insurance carrier, these columns are filled in using different formats. Some require both the To and From dates to be listed in six-digit format: (MM/DD/YY). Some require just the From date to be listed or just the To date. If the same procedure was provided multiple times on a single date, the specific date is entered once and the number of procedures is listed in form locator 24G.

Form Locator 24B: Place of Service   Place of service in form locator 24B is a mandatory field to be completed because it describes the place where the procedure or service was performed. This place could be many places, such as the physician's office, hospital, emergency department, skilled nursing facility, or even the patient's home. A code is used (see following list) to indicate the place of service.

Note that the CMS has stated that the place of service must also be fully written out in form locator 32 if the place of service is other than the physician's office. Consider this example: The patient was an inpatient (hospital) and the physician saw the patient in the hospital for an evaluation and management service. Therefore, the code 21 (see following list) would be entered in form locator 24B and the hospital address entered in form locator 32 with 9 digit zip code.

Common place of service codes include the following:

11	Physician's office
12	Private residence
13	Assisted living facility
20	Urgent care facility
21	Inpatient hospital
22	Outpatient hospital
23	Hospital emergency department
24	Ambulatory surgical center
25	Birthing center
26	Military treatment facility
31	Skilled nursing facility
34	Hospice
81	Independent laboratory.

Form Locator 24C: EMG (Emergency)   Form locator 24C is not required by Medicare.

Form Locator 24D: Procedures, Services, or Supplies   In form locator 24D, enter the CPT or HCPCS codes used to identify the procedures, services, or supplies provided. Modifiers are also listed in form locator 24D. If there are more than three modifiers used, list −99 here and enter the modifiers in form locator 19.

Form Locator 24E: Diagnosis Code (Pointer)   Form locator 24E indicates the number (1 through 8) of the diagnosis code listed in form locator 21 as it relates to each service or procedure. If there is more than one diagnosis attached to a single procedure or service, list the primary diagnosis first. The diagnosis pointer refers to the line number from form locator 21 that relates to the reason the service was performed.

Form Locator 24F: Charges   Form locator 24F lists the charges that are assigned to each CPT or HCPCS code listed. The amount should be entered without a decimal point or dollar sign. If multiple units are entered in 24G, the charges should reflect the amount of the procedure times the number of units. Charges should be updated on a regular basis to follow appropriate billing guidelines.

Form Locator 24G: Days or Units   Enter the number of units per procedure or service provided to a patient in form locator 24G. If billing for anesthesia, the amount entered should be entered in minutes and calculated accordingly. If billing for multiple services, such as liters of oxygen, list the actual number of liters. If multiple units are entered in 24G, the charges should reflect the amount of the procedure multiplied by the number of units.

When required by payers to provide the National Drug Code (NDC) units in addition to the HCPCS units, enter the applicable NDC units' qualifier and related units in the shaded line above the NDC qualifier and code. The following qualifiers are to be used when reporting NDC units:

F2	International Unit	ML	Milliliter
GR	Gram	UN	Unit

Form Locator 24H: EPSDT Family Plan   Form locator 24H is used to identify whether the patient is receiving services through Medicaid's Early and Periodic Screening, Diagnosis, and Treatment (EPSDT) program. If there is no requirement (e.g., state requirement) to report a reason code for EPSDT, enter "Y" for YES or "N" for No only in the unshaded area.

If there is a requirement to report a reason code for EPDST, enter the appropriate reason code as noted below. (A "Y" or "N" response is not entered with a code.) The two-character code is right justified in the top shaded area of the field.

The following codes for EPSDT are used in the electronic 837 Professional 4010A1:

AV   Available—Not used (Patient refused referral.)

S2   Under treatment (Patient is currently under treatment for referred diagnostic or corrective health problem.)

ST   New service requested (Referral to another provider for diagnostic or corrective treatment/scheduled for another appointment with screening provider for diagnostic or corrective treatment for at least one health problem identified during an initial or periodic screening service, not including dental referrals.)

NU   Not used (Used when no EPSDT patient referral was given.)

Form Locator 24I: ID Qualifier   Enter in the shaded area of form locator 24I the qualifier identifying whether the number is a non-NPI number. The other ID number of the rendering provider is then reported in form locator 24J in the shaded area. The NUCC defines the following qualifiers, which are the same as those listed in form locator 17a.

The rendering provider is the person or company (laboratory or other facility) who rendered or supervised the care. In the case where a substitute provider was used, enter that provider's information here. Report the identification number in form locator 24I and 24J only when different from data recorded in form locators 33a and 33b.

Form Locator 24J: Rendering Provider   The individual rendering the service is reported in form locator 24J. Enter the non-NPI ID number in the shaded area of the field. Enter the NPI number in the unshaded area of the field.

Report the identification number in form locators 24I and 24J only when different from data recorded in form locators 33a and 33b.

Form Locator 25: Federal Tax I.D. Number   List in form locator 25 the physician's federal tax I.D. number or his employer identification number (EIN). Do not enter hyphens with numbers. The appropriate selection should be marked and the corresponding number entered.

Form Locator 26: Patient's Account Number   In form locator 26, enter the patient account number assigned in the medical office. The computer system used in the office will generate the number and it should be entered on the claim. This in turn will allow for the account number to appear on the Explanation of Benefits (EOB) form, which makes it easier to locate the correct patient to post insurance payments.

Form Locator 27: Accept Assignment?   Form locator 27 is used to indicate whether or not the physician accepts assignment on this claim. If the physician does accept assignment and the patient has signed form locator 13, the insurance carrier will pay the physician directly for services provided. If the physician does not accept assignment, the insurance carrier will send the reimbursement to the patient.

Form Locator 28: Total Charge   Form locator 28 lists the total of charges, added together from those listed in form locator 24F. The charges should be checked for accuracy to ensure proper reimbursement. Do not use decimal points or dollar signs in this entry.

Form Locator 29: Amount Paid   Form locator 29 indicates the amount paid on this claim. This amount is usually added after the primary EOB is received and payment is posted. The CMS-1500 claim form instructions indicate that form locator 29 should be completed by entering "the total amount the patient paid on the covered services." For Medicare purposes, providers are reminded that entering **any** amount in form locator 29 on assigned claims will result in Medicare sending *partial or full reimbursement directly to the patient instead of the provider.* This is done under the assumption that the patient has already paid the provider for services that could have been covered by Medicare. Should Medicare send monies to the beneficiary based on an incorrect amount being entered into form locator 29, the provider will become responsible for seeking collection of any corrected amounts directly from the patient. *Providers can avoid having incorrect monies sent to the patient by leaving form locator 29 BLANK unless the patient has already paid them for covered services that are over and beyond copayments, deductibles, and noncovered services.* Do not use decimal points or dollar signs in this entry.

Form Locator 30: Balance Due   When Medicare is primary this form locator is left blank. When billing the secondary carrier, form locator 30 is used to record the difference between the amounts in form locators 28 and 29. This amount is the balance due on this particular claim. Do not use decimal points or dollar signs in this entry.

Form Locator 31: Signature of Physician or Supplier Including Degrees or Credentials   Form locator 31 identifies the name of the physician or supplier who has provided the services to the patient along with her credentials (M.D., PA-C, or NP).

If a paper claim is submitted, enter the physician or supplier's name, signature of the physician's or supplier's representative, or "Signature on File" or "SOF." Enter the six-digit date (MM/DD/YY), eight-digit date (MM/DD/CCYY), or alphanumeric date. A signature stamp may be used instead of a written signature. The stamp must leave a clear, nonsmeared image on the claim form.

Form Locator 32: Name and Address of Facility Where Services Were Rendered   Form locator 32 identifies the name of the facility where services were provided. Enter the name, address, 9 digit zip code, and NPI number 06 the facility where the service was provided. When more than one facility is used, a separate CMS-1500 claim form should be used.

Form Locator 32a: NPI Number   Enter the NPI number of the service facility location in form locator 32a.

Form Locator 32b: Other ID Number   Enter the two-digit qualifier identifying the non-NPI number followed by the ID number. Do not enter a space, hyphen, or other separator between the qualifier and number. The NUCC qualifiers are listed under form locator 17a.

Form Locator 33: Billing Provider Information and Phone Number   Enter the provider's or supplier's billing name, address, zip code, and phone number in form locator 33. The phone number is to be entered in the area to the right of the field title. Enter the name and address information in the following format:

First line: Name
Second line: Address
Third line: City, state, and zip code.

Form Locator 33a: NPI Number   Enter the NPI number of the billing provider in form locator 33a. The NPI number refers to the HIPAA National Provider Identifier number, which allows for the entry of 10 characters.

Form Locator 33b: Other ID Number Enter the NPI number. Do not enter a space, hyphen, or other separator between the qualifier and number. For the qualifier number, refer to form locator 17a.

Filing Guidelines

The rules and regulations for Medicare claims are complex. The MOS must be familiar with the rules and regulations for the provider's Medicare carrier. For instance, a medical necessity claim can be denied if it is billed too often during the allowed time period.

Local Coverage Determination (LCD)

Local Coverage Determinations (LCDs) are notices sent to physicians on a regular basis that contain detailed and updated information about the coding and medical necessity of a specific service.

Medicare Remittance Notice

If the Medicare claims processing computer determines that payment is due on a claim, the beneficiary or provider will receive payment in approximately 14 days for electronic claims and 29 days from the date of receipt for paper claims. The Medicare contractor (carrier) sends Medicare patients a **Medicare Summary Notice (MSN)** every 30 days itemizing what services were billed to Medicare by the provider, the amount Medicare paid, and the amount the beneficiary is responsible for paying the provider, if any.

Providers will receive a **Medicare Remittance Notice (MRN)** from a Medicare contractor on assigned claims. A Medicare Remittance notice is received electronically. It informs the provider what payment he will receive, what adjustments were made, and what the patient owes. It will also notify the provider if the claim has been forwarded to a Medigap payer.

Complete a Medicare claim based on the information provided below. To complete this exercise, copy the CMS-1500 form provided in Appendix D or download it from the CD-ROM that accompanies this text.

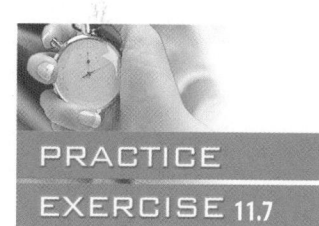

PRACTICE EXERCISE 11.7

Physician Information:

Physician Name:	Mallard and Associates, P.A.
	J.D. Mallard, M.D.
License Number:	TX54308
Address:	19333 Forrest Haven
	Dallas, TX 12345-2222
Phone Number:	214-555-5040

Group Identification Numbers

Group PIN:	M23548711
Group NPI:	7777788888
Referring Physician:	William F. Bonner, M.D.

Dr. William F. Bonner Identification Numbers

UPIN:	465922113
NPI:	1111199999

(continued)

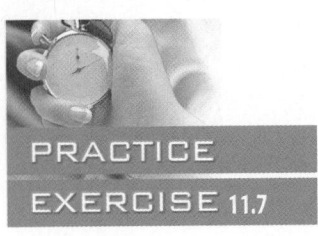

PRACTICE
EXERCISE 11.7

(continued)

Dr. J. D. Mallard Identification Numbers
EIN: 72-5727222
NPI: 8888877777
UPIN: 234665212

Patient Information Form:

Name: Your Name
                            1884 Dallas Way
                            Dallas, TX 12345
Phone Number: 972-555-4572
Social Secondary number: 145-87-5988
DOB: 06/25/44
SEX: Female, Single
Patient Account Number: Your Name (1st three letters of your last
                            name and 1st two letters of first name)
Employer: Allied Health Corporation
Insurance Carrier: Medicare
Insurance Address: P.O. Box 3463
                            Dallas, TX 75007
Insurance ID number: 145-87-5988A

Patient Encounter Form:

Date: Today's date
Date of first symptoms: Two days ago
CC: Patient complaining of abdominal pain
                            (789.00)
Lungs: Normal
Heart: Normal
Abdomen: Normal
Pelvic: Normal
Chest x-ray: 2 Views—Normal
ECG: Normal
DX: Abdominal Pain (789.00)

List of Fees for Services:

Date: Today's date
DX: Abdominal Pain (789.00), Hypertension 401.9
99203:   Expanded problem focused history,
                            examination, and MDM of low
                            complexity—$80.00, Diagnosis: 789.00
71020:   Radiological Exam, chest, frontal and lateral—
                            $75.00, Diagnosis: 789.00
93000:   Electrocardiogram, routine ECG with at least
                            12 leads with interpretation and report
                            $65.00, Diagnosis: 401.9
TOTAL CHARGES: $220.00

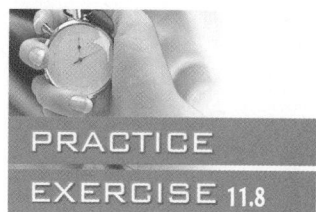

Utilizing the information in Practice Exercise 11.7 along with the following Medigap information, complete a CMS-1500 form for supplemental insurance. Copy the CMS-1500 form provided in Appendix D or download it from the CD-ROM that accompanies this text.

PRACTICE
EXERCISE 11.8

Medigap: United Health Care
              123 My Street
              Baltimore, MD 21204
              MG number 223546721

Medicare Fraud and Abuse

Medicare fraud and abuse affects the whole population. Fraud is a ploy to receive unearned reimbursement for services not rendered. The funds come from the taxes that each of us contribute. This in turn leads to increased Medicare premiums and less payment to the provider. As a result, providers do not choose to participate in the Medicare programs.

Medicare Fraud

Medicare fraud is defined by CMS as "Knowingly and willfully executing, or attempting to execute a scheme or artifice to defraud any health care benefit program or to obtain, by means of false or fraudulent pretenses, representations, or promises, any of the money or property owned by, or under the custody or control of, any health care benefit program." Figure 11.2 illustrates the four most common types of Medicare fraud.

Inappropriate actions or behaviors against the Medicare program that are identified by the provider but not remedied may be considered fraudulent by Medicare. All healthcare providers who participate in the Medicare program are expected to furnish and report services in accordance with the established regulations and policies.

Fraud Scenarios
The following are examples of fraud scenarios:

■ A clinical laboratory receives orders from a physician for specific clinical laboratory tests. The lab performs and bills for the tests indicated on the order, but then also bills for additional tests that were not ordered or rendered.

1. Billing for services that were not rendered.
2. Misrepresenting as medically necessary any noncovered or screening services by reporting covered procedure/revenue codes.
3. Signing blank records or certification forms or falsifying information on records or certification forms for the sole purpose of obtaining payment.
4. Consistently using procedure/revenue codes that describe more extensive services than those actually performed.

Figure 11.2

The four most common types of Medicare fraud.

- A patient recruiter convinces unsuspecting beneficiaries to reveal their Medicare numbers to him. The recruiter then sells the Medicare numbers to a fictitious provider who, in turn, bills for services/items that were never furnished. (Providers should ensure that only the services/items they order are furnished.)
- Nursing home patients are offered free exercise and/or social activities. However, the free services are billed to Medicare as covered partial hospitalization services at a community mental health center or as covered physical therapy at a rehabilitation facility.
- A durable medical equipment supplier has a financial arrangement with a physician who completes certificates of medical necessity (CMNs) for patients he has never treated. The completed CMNs are used to falsely document the medical necessity of equipment given to patients who do not need the equipment. A physician unwittingly signs blank certification forms for a home health agency that falsely represents that skilled nursing services are needed for patients who would not have qualified for home health services. (In these two scenarios, both providers are committing Medicare fraud. The durable medical equipment company committed fraud by filing false prescriptions and the physician committed fraud by signing incomplete or blank prescription forms for the purpose of obtaining Medicare payments.
- A physician routinely bills for high-level evaluation and management services procedure codes although many of the visits he furnishes do not meet the requirements for the codes reported.
- A hospital falsely reported pneumonia as the diagnosis for a majority of the inpatient hospital stays billed to Medicare. As a result, their diagnostic-related group payment was significantly higher than it should have been.

Be aware of other types of Medicare fraud:

- Using an incorrect or invalid provider number in order to be paid or to be paid at a higher rate of reimbursement.
- Selling or sharing Medicare health insurance claim numbers so that false Medicare claims can be filed.
- Routinely waiving coinsurance and/or deductibles for Medicare patients when no effort has been made to collect the amounts due or when the patient *does* have the ability to pay.
- Falsifying information on applications, medical records, billings statements, and/or cost reports, or on any document filed with the government.
- Offering, accepting, or soliciting bribes, rebates, or kickbacks.

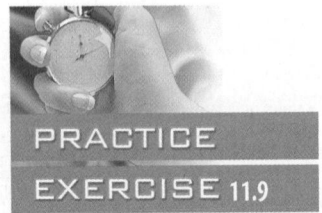

PRACTICE EXERCISE 11.9

Identify whether each of the providers in the following situations is guilty of upcoding, fraud, or abuse:

1. A radiologist routinely bills for chest x-rays with two views, although most of the chest x-rays performed are for single views.

2. A fictitious provider bills for services that were never furnished.

3. A physician uses a nonphysician practitioner to perform follow-up visits, but bills the practitioner's services as comprehensive initial evaluations.

(continued)

Identify whether each of the providers in the following situations is guilty of misrepresentation in terms of medically necessary, noncovered, or screening services:

4. A home health agency bills for covered home health services for an unqualified patient.

5. An ambulance company bills for emergency transportation for scheduled trips from a nursing home to a clinic.

6. A physician falsifies the diagnosis for a service that would otherwise be denied coverage if it were correctly reported.

7. Which of the following definitions is the correct definition of *nonrendered services*?

   A. Services/items furnished to a patient but not billed to Medicare.
   B. Noncovered services under Medicare.
   C. Services/items not furnished to a patient but billed to Medicare.

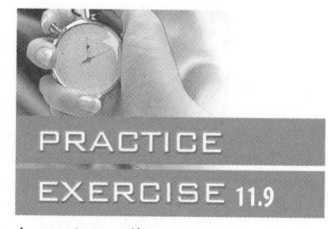

PRACTICE EXERCISE 11.9

(continued)

Medicare Abuse

Medicare abuse is legally defined by CMS as "Abuse may, directly or indirectly, result in unnecessary costs to the Medicare or Medicaid program, improper payment for services which fail to meet professionally recognized standards of care, or that are medically unnecessary. . . . Abuse involves payment for items or services when there is no legal entitlement to that payment and the provider has not knowingly and/or intentionally misrepresented facts to obtain payment."

The following are the two common types of Medicare abuse:

- Billing for services/items in excess of those needed by the patient
- Routinely filing duplicate claims, even if it does not result in duplicate payment.

Abuse Scenarios

The following are examples of Medicare abuse scenarios:

- Laboratory equipment is calibrated to run additional indices with every CBC test. Physician orders may only be for a CBC, but claims filed to Medicare include charges for the CBC and the additional indices. A hospital has a standard protocol that requires all patients admitted through the emergency room to have the following tests performed, regardless of the patient's condition: EKG, chest x-ray, urinalysis, and lab panel. This is abuse; not all patients require these tests.
- A provider's electronic billing program automatically refiles their claims if payment is not received within a 3-week period from the submission date.
- A hospital reports salaries paid to its administrators that have been determined to be excessive in prior cost report settlements.
- An outpatient rehabilitation facility includes noncovered charges in its "allowable costs" section of the cost report.

Protecting Against Medicare Fraud and Abuse

An important step in protecting the office from Medicare fraud and abuse is knowing when and how the practice may be liable as a provider. Keep these three points in mind when considering liability:

1. Providers are liable for Medicare fraud when their intent to purposely obtain money or property owned by Medicare through false or fraudulent pretenses has been clearly determined.
2. Providers are liable for Medicare abuse for all claims submitted that violate the Medicare program guidelines.
3. Providers may also be held responsible for fraudulent or abusive claims submitted where they are listed as referring physicians for services performed such as claims submitted by clinical laboratories.

Provider Liability Cases

Consider the following situations and discussions about provider liability:

■ **Q:** An external billing service set up as the payee of the provider (on Medicare's file) commits fraud by billing for additional services not rendered by the provider. Is the provider liable?
A: The provider would be liable for the Medicare fraud committed by the billing service in this case if her intent to commit fraud had definitely been established by the results of an investigation. If that were the case, the provider would be responsible for returning all overpayments to Medicare and may also be criminally liable.

■ **Q:** An employee of a provider commits fraud without the provider knowing it. Is the provider liable?
A: All providers are responsible for the actions of their employees. Prosecution of the provider in this case for his employee's Medicare fraud is unlikely if the provider's lack of intent has been definitely established by the results of an investigation. The provider will, however, be responsible for returning all overpayments to Medicare.

■ **Q:** A physician refers a patient to another provider for diagnostic tests. The other provider bills medically unnecessary services as covered services for the referred patient. Is the referring physician liable?
A: The referring physician, in this case, is not liable for the other provider's Medicare fraud as long as her referral information concerning the medical necessity of the test is appropriately documented.

■ **Q:** A provider uses incorrect billing procedures when billing Medicare for services that result in overpayment by Medicare. Is the provider liable?
A: Providers are responsible for incorrect billing practices. Providers are expected to correct mistakes and return overpaid monies to Medicare. If providers fail to correct mistakes and return overpaid monies, they may be suspected of fraud.

A provider's actions may be considered fraudulent and the provider would be considered liable if:

■ Claims are submitted that contain mistakes resulting in an overpayment.
■ Claims are submitted in which the provider intentionally "upcoded" charges.
■ Claims are submitted that contain mistakes resulting in an overpayment that the provider identifies but does not correct.

The Department of Health and Human Services (DHHS), which includes the CMS and the Office of Inspector General, has the authority to impose remedial action or administrative "sanctions" against individuals who consistently fail to comply with Medicare law or are deemed abusive to the Medicare program. Sanctions include:

- Provider education and warning
- Revocation of assignment privileges
- Withholding of provider's Medicare payments and recovery of Medicare's overpayments
- Exclusion of provider from the Medicare program
- Posting of provider's name on national Sanctioned Provider list that is sponsored by the U.S. government.

The penalties that may be imposed on individuals and/or entities that are convicted include loss of medical license; criminal penalties, fines, restitution, and/or imprisonment; and civil penalties, plus triple damages.

Chapter Summary

- Medicare is divided into two main programs: Medicare Part A, which is hospital insurance, and Medicare Part B, which is medical insurance.
- The fee-for-service method is a method of charging for healthcare services under which each procedure is based on a specific amount of reimbursement. Medicare determines their fees for service using the resource-based relative value scale reimbursement method.
- Recording the information from the Medicare card accurately is extremely important because that information will be used on many claims forms and medical documentation materials throughout the patient's history with the facility.
- A provider may choose to participate or not participate in the Medicare program. Medicare reimbursement depends on participation and non-participation.
- Medigap is a supplemental insurance sponsored by Medicare. It is an optional policy available to individuals who qualify for Medicare.
- For Medicare Part A the UB-04 is used for filing claims. The CMS-1500 is used for Medicare Part B.
- Medicare Fraud is knowingly and willfully executing, or attempting to execute a scheme to defraud any health care benefit program. Medicare abuse involves payment for items or services when there is no legal entitlement.

Chapter Review

True/False

Identify the statement as true (T) or false (F).

_____ **1.** The Medicare 2007 deductible for Part B is $200.00.

_____ **2.** A intermediary is a company that is paid to process claims for Medicare Part A.

_____ **3.** The medical office specialist should check patients' Medicare eligibility each time an appointment is made.

_____ **4.** Care in a skilled nursing facility is covered under Medicare Part B.

_____ **5.** Medicare Part A is administered by the CMS.

_____ **6.** The benefit period Medicare Part A is the period during which a patient is insured.

_____ **7.** Medicare Part A provides coverage for physician services and procedures.

_____ **8.** Medicare Part B provides coverage for durable medical equipment.

_____ **9.** Medicare covers an annual physical examination.

_____ **10.** Medicare Part B covers eyeglasses.

_____ **11.** Form locator 11 on the CMS-1500 form must be completed.

Multiple Choice

Identify the letter of the choice that best completes the statement or answers the question.

_____ **1.** Individuals who are over age 65 who do not receive Social Security benefits may enroll in Medicare Part A by:
   a. paying a deductible.
   b. paying into a Medical Savings account.
   c. paying a premium.
   d. enrolling in a Medicare HMO.

_____ **2.** Under the Medicare program, a nonparticipating, non-accepting assignment physician may not bill more than 115% of:
   a. the Medicare approved amount from the MFS.
   b. the Medicare limiting charge on the non-par Medicare Fee Schedule.
   c. either a or b, whichever is lower.
   d. neither a nor b.

_____ **3.** What percentage of the fee on the Medicare Fee Schedule is the limiting charge?
   a. 115%   c. 28.85%
   b. 100%   d. 80%

_____ **4.** Under the Medicare program, if the approved amount for a procedure is $100.00, the participating provider will be paid $100.00 (by Medicare and the patient), and the nonparticipating provider who accepts assignment will be paid:
   a. $115.00   c. $95.00
   b. $100.00   d. $80.00

Completion

Complete each sentence or statement.

1. People who are entitled to Medicare Part A benefits automatically qualify for Medicare _____.

2. When a patient is over age 65 and employed, the employer's group health plan, not Medicare, is the _____ plan.

3. If an individual is receiving coverage under a COBRA case as well as Medicare, the Medicare plan is the _____ payer.

4. What does CMS mean? _____

5. Under the rules of the Medicare program, a patient may sign a _____ release form.

6. Physicians who participate in the Medicare program can bill patients for services that are _____ from coverage.

7. _____ includes benefits of Medicare Part A and Medicare Part B.

8. The _____ form is used to file Medicare Part B claims.

9. _____ insurance coverage is offered under the original Medicare plan.

10. The _____ plan is supplemental to Medicare.

11. For Medicare to determine if the patient has been notified in advance that he will be responsible for payment, a(N) _____ modifier is used with the procedure.

12. If the patient refuses to sign the ABN for a nonassigned claim, use a (N) _____ modifier.

13. TRHCA is the abbreviation for _____.

14. The turnaround time for paper claims is _____, and for electronic claims is _____.

15. CMS has stated that the place of service must also be fully written out in form locator _____ .

Resources

Trailblazer Health Enterprises, LLC: *www.trailblazerhealth.com*

Chapter 12 Medicaid Medical Billing

Chapter Objectives

After reading this chapter, the student should be able to:

1. Understand the requirements for qualifying to receive Medicaid benefits.
2. Determine the schedule of benefits the Medicaid recipient will receive.
3. Discuss the method of verifying Medicaid benefits.
4. Submit a Medicaid claim and decipher claim status.

Key Terms

Aid to Families with Dependent Children (AFDC)
categorically needy
early and periodic screening, diagnostic, and treatment (EPSDT)
Federal Medical Assistance Percentages (FMAP) program

medically needy
Medi-Medi
payer of last resort
Programs for All-Inclusive Care for the Elderly (PACE)
restricted status
spend-down program

State Children's Health Insurance Program (SCHIP)
Supplemental Security Income (SSI)
Temporary Assistance for Need Families (TANF)
welfare reform bill

Case Study
Medicaid

The office manager, Darla, had received a notification from the state Medicaid program that fraudulent use of Medicaid cards was on the rise. As a result, all patients were to show a picture ID along with their Medicaid card. Darla had announced this new policy at the last staff meeting.

While Ginger was working as the receptionist, a patient arrived and showed her Medicaid card. Ginger explained that she needed to see picture ID due to increased fraud. The patient became indignant and refused to comply because she felt she was being accused of doing something illegal. Ginger asked Darla to explain the situation to the patient.

Questions

1. Should the patient be required to comply with the new policy in order to be seen by the physician? Why?

2. Could Ginger have handled the situation differently?

3. What should Darla tell the patient in order to calm her down?

Introduction

Title XIX of the Social Security Act is a federal/state entitlement program that pays for medical assistance for certain individuals and families with low incomes and resources. This program, known as Medicaid, became law in 1965 as a cooperative venture jointly funded by the federal and state governments to assist states in furnishing medical assistance to eligible needy persons. The federal government makes payments to states under the **Federal Medical Assistance Percentages (FMAP) program**. Medicaid is the largest source of funding for medical and health-related services for America's low-income individuals, some who may have no medical insurance or inadequate medical insurance. Providers choose to participate in the Medicaid program. Although the federal government establishes general guidelines for the program, specific program requirements are actually established by each state. Whether or not a person is eligible for Medicaid will depend on the state where he or she resides.

Medicaid Guidelines

Within broad national guidelines established by federal statutes, regulations, and policies, each state:

1. Establishes its own eligibility standards
2. Determines the type, amount, duration, and scope of services
3. Sets the rate of payment for services
4. Administers its own program.

Medicaid policies for eligibility, services, and payment are complex and vary considerably, even among states of similar size or geographic proximity. Thus, a person who is eligible for Medicaid in one state may not be eligible in another state, and the services provided by one state may differ considerably in amount, duration, or scope from services provided in a similar or neighboring state. In addition, state legislatures may change Medicaid eligibility, services, and/or reimbursement during any given year. Most Medicaid plans do not require a premium.

Eligibility Groups

States are required to include certain types of individuals or eligibility groups under their Medicaid plans, and they may include others. States' eligibility groups include the following:

1. Categorically needy
2. Medically needy
3. Special groups.

Categorically Needy

Persons who qualify as categorically needy under the Medicaid program include the following:

- Families who meet states' Aid to Families with Dependent Children (AFDC) eligibility requirements on July 16, 1996.
- Pregnant women and children under age 6 whose family income is at or below 133% of the federal poverty level (Services to these pregnant women are limited to those related to pregnancy, complications of pregnancy, delivery, and postpartum care).
- Children ages 6 to 19 with family income up to 100% of the federal poverty level.
- Caretakers (relatives or legal guardians who take care of children under age 18 (or 19 if still in high school).
- **Supplemental Security Income (SSI)** SSI is a federal income supplement program funded by general tax revenues designed to help the elderly and people who are blind or have a disability and who have little or no income.
- Individuals and couples who are living in medical institutions and who have monthly income up to 300% of the SSI income standard (federal benefit rate).

Medically Needy

People who are termed "medically needy" have too much money (and in some cases resources such as savings accounts) to be categorized as "categorically needy." If a state has a medically needy program, it must include pregnant women through a 60-day postpartum period, children under age 18, certain newborns for 1 year, and certain protected people who are blind.

The medically needy (MN) option allows states to extend Medicaid eligibility to additional people. These people would be eligible for Medicaid under one of the mandatory or optional groups, except that their income and/or resources are above the eligibility level set by their state. Persons may qualify immediately or may spend down by incurring medical expenses that reduce their income to or below their state's MN income level. A **spend-down program** is one in which the individual is required to spend a portion of her income or resources until she is at or below the state's income level. The concept is similar to an annual deductible, except that it resets at the beginning of every month. Each month, the enrollee pays a portion of incurred medical bills, up to a certain amount, before the Medicaid fee schedule takes effect and Medicaid takes over the payments.

Medicaid eligibility and benefit provisions for the medically needy do not have to be as extensive as for the categorically needy and, in fact, they may be quite restrictive.

Example

A patient who has a spend down of $100.00 per month visits the physician on June 5 and the fee is $75.00. The patient is responsible for the $75.00. Ten days later, on June 15, the patient returns to the physician and the fee is $75.00. The patient is responsible for $25.00 and Medicaid will pay the remaining $50.00. At the beginning of July, the patient is again responsible for $100.00 of medical services incurred during July.

Federal matching funds are available for MN programs. However, if a state elects to have a MN program, the federal government requires that certain *groups* and certain *services* must be included; that is, children under age 19 and pregnant women who are medically needy must be covered, and prenatal and delivery care for pregnant women, as well as ambulatory care for children, must be provided. A state may elect to provide MN eligibility to certain additional groups and may elect to provide certain additional services within its MN program.

Special Groups

States' eligibility groups may also include immigrants, families that need temporary assistance, and children with disabilities.

Immigrants

The Personal Responsibility and Work Opportunity Reconciliation Act of 1996 (Public Law 104-193), known as the **welfare reform bill**, made restrictive changes regarding eligibility for SSI coverage that impacted the Medicaid program. For example, legal resident aliens and other qualified aliens who entered the United States on or after August 22, 1996, are ineligible for Medicaid for 5 years. Medicaid coverage for most aliens entering before that date and coverage for those eligible after the 5-year ban are state options; emergency services, however, are mandatory for both of these alien coverage groups. For aliens who lose SSI benefits because of the new restrictions regarding SSI coverage, Medicaid can continue only if these persons can be covered for Medicaid under some other eligibility status (again with the exception of emergency services, which are mandatory). The welfare reform bill also affected a number of children with disabilities, who lost SSI as a result of the restrictive changes; however, their eligibility for Medicaid was reinstituted by the Balanced Budget Act.

TANF

Welfare reform also repealed the open-ended federal entitlement program known as **Aid to Families with Dependent Children (AFDC)** and replaced it with **Temporary Assistance for Needy Families (TANF)**, which provides states with grants to be spent on time-limited cash assistance. TANF generally limits a family's lifetime cash welfare benefits to a maximum of 5 years and permits states to impose a wide range of other requirements as well—in particular, those related to employment. Although most persons covered by TANF will receive Medicaid, it is not required by law. Eligibility for TANF is determined at the county level. The following questions are taken into account:

- Is the family's income below set limits?
- Are the family's resources (including property) equal to or less than set limits?
- Is there at least one child under 18 in the household?
- Is at least one parent unemployed, incapacitated, or absent from the home?
- Does the individual have a Social Security number and birth certificate?
- Does the individual receive adoptive or foster care assistance?

State Children's Health Insurance Program

Title XXI of the Social Security Act, known as the **State Children's Health Insurance Program (SCHIP)**, is a new program initiated by the Balanced Budget Act (BBA) of 1997. In addition to allowing states to craft or expand an existing state insurance program, SCHIP provides more federal funds for states to expand Medicaid eligibility to include a greater number of children who are currently uninsured. With certain exceptions, these are low-income children who would not qualify for Medicaid based on the plan that was in effect on April 15, 1997. Funds from SCHIP also may be used to provide medical assistance to children during a presumptive eligibility period for Medicaid. This is one of several options from which states may select to provide healthcare coverage for more children, as prescribed within the BBA's Title XXI program.

Medicaid coverage may begin as early as the third month prior to application—if the person would have been eligible for Medicaid had he or she applied during that time. Medicaid coverage generally stops at the end of the month in which a person no longer meets the criteria of any Medicaid eligibility group. The BBA allows states to provide 12 months (6 months in Texas) of continuous Medicaid coverage (without reevaluation) for eligible children under the age of 19. Not all Medicaid plans require the beneficiary to pay a premium.

The Ticket to Work and Work Incentives Improvement Act of 1999 (Public Law 106-170) provides or continues Medicaid coverage to certain beneficiaries with disabilities who work despite their disabilities. Those with higher incomes may pay a sliding scale premium based on income.

Scope of Medicaid Services

Title XIX of the Social Security Act allows considerable flexibility within the states' Medicaid plans. However, some federal requirements are mandatory if federal matching funds are to be received. A state's Medicaid program *must* offer medical assistance for certain *basic* services to most categorically needy populations. These services generally include the following:

- Inpatient hospital services
- Outpatient hospital services
- Prenatal care
- Vaccines for children
- Physician services
- Nursing facility services for persons age 21 or older
- Family planning services and supplies
- Rural health clinic services
- Home health care for persons eligible for skilled nursing services
- Laboratory and x-ray services
- Pediatric and family nurse practitioner services
- Nurse-midwife services
- Federally qualified health center (FQHC) services and the ambulatory services of an FQHC that would be available in other settings
- **Early and periodic screening, diagnostic, and treatment (EPSDT)** services for children under age 21.

States may also receive federal matching funds to provide certain *optional* services. The following are the most common of the 34 currently approved optional Medicaid services:

- Diagnostic services
- Clinic services
- Intermediate care facilities for people with mental retardation

- Prescribed drugs and prosthetic devices
- Optometrist services and eyeglasses
- Nursing facility services for children under age 21
- Transportation services
- Rehabilitation and physical therapy services
- Home and community-based care to certain persons with chronic impairments.

PACE

The BBA included a state option known as **Programs of All-Inclusive Care for the Elderly (PACE)**. PACE provides an alternative to institutional care for persons age 55 or older who require a nursing facility level of care. The PACE team offers and manages all health, medical, and social services and mobilizes other services as needed to provide preventive, rehabilitative, curative, and supportive care. This care, provided in day health centers, homes, hospitals, and nursing homes, helps the person maintain independence, dignity, and quality of life. PACE functions within the Medicare program as well. Regardless of source of payment, PACE providers receive payment only through the PACE agreement and must make available all items and services covered under both Titles XVIII and XIX, without amount, duration, or scope limitations and without application of any deductibles, copayments, or other cost sharing. The individuals enrolled in PACE receive benefits solely through the PACE program.

Amount and Duration of Medicaid Services

Within broad federal guidelines and certain limitations, states determine the amount and duration of services offered under their Medicaid programs. States may limit, for example, the number of days of hospital care or the number of physician visits covered. Two restrictions apply: (1) Limits must result in a sufficient level of services to reasonably achieve the purpose of the benefits, and (2) limits on benefits may not discriminate among beneficiaries based on medical diagnosis or condition.

In general, states are required to provide comparable amounts, duration, and scope of services to all categorically needy and categorically related eligible persons, with two important exceptions:

1. Medically necessary healthcare services that are identified under the EPSDT program for eligible children under age 21, and that are within the scope of mandatory or optional services under federal law, must be covered even if those services are not included as part of the covered services in that state's plan. For instance, in Texas, EPSDT is known as Texas Health Steps. This provides healthcare benefits to children under age 21 who are enrolled in Medicaid. States are required by federal law to inform all Medicaid-eligible persons in the state who are under age 21 of the availability of EPSDT and immunizations. Patients are not charged a fee for EPSDT services; however, some families do pay a premium. This program emphasizes preventive care. Health screening (known as well-child checkup) for medical, vision, hearing, and dental are performed at regular intervals.

2. States may request "waivers" to pay for otherwise uncovered home and community-based services (HCBS) for Medicaid-eligible persons who might otherwise be institutionalized. As long as the services are cost effective, states have few limitations on the services that may be covered under these waivers (except that, other than as a part of respite care, states may not provide room and board for the beneficiaries). With certain exceptions, a state's Medicaid program must allow beneficiaries to have some informed choices among participating providers of health care and to receive quality care that is appropriate and timely.

Payment for Medicaid Services

Medicaid operates as a vendor payment program. States may pay healthcare providers directly on a fee-for-service basis, or states may pay for Medicaid services through various prepayment arrangements, such as health maintenance organizations (HMOs). If Medicaid does not cover a service, the patient may be billed if the following conditions have been met:

- The physician informed the patient before the service was performed that the procedure was not covered by Medicaid.
- The medical office specialist had the patient sign an advanced beneficiary notice form before the service was rendered, which states the amount of the procedure and why it will not be covered.

If a claim is denied by Medicaid for the following reasons, the physician may not bill the patient for the amount:

- Necessary preauthorization was not obtained prior to the procedure.
- The service was not medically necessary.
- The claim was not filed within the allotted time period.

Within federally imposed upper limits and specific restrictions, each state, for the most part, has broad discretion in determining the payment methodology and payment rate for services. Generally, payment rates must be sufficient to enlist enough providers so that covered services are available at least to the extent that comparable care and services are available to the general population within that geographic area. Providers participating in Medicaid must accept Medicaid payment rates as payment in full; that is, providers are not allowed to bill patients for the unpaid balance. States must make additional payments to qualified hospitals that provide inpatient services to a disproportionate number of Medicaid beneficiaries and/or to other low-income or uninsured persons under what is known as the *disproportionate share hospital* (DSH) adjustment.

States may impose nominal deductibles, coinsurance, or copayments on some Medicaid beneficiaries for certain services. The following Medicaid beneficiaries, however, must be excluded from cost sharing: pregnant women, children under age 18, and hospital or nursing home patients who are expected to contribute most of their income to institutional care. In addition, all Medicaid beneficiaries must be exempt from copayments for emergency services and family planning services.

The federal government also reimburses states for 100% of the cost of services provided through facilities of the Indian Health Service, provides financial help to the 12 states that furnish the highest number of emergency services to undocumented aliens, and shares in each state's expenditures for the administration of the Medicaid program. Most administrative costs are matched at 50%, although higher percentages are paid for certain activities and functions, such as development of mechanized claims processing systems.

Except for the SCHIP program, the Qualifying Individuals (QI) program, and DSH payments, federal payments to states for medical assistance have no set limit (cap). Rather, the federal government matches (at FMAP rates) state expenditures for the mandatory services, as well as for the optional services that the individual state decides to cover for eligible beneficiaries, and matches (at the appropriate administrative rate) all necessary and proper administrative costs. The Balanced Budget Refinement Act of 1999 increased the amount that certain states and the territories can spend on DSH and SCHIP payments, respectively.

Medicaid Summary and Trends

Medicaid was initially formulated as a medical care extension of federally funded programs that provided cash income assistance to the poor, with an emphasis on dependent children and their mothers, people with disabilities, and the elderly. Over the years, however, Medicaid eligibility has been incrementally expanded beyond its original ties with eligibility for cash programs. Legislation in the late 1980s assured Medicaid coverage to an expanded number of low-income pregnant women, poor children, and to some Medicare beneficiaries who are not eligible for any cash assistance programs. Legislative changes also focused on increased access, better quality of care, specific benefits, enhanced outreach programs, and fewer limits on services.

In most years since its inception, Medicaid has had very rapid growth in expenditures. This rapid growth has been due primarily to the following factors:

- The increase in size of the Medicaid-covered populations as a result of federal mandates, population growth, and economic recessions.
- The expanded coverage and utilization of services.
- The DSH payment program, coupled with its inappropriate use to increase federal payments to states.
- The increase in the number of very old people and people with disabilities who require extensive acute and/or long-term health care and various related services.
- The results of technological advances to keep a greater number of very low-birth-weight babies and other critically ill or severely injured persons alive and in need of continued extensive and very costly care.
- The increase in drug costs and the availability of new expensive drugs.
- The increase in payment rates to providers of healthcare services, when compared to general inflation.

Another significant development in Medicaid is the growth in managed care as an alternative service delivery concept different from the traditional fee-for-service system. Under managed care systems, HMOs, prepaid health plans (PHPs), or comparable entities agree to provide a specific set of services to Medicaid enrollees, usually in return for a predetermined periodic payment per enrollee. Managed care programs seek to enhance access to quality care in a cost-effective manner. Waivers may provide the states with greater flexibility in the design and implementation of their Medicaid managed care programs. Waiver authority under Sections 1915(b) and 1115 of the Social Security Act is an important part of the Medicaid program. Section 1915(b) waivers allow states to develop innovative healthcare delivery or reimbursement systems. Section 1115 waivers allow statewide healthcare reform experimental demonstrations to cover uninsured populations and to test new delivery systems without increasing costs. Finally, the BBA provided states with a new option to use managed care.

The Medicaid–Medicare Relationship (MEDI-MEDI)

Medicare beneficiaries who have low incomes and limited resources may also receive help from the Medicaid program. For such persons who are eligible for full Medicaid coverage, the Medicare healthcare coverage is supplemented by services that are available under their state's Medicaid program, according to eligibility category. These additional services are known as **Medi-Medi** and may include nursing facility care beyond the 100-day limit covered by Medicare, prescription drugs, eyeglasses, and hearing aids. For persons enrolled in both programs, any services that are covered by Medicare are paid for by the Medicare program before any payments are made by the Medicaid program, since Medicaid is always the **payer of last resort**. CMS estimates that Medicaid currently provides some level of supplemental health coverage for about 6.5 million Medicare beneficiaries. Medicaid pays last on a claim when a patient has other effective insurance coverage.

Medicaid Managed Care

Managed care refers to a health system in which a network of healthcare providers agree to coordinate and provide health care to a population in exchange for a specific payment per person. Two different managed care models are:

- HMOs, which receive a monthly "capitation" payment for each person enrolled based on an average projection of medical expenses for the typical patient.
- Primary care case management, which is a noncapitated model. Each PCCM participant is assigned to a single primary care provider (PCP) who must authorize most other services, such as specialty physician care, before Medicaid can reimburse the specialty physician care. The state sets up physician networks and contracts directly with providers. Providers receive fee-for-service reimbursement, plus PCPs receive a small monthly case management fee for each patient.

Managed care programs are intended to reduce service fragmentation, increase access to care, reduce costs, and stimulate the development of more appropriate use of services. Medicaid clients are required to select a primary care provider. The PCP serves as the *medical home* and is responsible for 24-hour coverage when the patient requires access or care coordination. The medical home potentially gives enrollees a provider who knows their needs and can coordinate their health care. PCPs provide preventive checkups, treat the majority of conditions that enrollees experience, and refer the patient out of office for specialty care when necessary. The medical home was intended as a method for delivering coordinated care and a means to control costs. Some managed care Medicaid programs are designed to integrate delivery of acute and long-term care services through a managed care system. Participants receive all Medicaid services from their choice of HMOs. The HMOs provide all Medicaid primary, acute, and long-term care services through one service delivery system. This includes ensuring that each Medicaid-only member has a primary care doctor. Other acute care services include specialists, home health, medical equipment, laboratory, x-ray, and hospital services. If enrollees meet the medical necessity criteria to be in a nursing facility, they may choose to receive community-based alternatives and waiver services.

Enrollees with complex medical conditions are assigned a care coordinator, an HMO employee who is responsible for coordinating acute and long-term care services. The care coordinator develops an individual plan of care with the enrollee, family members, and providers, and can authorize services. The emphasis is on providing home and community-based services to avoid the need for institutionalization.

Medicaid Verification

Medicaid cards or coupons may be issued to qualified individuals. Some states issue cards twice a month, some once a month, and others every 2 months or every 6 months. Most states are changing to electronic verification of eligibility. Patients' eligibility should be checked *prior to each time they see the physician.* Many states provide both on-line and telephone verification systems. The medical office specialist should always verify patient eligibility because it may change on a monthly basis. During the verification process check to see if the patient is on **restricted status**, which requires him to see a specific physician (e.g., PCP) and/or pharmacy.

Medicaid Claims Filing

For claims payment to be considered, providers must adhere to the time limits described in this section. Claims received after the time limits have expired are not payable because the Medicaid program does not provide coverage for late claims.

Unless otherwise stated below, claims must be received within 95 days from each date of service (DOS). A 95- or 180-day filing deadline that falls on a weekend or holiday is extended to the next business day following the weekend or holiday.

For submission of prior authorization requests, refer to the specific Medicaid manual section for that program.

Time Limits for Submitting Claims

Review the following time limits for submitting claims:

- Inpatient claims filed by the hospital must be received by Medicaid within 95 days from the discharge date.
- Although not recommended, hospitals reimbursed according to diagnostic-related group (DRG) payment methodology may submit an interim claim if the client has been in the facility 30 consecutive days or longer. A total stay claim is needed to ensure accurate calculation for potential outlier payments for people younger than age 21.
- Children's hospitals reimbursed according to Tax Equity and Fiscal Responsibility Act (TEFRA) methodology may submit interim claims before discharge and must submit an interim claim if the client remains in the hospital past the hospital's fiscal year-end.
- When medical services are rendered to a Medicaid client, claims must be received within 95 days of the DOS. The date of service is the date the service is provided or performed. If the provider's enrollment is not complete, the claim will be denied. However, by ensuring that the claims are received within the 95-day filing limit, the provider has established the right to appeal for reimbursement once the enrollment process has been completed. To be considered

for payment, an appeal must be received within 180 days of the date of denial notification.

Appeal Time Limits

All appeals of denied claims and requests for adjustments on paid claims must be received within 180 days from the date of disposition, the date of the Remittance and Status (R&S) report on which that

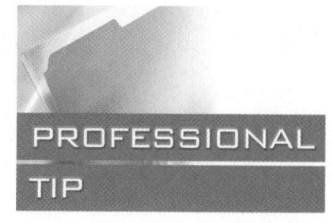

If a problem occurs with provider enrollment and the process is expected to take more than 180 days to complete, the original claims must be resubmitted and received before the 180-day appeals deadline has lapsed. Although this results in another denial of the claim, it will reestablish the provider's right to appeal.

PROFESSIONAL
TIP

claim appears. As mentioned earlier, if the 180-day appeal deadline falls on a weekend or holiday, the deadline will be extended to the next business day.

Claims with Incomplete Information and Zero Paid Claims

Claims lacking the information necessary for processing are listed on the R&S report with an explanation of benefits (EOB) code requesting the missing information. Providers must resubmit a signed, completed/corrected claim with a copy of the R&S on which the denied claim appears within 180 days from the date of the R&S to be considered for payment.

Newborn Claim Hints

When filing a claim for a newborn, if the mother's name is "Jane Jones," use "Boy Jane Jones" for a male child and a "Girl Jane Jones" for a female child.

Enter "Boy Jane" or "Girl Jane" in first name field and "Jones" in last name field. Always use "Boy" or "Girl" first and then the mother's full name. An exact match must be submitted or the claim will not be processed. Do **not** use "NBM" for newborn male or "NBF" for newborn female.

Medicaid participating physicians file claims using the CMS-1500 claim form. Medicaid participating hospitals and other inpatient facilities file claims using the UB-04. Healthcare Common Procedure Coding System (HCPCS) codes are required for both claim forms.

Completing the CMS-1500 Form for Medicaid (Primary)

This section reviews each form locator on the CMS-1500 and what information should be entered when filing a Medicaid claim.

Form Locator 1: Type of Insurance   Mark the Medicaid box with an X.

Form Locator 1a: Insured's ID Number   Enter the Medicaid number.

Form Locator 2: Patient's Name   Enter the name of the patient that received services in form locator 2. Input last name, first name, and middle name or initial. *The spelling should match the insurance card exactly.* If the name on the card is misspelled, then the name in the computer should be misspelled until the patient provides a new card with the correct spelling.

Form Locator 3: Patient's Date of Birth and Sex   In form locator 3, enter the patient's date of birth and sex/gender. The date of birth is entered using the eight-digit format: MMDDCCYY. The patient's sex/gender is identified as either male or female.

Form Locator 4: Insured's Name   Leave blank.

Form Locator 5: Patient's Address   Form locator 5 lists the patient's home address and telephone number. This information is taken from the patient information form when the patient registers in the office. The address should include the street name and number, city, state (two-letter abbreviations), zip code, and telephone number. Do not use commas, periods, or other punctuation in the address. When entering a nine-digit zip code, include the hyphen. Do not use a hyphen or space as a separator within the telephone number.

Form Locator 6: Patient's Relationship to the Insured   Mark an X in the Self box for relationship to the insured, unless the claim is for a newborn, then choose Child.

Form Locator 7: Insured's Address   Leave blank.

Form Locator 8: Patient Status   Enter the marital status of the patient.

Form Locators 9a–d: Other Insured's Name   Leave blank (since Medicaid is the "payer of last resort").

Form Locators 10a–c: Is Patient's Condition Related To?   Enter an X in the correct box.

Form Locator 10d: Reserved for Local Use   Form locator 10d is used by different insurance carriers for different reasons. One example of use would be a specific insurance carrier requiring the word "Attachment" to be placed here in the event that there are paper attachments with the claim. When required by payers to provide the subset of condition codes approved by the National Uniform Claim Committee (NUCC), enter the condition code in this field.

Form Locator 11: Insured's Policy Group or FECA Number   Enter the word "None."

Form Locators 11a–d: Insured's Date of Birth and Sex   Leave blank.

Form Locator 12: Patient's or Authorized Person's Signature   Form locator 12 is where the patient or guarantor signs to allow the release of any medical information to the insurance company for billing purposes. This release is only valid for billing information. Any other request for records require a formal release of information form to be signed by the patient or guarantor. This signature is good for 1 year from the date it is signed and should be updated annually. When submitting claims the words "Signature on File" or "SOF" may be added here in place of a signature. The actual patient signature must then be on file in the patient's chart. Enter the date in the six-digit format (MM/DD/YY) or eight-digit format (MM/DD/CCYY). If there is no signature on file, leave blank or enter "No Signature on File."

Form Locator 13: Insured's or Authorized Person's Signature   Form locator 13 is where the patient or insured signs to authorize the insurance company to reimburse the physician or supplier directly. As stated for form locator 12, the words "Signature on File" or "SOF" may be added here in place of a written signature when filing claims. If there is no signature on file, leave blank or enter "No Signature on File."

Form Locator 14: Date of Current: Illness, Injury, Pregnancy   Use form locator 14 to indicate the first date of the current illness, injury, or pregnancy. The date should be entered in the six-digit (MM/DD/YY) or eight-digit format (MM/DD/CCYY). For a pregnancy, the first day of the woman's last menstrual period (LMP) is used. If this information is not known, leave blank.

Form Locator 15: If Patient Has Had Same or Similar Illness   Use form locator 15 to indicate the first date of treatment for the same or a similar illness in the past. The date should be entered in the six-digit (MM/DD/YY) or eight-digit format (MM/DD/CCYY). If the information is not known, leave blank.

Form Locator 16: Dates Patient Unable to Work in Current Occupation   Form locator 16 indicates the dates the patient is unable to work due to his illness or injury. These dates will be required when filing workers' compensation or disability claims. The dates should be entered in the six-digit (MM/DD/YY) or eight-digit format (MM/DD/CCYY). If the information is not required, leave blank.

Form Locator 17: Name of Referring Provider or Other Source   Form locator 17 asks for the name of the physician referring the patient. Some insurance companies require this information to be on a claim. The information entered should include the physician's last name, first name, and credentials. If multiple providers are involved, enter one provider using the following priority order:

1. Referring provider

2. Ordering provider

3. Supervising provider.

If there is no referring physician, leave blank.

Form Locator 17a: ID Number of Referring Physician   The ID number of the referring, ordering, or supervising provider is reported in form locator 17a in the shaded area. The qualifier indicating what the number represents is reported in the qualifier field to the immediate right of the "17a." The National Uniform Claim Committee (NUCC) defines the following qualifiers:

0B	State license number
1B	Blue Shield provider number
1C	Medicare provider number
1D	Medicaid provider number
1G	Provider UPIN number
1H	TRICARE/CHAMPUS identification number
E1	Employer identification number
G2	Provider commercial number
LU	Location number
N5	Provider plan network identification number
SY	Social Security number (Note: The Social Security number may not be used for Medicare.)
X5	State industrial accident provider number
ZZ	Provider taxonomy (Taxonomy codes, also known as specialty codes, identify a provider's specialty category.).

The non-National Provider Identifier (NPI) number of the referring, ordering, or supervising provider refers to the payer-assigned unique identifier of the professional. This field allows for the entry of 2 characters in the qualifier field and 17 characters in the Other ID Number field.

Form Locator 17b: NPI (Number)   Enter the NPI number of the referring, ordering, or supervising provider in form locator 17b. The NPI number refers to the HIPAA National Provider Identifier number, which is a 10-digit number.

Form Locator 18: Hospitalization Dates Related to Current Services   Enter the dates the patient has been hospitalized in relation to the current services in form locator 18. If the patient has been discharged from the hospital, the dates should include the day admitted and the day discharged. If the patient is still hospitalized only include the day admitted. The dates should be entered in the six-digit (MM/DD/YY) or the eight-digit format (MM/DD/CCYY). If the patient has not been hospitalized, leave blank.

Form Locator 19: Reserved for Local Use   Form locator 19 is a conditional entry. Enter additional modifiers, dates, narrative, and information.

Form Locator 20: Outside Lab   Form locator 20 is used to indicate if lab work was done that was performed outside the office. A YES answer indicates that an entity other than the entity billing for the service performed the purchased services. If YES is chosen, enter the purchased price under Charges. When YES is chosen, form locator 32 must be completed. When billing for multiple purchased services, each service should be submitted on a separate claim form. Only one box can be marked. A NO answer indicates that no purchased services are included on the claim.

When the answer is YES the dollar amount must be entered in the $ Charges area. There is a limit of nine characters.

Form Locator 21: Diagnosis or Nature of Illness or Injury   In form locator 21, the ICD-9 codes for the diagnoses applied to this claim are entered. At least one code must be entered and up to four codes can be used on the claim. They are placed in order of precedence; with line 1 being the primary diagnosis and so forth. No written diagnoses are used on a claim form. The ICD-9 codes should be checked for medical necessity to make sure they are used appropriately with the CPT® codes used in form locator 24D. Relate lines 1, 2, 3, and 4 to the lines of service in 24E by line number.

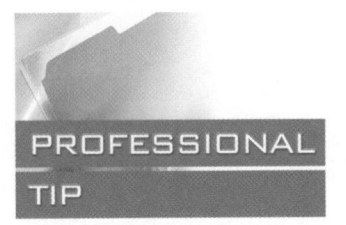

PROFESSIONAL TIP

Always make sure that the ICD-9 codes used are the most recent, up-to-date codes utilized to avoid denials. Codes used should be coded to the highest level of specificity.

Form Locator 22: Medicaid Resubmission Code   If required, form locator 22 is where the Medicaid resubmission code used for Medicaid claims is entered. List the original reference number and the code for resubmitted claims.

Example

22. Medicaid Resubmission Code 123	ORIGINAL REF NO. ABC1234567890

Form Locator 23: Prior Authorization Number   Some insurance plans, such as those of HMOs, EPOs, and preferred provider organizations (PPOs), require a prior authorization number. If required, when preauthorization is obtained from an insurance company for services, the number assigned is input in form locator 23. Also, HMO required referral numbers are input in this form locator. Any of the following can be entered here: prior authorization number, referral

CPT is a registered trademark of the American Medical Association.

number, mammography precertification number, or Clinical Laboratory Improvement Amendments (CLIA) number, as assigned by the payer for the current service. Do not enter hyphens or spaces within the number. If prior authorization is required and is omitted, the claim will be denied. If no prior authorization is required, leave blank.

Section 24

The six service lines in Section 24 have been divided horizontally to accommodate submission of both the NPI and another/proprietary identifier during the NPI transition and to accommodate the submission of supplemental information to support the billed service. The top area of the six service lines is shaded and is the location for reporting supplemental information. (It is not intended to allow the billing of 12 lines of service.)

The supplemental information is to be placed in the shaded section of 24A through 24G as defined in each item number. Providers must verify this supplemental information with the payer.

The following types of supplemental information can be entered in the shaded lines of Section 24:

- Anesthesia duration in hours and/or minutes with start and end times
- Narrative description of unspecified codes
- NDCs for drugs
- Vendor product number from the Health Industry Business Communication Council (HIBCC)
- Product number from the Health Care Uniform Code Council—Global Trade Item Number (GTIN), formerly Universal Product Code (UPC) for products
- Contract rate.

The following qualifiers are used when reporting these services:

7	Anesthesia information
ZZ	Narrative description of unspecified code
N4	NDCs
VP	Vendor product number from the HIBCC labeling standard
OZ	Product number from the Health Care Uniform Code Council (GTIN)
CTR	Contract rate.

If required to report other supplemental information not listed above, follow payer instructions for the use of a qualifier for the information being reported. When reporting a service that does not have a qualifier, enter two blank spaces before entering the information. To enter supplemental information, begin at 24A by entering the qualifier and then the information. Do not enter a space between the qualifier and the number/code/information. Do not enter hyphens or spaces within the number/code.

Form Locator 24A: Dates of Service   In form locator 24A, enter the dates of service for the services provided. Depending on the insurance carrier, these columns are filled in using different formats. Some require both the To and From dates to be listed in six-digit format (MM/DD/YY). Some require just the From date to be listed or just the To date. If the same procedure was provided multiple times on a single date, the specific date is entered once and the number of procedures is listed in form locator 24G.

Form Locator 24B: Place of Service   Place of service in form locator 24B is a mandatory field to be completed because it describes the place where the procedure or service was performed. This place could be many places, such as the physician's office, hospital, emergency department, skilled nursing facility, or even the patient's home. A code is used (see following list) to indicate the place of service.

Note that the CMS has stated that the place of service must also be fully written out in form locator 32 if the place of service is other than the physician's office. Consider this example: The patient was an inpatient (hospital) and the physician saw the patient in the hospital for an evaluation and management service. Therefore, the code 21 (see following list) would be entered in form locator 24B and the hospital address entered in form locator 32.

Common place of service codes include the following:

11	Physician's office
12	Private residence
13	Assisted living facility
20	Urgent care facility
21	Inpatient hospital
22	Outpatient hospital
23	Hospital emergency department
24	Ambulatory surgical center
25	Birthing center
26	Military treatment facility
31	Skilled nursing facility
34	Hospice
81	Independent laboratory.

Form Locator 24C: EMG (Emergency)   This form locator should be marked with a Y for YES or left blank for NO. The definition of an emergency is defined by either federal or state regulations or programs and/or payer contracts.

Form Locator 24D: Procedures, Services, or Supplies   In form locator 24D, enter the CPT or HCPCS codes used to identify the procedures, services, or supplies provided. Modifiers are also listed in form locator 24D. If more than three modifiers are used, list 99 here and enter the modifiers in form locator 19.

Form Locator 24E: Diagnosis Code (Pointer)   Form locator 24E indicates the number (1, 2, 3, and 4) of the diagnosis code listed in form locator 21 as it relates to each service or procedure. If more than one diagnosis is attached to a single procedure or service, list the primary diagnosis first.

Form Locator 24F: Charges   Form locator 24F lists the charges that are assigned to each CPT or HCPCS code listed. The amount should be entered without a decimal point or dollar sign. If multiple units are entered in form locator 24G, the charges should reflect the amount of the procedure times the number of units. Charges should be updated on a regular basis to follow appropriate billing guidelines.

Form Locator 24G: Days or Units   Enter the number of units per procedure or service provided to a patient in form locator 24G. If billing for anesthesia, the amount entered should be entered in minutes and calculated accordingly. If billing for multiple services, such as liters of oxygen, list the actual number of liters. If multiple units are entered in 24G, the charges should reflect the amount of the procedure multiplied by the number of units.

When required by payers to provide the National Drug Code (NDC) units in addition to the HCPCS units, enter the applicable NDC units' qualifier and related units in the shaded line following the NDC qualifier and code. The following qualifiers are to be used when reporting NDC units:

F2   International Unit   ML   Milliliter
GR   Gram   UN   Unit

Form Locator 24H: EPSDT Family Plan   Form locator 24H is used to identify whether the patient is receiving services through Medicaid's EPSDT program. If there is no requirement (e.g., state requirement) to report a reason code for EPSDT, enter "Y" for YES or "N" for NO only.

If there is a requirement to report a reason code for EPDST, enter the appropriate reason code as noted below. (A "Y" or "N" response is not entered with a code.) The two-character code is right justified in the top shaded area of the field.

The following codes for EPSDT are used:

AV   Available—Not used (Patient refused referral.)
S2   Under treatment (Patient is currently under treatment for referred diagnostic or corrective health problem.)
ST   New service requested (Referral to another provider for diagnostic or corrective treatment/scheduled for another appointment with screening provider for diagnostic or corrective treatment for at least one health problem identified during an initial or periodic screening service, not including dental referrals.)
NU   Not used (Used when no EPSDT patient referral was given.)

If the service is for family planning, enter "Y" for YES or "N" for NO in the bottom, unshaded area of the field.

Form Locator 24I: ID Qualifier   Enter in the shaded area of form locator 24I the qualifier identifying whether the number is a non-NPI number. The other ID number of the rendering provider is then reported in form locator 24J in the shaded area. Refer back to form locator 17a for a list of qualifiers.

Form Locator 24J: Rendering Provider   The individual rendering the service is reported in form locator 24J. Enter the non-NPI ID number in the shaded area of the field. Enter the NPI number in the unshaded area of the field.

The Rendering Provider is the person or company (laboratory or other facility) who rendered or supervised the care. In the case where a substitute provider was used, enter that provider's information here. Report the Identification Number in form locator 24I and 24J only when different from data recorded in form locators 33a and 33b.

Form Locator 25: Federal Tax I.D. Number   List in form locator 25 the physician's federal tax I.D. number or his employer identification number (EIN). Do not enter hyphens with numbers. The appropriate selection should be marked and the corresponding number entered.

Form Locator 26: Patient's Account Number   In form locator 26, enter the patient account number assigned in the medical office. The computer system used in the office will generate the number and it should be entered on the claim. This in turn will allow for the account number to appear on the

Explanation of Benefits (EOB) form, which makes it easier to locate the correct patient to post insurance payments.

Form Locator 27: Accept Assignment?   Form locator 27 is used to indicate whether or not the physician accepts assignment on this claim. If the physician does accept assignment and the patient has signed form locator 13, the insurance carrier will pay the physician directly for services provided. If the physician does not accept assignment, the insurance carrier will send the reimbursement to the patient.

Form Locator 28: Total Charge   Form locator 28 lists the total of charges, added together from those listed in form locator 24F. The charges should be checked for accuracy to ensure proper reimbursement. Do not use decimal points or dollar signs in this entry.

Form Locator 29: Amount Paid   Form locator 29 indicates the amount paid on this claim. This amount is usually added after the primary EOB is received and payment is posted. A secondary claim is printed to be sent to the secondary insurance carrier along with a copy of the primary insurance carrier's EOB. Do not use decimal points or dollar signs in this entry.

Form Locator 30: Balance Due   Because Medicaid is the payer of last resort, this form locator is left blank.

Form Locator 31: Signature of Physician or Supplier Including Degrees or Credentials   Form locator 31 identifies the name of the physician or supplier who has provided the services to the patient along with her credentials (M.D., PA-C, or NP).

If a paper claim is submitted, enter the signature of the physician's or supplier's representative, or "Signature on File" or "SOF." Enter the six-digit date (MM/DD/YY), eight-digit date (MM/DD/CCYY), or alphanumeric date. A signature stamp may be used instead of a written signature. The stamp must leave a clear, nonsmeared image on the claim form.

Form Locator 32: Name and Address of Facility Where Services Were Rendered   Form locator 32 identifies the name of the facility where services were provided. Enter the name, address, zip code, and NPI number when billing for purchased diagnostic tests. When more than one supplier is used, a separate CMS-1500 claim form should be used for each supplier.

Form Locator 32a: NPI Number   Enter the NPI number of the service facility location in form locator 32a.

Form Locator 32b: Other ID Number   Enter the two-digit qualifier identifying the non-NPI number followed by the ID number. Do not enter a space, hyphen, or other separator between the qualifier and number. Refer back to form locator 17a for a list of qualifiers.

Form Locator 33: Billing Provider Information and Phone Number   Enter the provider's or supplier's billing name, address, zip code, and phone number in form locator 33. The phone number is to be entered in the area to the right of the field title. Enter the name and address information in the following format:

First line: Name
Second line: Address
Third line: City, state, and zip code.

Form Locator 33a: NPI Number   Enter the NPI number of the billing provider in form locator 33a. The NPI number refers to the HIPAA National Provider Identifier number, which allows for the entry of 10 characters.

For Locator 33b: Other ID Number   Enter the two-digit qualifier identifying the non-NPI number followed by the ID number. Do not enter a space, hyphen, or other separator between the qualifier and number. Refer back to form locator 17a for a list of qualifiers.

The non-NPI ID number of the billing provider refers to the payer-assigned unique identifier of the professional.

Practice Exercises

Complete Practice Exercises 12.1 through 12.4 by completing a CMS-1500 claim form using the patient information forms and encounter forms provided.

The information for the provider's practice is as follows:

Allied Medical Center
1933 E. Frankford Rd.
Carrollton, TX 12345
972-555-5482
Tax ID: 75-1234567

Samantha E. Smith, M.D.   NPI: 1234567890   Medicaid PIN: S1750

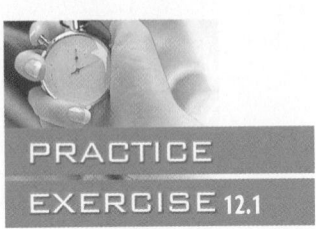

Fill out the CMS-1500 form based on the information given here. To complete this exercise, copy the CMS-1500 form provided in Appendix D or download it from the CD-ROM that accompanies this text.

Capital City Medical—123 Unknown BLVD, Capital City, NY 12345-2222 (555)555-1234 Phil Wells, MD, Mannie Mends, MD, Bette R. Soone, MD	Patient Information Form Tax ID: 75-0246810 Group NPI: 1513171216

Patient Information:

Name: (Last, First) _Shelton, Margaret_   ❑ Male   ☒ Female   Birth Date: _03/25/2007_

Address: _12 Bonnie Ln Dallas, TX 12345_   Phone: (214) 555-1212

Social Security Number: _258749633_   Full-Time Student: ❑ Yes   ☒ No

Marital Status: ☒ Single   ❑ Married   ❑ Divorced   ❑ Other

- -

Employment:

Employer: _____   Phone: ( ) _____

Address: _____

Condition Related to: ❑ Auto Accident   ❑ Employment   ❑ Other Accident

Date of Accident: _____   State _____

Emergency Contact: _Sheila Shelton, Mother_   **Phone:** (214) 555-6958

- -

Primary Insurance: _Medicaid_   Phone: (800) 333-4563

Address: _P.O. Box 200555, Austin, TX 12345_

Insurance Policyholder's Name: _Shelton, Margaret_   ❑ M ❑ F DOB: _____

Address: _Same_

Phone: _Same_   Relationship to Insured: ☒ Self ❑ Spouse ❑ Child ❑ Other

Employer: _____   Phone: ( ) _____

Employer's Address: _____

Policy/ID No: _558479630_   Group No: _____ Percent Covered: _100_ %, Copay Amt: $____

- -

Secondary Insurance: _____   Phone: ( ) _____

Address: _____

Insurance Policyholder's Name: _____   ❑ M ❑ F DOB: _____

Address: _____

Phone: _____ Relationship to Insured: ❑ Self ❑ Spouse ❑ Child ❑ Other

Employer: _____   Phone: ( ) _____

Employer's Address: _____

Policy/ID No: _____ Group No: _____ Percent Covered: ____%, Copay Amt: $____

- -

Reason for Visit: Routine well-child examination

Known Allergies: _____

Were you referred here? If so, by whom?: _____

(continued)

(continued)

ALLIED MEDICAL CENTER

Patient: Shelton, Margaret   **Chart#:**   **Date:** Today's date
Address: 12 Bonnie Lane, Dallas, TX 12345   **Phone:** 214-555-1212

Code	Description		Fee
	New Patient Codes		
99201	New Patient Focused		
99202	New Patient Expanded		
99203	New Patient Complete Physical		
99204	New Patient Comprehensive		
	Established Patient Codes		
99213	Established Patient Expanded		
99214	Established Patient Routine	✕	95.00
99215	Established Patient Complex		
99211	Established Patient Minimal		
99212	Established Patient Focused		
	Procedures		
85007	Manual WBC		
85651	ESR-Erythrocyte Sed Rate		
86403	Strep Test, Rapid		
86585	Tine Test		
87072	Strep Culture		
87086	Urine Culture		
93000	Electrocardiogram-ECG-Intrp/Rprt		
93015	Treadmill Stress Test		
90471	Injection		
90707	MMR Vaccination		
	Other Codes:		

DIAGNOSIS: V20.2

NOTES/REMARKS:

Today's Charges: 95.00

Next Appt: **Amt Paid:**   0.00

Check the accuracy of your work by comparing your claim form to the completed claim form in Appendix J.

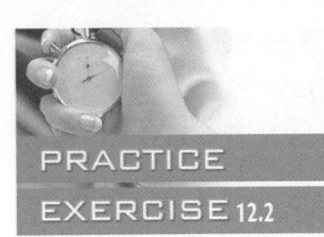

Fill out the CMS-1500 form based on the information given here. To complete this exercise, copy the CMS-1500 form provided in Appendix D or download it from the CD-ROM that accompanies this text.

Capital City Medical—123 Unknown BLVD, Capital City, NY 12345-2222 (555)555-1234	Patient Information Form
	Tax ID: 75-0246810
Phil Wells, MD, Mannie Mends, MD, Bette R. Soone, MD	Group NPI: 1513171216

Patient Information:

Name: (Last, First) Churchill, Shawn L.   ☒ Male   ☐ Female   Birth Date: 07/29/2005

Address: 6580 Belt Line Road, #12B, Plano, TX 12345   Phone: (469) 555-7406

Social Security Number: 258-30-7444   Full-Time Student: ☐ Yes   ☒ No

Marital Status: ☒ Single   ☐ Married   ☐ Divorced   ☐ Other

Employment:

Employer: _____ Phone: ( ) _____

Address: _____

Condition Related to: ☐ Auto Accident   ☐ Employment   ☐ Other Accident

Date of Accident: _____ State _____

Emergency Contact: Edward Churchill, father   **Phone:** (214) 555-8652

Primary Insurance: Medicaid   Phone: (800) 333-4563

Address: P.O. Box 200555, Austin, TX 12345

Insurance Policyholder's Name: Same as patient   ☐ M ☐ F DOB: _____

Address: _____

Phone: _____ Relationship to Insured: ☒ Self ☐ Spouse ☐ Child ☐ Other

Employer: _____ Phone: ( ) _____

Employer's Address: _____

Policy/ID No: 599630014   Group No: _____ Percent Covered: 100 %, Copay Amt: $____

Secondary Insurance: _____ Phone: ( ) _____

Address: _____

Insurance Policyholder's Name: _____ ☐ M ☐ F DOB: _____

Address: _____

Phone: _____ Relationship to Insured: ☐ Self ☐ Spouse ☐ Child ☐ Other

Employer: _____ Phone: ( ) _____

Employer's Address: _____

Policy/ID No: _____ Group No: _____ Percent Covered: ____%, Copay Amt: $____

Reason for Visit: Flu shot

Known Allergies: Feather

Were you referred here? If so, by whom?: _____

(continued)

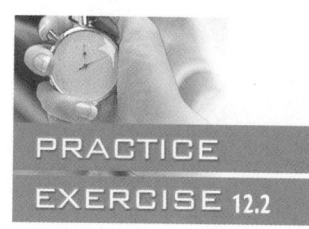

PRACTICE EXERCISE 12.2

(continued)

ALLIED MEDICAL CENTER

Patient: Churchill, Shawn L.   **Chart#:**   **Date:** Today's date

Address: 6580 Belt Line Road, #12B, Plano, TX 12345   **Phone:** 469-555-7406

Code	Description	Fee
	New Patient Codes	
99201	New Patient Focused	
99202	New Patient Expanded	
99203	New Patient Complete Physical	
99204	New Patient Comprehensive	
	Established Patient Codes	
99213	Established Patient Expanded	
99214	Established Patient Routine	
99215	Established Patient Complex	
99211	Established Patient Minimal	
99212	Established Patient Focused	
	Procedures	
85007	Manual WBC	
85651	ESR-Erythrocyte Sed Rate	
86403	Strep Test, Rapid	
86585	Tine Test	
87072	Strep Culture	
87086	Urine Culture	
93000	Electrocardiogram-ECG-Intrp/Rprt	
93015	Treadmill Stress Test	
90471	Injection	✕ 5.00
90707	MMR Vaccination	
	Other Codes: 90658 FLU VACCINE	✕ 15.00

DIAGNOSIS: V04.81

NOTES/REMARKS:

Next Appt:

Today's Charges: 20.00

Amt Paid: 0.00

Check the accuracy of your work by comparing your claim form to the completed claim form in Appendix J.

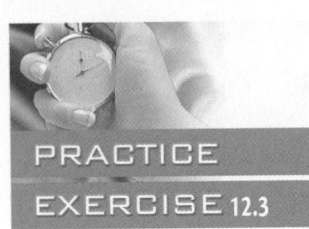

PRACTICE
EXERCISE 12.3

Fill out the CMS-1500 form based on the information given here. To complete this exercise, copy the CMS-1500 form provided in Appendix D or download it from the CD-ROM that accompanies this text.

Capital City Medical—123 Unknown BLVD, Capital City, NY 12345-2222 (555)555-1234 Phil Wells, MD, Mannie Mends, MD, Bette R. Soone, MD	Patient Information Form Tax ID: 75-0246810 Group NPI: 1513171216

Patient Information:

Name: (Last, First) <u>Bradford, Luella M.</u>   ❑ Male   ☒ Female   Birth Date: <u>03/17/1988</u>

Address: <u>2594-B Lovers Lane, Dallas, TX 12345</u>   Phone: (214) <u>555-0147</u>

Social Security Number: <u>987-25-6301</u>   Full-Time Student: ❑ Yes   ☒ No

Marital Status: ☒ Single   ❑ Married   ❑ Divorced   ❑ Other

Employment:

Employer: <u>None</u>   Phone: ( ) _____

Address: _____

Condition Related to: ❑ Auto Accident   ❑ Employment   ❑ Other Accident

Date of Accident: _____ State _____

Emergency Contact: <u>Mary Beth Bradford, mother</u>   **Phone:** (972) <u>555-8733</u>

Primary Insurance: <u>Americaid</u>   Phone: (800) <u>600-4441</u>

Address: <u>P.O. Box 61117, Virginia Beach, VA 12345</u>

Insurance Policyholder's Name: <u>Same as patient</u>   ❑ M ❑ F DOB: _____

Address: _____

Phone: _____ Relationship to Insured: ☒ Self ❑ Spouse ❑ Child ❑ Other

Employer: _____ Phone: ( ) _____

Employer's Address: _____

Policy/ID No: <u>515301607</u>   Group No: <u>T3AM</u> Percent Covered: ___%, Copay Amt: $<u>5</u>

Secondary Insurance: _____   Phone: ( ) _____

Address: _____

Insurance Policyholder's Name: _____   ❑ M ❑ F DOB: _____

Address: _____

Phone: _____ Relationship to Insured: ❑ Self ❑ Spouse ❑ Child ❑ Other

Employer: _____ Phone: ( ) _____

Employer's Address: _____

Policy/ID No: _____ Group No: _____ Percent Covered: ___%, Copay Amt: $___

Reason for Visit: <u>Pregnancy Test</u>

Known Allergies: _____

Were you referred here? If so, by whom?: _____

(continued)

ALLIED MEDICAL CENTER

Patient: Bradford, Luella   **Chart#:**   **Date:** Today's date
Address: 2594-B Lovers Lane, Dallas, TX 12345   **Phone:** 214-555-0147

Code	Description	Fee
	New Patient Codes	
99201	New Patient Focused	
99202	New Patient Expanded	
99203	New Patient Complete Physical	
99204	New Patient Comprehensive	
	Established Patient Codes	
99213	Established Patient Expanded	
99214	Established Patient Routine	
99215	Established Patient Complex	
99211	Established Patient Minimal	
99212	Established Patient Focused	
	Procedures	
85007	Manual WBC	
85651	ESR-Erythrocyte Sed Rate	
86403	Strep Test, Rapid	
86585	Tine Test	
87072	Strep Culture	
87086	Urine Culture	
93000	Electrocardiogram-ECG-Intrp/Rprt	
93015	Treadmill Stress Test	
90471	Injection	
90707	MMR Vaccination	
	Other Codes: 81025 Urine pregnancy test	✕ 20.00

DIAGNOSIS: V72.40 Pregnancy Test

NOTES/REMARKS:

Next Appt:

Today's Charges: 20.00
Amt Paid: 5.00

Check the accuracy of your work by comparing your claim form to the completed claim form in Appendix J.

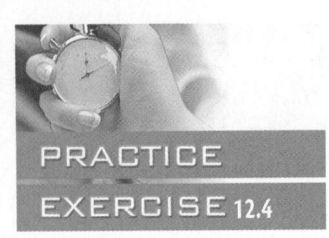

Fill out the CMS-1500 form based on the information given here. To complete this exercise, copy the CMS-1500 form provided in Appendix D or download it from the CD-ROM that accompanies this text.

Capital City Medical—123 Unknown BLVD, Capital City, NY 12345-2222 (555)555-1234	Patient Information Form
	Tax ID: 75-0246810
Phil Wells, MD, Mannie Mends, MD, Bette R. Soone, MD	Group NPI: 1513171216

Patient Information:

Name: (Last, First) Nguyen, Thuy   ☐ Male   ☒ Female   Birth Date: 05/01/2007

Address: 7619 Chattington Lane, Dallas, TX 12345   Phone: (214) 555-6488

Social Security Number: 321-65-9872   Full-Time Student: ☐ Yes   ☒ No

Marital Status: ☒ Single   ☐ Married   ☐ Divorced   ☐ Other

Employment:

Employer: _____   Phone: ( ) _____

Address: _____

Condition Related to: ☐ Auto Accident   ☐ Employment   ☐ Other Accident

Date of Accident: _____ State _____

Emergency Contact: Josie Thuy, mother   **Phone:** (800) 333-4563

Primary Insurance: Medicaid   Phone: _____

Address: P.O. Box 200555, Austin, TX 12345

Insurance Policyholder's Name: Same   ☐ M ☐ F DOB: _____

Address: _____

Phone: _____ Relationship to Insured: ☒ Self ☐ Spouse ☐ Child ☐ Other

Employer: _____   Phone: ( ) _____

Employer's Address: _____

Policy/ID No: 999528741   Group No: _____ Percent Covered: 100 %, Copay Amt: $____

Secondary Insurance: _____ Phone: ( ) _____

Address: _____

Insurance Policyholder's Name: _____   ☐ M ☐ F DOB: _____

Address: _____

Phone: _____ Relationship to Insured: ☐ Self ☐ Spouse ☐ Child ☐ Other

Employer: _____   Phone: ( ) _____

Employer's Address: _____

Policy/ID No: _____   Group No: _____ Percent Covered: ____%, Copay Amt: $____

Reason for Visit: Low birth weight

Known Allergies: _____

Were you referred here? If so, by whom?: _____

(continued)

ALLIED MEDICAL CENTER

Patient: Nguyen, Thuy **Chart#:** **Date:** Today's date
Address: 7619 Chattington Lane, Dallas, TX 12345 **Phone:** 214-555-6488

Code	Description	Fee
	New Patient Codes	
99201	New Patient Focused	
99202	New Patient Expanded	
99203	New Patient Complete Physical	
99204	New Patient Comprehensive	
	Established Patient Codes	
99213	Established Patient Expanded	
99214	Established Patient Routine	
99215	Established Patient Complex	
99211	Established Patient Minimal	
99212	Established Patient Focused	
	Procedures	
85007	Manual WBC	
85651	ESR-Erythrocyte Sed Rate	
86403	Strep Test, Rapid	
86585	Tine Test	
87072	Strep Culture	
87086	Urine Culture	
93000	Electrocardiogram-ECG-Intrp/Rprt	
93015	Treadmill Stress Test	
90471	Injection	
90707	MMR Vaccination	
	Other Codes: 99382 NP 1–4 yrs old	✕ 175.00

DIAGNOSIS: V21.35 Low Birth Weight

NOTES/REMARKS:

Today's Charges: 175.00

Next Appt: **Amt Paid:** 0.00

Check the accuracy of your work by comparing your claim form to the completed claim form in Appendix J.

Chapter Summary

- Medicaid is the largest source of funding for medical and health-related services for America's poorest people. The Medicaid program provides medical benefits to groups of low-income people, some of whom may have no medical insurance or inadequate medical insurance.
- States may pay healthcare providers directly on a fee-for-service basis, or states may pay for Medicaid services through various prepayment arrangements, such as HMOs.
- If Medicaid does not cover a service, the patient may be billed if certain conditions have been met.
- A significant development in Medicaid is the growth in managed care as an alternative service delivery concept different from the traditional fee-for-service system.
- For claims payment to be considered, providers must adhere to claim filing time limits.
- All appeals of denied claims and requests for adjustments on paid claims must be received within 180 days from the date of disposition, the date of the Remittance and Status (R&S) report on which that claim appears.
- Claims lacking the information necessary for processing are listed on the R&S report with an explanation of benefits (EOB) code requesting the missing information. Providers must resubmit a signed, completed/corrected claim with a copy of the R&S on which the denied claim appears within 180 days from the date of the R&S to be considered for payment.
- When filing a claim for a newborn, if the mother's name is "Jane Jones," use "Boy Jane Jones" for a male child and a "Girl Jane Jones" for a female child.
- Medicaid participating physicians file claims using the CMS-1500 claim form. Medicaid participating hospitals and other inpatient facilities file claims using the UB-04. Healthcare Common Procedure Coding System (HCPCS) codes are required for both claim forms.

Chapter Review

True/False

Identify the statement as true (T) or false (F).

_____ 1. Under the payer-of-last-resort regulation, Medicaid pays last on a claim when a patient has other effective insurance coverage.

_____ 2. The medical office specialist should check patients' Medicaid eligibility *prior to each time they see the physician.*

_____ 3. Under a Medicaid spend-down program, individuals are required to spend all of their discretionary income on health costs before Medicaid begins to contribute.

_____ **4.** Children under 6 years old who meet TANF requirements or whose family income is below 133% of the poverty level must be offered state Medicaid benefits.

_____ **5.** A person eligible for Medicaid in a given state is also eligible in all states that border on that state.

_____ **6.** Individuals receiving financial assistance under TANF due to low incomes and few resources must be covered by state Medicaid programs.

_____ **7.** TANF is the abbreviation for Temporary Assistance for Needy Families.

_____ **8.** Inpatient claims filed by the hospital must be received by Medicaid within 95 days from the discharge date.

_____ **9.** All appeals of denied claims and request for adjustments on paid claims must be received within 180 days from the date of the R&S Report.

_____ **10.** The federal government makes payments to states under the Federal Medical Assistance Percentages (FMAP) program.

_____ **11.** Immigrants are automatically excluded from state medical programs.

_____ **12.** The managed care PCP serves as the medical home and the liaison between the Medicaid recipient and the state.

Multiple Choice

Identify the letter of the choice that best completes the statement or answers the question.

_____ **1.** Within broad national guidelines established by federal statutes, regulations, and policies, each state:
   a. follows the Medicare eligibility standards.
   b. receives the type, amount, duration, and scope of services.
   c. sets the rate of payment to receive from the federal government.
   d. administers its own program.

_____ **2.** States' eligibility groups will be considered one of the following:
   a. income needy
   b. medically needy
   c. geographic groups
   d. education level

_____ **3.** If a state has a medically needy program, it must include:
   a. college students that qualify for financial aid.
   b. pregnant women.
   c. children under age 18.
   d. certain protected elderly persons.

_____ **4.** Which of the following provides states with grants to be spent on time-limited cash assistance?
   a. TANF   c. CMS
   b. SIS   d. welfare reform

_____ **5.** Medi-Medi benefits may include:
   a. hospital care beyond the 100-day limit covered by Medicare.
   b. over-the-counter drugs.
   c. eyeglasses and hearing aids.
   d. orthopedic care.

_____ **6.** When filing a claim for a male newborn, if the mother's name is "Jane Jones," then the claim would be filed as:
   a. Boy Jane Jones.
   b. Jane Jones Boy.
   c. Jones, Jane Boy.
   d. Jones, Baby Boy.

Completion

Complete each sentence or statement.

1. Medicaid, by law, is the _____ of last resort.

2. The _____ program under Medicaid offers health insurance coverage for uninsured children.

3. Persons may qualify immediately or may _____ by incurring medical expenses that reduce their income to or below their state's MN income level.

4. _____ determine the amount and duration of services offered under their Medicaid programs.

5. Two different managed care models are _____ and _____.

6. An R&S report is the _____ and _____ report.

For Additional Practice

Use the following information to complete a CMS-1500 form.

Physician Information:	Charles H. Borden, M.D.
	980 Frederick Road
	Dallas, TX 12345
Phone:	899-555-2276
EIN:	22-9872767
Professional License:	TX2056
UPIN:	3468923
Medicaid PIN:	K00J879
NPI:	1234568901

Patient Information:	Katherine Becker
	254 Pleasure Avenue
	Dallas TX 12345
	999-555-3457
DOB:	06/23/1954
Social Security number:	968-34-0025
Patient Account:	12358
Status:	Married
Sex:	Female
Patient's Insurance	Medicaid ID# 5555211106
Information:	1123 High Point
	Dallas, TX 12345
	800-973-1123

Date of Service: Today's date

CC: Patient CC of back pain. Leaned over to pick up 2-yr-old toddler and felt sharp pain in low back.

DX: Lumbar Sprain 847.2

99203—NP Office Visit, Problem focused-history and examination, straightforward decision making $85.00, DX code: 847.2

Plan: Rx for Relafen one tab daily. Return in one week.

Resources

Medicaid Billing/Claim Handbook: *www.oms.nysed.gov/medicaid/guidebook/ guideboo.htm*

Chapter 13 TRICARE Medical Billing

Chapter Objectives

After reading this chapter, the student should be able to:

1. Determine eligibility for TRICARE participants.

2. Identify different types of benefits available to veterans and their family members.

3. Submit claims to TRICARE using the CMS-1500 and the UB-04 (CMS-1450) form.

Key Terms

beneficiary
catastrophic cap
Civilian Health and Medical Program of the Uniformed Services (CHAMPUS)
Civilian Health and Medical Program of the Department of Veterans Affairs (CHAMPVA)
cost share

Defense Enrollment Eligibility Reporting System (DEERS)
military treatment facility (MTF)
nonavailability statement (NAS)
Palmetto Government Benefits Administrators (PGBA)
primary care manager (PCM)
sponsor

TRICARE
TRICARE Extra
TRICARE Prime
TRICARE Prime Remote (TPR)
TRICARE Prime Remote for Active Duty Family Members (TPRADFM)
TRICARE Senior Prime
TRICARE Standard
Wisconsin Physicians Services (WPS)

Case Study
TRICARE

Kerry Kosh had a new patient appointment with Dr. Lader. She is covered by TRICARE under the sponsorship of her husband, Carl. She presented her insurance card.

At the visit, the doctor gave Kerry three prescriptions for long-term medications. Each prescription was written for a year's worth of refills. As the Medical Assistant handed the prescriptions to Kerry, she noticed the number of refills. She told the patient that she could mail the prescriptions to the military base that was approximately 40 miles away, but that she probably wouldn't receive the refills for more than a week. She then offered to call in a week's worth of medications to a local pharmacy.

Questions

1. What is the term used for the policyholder of a TRICARE plan?

2. What would be the advantage of sending the prescriptions to the military base?

3. How does this show the concern for the patient's healthcare by the Medical Assistant?

392 Section V Government Medical Billing

Introduction

TRICARE is the Department of Defense (DoD) medical entitlement program that covers medically necessary care for eligible uniformed services beneficiaries (active duty, retirees, family members, and survivors). In this chapter, you will learn how to determine eligibility for TRICARE participants and how to file claims under the TRICARE program.

TRICARE

The U.S. Congress created the **Civilian Health and Medical Program of the Uniformed Services (CHAMPUS)** in 1966 under Public Law 89-614 because individuals in the military were finding it increasingly difficult to pay for the medical care required by their families. CHAMPUS was a congressionally funded comprehensive health benefits program. Beginning in 1988 CHAMPUS beneficiaries had a choice of retaining their benefits under CHAMPUS or enrolling in a managed care plan called CHAMPUS Prima, a plan to control escalating medical costs and standardize benefits for active duty families, military retirees, and their dependents. In January 1994, TRICARE became the new title for CHAMPUS. Individuals can choose from five different TRICARE health plans:

1. **TRICARE Standard** is a fee-for-service, cost-sharing type of option.
2. **TRICARE Prime** is a health maintenance organization (HMO) type of option.
3. **TRICARE Prime Remote (TPR)** is another type of HMO option.
4. **TRICARE Extra** is a preferred provider organization (PPO) type of option.
5. **TRICARE Senior Prime** is a program for Medicare-eligible beneficiaries ages 65 and older.

Eligible TRICARE beneficiaries may receive care at either a **military treatment facility (MTF)** or from TRICARE-authorized civilian providers. Authorization of civilian providers is discussed in a later section.

TRICARE Eligibility

An individual who qualifies for TRICARE is known as a **beneficiary**; the active duty service member is called the **sponsor**. A person who is retired from a career in the armed forces is known as a *service retiree* or *military retiree* and remains in the TRICARE program until age 65, at which time the individual becomes eligible for the Medicare program. At that point Medicare becomes the primary insurance policy and TRICARE is the secondary policy. No further family benefits are provided in the event that an active duty military person served from 4 to 6 years and then chose to leave the armed services, thereby giving up a military career. **Civilian Health and Medical Program of the Department of Veterans Affairs (CHAMPVA)** beneficiaries are not eligible for TRICARE. CHAMPVA is for veterans with 100% service-related disabilities and their families.

To be eligible for TRICARE, all uniformed services sponsors and family members must be enrolled in the **Defense Enrollment Eligibility Reporting System (DEERS)**. Sponsors needing to enroll themselves or family members may contact or visit their personnel office, their nearest identification card–issuing facility, or the Defense Manpower Data Center Support Office (DSO). A TRICARE beneficiary may check status by contacting the nearest personnel office of any branch of the service or by calling the toll-free number of the DEERS center.

The Patient's Financial Responsibilities

The TRICARE fiscal year begins October 1 and ends September 30. TRICARE's treatment of deductibles is different from that of most other healthcare programs. The medical office specialist (MOS) should be aware of these differences when collecting deductibles. Generally, insurance deductibles renew (or start over) on January 1; however, because of the TRICARE fiscal year, TRICARE deductibles renew on October 1 each year. Another way TRICARE differs from other health plans is that instead of *coinsurance*, TRICARE uses the term **cost share** to refer to the charges that are the responsibility of the patient.

Other differences are discussed later in the discussion of how to complete the CMS-1500 form.

Timely Filing

Professional and institutional TRICARE claims must be submitted within 30 days from the date of service, or inpatient discharge date, but no later than 1 year from the date of service or discharge. Claims older than 1 year must be submitted with a detailed explanation why the claim is being filed late. Each case is reviewed by a claims processor and given individual consideration.

Penalties and Interest Charges

Penalties or interest charges cannot be billed to a beneficiary by a physician or supplier due to TRICARE's failure to make payment on a timely basis.

Authorized Providers

An authorized provider may treat a TRICARE Standard patient. This means that the provider is qualified to provide certain health benefits to TRICARE beneficiaries and can be reimbursed by TRICARE for its share of costs for medical benefits. Only "certified" providers, that is, those who have passed a credentialing process, can be authorized by TRICARE. Beneficiaries who use nonauthorized providers may be responsible for their entire bill and there are no legal limits on the amounts these providers can bill beneficiaries. Examples of nonauthorized providers are most chiropractors and acupuncturists and those physicians who do not meet state licensing or training requirements or were rejected for authorization by TRICARE. Authorized providers include:

- Doctor of medicine (MD)
- Doctor of osteopathy (DO)
- Doctor of dental surgery (DDS)
- Doctor of dental medicine (DDM)
- Doctor of podiatry (DPM)
- Doctor of optometry (DO)
- Psychologist (PhD).

Other authorized nonphysician providers include audiologists, certified nurse midwives, clinical social workers, licensed practical nurses, licensed vocational nurses, registered nurses, registered physical therapists, and speech therapists.

A participating provider is assigned a personal identification number (PIN) and agrees to accept the TRICARE allowable charge in full for services, which is the Medicare fee. A nonparticipating provider cannot charge more than 115% of the TRICARE allowed charge (Medicare fee).

Preauthorization

TRICARE enforces certain referral and preauthorization requirements for TRICARE Standard patients when specialty care or hospitalization is necessary. A military treatment facility must be used if services are available; otherwise, a **nonavailability statement (NAS)** must be obtained so that the patient may see a civilian provider. NAS request forms are submitted electronically to the DEERS database prior to any treatment by a civilian provider. An NAS request is an electronic document stating that the service the patient requires is not available at the nearby MTF. Once approved by DEERS, NASs are valid for 30 days after they are issued and for 15 days after hospital discharge for treatment related to the original condition. If a NAS is not filed and approved, TRICARE will not pay any claims associated with the non-MTF treatment.

A healthcare finder (HCF) will assist the patient with a referral or preauthorization process. HCFs are available at TRICARE service centers along with beneficiary representatives.

All admissions, ambulatory surgical procedures, and other selected procedures require preauthorization. Certain types of healthcare services require prior approval from the TRICARE health contractor, including:

- Arthroscopy
- Breast mass or tumor removal
- Cardiac catheterization
- Cataract removal
- Cystoscopy
- Dental care
- Dilation and curettage (D&C)
- Durable medical equipment (DME) purchases
- Gastrointestinal endoscopy
- Gynecologic laparoscopy
- Hernia repair
- Laparoscopic cholecystectomy
- Ligation or transection of fallopian tubes
- Magnetic resonance imaging (MRI) services
- Mental health care
- Myringotomy or tympanostomy
- Neuroplasty
- Rhinoplasty or septoplasty
- Strabismus repair
- Tonsillectomy and adenoidectomy
- Physical therapy.

TRICARE Standard

Military families may receive services at an MTF, but the services offered vary by facility and first priority is given to active duty members. So TRICARE Standard has been developed as a fee-for-service program that covers medical services provided by a civilian physician when the individual cannot receive treatment from an MTF. When an individual has to seek care from a civilian provider, the TRICARE Standard benefits go into effect.

Under TRICARE Standard, medical expenses are shared between TRICARE and the beneficiary. Most enrollees pay an annual deductible. In addition to the deductible, families of active duty members pay 20% of outpatient charges. Retirees and their families, former spouses, and families of deceased personnel pay a 25% cost share for outpatient services. If a beneficiary is treated by a provider who does not accept assignment, he or she is also responsible for the provider's additional charges up to 115% of the allowable charge (i.e., the limiting charge; see Chapter 11). Patient cost share payments are subject to an annual **catastrophic cap** (i.e., a limit on the total medical expenses) that beneficiaries are required to pay within 1 year. For active duty families, the annual cap is $1,000.00; for all other beneficiaries the limit is $7,500.00. Once this cap has been met, TRICARE pays 100% of additional charges for that year.

The following is a list of services that are *not* covered under the TRICARE Standard plan:

- Chiropractic care
- Cosmetic surgery
- Custodial care
- Unproven procedures or treatments
- Routine physical examinations
- Routine foot care.

If a TRICARE Standard beneficiary needs treatment that is not available at an MTF, the person must file an NAS with DEERS as discussed earlier.

TRICARE Prime

TRICARE Prime is a managed care plan, similar to an HMO. In addition to most of the benefits offered by TRICARE Standard, the program offers additional preventive care, including routine physical examinations.

The TRICARE Prime option requires enrollment. After enrolling in the plan, each individual is assigned a **primary care manager (PCM)** who coordinates and manages that patient's medical care. The PCM may be a single military or civilian provider or a group of providers. All referrals for specialty care must be arranged by the PCM to avoid point-of-service charges.

TRICARE Prime enrollees receive the majority of their healthcare services from MTFs and they receive priority at these facilities. TRICARE Prime results in fewer out-of-pocket costs than any other TRICARE option. Active duty members and their families do not pay enrollment fees, annual deductibles, or copayments for care provided within the TRICARE network.

Retired service members may also take advantage of the TRICARE Prime plan, but they must pay an annual enrollment fee of $230.00 for an individual or $460.00 for a family, and minimal copays apply for care within the TRICARE network. TRICARE Prime also offers a "point-of-service" option for care received outside of the TRICARE Prime network, but point-of-service care requires payment of significant out-of-pocket costs. Visits to civilian network providers require a $6.00 or $12.00 copayment, depending on the grade (military rank; e.g., E4) of the sponsor. Charges for visits to providers outside the TRICARE Prime network are paid 50% by TRICARE and 50% by the beneficiary.

TRICARE Prime enrollees are guaranteed certain access standards for care, as listed in Table 13.1.

Table 13.1	Access Standards for TRICARE Prime Enrollees			
	Urgent Care	Routine Care	Referred Specialty Care	Wellness/Preventive Care
Appointment wait time	Not to exceed 24 hours	Not to exceed 7 days	Not to exceed 4 weeks	Not to exceed 4 weeks
Drive time	Within 30 minutes of home	Within 60 minutes of home	Within 60 minutes of home	Within 60 minutes of home

Wait time in office: Not to exceed 30 minutes for nonemergency situations.

TRICARE Prime Remote

TRICARE Prime Remote (TPR) is a healthcare program for active duty service members who are assigned to permanent duty stations that are not near sources of military care, typically 50 miles or more from a military treatment facility. TPR is offered in the 50 United States only and requires enrollment. **TRICARE Prime Remote for Active Duty Family Members (TPRADFM)** is the TPR benefit that is available only to family members of active duty personnel—retirees and others are not eligible. TPRADFM also requires enrollment and has benefits and program requirements similar to those of TPR. The benefits under TRICARE Prime Remote are the same as TRICARE Prime, and there are no out-of-pocket costs for TPR or TPRADFM enrollees.

Enrollees must select or be assigned a local PCM. If no network PCMs are available in the area, beneficiaries may use any TRICARE-authorized provider for primary care. PCMs provide preventive services, care for routine illnesses or injuries, and manage referrals to specialists or hospitals if needed.

All specialty care must be coordinated through the TRICARE regional health care finder. Network PCMs will coordinate specialty care directly with the regional HCF. The regional HCF will coordinate active duty TRICARE Prime Remote specialty care referrals through the service point of contact (SPOC) to determine if the specialty care must be received from a military provider for a "fitness for duty" determination. Specialty care referrals for TPR active duty family members are managed by the HCF and are not coordinated through the SPOC.

TRICARE Extra

Because active duty personnel and TRICARE Prime enrollees receive priority at MTFs, some family members of active duty personnel and retirees under age 65 and their family members may opt for TRICARE Extra. TRICARE Extra is an alternative managed care plan to TRICARE Prime that allows individuals who do not have priority at an MTF to receive services primarily from civilian facilities and physicians rather than from military facilities. Active duty service members are not eligible for TRICARE Extra. Because it is a managed care plan, eligible individuals must receive healthcare services from a select network of healthcare professionals.

TRICARE Extra is more expensive than TRICARE Prime, but less costly than TRICARE Standard. There is no enrollment fee, but there is an annual deductible of $150.00

Table 13.2	A Brief Comparison of TRICARE Plans	
	TRICARE Standard/Extra	**TRICARE Prime/Prime Remote**
Type of program	A fee-for-service program with the option of using a preferred provider network under the TRICARE Extra benefit	A managed care program, similar to an HMO
Availability	Throughout the United States and overseas	Only available in TRICARE Prime service areas (PSAs); active duty families eligible for TRICARE Prime Remote can enroll outside a PSA
Enrollment	Not required	Required
Enrollment fees	No fee	*Active duty families:* None *Retirees/others:* $230.00/individual $460.00/family
Costs	Deductibles and 20–25% cost shares; 5% discount for using network providers	*Active duty families:* None *Retirees/others:* Small copays per service
Provider choices	Any TRICARE authorized provider (generally, any state licensed medical provider)	Limited to MTFs and TRICARE network providers
MTF priority	Only limited space-availability access	Priority access to MTFs
Primary care managers	No designated PCM required	All care is coordinated through a designated PCM
Referral and authorization requirements	No referrals required; only a few types of services require prior authorization	Most care requires referral by the PCM; there are more authorization requirements than TRICARE Standard/Extra
Clinical preventive care	Limited benefits compared to Prime	Various preventive benefits such as routine eye exams and routine preventive care exams

for an individual and $300.00 for a family. TRICARE Extra beneficiaries pay 15% for civilian outpatient charges (5% less than TRICARE Standard enrollees). Beneficiaries are not subject to additional charges of up to 115% of the allowable charge, since participating physicians agree to accept TRICARE's fee schedule.

A brief comparison of the four TRICARE plans discussed thus far is shown in Table 13.2. Sample military ID cards and TRICARE cards are shown in Figure 13.1.

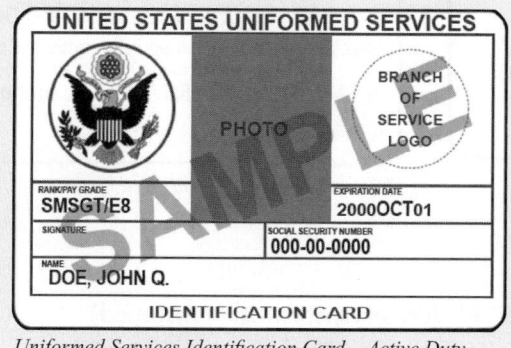

Uniformed Services Identification Card - Active Duty

Figure 13.1

Sample military and TRICARE patient cards.

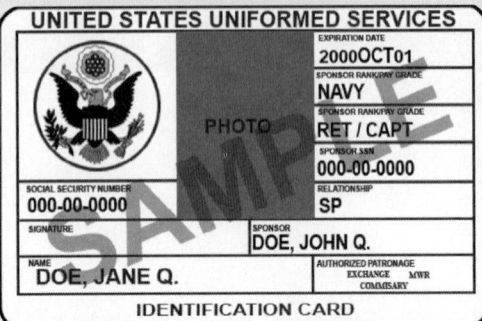

Uniformed Services Identification Card - Active Duty
Family Member

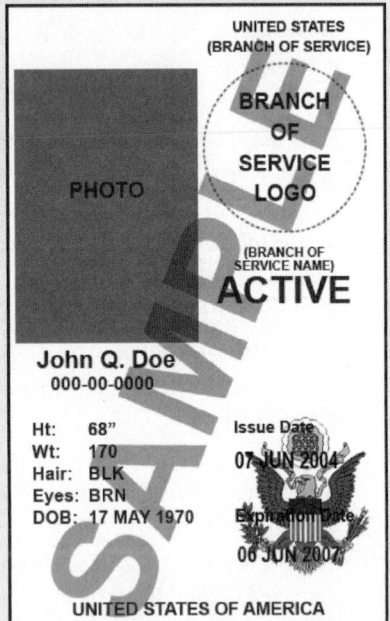

Common Access Card

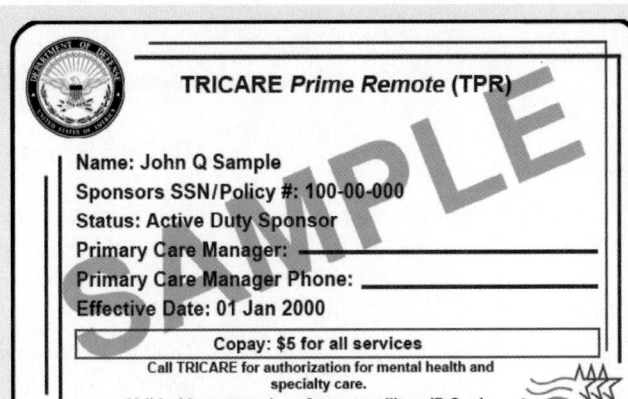

TRICARE Prime Remote (TPR) Card

TRICARE: The World's Best Health Care
for the World's Best Military
TRICARE PRIME

Name: John Q Sample
Status: Active Duty Sponsor
Primary Care Manager:_____
Primary Care Manager Phone:_____
Effective Date: 01 Jan 2000

Valid with presentation of current military ID Card
Contact your personnel office if any of
the above information is incorrect

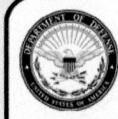

TRICARE Prime Card

TRICARE — The World's Best Health Care
For the World's Best Military

TRICARE Reserve Select

TRS Member   John Q Doe

Effective Date   01/01/2005

Covered Person   Susie Q. Doe

The TRS identification number is the
TRS member's Social Security Number.

www.tricare.osd.mil

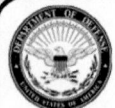

TRICARE Reserve Select Card front

This card is not a guarantee of coverage. Coverage under TRS is separate
from any medical coverage indicated on the military identification card. TRS
benefits are available from TRICARE-authorized providers and TRICARE
Network providers. Pre-certification is required for inpatient mental health
and selected regionally-determined procedures.

TRICARE Regional Contractor   888-TRIWEST
                               www.triwest.com
TRICARE Retail Pharmacy   866-363-8779
TRICARE Mail Order Pharmacy   866-DOD-TMOP
http://member.express.scripts.com/dodCustom/welcome.do

In EMERGENCY—dial 911 or go to the nearest emergency
medical facility

TRICARE Reserve Select Card back

Figure 13.1   Sample military and TRICARE patient cards. (continued)

TRICARE Senior Prime

Individuals over the age of 65 who are eligible for Medicare and TRICARE may receive health care at a military treatment facility. Benefits offered through TRICARE Senior Prime, also known as TRICARE for Life, are similar to those of a Medicare HMO, with an emphasis on preventive and wellness services. Prescription drug benefits are also included in TRICARE Senior Prime.

All enrollees in TRICARE Senior Prime must be enrolled in Medicare Parts A and B and must have Part B premiums deducted from their Social Security checks. Other than Medicare costs, TRICARE Senior Prime beneficiaries pay no enrollment fees and no cost share fees for inpatient or outpatient care at a military facility. Treatment at a civilian network facility costs $12.00 for outpatient care and $11.00 per day for inpatient treatment. Beneficiaries can also choose to use Medicare providers. TRICARE acts as a second payer to Medicare for benefits payable by both Medicare and TRICARE. Claims will automatically be forwarded to TRICARE after Medicare pays. TRICARE is the primary payer if benefits are not covered under Medicare, such as pharmacy benefits.

CHAMPVA

CHAMPVA is a comprehensive healthcare program in which the Veterans Affairs (VA) shares the cost of covered healthcare services and supplies with veterans with 100% service-related disabilities and their families. The program is administered by the Health Administration Center, which has offices in Denver, Colorado.

Due to the similarity between CHAMPVA and the DoD TRICARE program, the two are often mistaken for each other. CHAMPVA is a Department of Veterans Affairs program, whereas TRICARE is a regionally managed healthcare program for active duty and retired members of the uniformed services, their families, and survivors. An eligible CHAMPVA sponsor may be entitled to receive medical care through the VA healthcare system based on his own veteran status. Additionally, as the result of a recent policy change, if the eligible CHAMPVA sponsor is the spouse of another eligible CHAMPVA sponsor, both may now be eligible for CHAMPVA benefits. In each instance where the eligible spouse requires medical attention, she may choose the VA healthcare system or coverage under CHAMPVA for her healthcare needs.

Veterans requesting medical care through the VA healthcare system should first seek to obtain care in VA facilities. Sometimes, however, VA facilities cannot provide the necessary medical care and services. In such cases, the VA may authorize medical care provided in the community for those veterans who meet the eligibility requirements. The VA authorization will specify:

- Medical services approved by the VA
- Length of period for treatment
- Amount the VA will pay.

Each individual veteran's eligibility status and medical care needs are reviewed to decide whether community treatment can be approved. All VA authorized services *must be approved* before the veteran receives treatment. However, it may not be possible to contact the VA prior to treatment in life-threatening emergency situations.

CHAMPVA is always the last payer after Medicare and any other health insurance.

Submitting Claims to TRICARE

Physicians submit paper claims to TRICARE using the CMS-1500 form. Hospitals and other inpatient facilities submit paper claims on the UB-04 (CMS-1450) claim form. Figure 13.2 lists the information that must be on the submitted claim form. Paper claims submission addresses vary depending on the provider's location. To determine the appropriate claims mailing address, the MOS should visit www.tricareonline.com on the Internet. **Wisconsin Physicians Service (WPS)** is the claims processor for all TRICARE Senior Prime claims. The Medicare provider submits a claim to Medicare first. After adjudicating the claim, Medicare will forward the claim to WPS TRICARE for Life.

Claims for CHAMPVA patients are sent electronically through the VA's clearinghouse, Emdeon© Envoy, or submitted on paper. Paper claims for CHAMPVA are submitted to the Fee Department of the VA Facility that authorized payment of services in advance or to VA Health Administration Center, CHAMPVA, P.O. Box 65024, Denver, Colorado 80206-9024.

Health Net Federal Services, Inc., care of **Palmetto Government Benefits Administrators (PGBA)**, is the TRICARE claims payer for the northern region of the United States. PGBA provides an online claims submission program, called XPressClaim, that is easy to use, fast, and free of charge. Claims can be submitted while the patient is still in the office. Submitting claims electronically with this program offers providers the following advantages:

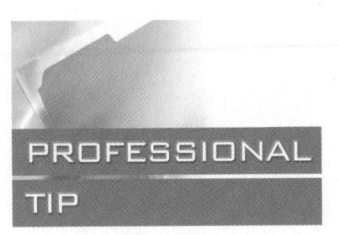

The term *sponsor* refers to the member who is/was active in the military. The terms *beneficiary* and *patient* are synonymous.

- Direct transmission to PGBA (no clearinghouse, billing services, or bulletin boards)
- An immediate online claims acceptance or rejection report
- Time-saving online correction of claims prior to being sent to PGBA
- Processing and payment in a shorter period of time.

Figure 13.2

Information that must appear on the submitted TRICARE claim form.

All claims must include the following information:

- Patient's name as it appears on his or her military ID card
- Sponsor's Social Security number (SSN)
- Patient's date of birth
- Other health insurance (OHI) information
- Appropriate HCPCS, CPT, and ICD-9 codes on CMS-1500 claim forms
- Appropriate HCPCS, CPT, ICD-9, and revenue codes on UB-04 claim forms
- Admitting diagnosis on UB-04 claim forms

- Care approval number, if applicable
- Provider's tax ID number or SSN
- Referring physician
- Rendering physician
- Beneficiary's signature (or indicate "signature on file" if the beneficiary's signature is on a "release of information" document)
- The provider's or representative's signature

All professional charges must be submitted on a CMS-1500 claim form according to TRICARE guidelines. It is not necessary to complete all locators on the claim form.

> To register for online CMS-1500 claim submission through XPressClaim, providers can go online to www.mytricare.com. The site has a demo available to show how easy it is to submit a claim.

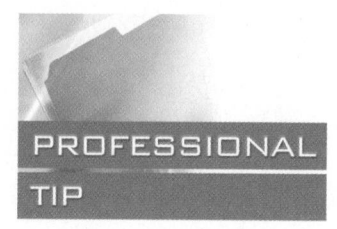

PROFESSIONAL TIP

Completing the CMS-1500 Form for TRICARE (Primary)

This section reviews each form locator on the CMS-1500 and what information should be entered when filing a TRICARE claim.

Form Locator 1: Type of Insurance   Mark an X in the TRICARE/CHAMPUS box.

Form Locator 1a: Insured's ID Number   Enter the sponsor's Social Security number.

Form Locator 2: Patient's Name   Enter the patient's full name: last name, first name, and middle initial exactly as on the patient's TRICARE card.

Form Locator 3: Patient's Date of Birth and Sex   Enter the date of birth and sex/gender. The date of birth is entered using the eight-digit format: MM/DD/CCYY. The patient's sex/gender is identified as either male or female.

Form Locator 4: Insured's Name   Enter the sponsor's name.

Form Locator 5: Patient's Address   Enter the patient's home address. This information is taken from the patient information form when the patient register's in the office. The address should include the street name and number, city, state (two-letter abbreviations), and zip code. Do not use commas, periods, or other punctuation in the address. When entering a nine-digit zip code, include the hyphen. Do not use a hyphen or space as a separator within the telephone number.

Form Locator 6: Patient's Relationship to the Insured   Mark an X in the appropriate box for relationship to the insured.

Form Locator 7: Insured's Address   Enter the sponsor's military address.

Form Locator 8: Patient Status   Enter the marital status of the patient.

Form Locators 9a–d: Other Insured's Name   Leave blank unless patient has Medicaid, in which case, "Medicaid" would be entered.

Form Locators 10a–c: Is Patient's Condition Related To?   Enter an X in the correct box.

Form Locator 10d: Reserved for Local Use   Leave blank.

Form Locator 11: Insured's Policy Group or FECA Number   Enter the word "None."

Form Locators 11a–d: Insured's Date of Birth and Sex   If the patient is other than the sponsor, enter the sponsor's date of birth and gender.

Form Locators 12 and 13: Patient's or Authorized Person's Signature   Form locator 12 is where the patient or guarantor signs to allow the release of any medical information to the insurance company for billing purposes. This release is only valid for billing information. Any other request for records requires a formal release of information form to be signed by the patient or guarantor. This signature is good for 1 year from the date it is signed and should be updated annually. When submitting claims the words "Signature on File" or "SOF" may be added here in place of a signature. The actual patient signature must then be on file in the patient's chart. Enter the date in the six-digit format (MM/DD/YY) or eight-digit format (MM/DD/CCYY). If there is no signature on file, leave blank or enter "No Signature on File."

Form Locator 14: Date of Current: Illness, Injury, Pregnancy   Enter the date of service and, if applicable, last menstrual period.

Form Locator 15: If Patient Has Had Same or Similar Illness   Leave blank.

Form Locator 16: Dates Patient Unable to Work in Current Occupation   Leave blank.

Form Locator 17: Name of Referring Provider or Other Source   Enter the name of the ordering or referring physician. The information entered should include the physician's last name, first name, and credentials. If multiple providers are involved, enter one provider using the following priority order:

1. Referring provider

2. Ordering provider

3. Supervising provider.

If there is no referring physician, leave blank.

Form Locator 17a: ID Number of Referring Physician   Leave blank.

Form Locator 17b: NPI Number   Enter the NPI of the provider listed in form locator 17. The NPI number refers to the HIPAA National Provider Identifier number, which is a 10-digit number.

Form Locator 18: Hospitalization Dates Related to Current Services   Enter the dates the patient has been hospitalized in relation to the current services in form locator 18. If the patient has been discharged from the hospital, the dates should include the day admitted and the day discharged. If the patient is still hospitalized only include the day admitted. The dates should be entered in the six-digit (MM/DD/YY) or the eight-digit format (MM/DD/CCYY). If the patient has not been hospitalized, leave blank.

Form Locator 19: Reserved for Local Use   Form locator 19 is a conditional entry. Enter additional modifiers, dates, and narrative or other information. When an independent physical or occupational therapist or podiatrist providing routine foot care submits claims, enter the six-digit date the patient was last seen by their attending physician with the NPI of the attending physician. The attending physician is the individual who wrote the prescription for the treatment. For physical and occupational therapists, entering this information certifies that the required physician certification is being kept on file. Do not enter a space, hyphen, or other separator between the qualifier code and the number.

Form Locator 20: Outside Lab   Complete this field when billing for diagnostic tests subject to purchase price limitations. Enter the purchase price under charges if the "Yes" block is checked. A "Yes" check indicates that an entity other than the entity billing for the service performed the diagnostic test. A "No" check indicates "no purchased tests are included on the claim." When "Yes" is marked, locator 32 shall be completed.

Form Locator 21: Diagnosis or Nature of Illness or Injury   In form locator 21, the ICD-9 codes for the diagnoses applied to this claim are entered. At least one code must be entered and up to four codes can be used on claim. They are placed in order of precedence, with line 1 being the primary diagnosis and so forth. No written diagnoses are used on a claim form. The ICD-9 codes should be checked for medical necessity to make sure they are used appropriately with the CPT® codes used in form locator 24D. Relate lines 1, 2, 3, and 4 to the lines of service in 24E by line number.

Form Locator 22: Medicaid Resubmission Code   Leave blank.

Form Locator 23: Prior Authorization Number   Some insurance plans, such as those of HMOs, exclusive provider organizations (EPOs), and preferred provider organizations (PPOs), require a prior authorization number. If required, when preauthorization is obtained from an insurance company for services, the number assigned is input in form locator 23. Also, HMO required referral numbers are input in this form locator. Any of the following can be entered here: prior authorization number, referral number, mammography precertification number, or Clinical Laboratory Improvement Amendments (CLIA)10-digit number, as assigned by the payer for the current service. Do not enter hyphens or spaces within the number. If prior authorization is required and is omitted, the claim will be denied. If no prior authorization is required, leave blank.

Form Locator 24a: Dates of Service   Enter dates of service for medical care. If service begins and ends on the same date enter the date in both the From and To blocks in eight-digit format (MM/DD/CCYY).

Form Locator 24b: Place of Service   Enter the place of service code where services were rendered. Common place of service codes include the following:

11	Physician's office
12	Private residence
13	Assisted living facility
20	Urgent care facility
21	Inpatient hospital
22	Outpatient hospital
23	Hospital emergency department
24	Ambulatory surgical center
25	Birthing center
26	Military treatment facility
31	Skilled nursing facility
34	Hospice
81	Independent laboratory.

Form Locator 24C: EMG (Emergency)   This form locator should be marked with a Y for YES or left blank for NO. The definition of an emergency is defined by either federal or state regulations or programs or payer contracts.

Form Locator 24D: Procedures, Services, or Supplies   In form locator 24D, enter the CPT or HCPCS codes used to identify the procedures, services, or supplies provided. Modifiers are also listed in form locator 24D. If more than three modifiers are used, list 99 here and enter the modifiers in form locator 19.

Form Locator 24E: Diagnosis Code (Pointer)   Form locator 24E indicates the number (1, 2, 3, and 4) of the diagnosis code listed in form locator 21 as it relates to each service or procedure. If more than one diagnosis is attached to a single procedure or service, list the primary diagnosis first.

Form Locator 24F: Charges   Form locator 24F lists the charges that are assigned to each CPT or HCPCS code listed. The amount should be entered without a decimal point or dollar sign. If multiple units are entered in form locator 24G, the charges should reflect the amount of the procedure times the number of units. Charges should be updated on a regular basis to follow appropriate billing guidelines.

Form Locator 24G: Days or Units   Enter the number of units per procedure or service provided to a patient in form locator 24G. If billing for anesthesia, the amount entered should be entered in minutes and calculated accordingly. If billing for multiple services, such as liters of oxygen, list the actual number of liters. If multiple units are entered in 24G, the charges should reflect the amount of the procedure multiplied by the number of units.

Form Locator 24H: EPSDT Family Plan   Leave blank.

Form Locator 24I: ID Qualifier   Leave blank.

Form Locator 24J: Rendering Provider   The individual rendering the service is reported in form locator 24J. Enter the NPI number in the unshaded area of the field.

   The rendering provider is the person or company (laboratory or other facility) who rendered or supervised the care. In the case where a substitute provider was used, enter that provider's information here. Report the identification number in form locator 24J only when different from data recorded in form locators 33a and 33b.

Form Locator 25: Federal Tax I.D. Number   List in form locator 25 the physician's federal tax I.D. number or his employer identification number (EIN). Do not enter hyphens with numbers. The appropriate selection should be marked and the corresponding number entered.

Form Locator 26: Patient's Account Number   In form locator 26, enter the patient account number assigned in the medical office. The computer system used in the office will generate the number and it should be entered on the claim. This in turn will allow for the account number to appear on the Explanation of Benefits (EOB) form, which makes it easier to locate the correct patient to post insurance payments.

Form Locator 27: Accept Assignment?   Form locator 27 is used to indicate whether or not the physician accepts assignment on this claim. If the physician does accept assignment and the patient has signed form locator 13, the insurance carrier will pay the physician directly for services provided. If the physician does not accept assignment, the insurance carrier will send the reimbursement to the patient.

Form Locator 28: Total Charge   Form locator 28 lists the total of charges, added together from those listed in form locator 24F. The charges should be checked for accuracy to ensure proper reimbursement. Do not use decimal points or dollar signs in this entry.

Form Locator 29: Amount Paid   Form locator 29 indicates the amount paid on this claim. This amount is usually added after the primary EOB is received and payment is posted. A secondary claim is printed to be sent to the secondary insurance carrier along with a copy of the primary insurance carrier's EOB. Do not use decimal points or dollar signs in this entry.

Form Locator 30: Balance Due   This form locator is left blank.

Form Locator 31: Signature of Physician or Supplier Including Degrees or Credentials   Form locator 31 identifies the name of the physician or supplier who has provided the services to the patient along with her credentials (M.D., PA-C, or NP). If a paper claim is submitted, enter the signature of the physician's or supplier's representative, or "Signature on File" or "SOF." Enter the six-digit date (MM/DD/YY), eight-digit date (MM/DD/CCYY), or alphanumeric date. A signature stamp may be used instead of a written signature. The stamp must leave a clear, nonsmeared image on the claim form.

Form Locator 32: Name and Address of Facility Where Services Were Rendered Form locator 32 identifies the name of the facility where services were provided. Enter the name, address, zip code, and NPI number when billing for purchased diagnostic tests. When more than one supplier is used, a separate CMS-1500 claim form should be used for each supplier.

Form Locator 32a: NPI Number Enter the NPI number of the service facility location in form locator 32a.

Form Locator 32b: Other ID Number Leave blank.

Form Locator 33: Billing Provider Information and Phone Number Enter the provider's or supplier's billing name, address, zip code, and phone number in form locator 33. The phone number is to be entered in the area to the right of the field title. Enter the name and address information in the following format:

First line: Name
Second line: Address
Third line: City, state, and zip code.

Form Locator 33a: NPI Number Enter the NPI number of the billing provider in form locator 33a. The NPI number refers to the HIPAA National Provider Identifier number, which allows for the entry of 10 characters.

For Locator 33b: Other ID Number Enter the TRICARE PIN.

Fill out the CMS-1500 form based on the information given here. To complete this exercise, copy the CMS-1500 form provided in Appendix D or download it from the CD-ROM that accompanies this text.

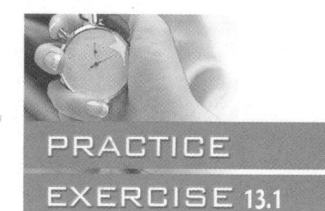

PRACTICE
EXERCISE 13.1

Physician Information:	Charles H. Borden, M.D.
	980 Frederick Road
	Dallas, TX 12345
Phone:	899-555-2276
EIN:	22-9872767
Professional License:	TX2056
UPIN:	3468923
TRICARE PIN:	9856471
NPI:	7536982014
Patient Information:	Barbara Cook
	8742 Fairview Road
	Dallas TX 12345
	999-555-3457
DOB:	06/18/1972
Social Security number:	885-26-3341
Patient Account:	COOBA
Status:	Married
Sex:	Female

(continued)

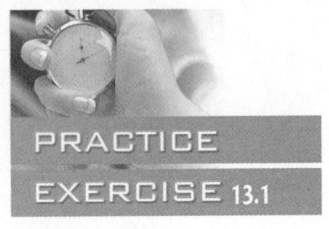

**PRACTICE
EXERCISE 13.1**

(continued)

Patient's Insurance Information:	TRICARE
Spouse's Information:	Christopher F. Cook P.O. Box 5431 Fort Dix, NJ 12345 555-124-8947
Insured's (Sponsor) Social Security number: Today's Date	603-87-9521
CC:	Influenza with Bronchitis
DX:	487.1
99213 Established Patient:	Problem focused history and examination, straightforward decision making $85.00 DX: 487.1
Accepting assignment	

Check the accuracy of your work by comparing your claim form to the completed claim form in Appendix J.

Confidential and Sensitive Information

Claims examiners who review claims for sensitive and confidential information stamp "CONFIDENTIAL" on the face of each claim form containing such information. The claim is treated as a confidential situation throughout the claims adjudication process. The examiner stamps both the envelope being mailed to the beneficiary and the provided return envelope "CONFIDENTIAL" when a claim is returned for additional information or because an incorrect claim form was used. PGBA employees do not provide information to parents or guardians of minors or persons who are unable to make healthcare decisions for themselves when the services are related to the following diagnoses:

- Alcoholism
- Abortion
- Drug abuse
- Venereal disease
- HIV.

Chapter Summary

- In January 1994 TRICARE became the new title for CHAMPUS. Individuals can choose from five different TRICARE health plans: (1) TRICARE Standard, a fee-for-service, cost-sharing type of option; (2) TRICARE Prime, an HMO type of option; (3) TRICARE Prime Remote (TPR), another type of HMO option; (4) TRICARE Extra, a PPO type of option; or (5) TRICARE Senior Prime, a program for Medicare-eligible beneficiaries ages 65 and older.

- Only certified providers, that is, those who have passed a credentialing process, can be authorized by TRICARE.
- Physicians submit paper claims to TRICARE using the CMS-1500 form. Hospitals and other inpatient facilities submit paper claims on the UB-04 (CMS-1450) claim form. The mailing address for claims varies depending on the provider's geographic location.
- Professional and institutional TRICARE claims must be submitted within 30 days from the date of service, or inpatient discharge date, but no later than 1 year from the date of service or discharge.

Chapter Review

True/ False

Identify the statement as true (T) or false (F).

_____ **1.** A nonavailability statement in the TRICARE program excuses the beneficiary from paying the cost share.

_____ **2.** In the TRICARE and CHAMPVA programs, cost share has the same meaning as coinsurance.

_____ **3.** The TRICARE program serves families of veterans with 100% service-related disability.

_____ **4.** TRICARE participating provider charges generally follow the Medicare Fee Schedule.

_____ **5.** It is not necessary to complete all form locators on the CMS-1500 form when completing a TRICARE claim.

Multiple Choice

Identify the letter of the choice that best completes the statement or answers the question.

_____ **1.** The TRICARE program that offers fee-for-service coverage is:
  - a. TRICARE Standard.
  - b. TRICARE Prime.
  - c. TRICARE Extra.
  - d. none of the above.

_____ **2.** The TRICARE program that offers an alternative managed care plan to TRICARE Prime with no enrollment fee is:
  - a. TRICARE Standard.
  - b. TRICARE Extra.
  - c. CHAMPUS.
  - d. CHAMPVA.

_____ **3.** TRICARE Standard is a:
  - a. fee-for-service plan.
  - b. capitated plan.
  - c. managed care organization.
  - d. program for children of veterans.

_____ **4.** A service that is not covered under TRICARE standard is:
   a. chiropractic care.
   b. cosmetic surgery.
   c. routine physical examinations.
   d. all of the above

_____ **5.** Professional and institutional TRICARE claims must be submitted to PGBA within how many days from the date of service, or inpatient discharge date.
   a. 60 days   c. 120 days
   b. 30 days   d. 180 days

Completion

Complete each sentence or statement.

1. The _____ manager is the provider who coordinates care of TRICARE beneficiaries.

2. The worldwide database of TRICARE and CHAMPVA beneficiaries is _____.

3. The TRICARE fiscal year begins _____ and ends _____.

4. An online claims submission program provided by PGBA is called _____.

5. A TRICARE beneficiary who lives within a certain distance of a military hospital must file a(n) _____ before entering a civilian hospital for inpatient non-emergency care.

6. TRICARE physician charges are filed using the _____ claim form.

7. Paper claims for CHAMPVA are submitted to the _____ department of the VA Health Administration Center.

8. All enrollees in TRICARE _____ must be enrolled in Medicare parts A and B.

9. TRICARE _____ and _____ require enrollment.

10. Active duty service members who are not near sources of military care qualify for _____.

Resources

TRICARE—U.S. Department of Defense Military Health System: *www.tricare.mil/provider.aspx*
TRICARE—Military: Explanation of Benefits: *www.tricare.mil/eob/*

Accounts Receivable

Receivables are the strength and stability of any growing practice. Accounts receivables include monies owed to a practice by both payers and patients. Chapter 14 presents a thorough understanding of the Explanation of Benefits (EOB) and the Electronic Remittance Advice (ERA). With this information in hand, the medical office specialist can post payment, apply write-offs, and bill patients correctly. With a clear understanding of these documents, the medical office specialist will be able to resolve any payment issues with the payer, adjust patients' accounts, and collect balances due from patients.

In the medical office facility, it is not uncommon for the medical office specialist to receive denial notices from insurance carriers. Therefore, it is important for the medical office specialist to be familiar with medical records, verification of benefits forms, precertification/preauthorization/referral requirements, and the appeals process for each insurance carrier with which the provider contracts. Chapter 15 provides the student with the knowledge required to submit additional clinical and other pertinent information to an insurance carrier to overturn a denied or downcoded claim by the payer.

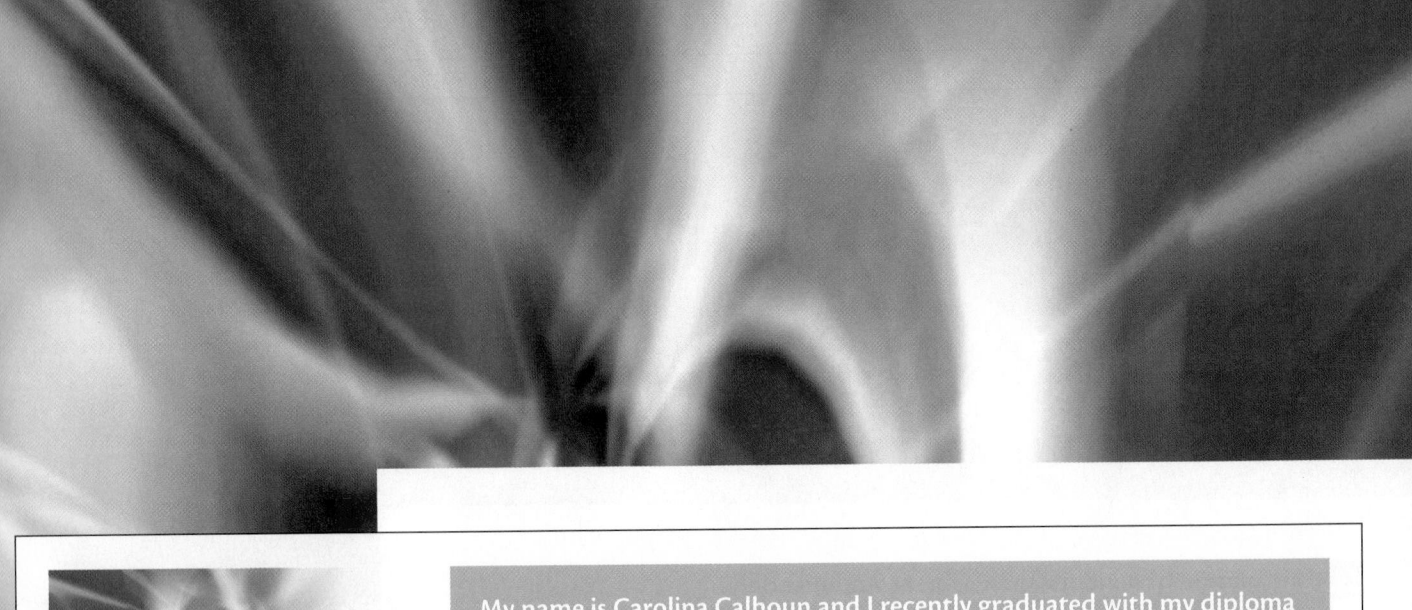

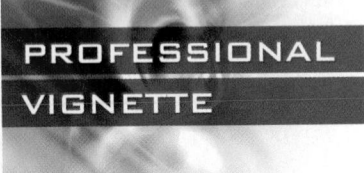

PROFESSIONAL VIGNETTE

My name is Carolina Calhoun and I recently graduated with my diploma in medical insurance billing and coding. I had previously worked as a manager in retail, but needed to find a new career direction due to a disability with my voice. A family member who works in medical coding suggested this field to me. I've always been interested in the medical field, so I jumped at the opportunity.

I enjoyed all aspects of my education and became really inspired by all the challenges that Medicare and other insurances present. For my externship, I worked in a hospital lab performing insurance verification and following up on denied claims. Thousands of claims were being denied due to improper diagnoses. I called the physician offices who had ordered the lab tests to get more appropriate diagnoses. For example, they may have ordered a PSA test but indicated the patient's chronic diabetes as the diagnosis, rather than the immediate problem that gave rise to the PSA. I had to obtain the correct diagnosis and resubmit the claim.

I have been actively involved in the local chapter of a national coder's association, and hope to start a chapter closer to my home. Now that I'm done with school, I am preparing for my certification exam and looking for permanent employment in my new field. I hope to be very successful in my new career.

Chapter 14 Explanation of Benefits and Payment Adjudication

Chapter Objectives

After reading this chapter, the student should be able to:

1. Define the steps for filing a medical claim.
2. Understand the importance of the Explanation of Benefits and Electronic Remittance Advice forms.
3. Calculate accurate payment by a carrier or third-party payer.
4. Make adjustments to patient accounts.
5. Review reason codes.
6. Describe different types of hospital reimbursement.

Key Terms

adjudication
adjustment
allowed charges
appeal
balance billing
capitation plan
charge-based fees
conversion factor
coordination of benefits (COB)
Electronic Remittance Advice (ERA)
excluded services
Explanation of Benefits (EOB)

Geographic Practice Cost Index (GPCI)
lifetime maximum
manual review
Medicare conversion factor (MCF)
Medicare Fee Schedule (MFS)
nationally uniform relative value
out-of-pocket expenses
pending claim
per member per month (PMPM)

reason codes/remark codes
relative value unit (RVU)
resource-based fees
resource-based relative value scale (RBRVS)
retention schedule
turnaround time
usual, customary, and reasonable (UCR)
withhold
write-offs

Case Study
Explanation
of Benefits
and Payment
Adjudication

Henry, the billing supervisor, noticed that Gloria, the biller responsible for sending out patient statements, had charged several patients for the balance that insurance had not paid. In discussing this with Gloria, Henry realized that she hadn't been properly trained regarding balance billing. He explained that in most managed care plans, the difference between the amount billed and the amount allowed by the insurer was to be entered as an adjustment and not billed to the patient.

Questions

1. What should be done regarding the patients who were incorrectly sent a statement?

2. How could Henry have prevented this error from occuring?

3. Is balance billing allowed in non-managed care plans?

Introduction

Understanding the Explanation of Benefits (EOB) or the remittance advice supplied by the payer allows the medical office specialist to post payments, apply write-offs, and bill patients correctly. The adjustment reason codes on an EOB inform the medical office specialist (MOS) about the reason for the denial, amount due from the patient, incorrect coding, etc. With a clear understanding of this remittance, the MOS will be able to resolve any payment issues with the payer, adjust patient accounts, and collect balances due from patients. In this manner, the accounts receivable will show a true reflection of balances owed the practice, which will affect the collection process. Accounts receivable represent monies owed to a provider by insurance carriers or the patient/insured. These payments are applied to the patient's account to reduce the overall balance due. The MOS is trained in communicating with patients to help resolve billing issues, such as amounts of copayments and collecting for deductibles. Accounts receivables are the strength and stability of any growing practice.

Steps for Filing a Medical Claim

An **Explanation of Benefits (EOB)** is a notification form sent from the insurance carrier to the patient and the healthcare provider (if the provider accepted assignment) after an insurance claim has been processed. If the provider has not accepted assignment, the payment and the EOB is sent to the patient. The form states the status of the claim; that is, whether it is paid, pending, rejected, or denied. However, before an EOB is received, the MOS is responsible for completing many steps, including:

1. Obtaining a correct and complete patient information form
2. Verifying patient insurance benefits
3. Obtaining signatures on the proper forms (release of information and assignment of benefits)
4. Entering computer data
5. Preparing encounter forms
6. Preparing sign-in sheets
7. Posting (entering into the computer) charges and diagnoses, as noted on the encounter form
8. Submitting a "clean claim."

Rejected or delayed insurance claims are expensive for the medical facility because resubmitting a claim means that work is being done a "second time." Dealing with insurance claims that a third-party payer denies, downcodes, or requests more information on ultimately affects the financial status of the practice. Practices are successful if their **turnaround time** (the amount of time it takes for the insurance carrier to process the claim) is within a reasonable period depending on the payer. A continuing cash flow results in a successful practice.

In reality, gathering the information required on a medical claim begins when the patient first enters the physician's office or hospital. Data used to complete locators 1 through 14 on the CMS-1500 and locators 8–11, 50, 58–62, and 65 on the UB-04 is collected during patient registration (Figures 14.1 and 14.2). The patient's proof of insurance and identification information is photocopied (Figure 14.3). Signatures are

1. MEDICARE MEDICAID TRICARE CHAMPVA GROUP FECA OTHER	1a. INSURED'S I.D. NUMBER (For Program in Item 1)
CHAMPUS HEALTH PLAN BLK LUNG	
☐(Medicare #) ☐(Medicaid #) ☐(Sponsor's SSN) ☐(Member ID#) ☐(SSN or ID) ☐(SSN) ☐(ID)	

2. PATIENT'S NAME (Last Name, First Name, Middle Initial) | 3. PATIENT'S BIRTH DATE SEX MM DD YY M☐ F☐ | 4. INSURED'S NAME (Last Name, First Name, Middle Initial)

5. PATIENT'S ADDRESS (No, Street) | 6. PATIENT RELATIONSHIP TO INSURED Self☐ Spouse☐ Child☐ Other☐ | 7. INSURED'S ADDRESS (No, Street)

CITY STATE | 8. PATIENT STATUS Single☐ Married☐ Other☐ | CITY STATE

ZIP CODE TELEPHONE (Include Area Code) ( ) | Full-Time Part-Time Employed☐ Student☐ Student☐ | ZIP CODE TELEPHONE (Include Area Code) ( )

9. OTHER INSURED'S NAME (Last Name, First Name, Middle Initial) | 10. IS PATIENT'S CONDITION RELATED TO: | 11. INSURED'S POLICY GROUP OR FECA NUMBER

a. OTHER INSURED'S POLICY OR GROUP NUMBER | a. EMPLOYMENT? (Current or Previous) ☐YES ☐NO | a. INSURED'S DATE OF BIRTH MM DD YY SEX M☐ F☐

b. OTHER INSURED'S DATE OF BIRTH SEX MM DD YY M☐ F☐ | b. AUTO ACCIDENT? PLACE (State) ☐YES ☐NO ☐ | b. EMPLOYER'S NAME OR SCHOOL NAME

c. EMPLOYER'S NAME OR SCHOOL NAME | c. OTHER ACCIDENT? ☐YES ☐NO | c. INSURANCE PLAN NAME OR PROGRAM NAME

d. INSURANCE PLAN NAME OR PROGRAM NAME | 10d. RESERVED FOR LOCAL USE | d. IS THERE ANOTHER HEALTH BENEFIT PLAN? ☐YES ☐NO If yes, return to and complete item 9 a-d

READ BACK OF FORM BEFORE COMPLETING & SIGNING THIS FORM.
12. PATIENT'S OR AUTHORIZED PERSON'S SIGNATURE I authorize the release of any medical or other information necessary to process this claim. I also request payment of government benefits either to myself or to the party who accepts assignment below.
SIGNED _____ DATE _____ | 13. INSURED'S OR AUTHORIZED PERSON'S SIGNATURE I authorize payment of medical benefits to the undersigned physician or supplier for services described below.
SIGNED _____

14. DATE OF CURRENT MM DD YY ◄ ILLNESS (First symptom) OR INJURY (Accident) OR PREGNANCY (LMP) | 15. IF PATIENT HAS HAD SAME OR SIMILAR ILLNESS, GIVE FIRST DATE MM DD YY | 16. DATES PATIENT UNABLE TO WORK IN CURRENT OCCUPATION FROM MM DD YY TO MM DD YY

PATIENT AND INSURED INFORMATION

Figure 14.1 Locators on the CMS-1500 claim form that are gathered during the patient registration process.

8 PATIENT NAME a	9 PATIENT ADDRESS a
b	b c d e
10 BIRTHDATE	11 SEX	12 DATE	ADMISSION 13 HR 14 TYPE 15 SRO	16 DHR	17 STAT	18 19 20 21	CONDITION CODES 22 23 24 25 26 27 28	29 ACCT 30 STATE

50 PAYER NAME	51 HEALTH PLAN ID	52	53	54 PRIOR PAYMENTS	55 EST. AMOUNT DUE	56 NPI
						57 OTHER PRV. ID
58 INSURED'S NAME	59 P. REL	60 INSURED'S UNIQUE ID	61 GROUP NAME	62 INSURANCE GROUP NO.

Figure 14.2 Locators on the UB-04 claim form that are gathered during the patient registration process.

Example: Driver's license

TEXAS
DEPARTMENT OF PUBLIC SAFETY
DRIVER LICENSE

01-02-97
12345678
HT: 5-10
EYES

Driver License Number

12345678
DOB: 01-02-70
EXPIRES: 01-02-04
REST:
END:
HT: 5-04
EYES: BRN
SEX: F

SAMPLE,IMA
2120 OLD MAIN STREET
ANYTOWN TX 12345-0010

Ima Sample

Example: United States passport

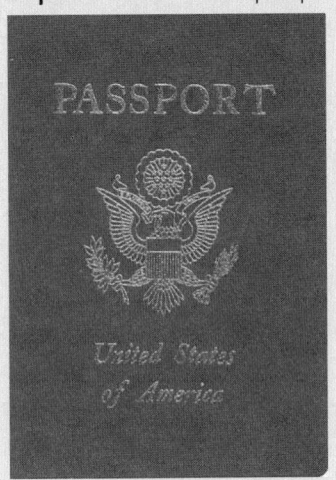

PASSPORT

United States
of America

Example: Insurance carrier ID card

CIGNA

Connecticut General Life Insurance Co.

Account	**3173952**	**Network**
Issuer (80842)		Copays:
ID:	**444551129 01**	PCP Visit $15
Name:	**Sue Smith**	Specialist $15
Coverage Effective Date: 01/01/2003		Hospital ER$50
		Urgent Care$50
PCP:	**Richard Cook**	
PCP Phone:	972-881-6000	

WWW. CIGNA.COM

You may be asked to present this card when you receive care. The card does not guarantee coverage. You must comply with all terms and conditions of the plan. Willful misuse of this card is considered fraud.

IN AN EMERGENCY: Seek care immediately. Go directly to the nearest emergency facility or call 911. If you have selected a PCP, call your PCP (or have someone call for you) as soon as possible for further assistance and directions on follow-up care. When possible, you should call your PCP within 48 hours.

CIGNA Claims: P.O. Box 180000, Chattanooga, TN 37000-7000

Member Services: 800-222-6222   Mental Health/Substance Abuse: 800-333-6333

Back of Insurance card

UnitedHealthcare

myuhc.com
PAID Prescriptions LLC
RX Bin 610000 UHEALTH

MICHAEL SMITH
Member # 123-45-6789

THRUPOINT, INC.

Group # 700000
COPAY: Office Visit $10 ER $50
  Rx $10Gn/$15Br/$25NF

Electronic Claims Payer ID 80000

Call toll-free 800-555-1111 for Member Services

**UnitedHealthcare
Options PPO
Effective 01/01/03**

MTH

BlueCross BlueShield Of the National Capital Area		Capital Care
ADM. CERT	**BC PLAN DBC**	**PRE-CERT**

9999999	**DC000**
Identification No.	Group
JOHN BROWN	
Member Name	
A1234567	**01/11/61**
Physician Number	Member Date of Birth
MARION WELBY, M.D.	
Physician Name	
PS $10 ER $25 UC $10 IPO Di	
Copay Rider Information	

Figure 14.3   **Photocopy the patient's proof of insurance and identification information (samples are only representations and not actual health insurance cards).**

required as policies and procedures are explained to the patient. It is the medical office specialist's responsibility to see that all patient, guarantor, and insurance information is in order and that all forms are completed before the patient is seen by the physician.

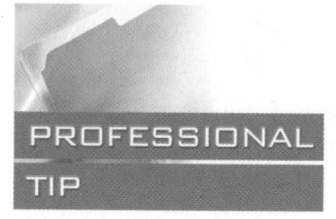

Always ask for a patient's passport, green card, driver's license, or government ID to keep on file. It is standard to make a copy of all requested identification.

During the patient's care all procedures and tests are documented on an encounter form or electronically. The physician will document the diagnosis after the visit or after test results have been received. All data is then integrated onto the claim form. The claim form is submitted to the carrier for payment.

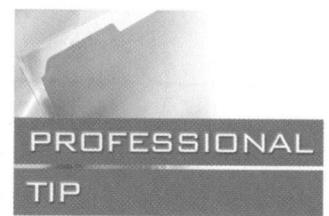

Always make a copy (front and back) of the patient's insurance ID card and file it in the patient's medical chart. It is a good idea to date stamp each copy to keep track of old and new cards.

Claims Process

The insurance carrier's decision regarding whether or not to pay a claim is called adjudication. **Adjudication** is the act of processing a claim that consists of edits, review, and determination (Figure 14.4). Once the insurance carrier receives a claim from the physician or healthcare facility it is processed. The initial review of each claim consists of computer edits that screen the basic data on the claim form. The claim is edited to check for billing errors (such as a policy ID number missing). A claim examiner will check that the diagnosis and CPT® codes are linked when reviewing claims. The diagnosis and procedures are reviewed to be sure the treatment was medically necessary, which means appropriate for the diagnosis. Medical review examiners are part of the third-party payer's staff and they verify the medical necessity of providers' reported procedures.

The claim may be denied if the reported procedure does not match the diagnosis code. The examiner determines if the claim is payable, and a payment decision is made. The claims examiner then pays, denies, or partially pays the claim. A claim that is removed from a payer's automated processing system is sent for **manual review**. When a claim is pulled for manual review, the provider may be asked to submit clinical documentation to support the claim. A carrier's manual review may result in a claim denial due to three reasons: (1) lack of required preauthorization, (2) lack of medical necessity, and (3) lack of eligibility for a reported procedure. The carrier then makes a determination to pay the claim (or not) and provides an EOB to the provider and the insured.

To use an extreme example, suppose the codes on the insurance claim form indicate the patient has a broken arm and the treatment given was removal of the tonsils. Because removing the tonsils is not a medically necessary treatment for a broken arm, the claim would be denied. If the patient were instead treated with a cast for the broken arm, it would suit the diagnosis and would be considered medically necessary.

A carrier will "downcode" a claim if it is determined to not be medically necessary at the level reported. Downcoding is also referred to as "medical necessity reduction."

CPT is a registered trademark of the American Medical Association.

Figure 14.4

Steps of adjudication.

1. Insurance carrier receives insurance claim form.
2. Claims department processes the information to determine what benefits are due according to the patient's policy.
3. First items checked are the patient's and insured's policy identification numbers (refer to patient information form).
4. Correct spelling of names and use of names as they appear in the insurance carrier's master file are essential.
5. A claims specialist reviews the claim.
6. Procedure codes are compared with the patient's policy schedule of benefits to see whether the reported services are covered.
7. Procedure codes and diagnostic codes are compared to see whether services were medically necessary.
8. The amount the policy covers for each service, generally called the allowed charge or allowable charge, is determined according to the policy's guidelines.
9. If the patient or insured must pay a deductible and/or coinsurance, *that amount is subtracted from the allowed charge.*
10. The remainder is the amount due to the provider.
11. The insurance carrier then issues the benefit payment (check) along with an EOB.
12. An EOB is sent to *both* the policyholder and the provider. Even if no benefit or payment is due from the insurance carrier, an EOB is sent out.

Special note: Completion of this process may be delayed by errors on the insurance claim form. Incomplete or inaccurate insurance claim forms are retained and a letter is sent asking for additional information. Payment is withheld until problems are resolved.

After the claim has gone through the adjudication process and a claim has been downcoded or denied, an **appeal** may be submitted to the insurance carrier by participating providers (PARs). The person requesting an appeal is referred to as the *claimant.* These claims need to be reviewed and appealed for reconsideration. The appeals process is done in writing and may include documents such as operative reports or x-rays to aid in determining medical necessity. The MOS must evaluate the claim to see if the claim needs resubmitting or if an appeal letter must be written to appeal a claim. If a carrier has continued to deny all of the practice's appeal requests, the provider can file a request to the state insurance commissioner for assistance. The state insurance commissioner has regulatory control over insurance carriers and will assist in insurance appeals or disputes.

Any precautions that can be taken when submitting claims to carriers should be taken to ensure that claims are not denied due to medical necessity reduction. If a claim is denied due to lack of medical necessity, the provider must refund any payment made on the claim by the payer and the patient. Denials are a challenge for healthcare providers because of the loss of revenue, which includes lost resources and time. Healthcare providers work diligently to improve the management of medical necessity denials. The priority here is to prevent a denial from ever occurring by proving that the procedure or treatment is medically necessary. The MOS who is posting EOBs needs to be aware of downcoding by the payer and take appropriate action.

The claims department compares the fees to the schedule of benefits in the patient's policy and determines the amount of benefit to be paid on the claim. After adjudication is completed and the claim is deemed payable, an Explanation of Benefits is forwarded to the provider with payment.

Determining the Fees

Providers have different methods in determining their fee structure (the amount charged for each procedure performed). As stated by the American Medical Association (AMA), "Physicians have the right to establish their fees at a level which they believe fairly reflects the costs of providing a service and the value of the professional judgment." Two main methods are used for determining fees: charged-based and resource-based fee structures.

Charge-Based Fee Structure

Charge-based fees are the fees that many providers charge for similar services. To set their fees, providers begin with an analysis of their procedure codes. To determine if their fees are in range with other providers of the same specialty they may research a nationwide fee database. This information can be purchased by the provider to ascertain how fees compare to national averages. The database is divided into categories to indicate fees that are 25%, 50%, 75%, and 90% higher based on fees charged throughout the nation. A provider can decide if his usual fees should be on the high, low, or midpoint range.

Resource-Based Fee Structures

Resource-based fees are based on the following three factors:

1. How difficult it is for the provider to perform the procedure (work)
2. How much office overhead the procedure involves (practice expense)
3. The relative risk that the procedure presents to the patient and the provider (malpractice).

Third-party payers also establish the amount they will reimburse providers. Each payer will determine the **usual, customary, and reasonable (UCR)** fee they feel should be charged by the provider by determining the percentage of the published fee in the national database that they will pay.

History of the RBRVS

Due to rapidly rising expenditures in the Medicare program, in December 1985, Harvard University conducted a national study and submitted the final report in 1988. Previously, Medicare payments had been based on a Medicare-developed "reasonable fee schedule" that used historical charges. The Omnibus Budget Reconciliation Act (OBRA) of 1989 enacted a physician payment schedule based on a **resource-based relative value scale (RBRVS)**. This law called for the reasonable fee schedule to be gradually replaced by the RBRVS payment system because it fairly represented the resources used to perform the procedure or service.

On January 1, 1992, Medicare implemented the RBRVS system as the payment system to be used. The RBRVS replaced Medicare's 25-year-old "customary, prevailing, and reasonable" (CPR) charge system. This was the most sweeping and far-reaching change to the Medicare Part B payment system to date. In brief, RBRVS ranks physician services by assigning each a relative value. It replaced providers' consensus on fees, the historical charges, with a relative value based on resources.

Resource-Based Relative Value Scale (RBRVS)

A **relative value unit (RVU)** is a unit of measurement assigned to a medical service based on the relative skill and time required to perform it. The RBRVS system is composed of three elements measured in RVUs:

1. Nationally uniform relative value: This value is based on three cost elements, which are:

- *Provider's work:* the physician's individual effort (the largest cost element), which accounts for 52% of the total relative value for each service. The initial physician work RVUs were based on the results of the Harvard University study. The factors used to determine physician work include the time it takes to perform the service, the technical skill and physical effort, the required mental effort and judgment, and stress due to the potential risk to the patient. The physician's work relative values are updated each year to account for changes in medical practice. Also, the legislation enacting the RBRVS requires the Centers for Medicare and Medicaid Services (CMS) to review the whole scale at least every 5 years.
- *Practice expense:* the practice costs associated with delivering a physician service (overhead). The practice expense component of the RBRVS accounts for an average of 44% of the total relative value for each service. Until recently, practice expense RVUs were based on a formula using average Medicare-approved charges from 1991 (the year before the RBRVS was implemented) and the proportion of each specialty's revenue that is attributable to practice expenses. However, in January 1999, CMS began a transition to resource-based practice expense RVUs for each CPT code that differs based on the site of service. In 2002, the resource-based practice expenses were fully transitioned.
- *Professional liability insurance:* the professional liability insurance premium costs (malpractice). On January 1, 2000, CMS implemented the resource-based professional liability insurance (PLI) relative value units. The PLI component of the RBRVS accounts for an *average of* 4% of the total relative value for each service. The CMS began reviewing appropriate PLI relative values. With this implementation and final transition of the resource-based practice expense relative units on January 1, 2002, all components of the RBRVS became resource based.

To understand the uniform relative value, one must look at each value separately and place a measurement on it. For example, for each $1.00 of services, the work accounts for x amount, the PE (practice expense) accounts for x amount, and the malpractice accounts for x amount to equal the total of $1.00. A family practitioner who charges for a flu shot has relative values that are much lower than those of a cardiac surgeon who performs open heart surgery. For each value the number will be placed according to the provider's work performed, the cost to practice, and the cost of the malpractice insurance or liability risk to the patient.

2. Geographic Practice Cost Index (GPCI): This value is the number that is multiplied by each RVU to show the cost element for each value in that specific geographical location. Used by Medicare in their RBRVS payment systems, GPCIs are designed to represent the relative costs coupled with physician work, practice, and malpractice expenses in a Medicare area compared to the national average relative costs. However, in 1989 OBRA mandated that 25% of a physician's work payment be adjusted according to geographic earnings differences. The remaining 75% of the physician's work payment is to be the same for all areas. For example, it would cost more for work, for practice overhead, and for malpractice insurance in Manhattan, New York, than Waco, Texas. Under current law, changes in GPCIs do not impact total Medicare expenditures. Instead, GPCIs redistribute payments among Medicare payment localities.

3. Nationally uniform conversion factor: A **conversion factor** is a numerical factor (dollar amount) used to multiply or divide a quantity when converting from one system of units to another. This conversion factor is determined annually by the legislature and published in the *Federal Register*. It is used by Medicare to make adjustments according to the changes in the cost of living index. The **Medicare conversion factor (MCF)** is a national value, that converts the total RVUs into payment amounts for the purpose of reimbursing physicians for services provided. The conversion factor is updated every year by CMS and published in the *Federal Register*.

The 2006 Medicare Conversion Factor is $37.8975, which is the same as the 2005 conversion factor. The 2006 conversion factor was initially $36.1770, but aggressive lobbying by the AMA caused the conversion factor to be reset to the 2005 amount on February 9, 2006. The 2007 conversion factor still remains at $37.8975.

Determining the Medicare Fee

The relative value of each unit is multiplied by GPCIs for each Medicare locality and then translated into a dollar amount by an annually adjusted conversion factor. The **Medicare Fee Schedule (MFS)** is based on RBRVS fees. Therefore, the fees are based on the federal government's data of what each service costs.

When calculating the allowed Medicare fee for a physician, the formula is as follows:

1. Determine the procedure code for the service (CPT).
2. Use the RVUs for work, practice expense, and malpractice.
3. Use the GPCI for work, practice expense, and malpractice.
4. Multiply each RVU by each GPCI.
5. Add the three adjusted totals.
6. Multiply the total sum by the conversion factor.

Practice exercises follow that will help the student determine the Medicare allowed fees for the procedures listed. The relative values are also listed with the GPCI. Figure 14.5 demonstrates the calculations for procedure code 99203 using the locale of Dallas, Texas, with a 2007 conversion factor of $37.8975.

To complete Practice Exercises 14.1 and 14.2, determine the Medicare allowed fee for the geographical areas listed by using the GPCIs and conversion factors from Figures 14.6 and 14.7.

	RVU GPCI
WORK	$1.34 \times 1.010 = 1.3534$
PRACTICE EXPENSE	$1.13 \times 1.065 = 1.20345$
MALPRACTICE +	$0.10 \times 0.996 = 0.0996$
	TOTAL 2.65645

$2.65645 \times 37.8975 = 100.67281 = \$100.67$

Figure 14.5

Example of how to determine the Medicare allowed fee for procedure code 99203 for a physician in Dallas, Texas.

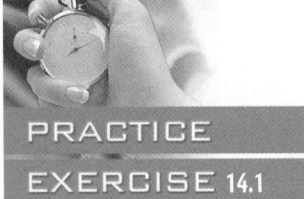

Figure 14.6

GPCIs and conversion factors.

Geographic Location	Work GPCI	Practice Expense GPCI	Malpractice Expense GPCI
Dallas, TX	1.010	1.065	0.996
Houston, TX	1.000	0.969	1.318
Ft. Worth, TX	1.000	0.981	0.996

Figure 14.7

Procedure codes and conversion factors.

CPT Description	Work RVU	Practice RVU	Malpractice RVU
99203 Office outpatient/new	1.34	1.13	0.10
99213 Office outpatient/established	0.67	0.70	0.04
23500 Treat clavicle fracture	2.08	3.66	0.31

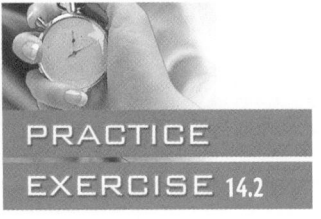

PRACTICE
EXERCISE 14.1

Determine the Medicare allowed fees for the procedures listed. Use the 2007 conversion factor of $37.8975.

	Dallas	Houston	Fort Worth
99203:	100.67		
99213:			
23500:			

On completion of this exercise, refer to Appendix J to check the accuracy of your work.

PRACTICE
EXERCISE 14.2

Determine the Medicare allowed fees for the procedures listed. Use the 2004 conversion factor of $37.3374.

	Dallas	Houston	Fort Worth
99203:			
99213:			
23500:			

On completion of this exercise, refer to Appendix J to check the accuracy of your work.

Other payers (insurance carriers) are switching to the resource-based fees rather than the charge-based fees that represented the providers' consensus on fees/charges. Debate surrounds the use of resource-based fees because physicians' malpractice insurance has increased so dramatically in the past few years. The increase in malpractice insurance is one of the main reasons why many providers are no longer able to practice medicine. The specialists who are affected the most are obstetricians and gynecologists, and orthopedic surgeons. If the RVU for malpractice were increased to accommodate the cost increase in the insurance, physicians' fees would greatly increase. In the president's state of the union address in 2003, he addressed this issue and asked Congress to put into law medical liability reform. This would help alleviate the high malpractice bills.

The MOS must be aware of and become familiar with payers' reimbursement calculations in order to review an EOB to determine if the payment amount is correct.

Allowed Charge

Allowed charges refer to the maximum allowed amount for a covered charge. Some payers refer to this as the *maximum allowed fee, allowed amount,* or *allowable charge*. This is the amount the payer will pay the provider for her service. An allowed charge also includes the amount that the patient will pay. The provider's usual charge for the procedure or service may be higher, equal to, or lower than the allowed charge.

> **Example**
>
> The allowed amount is $100.00 but within that allowed amount, the patient is responsible for 20% and the payer is responsible for 80%, equaling 100% of the allowed amount.
>
> Consider another example in which the allowed amount is $100.00. The payer will pay $75.00 of the allowed and the patient's copay is $25.00. Again the two payments equal 100% of the allowed amount.

The allowed amount a provider receives from the third-party payer depends on whether the provider is participating or not participating in the payer's plan. Participating providers agree by contract to accept the third-party payer's allowed charge.

If a provider is a PAR with the payer, she agrees to the fees and the rules that stipulate that the provider may not bill a patient for the part of the charge that the payer did not pay.

When an allowed charge has been set, the carrier never pays more than this amount to the provider. If the provider's usual charge is less than the insurance carrier's allowed charge, the carrier will pay the lower of the two. The payment is *always* based on the lower of the two, whether it is the provider's usual charge or the allowed charge. Figure 14.8 demonstrates that a provider should always review his usual charges annually to receive the highest reimbursement.

A non-PAR provider will only receive the allowed charge from the third-party payer and may bill the balance to the patient.

Provider A usual charge $200.00   Allowed amount/payer pays: $150.00

Provider B usual charge $125.00   Allowed amount $150.00/payer pays: $125.00

As the medical office specialist can see, Provider B lost $25.00 because his usual charge was too low.

Figure 14.8

A provider should always review usual charges annually to receive the highest reimbursement.

The physician charges	$200.00
Allowed amount	$175.00
	$25.00 (provider's write-off)
Allowed amount	$175.00
Medicare deductible	−$131.00 (subtract 2007 deductible)
	$ 44.00

$44.00 × 80% = $35.20 Medicare pays to provider

$44.00 × 20% = $8.80 + $131.00 (deductible) = $139.80 (total patient responsibility)

Figure 14.9

Example of an allowed charge for a provider who is participating with Medicare.

Payers' Policies

Figure 14.9 provides an example of an allowed charge for a provider who is participating with Medicare. Under Medicare Part B, reimbursement to a PAR provider will pay the physician 80% of the allowed amount *after the calendar year deductible has been satisfied.* The patient is responsible for 20%, which is her coinsurance.

A payer's policy has an allowed charge for each procedure. In Figure 14.10, the plan pays 100% of the provider's usual charges—*up to* the maximum allowed by the payer.

When a patient has a policy that requires coinsurance payments and the payer has a maximum allowed charge for each procedure, the patient is only responsible for the coinsurance of the maximum allowed charge if the provider is a PAR provider (Figure 14.11). If the provider is a non-PAR provider (Figure 14.12), the patient again is responsible for the difference between the provider's usual charge and the maximum allowed charge.

Figure 14.10

In this example, the plan pays 100% of the provider's usual charges, up to the maximum allowed by the payer.

Provider A—Participating

Provider's usual charge	$2000.00
Policy pays its allowed charge	$1500.00
Provider writes off the difference between the usual charge and the allowed amount	$500.00

Provider B—Nonparticipating

Provider's usual charge	$2000.00
Policy pays its allowed charge	$1500.00
Provider bills the patient for the difference between the usual and allowed charge.	$500.00
Provider B has no write-off.	

Figure 14.11

The patient is only responsible for the coinsurance of the maximum allowed charge if the provider is a PAR provider.

Provider A—Participating

Usual charge	$2000.00
Allowed charge	$1500.00
Policy pays 80% of the allowed charge	$1200.00
Patient responsible for the 20% of the allowed charge	$300.00
Provider writes off the difference between the usual and allowed charge	$500.00

Provider B—Nonparticipating

Usual charge	$2000.00
Allowed charge	$1500.00
Policy pays 80% of the allowed charge	$1200.00
Patient responsible for 20% of the allowed charge ($300.00) and the difference between the usual and allowed charge ($500.00)	$800.00
Provider B has no write-off.	

Figure 14.12

If the provider is a non-PAR provider, the patient is responsible for the difference between the provider's usual charge and the maximum allowed charge.

Calculate the financial responsibility of the patient, the amount the carrier will pay, and the amount the provider must write off.

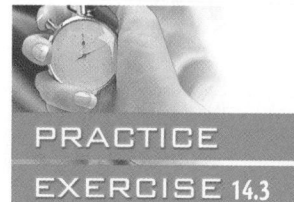

PRACTICE EXERCISE 14.3

1. Debbie Ducktails was seen in Dr. Musk's office today for knee pain. Total charges are $315.00. Allowed amount is $175.00. Benefits pay at 70%.

   Usual charge   _____

   Allowed charge   _____

   Policy pays _____ of the allowed charge, which is _____.

   Patient responsible for _____ of the allowed charge, which is _____.

   Provider writes off the difference between the usual and allowed charge: _____.

   _____   _____   _____
   Patient's responsibility   Write-off   Carrier pays

2. Kate Baird was seen in the doctor's office today for an ingrown toenail. Total charges are $200.00. Allowed amount is $135.00. Kate is subject to a deductible of $100.00. Once this is met, her benefits pay at 75%.

   Usual charge   _____

   Allowed charge   _____

   Deductible   _____

   Policy pays _____ of the allowed charge, which is _____.

   Patient responsible for _____ of the allowed charge, which is _____.

   Provider writes off the difference between the usual and allowed charge: _____.

   _____   _____   _____
   Patient's responsibility   Write-off   Carrier pays

3. Sue Smith is being seen in Dr. Sampson's office today for ear piercing. Total charges are $200.00. This fee is not covered by her insurance company.

   Usual charge   _____

   Allowed charge   _____

   Deductible   _____

(continued)

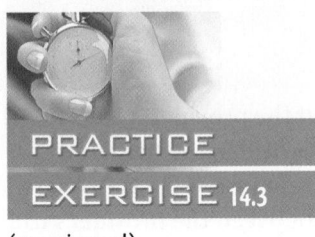

PRACTICE
EXERCISE 14.3
(continued)

Policy pays _____ of the allowed charge, which is _____.

Patient responsible for _____ of the allowed charge, which is _____.

Provider writes off the difference between the usual and allowed charge: _____.

_____	_____	_____
Patient's responsibility	Write-off	Carrier pays

4. Kalvin Combs is having outpatient surgery at the Baylor Medical Center. Kalvin is on an indemnity plan. Total charges are $1489.32. He is subject to a $250.00 deductible. Once the deductible is met, benefits pay at 80%.

Usual charge   _____

Allowed charge   _____

Deductible   _____

Policy pays _____ of the allowed charge, which is _____.

Patient responsible for _____ of the allowed charge, which is _____.

Provider writes off the difference between the usual and allowed charge: _____.

_____	_____	_____
Patient's responsibility	Write-off	Carrier pays

On completion of this exercise, refer to Appendix J to check the accuracy of your work.

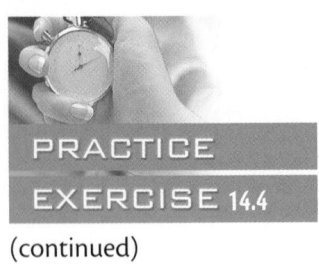

PRACTICE
EXERCISE 14.4
(continued)

Calculate the financial responsibility of the patient, the amount the carrier will pay, and the amount the provider must write off.

1. Annie Bates was seen in the doctor's office today for sinusitis. She is subject to her annual deductible of $150.00. Once her deductible is met, she must pay a copayment of $20.00. Today's total billed charges are $215.00. The allowed amount is $175.00.

Usual charge   _____

Allowed charge   _____

Deductible   _____

Policy pays _____ of the allowed charge, which is _____.

Patient responsible for the _____ of the allowed charge, which is _____.

Provider writes off the difference between the usual and allowed charge: _____.

_____	_____	_____
Patient's responsibility	Write-off	Carrier pays

2. Jessica Woods was seen in the office today for an allergic reaction to Allegra. She is subject to a $500.00 deductible, and today's charges total $217.00. Total allowed amount is $125.00.

    Usual charge   _____

    Allowed charge   _____

    Deductible   _____

    Policy pays _____ of the allowed charge, which is _____.

    Patient responsible for _____ of the allowed charge, which is _____.

    Provider writes off the difference between the usual and allowed charge: _____.

    _____   _____   _____
    Patient's responsibility   Write-off   Carrier pays

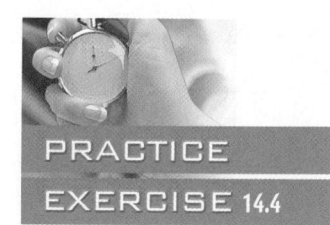

PRACTICE EXERCISE 14.4

(continued)

3. Melissa Jackson had outpatient surgery at Taylor Medical Center. Total charges are $3895.56. Allowed amount is $2956.18. Melissa is subject to a $500.00 deductible and her rate of benefit is 90%.

    Usual charge   _____

    Allowed charge   _____

    Deductible   _____

    Policy pays _____ of the allowed charge, which is _____.

    Patient responsible for _____ of the allowed charge, which is _____.

    Provider writes off the difference between the usual and allowed charge: _____.

    _____   _____   _____
    Patient's responsibility   Write-off   Carrier pays

4. Sara Tipping is seen in Dr. Smith's office today for hyperthyroidism. She is subject to a $20.00 copayment. Total charges are $85.00. Allowed amount is $65.00. Dr. Smith referred her for some lab work to be done at Ballard Laboratory, total lab charges are $175.00. Allowed amount is $125.00. These lab charges are subject to her deductible of $100.00 and paid at the 80% rate of benefit.

    Usual charge   _____

    Allowed charge   _____

    Deductible   _____

    Policy pays _____ of the allowed charge, which is _____.

    Patient responsible for _____ of the allowed charge, which is _____.

    Provider writes off the difference between the usual and allowed charge: _____.

    _____   _____   _____
    Patient's responsibility   Write-off   Carrier pays

On completion of this exercise, refer to Appendix J to check the accuracy of your work.

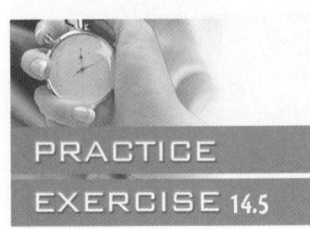

PRACTICE
EXERCISE 14.5
(continued)

Calculate the financial responsibility of the patient, the amount the carrier will pay, and the amount the provider must write off.

1. Jill Self was seen in Dr. Dancing's office today for the flu. She is subject to a $20.00 copayment. Total charges are $175.00. Allowed amount is $125.00.

    Usual charge   _____

    Allowed charge   _____

    Policy pays _____ of the allowed charge, which is _____.

    Patient responsible for the _____ of the allowed charge, which is _____.

    Provider writes off the difference between the usual and allowed charge: _____.

    _____   _____   _____
    Patient's responsibility   Write-off   Carrier pays

2. Tanya Taylor had outpatient surgery at Baylor Medical Center. Total charges are $726.25. Allowed amount is $558.16. She is subject to a $250.00 deductible. Once her deductible is met, benefits are paid at 80%.

    Usual charge   _____

    Allowed charge   _____

    Deductible   _____

    Policy pays _____ of the allowed charge, which is _____.

    Patient responsible for _____ of the allowed charge, which is _____.

    Provider writes off the difference between the usual and allowed charge: _____.

    _____   _____   _____
    Patient's responsibility   Write-off   Carrier pays

3. Angie Grant was having outpatient lab work done at the Duncan Laboratory facility. Total charges were $576.00. (This is an indemnity plan, so it is a fee-for-service plan.) Angie is subject to a $250.00 deductible. Once this is met, her benefits pay at 80%.

    Usual charge   _____

    Allowed charge   _____

    Deductible   _____

    Policy pays _____ of the allowed charge, which is _____.

    Patient responsible for _____ of the allowed charge, which is _____.

    Provider writes off the difference between the usual and allowed charge: _____.

    _____   _____   _____
    Patient's responsibility   Write-off   Carrier pays

4. Patricia Pegus is having a chest x-ray done at the Diagnostic Center in Dallas. Patricia is on an indemnity plan. Total charges today are $175.00. She is subject to a $100.00 deductible, and her benefits pay at 90%.

Usual charge   _____

Allowed charge   _____

Deductible   _____

Policy pays _____ of the allowed charge, which is _____.

Patient responsible for _____ of the allowed charge, which is _____.

Provider writes off the difference between the usual and allowed charge: _____.

_____   _____   _____
Patient's responsibility   Write-off   Carrier pays

PRACTICE EXERCISE 14.5

(continued)

On completion of this exercise, refer to Appendix J to check the accuracy of your work.

Capitation

When a provider enters into a **capitation plan** or contract with a carrier, the provider agrees to treat a number of members in that plan. The carrier in turn agrees to pay that provider based on a designated fee each month for each member in that plan. This is referred to as a **per member per month (PMPM)** fee. The member enrollment can change monthly. The payer sends the provider a list of the members at the beginning of the month with a check to pay for care for those members whether they are treated or not. The physician's incentive is to render as few services as possible in one sitting while still providing excellent medical care. The term *cap rate* means *capitation rate*. During the course of the year, some payers hold back or withhold a percentage of the provider's payment to pay or offset any additional costs that may be incurred for referrals, hospital admissions, or other services provided by the plan. At the end of the year, any **withhold** not used is distributed to providers as a bonus.

Consider this example of a capitation plan: A payer is negotiating with a physiatrist for physical therapy for its members. A list of procedures will be agreed on for services rendered under this contract. The payer sets a dollar amount for each member for physical therapy services listed. At the beginning of each month, the provider receives X amount of dollars for the members enrolled—whether they are seen or not.

Example

For physical therapy the provider would receive $30.00 for each member. The total members enrolled for the month equals 100. Therefore, the provider would receive $3000.00 at the beginning of each month.

Calculations of Patient Charges

The medical office specialist will determine the patient's charges at the time of service so he will know the dollar amount to collect from the patient. The employer often chooses the insurance for the employee, so the patient doesn't have a choice in the type of coverage she has. If choices are given, the insured has chosen her own insurance policy according to the deductible, copays, coinsurance, and excluded services. Depending on the medical plan, the insured may be required to make four types of payments: deductibles, copayments, coinsurance, and payments for excluded services. The MOS will know exactly what needs to be paid at the time of service after verifying the insured's insurance plan benefits.

Deductible

Many payers require policyholders or the insured to pay a certain amount of covered expenses to the provider before the insurance benefits begin. This amount is called the *deductible*. The reason it is called a *deductible* is because the payer deducts this specific amount from any charges billed before paying the bill.

> ### Example
>
> **A new patient is seen in a physician's office and the charge is $250.00. The patient's deductible is $200.00. When the MOS sends a claim for $250.00, the payer deducts the $200.00 and pays according to the contract on the $50.00 only.**

Some plans have individual deductibles, which must be met by each individual listed on the policy. Family deductibles are the combined amount for all individuals listed on the plan. The policy may state that a family deductible refers to at least three individuals. For the family deductible to be met, the total for all individuals listed on the policy must be met before the plan will pay for benefits.

Individual and family deductibles are a fixed dollar amount and are set by the insurance carrier. This information is stated in the insured's policy. One individual member of a family can meet a family deductible. When a deductible is required, it must be met before benefits from the carrier begin. The deductibles, copayments, and coinsurance that patients are required to pay are referred to as **out-of-pocket expenses**. Deductibles are set per calendar year. For example, each January the deductible amount is reset and must be satisfied (met) before insurance benefits pay out.

Maximum out-of-pocket expenses are determined by the payer and listed in the insured's policy. The payer will reimburse services at 100% once the maximum out-of pocket expenses have been met for the year. The policy may state, for example, that services will be paid at 100% after a $2500.00 maximum out-of-pocket limit has been met within the year. This benefit protects the insured from extreme financial losses due to high medical bills.

The **lifetime maximum** benefit specified in an insurance policy is different from out-of-pocket expenses because once the stated maximum has been met for a lifetime, no more benefits will be paid. The maximum benefit should be questioned at the time the MOS verifies the patient's insurance.

Copayments

A medical insurance plan may require a copay to be paid at the time of service. The copay is a set amount. Usually the copay is stated on the card. An example would be:

OV $15.00 (copay for office visit)
SP $35.00 (copay for specialist visit)
ER $100.00 (copay for emergency room visit)

Coinsurance

Many payers require coinsurance payments, which are a percentage of the contracted allowable charge. Here is an example: Medicare pays 80% of the MFS (Medicare Fee Schedule) to a participating provider after the deductible is met. The patient is responsible for 20% (which is the coinsurance amount) and the deductible if it has not been met.

Excluded Services

Excluded services are procedures or office visits that are not covered by the insurance carrier as defined in its policy. A medical insurance contract will usually state the medical services it does not cover. The physician's office may provide care for services that are not covered under a patient's policy. In this case, the patient is expected to pay at the time service is rendered. The medical office specialist is responsible for advising the patient about nonpayment before these services are rendered to discuss payment options. With some payers, such as Medicare, the MOS needs to have the patient sign a form stating that she is responsible for the noncovered service. Table 14.1 shows procedures that may not be covered under certain types of managed care plans. Because the employer customizes some plans offered to their employees, it is recommended that the patient's benefits always be verified.

Table 14.1	Common Benefits under Various Plans					
Plan Types	**Deductible**	**Copay**	**Coinsurance**	**Out of Pocket**	**Coinsurance Post OOP**
PPO (Managed Care)					
Office: PAR	—	20.00[a]	—	—	—
Office: Non–PAR[b]	250.00	—	30%	—	—
Outpatient and Inpatient: PAR[b]	250.00	—	20%	1,500.00	0%
Outpatient and Inpatient: Non-Par**	250.00	—	30%	2,500.00	0%
HMO (Managed Care)					
Office: PAR to PCP	—	20.00*	—	—	—
Office: Non-PAR to PCP[c]	—	—	—	—	—
Outpatient (referred by PCP)[b]		50.00	0%		
Inpatient (referred by PCP)[b]		100.00	0%		
INDEMNITY (NOT Managed Care)[d]	250.00		20%	1,500.00	0%

[a]Covers office visits and any lab or x-rays done in physician's office.
[b]Precertification required.
[c]All services must be authorized by primary care provider (PCP) or no benefits are available.
[d]No discounts on indemnity plans unless negotiated with the provider. UCR applies for charges billed.

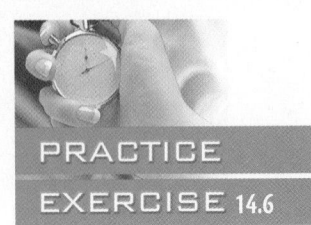

Using the information provided in the table below, calculate the patients' payment amounts.

CPT CODE	Provider's Charge	Adjustment	Allowed Amount
99212	$66.00	$12.00	$54.00
93040	44.00	8.00	36.00
99201	88.00	26.00	62.00
99204	108.00	33.00	75.00
97032	45.00	16.00	29.00
97110	45.00	16.00	29.00
99213	90.00	38.00	52.00
73630	88.00	16.00	72.00

1. Patient 1 charges 99213, 73630, and 97110. No deductible applies. Plan pays @ 80/20.

    Payer payment to provider _____

    Coinsurance _____

    Discount amount _____

2. Patient 2 charges 99212 and 73630. Deductible of $100.00 applies. Plan pays @ 80/20.

    Payer payment to provider _____

    Coinsurance _____

    Discount amount _____

3. Patient 3 charges 93040 and 97032. Deductible of $100.00 applies. Plan pays @ 90/10.

    Payer payment to provider _____

    Coinsurance _____

    Discount amount _____

4. Patient 4 charge 99201. Copay of $20.00 applies. Plan pays @ 100% after copay.

    Payer payment to provider _____

    Copayment _____

    Discount amount _____

5. Patient 5 charge 99204. Copay of $25.00 applies. Plan pays 100% after copay.

    Payer payment to provider _____

    Copayment _____

    Discount amount _____

On completion of this exercise, refer to Appendix J to check the accuracy of your work.

Balance Billing

Balance billing is the act of billing a patient for any dollar amount left after the insurance carrier has paid and any copayment has been met. Whether a provider can balance the bill depends on the payers' rules. This is why it is important for medical office specialists to know the rules of their payers, especially the payers with whom they have negotiated contracts. Patients may be responsible for the amount of the usual charge that exceeds the payer's allowed charge.

Non-PAR providers can demand payment in full from the patient rather than waiting for the insurance carrier to process claims based on the UCR amount offered by healthcare plans. Because this affects the noncontracted, non-network providers, the billed charges are the full responsibility of the patient. Although the patient may have insurance coverage, when the patient is treated by a non-par provider, the provider can charge her usual fee. The patient will be reimbursed by the payer according to the payer's allowed fees. Under an indemnity plan, the billed amount is subject to UCR fees. The amount denied or reduced can be balance billed to the patient. Because the provider has no contract with the carrier, there are no rules binding the provider to write any amount off of the patient's account.

Processing an Explanation of Benefits

An EOB states the status of a claim—whether it is paid, pending, rejected, or denied. The medical office specialist must review all EOBs and apply payment information to the patient's account.

An explanation will not always be accompanied by payment, but it will state the status of the claim. The claim may be pending waiting for additional information. A **pending claim** is one that is received but not processed by the carrier because additional information is needed or there is an error. For claims submitted electronically, the EOB is referred to as the **Electronic Remittance Advice (ERA)**. The EOB lists the patient, dates of services, types of service, and the charges filed on the insurance claim form. The EOB also describes how the amount of the benefit payment was determined. If claim forms were filed for more than one patient with the same insurance carrier at the same time, the provider's EOB may include information on more than one patient.

The format and contents of each EOB vary based on the benefit plan and the services provided. No universal form for explaining benefits is available. It has been a point of debate that all providers are required to use the CMS-1500 and the UB-04 standardized forms, yet carriers can customize their EOBs in any way. Terminology is also different on various EOBs. For example, some EOBs show the "Allowed Amount or Charge" and some EOBs read "Deducted Amount." The medical office specialist will eventually become accustomed to the carriers with whom the provider contracts, but should always review all EOBs carefully prior to entering data.

However, many terms and categories are common to all carriers. Insurance carriers often use codes on the EOB to refer to these terms or situations. These codes are called **reason codes** and **remark codes**. Usually these codes are explained on the face or back of the EOB. If one line is read at a time, the descriptions and calculations for each patient are easily understood. An EOB statement has three sections that explain how a claim was processed:

- *Service Information.* Identifies the provider (hospital or other facility, doctor, specialist or clinic), dates of service, and charges from the provider.

■ *Coverage Determination.* Summarizes the total deductions, charges not covered by the plan, and the amount the patient may owe the provider.

■ *Benefit Payment Information.* Indicates who was paid, how much, and when.

Information on an EOB

The following information appears on an EOB:

1. Account name: company name
2. Date the EOB statement was finalized
3. Member's or insured's name and ID number
4. Patient's identification number as it appears on his ID card
5. Number assigned to the claim
6. Name of the person who received the service (the patient)
7. Provider's name
8. Service description column, which indicates:
   - Dates of the services provided (DOS)
   - Procedures performed (CPT codes)
   - Total charge for each procedure
   - The portion of the bill not covered by the plan
   - The contractual allowed amount
   - Patient's copay
   - Patient's deductible or noncovered procedures or amounts
   - Patient's coinsurance
9. Total payment to the provider
10. The total amount that is the patient's responsibility to the provider of services.

Practice Exercises 14.7 through 14.9 provide examples of information shown on an EOB. Complete the tables using the payment information given.

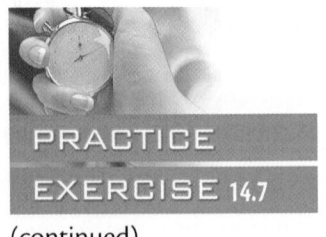

PRACTICE EXERCISE 14.7

(continued)

Complete the table and fill in the blanks using the payment information provided.

Physician Charges	Allowed Amounts	Insurance Pays	Deductible
$ 88.00	$66.00	80%	$150.00*
120.00	99.00		
90.00	81.00		

	Charge	Adjustment	Allowed	Deductible	Copay	Ins. Pays	Coinsurance
	$	$	$	$	$	$	$
	$	$	$	$	$	$	$
TOTALS	$	$	$	$	$	$	$

*Deductible not met.

BALANCE DUE FROM PATIENT:

Patient's Deductible: $_____

Patient's Coinsurance: $_____

TOTAL INSURANCE PAYMENT: $_____

TOTAL PHYSICIAN WRITE-OFF: $_____

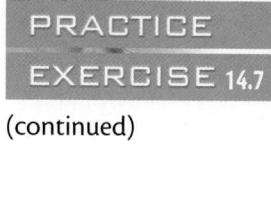

PRACTICE

EXERCISE 14.7

(continued)

On completion of this exercise, refer to Appendix J to check the accuracy of your work.

Complete the table and fill in the blanks using the payment information provided.

Physician Charges	Allowed Amounts	Insurance Pays	Deductible
$2000.00	85%	70%	$200.00*

PRACTICE

EXERCISE 14.8

	Charge	Adjustment	Allowed	Deductible	Copay	Ins. Pays	Coinsurance
	$	$	$	$	$	$	$
TOTALS	$	$	$	$	$	$	$

*$45.00 of deductible has been met.

BALANCE DUE FROM PATIENT:

Patient's Deductible: $_____

Patient's Coinsurance: $_____

TOTAL INSURANCE PAYMENT: $_____

TOTAL PROVIDER WRITE-OFF: $_____

On completion of this exercise, refer to Appendix J to check the accuracy of your work.

Complete the table and fill in the blanks using the payment information provided.

Physician Charges	Allowed Amounts	Insurance Pays	Deductible
$3875.00	80%	90%	$250.00*

PRACTICE

EXERCISE 14.9

	Charge	Adjustment	Allowed	Deductible	Copay	Ins. Pays	Coinsurance
	$	$	$	$	$	$	$
TOTALS	$	$	$	$	$	$	$

*Deductible has not been met.

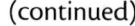

(continued)

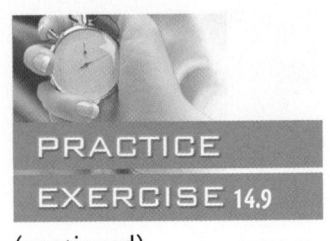

BALANCE DUE FROM PATIENT:

Patient's Deductible: $_____

Patient's Coinsurance: $_____

TOTAL INSURANCE PAYMENT $_____

TOTAL PROVIDER WRITE-OFF: $_____

On completion of this exercise, refer to Appendix J to check the accuracy of your work.

After receiving an EOB/ERA and posting payments to patients' accounts, the MOS must follow-up on unpaid claims. Follow-up can be done online or by making telephone calls. Figures 14.13 through 14.16 are ERAs showing the status of claims. Insurance companies have specific time frames, called a *claim turn-around time* (and specified in the provider's contract), in which a claim will be processed once it is received in their office.

Figure 14.13

Sample ERA showing status of rejected claims.

Title: Rejected Claims Report

Purpose: To let the submitter know which claims were rejected and the reason (sometimes, very cryptic) for the rejection.

Comment: None

03/02/09 ---

REJECTED CLAIMS for NAME OF DOCTOR MD—03/02/09

PATIENT	DATA in ERROR	DESCRIPTION
922387	97118	PROCCD INVALID FOR PAYER USE HCPC

Figure 14.14

Sample ERA showing status of settled claims.

Title: Claims Settlement Report

Purpose: To let the submitter know which claims were settled (not necessarily paid) by the insurance company.

Comment: Some insurance companies will return this report, not all.

03/02/09 ---

CLAIM SETTLEMENT for NAME OF DOCTOR MD—03/02/09

COMPLETED: EXPENSES INCURRED PRIOR TO COVERAGE

PATIENT	STATEMENT DATES		PAYER	TOTAL AMOUNT	
	FROM	THRU		CHARGES	PAID
911851	06/25/08–07/02/08		METROPOLITAN LIFE	$599.00	0.00
911879	08/13/08–08/18/08		METROPOLITAN LIFE	560.00	0.00

(continued)

COMPLETED: PAYMENT MADE ACCORDING TO PLAN PROVISIONS

PATIENT	STATEMENT DATES		PAYER	TOTAL AMOUNT	
	FROM	THRU		CHARGES	PAID
917914	10/27/08	–10/27/08	CIGNA	$274.00	0.00
917914	10/27/08	–10/27/08	CIGNA	274.00	0.00
917922	10/29/08	–10/31/08	CIGNA	560.00	0.00
917922	10/29/08	–10/31/08	CIGNA	560.00	0.00
917922	10/29/08	–10/31/08	CIGNA	560.00	0.00
917922	10/29/08	–10/31/08	CIGNA	560.00	0.00
917922	10/29/08	–10/31/08	CIGNA	560.00	0.00
917922	10/29/08	–10/31/08	CIGNA	560.00	0.00
917922	10/29/08	–10/31/08	CIGNA	560.00	0.00
917922	10/29/08	–10/31/08	CIGNA	560.00	0.00
917894	09/29/08	–09/29/08	CIGNA	274.00	0.00
917894	09/29/08	–09/29/08	CIGNA	274.00	0.00
917922	11/04/08	–11/06/08	CIGNA	553.00	0.00
917922	11/04/08	–11/06/08	CIGNA	553.00	0.00
917922	11/04/08	–11/06/08	CIGNA	553.00	0.00
917922	11/04/08	–11/06/08	CIGNA	553.00	0.00

COMPLETED: NO PAYMENT WILL BE MADE FOR THIS CLAIM

PATIENT	STATEMENT DATES		PAYER	TOTAL AMOUNT	
	FROM	THRU		CHARGES	PAID
911851	06/25/08	–07/02/08	METROPOLITAN LIFE	$599.00	0.00
911851	07/02/08	–07/02/08	METROPOLITAN LIFE	371.00	0.00
911879	08/13/08	–08/18/08	METROPOLITAN LIFE	560.00	0.00

Figure 14.14

Sample ERA showing status of settled claims. (continued)

Title: Zero Payment Report

Purpose: From insurance company to submitter. Claims that were fully processed and for which no payment will be made.

Comment: None

03/02/09 --

ZERO PAYMENT CLAIMS for NAME OF DOCTOR M.D.—03/02/09

CLAIM STATUS MESSAGE—COMPLETED: EXPENSES INCURRED PRIOR TO COVERAGE

PATIENT NAME	CONTROL NUMBER	STATEMENT DATES FROM THRU	TOTAL CHARGES
E LIU	911851	06/25/08–07/02/08	$599.00

Payer: METROPOLITAN LIFE (714)555-2500

| E LIU | 911879 | 08/13/08–08/18/08 | 560.00 |

Payer: METROPOLITAN LIFE (714)555-2500

Figure 14.15

Sample ERA showing status of claims for which no payment is forthcoming.

(continued)

Figure 14.15

Sample ERA showing status of claims for which no payment is forthcoming. (continued)

CLAIM STATUS MESSAGE—COMPLETED: NO PAYMENT WILL BE MADE FOR THIS CLAIM

PATIENT NAME	CONTROL NUMBER	STATEMENT DATES FROM THRU	TOTAL CHARGES
E LIU	911851	06/25/08–07/02/08	$599.00

Payer: METROPOLITAN LIFE (714)555-2500

| E LIU | 911851 | 07/02/08–07/02/08 | 371.00 |

Payer: METROPOLITAN LIFE (714)555-2500

| E LIU | 911879 | 08/13/08–08/18/08 | 560.00 |

Payer: METROPOLITAN LIFE (714)555-2500

Figure 14.16

Medicare remittance allowance.

Title: Medicare Remittance Advice

Purpose: To let the submitter know the disposition of Medicare claims.

Comment: Contact Medicare for an explanation of the codes.

06-18-09 MEDICARE CLAIMS SUBMITTED FOR DRJU—"Name of Provider"

06-18-1909 MEDICARE Remittance Advice for "Medicare Provider Number"

DEL DOTTO, EVA M	BILLED	ALLOWED	DED.	CoINS	PROV-PD	MC-ADJUST
04-16-09 21 1 99291	$250.00	$207.41	$41.48	$165.93	$ 42.59	CO42
04-17-09 21 1 99232	66.84	58.12	11.62	46.50	8.72	CO42
04-18-09 21 1 99232	66.84	58.12	11.62	46.50	8.72	CO42
CLAIM TOTALS:	383.68	323.65	64.72	258.93	60.03	

TRASVINA, CARMEN P	BILLED	ALLOWED	DED.	CoINS	PROV-PD	MC-ADJUST
02-20-09 11 1 99205	157.68				157.68	CO16
CLAIM TOTALS:	157.68				157.68	

FIGLIETTI, JOSEPH S	BILLED	ALLOWED	DED.	CoINS	PROV-PD	MC-ADJUST
04-16-09 11 1 95117	26.13	22.72	4.54		3.41	PR42
CLAIM TOTALS:	26.13	22.72	4.54	3.41		

WADE, DAVID M	BILLED	ALLOWED	DED.	CoINS	PROV-PD	MC-ADJUST
04-15-09 11 1 99213	49.71	45.89	9.18		3.82	PR42
CLAIM TOTALS:	49.71	45.89	9.18	3.82		

TOSCHI, DAVID R	BILLED	ALLOWED	DED.	CoINS	PROV-PD	MC-ADJUST
04-13-09 11 1 95117	26.13	22.72	4.54		3.41	PR42
04-13-09 11 1 9921325	49.71	45.89		9.18	3.82	PR42
CLAIM TOTALS:	75.84	68.61		13.72	7.23	

(continued)

SINGLETON, IRENE M	BILLED	ALLOWED	DED.	CoINS	PROV-PD	MC-ADJUST
04-13-09 11 1 99213	$ 49.71	45.89	9.18		3.82	PR42
CLAIM TOTALS:	49.71	45.89	9.18	3.82		

NELSON, MIRIAM	BILLED	ALLOWED	DED.	CoINS	PROV-PD	MC-ADJUST
01-12-09 11 1 9921425	74.23			74.23		CO18
01-12-09 11 1 94060	76.92			76.92		PR50
01-12-09 11 1 90724	4.76			4.76		COB18
01-12-09 11 2 J1040	11.34			11.34		CO18
01-12-09 11 2 J1040	11.34			11.34		CO18
CLAIM TOTALS:	178.59			178.59		

BROWER, JOHN R	BILLED	ALLOWED	DED.	CoINS	PROV-PD	MC-ADJUST
05-25-09 11 1 99213	49.71			49.71		CO18
05-25-09 11 2 J1040	11.34			11.34		CO18
05-25-09 11 2 J1040	11.34			11.34		CO18
05-25-09 11 2 J2010	6.52			6.52		CO18
CLAIM TOTALS:	78.91			78.91		

Figure 14.16

Medicare remittance allowance. (continued)

To apply your knowledge of EOBs and the method of calculating provider **write-offs** and patient financial responsibilities, complete Practice Exercises 14.10 through 14.13.

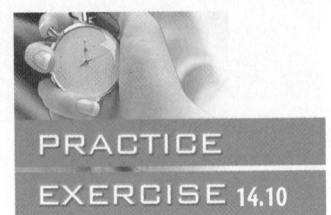

PRACTICE
EXERCISE 14.10

Complete the following Explanation of Benefits.

EXPLANATION OF BENEFITS

Today's Date

Payer's Name and Address

Aetna Insurance Company
P.O. Box 15999
New York, NY 12345

Provider's Name and Address

J.D. Mallard, M.D.
1933 East Frankford Road
Carrollton, TX 12345

This statement covers payments for the following patient(s):
Claim Detail Section (If there are numbers in the "REMARKS" column, see the Remarks Section for explanation)

Patient Name: Hughes, Patsy   **Patient Account Number:** Hugan0
Patient ID Number: **Insured's Name:** Andrew Hughes
Group Number: 55216
Provider Name: J.D. Mallard, M.D.   **Inventory Number:** 44562   **Claim Control Number:** 28971

Service Date(s)	Procedure	Charges	Adjustment	Allowed	Copay	Deduct/Not Covered	Coins	Paid Amt.	Provider Paid/Remarks
02/16/2008	97039	$50.00	$	$49.00	$0.00	$	$	80%	
02/16/2008	97042	65.00	65.00		0.00	00.00			
02/19/2008	97039	50.00		50.00	0.00			80%	
02/21/2008	97039	50.00		50.00		50.00		80%	03
TOTALS									

BALANCE DUE FROM PATIENT: PT'S DED/NOT COV $_____

PT'S COINS. $_____

031 Met Maximum Limit

PAYMENT SUMMARY SECTION (TOTALS)

Charges	Adjustment	Allowed	Copay	Deduct/Not Covered	Coins	Total Paid

Remarks: 031-Met Maximum Limit

On completion of this exercise, refer to Appendix J to check the accuracy of your work.

Complete the following Explanation of Benefits.

EXPLANATION OF BENEFITS

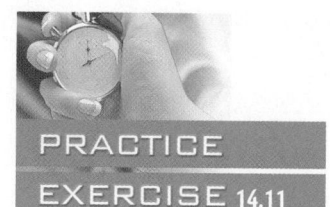

Today's Date

Payer's Name and Address

| Aetna Insurance Company |
| P.O. Box 15999 |
| New York, NY 12345 |

Provider's Name and Address

| J.D. Mallard, M.D. |
| 1933 East Frankford Road |
| Carrollton, TX 12345 |

This statement covers payments for the following patient(s):
Claim Detail Section (If there are numbers in the "REMARKS" column, see the Remarks Section for explanation.)

Patient Name: Hughes, Patsy   **Patient Account Number:** Hugan0
Patient ID Number: **Insured's Name:** Andrew Hughes
Group Number: 55216
Provider Name: J.D. Mallard, M.D.   **Inventory Number:** 44562   **Claim Control Number:** 28971

Service Date(s)	Procedure	Charges	Adjustment	Allowed	Copay	Deduct/Not Covered	Coins	Paid Amt.	Provider Paid/Remarks
01/02/2008	65542	$1500.00	$	$1200.00	$0.00	$300.00	$	80%	
TOTALS									

BALANCE DUE FROM PATIENT: PT'S DED/NOT COV $_____
PT'S COINS. $_____

PAYMENT SUMMARY SECTION (TOTALS)

Charges	Adjustment	Allowed	Copay	Deduct/Not Covered	Coins	Total Paid

Remarks:

On completion of this exercise, refer to Appendix J to check the accuracy of your work.

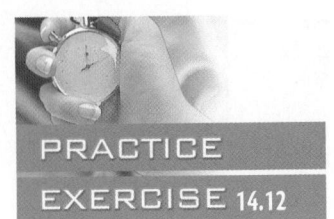

Complete the following Explanation of Benefits.

EXPLANATION OF BENEFITS

Today Date

Payer's Name and Address

| Aetna Insurance Company |
| P.O. Box 15999 |
| New York, NY 12345 |

Provider's Name and Address

| J.D. Mallard, M.D. |
| 1933 East Frankford Road |
| Carrollton, TX 12345 |

This statement covers payments for the following patient(s):
Claim Detail Section (If there are numbers in the "REMARKS" column, see the Remarks Section for explanation.)

Patient Name: Hughes, Patsy   **Patient Account Number:** Hugan0
Patient ID Number: **Insured's Name:** Andrew Hughes
Group Number: 55216
Provider Name: J.D. Mallard, M.D.   **Inventory Number:** 44562   **Claim Control Number:** 28971

Service Date(s)	Procedure	Charges	Adjustment	Allowed	Copay	Deduct/Not Covered	Coins	Paid Amt.	Provider Paid/Remarks
04/09/2008	99213	$100.00	$	$ 78.00	$25.00	$0.00	$0.00		
04/09/2008	80048	150.00		100.00					
04/09/2008	71020	78.00		56.00					
TOTALS									

BALANCE DUE FROM PATIENT: PT'S DED/NOT COV $_____

                                                        PT'S COINS. $_____

PAYMENT SUMMARY SECTION (TOTALS)

Charges	Adjustment	Allowed	Copay	Deduct/Not Covered	Coins	Total Paid

Remarks:

On completion of this exercise, refer to Appendix J to check the accuracy of your work.

Complete the following Explanation of Benefits.

EXPLANATION OF BENEFITS

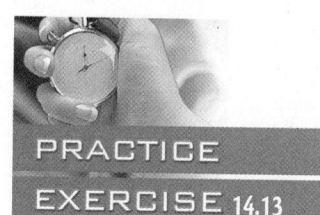

Today's Date

Payer's Name and Address

| Aetna Insurance Company |
| P.O. Box 15999 |
| New York, NY 12345 |

Provider's Name and Address

| J.D. Mallard, M.D. |
| 1933 East Frankford Road |
| Carrollton, TX 12345 |

This statement covers payments for the following patient(s):
Claim Detail Section (If there are numbers in the "REMARKS" column, see the Remarks Section for explanation.)

Patient Name: Hughes, Patsy   **Patient Account Number:** Hugan0
Patient ID Number: **Insured's Name:** Andrew Hughes
Group Number: 55216
Provider Name: J.D. Mallard, M.D.   **Inventory Number:** 44562   **Claim Control Number:** 28971

Service Date(s)	Procedure	Charges	Adjustment	Allowed	Copay	Deduct/Not Covered	Coins	Paid Amt.	Provider Paid/Remarks
05/02/2008	72149	$1300.00	$	$950.00	$0.00	$500.00	$	80%	
05/02/2008	94010	325.00		245.00	0.00			80%	
05/02/2008	99214	150.00		125.00	0.00			80%	
TOTALS									

BALANCE DUE FROM PATIENT: PT'S DED/NOT COV $_____

PT'S COINS. $_____

PAYMENT SUMMARY SECTION (TOTALS)

Charges	Adjustment	Allowed	Copay	Deduct/Not Covered	Coins	Total Paid

Remarks:

On completion of this exercise, refer to Appendix J to check the accuracy of your work.

Reviewing Claims Information

When the EOB arrives at the physician's office, the medical office specialist reviews it, checks all calculations, and makes sure that all charges submitted were processed and that the amounts paid are correct. If an error is found with the EOB, the MOS must research the interoffice information first. For example, the MOS should verify that the health insurance claim numbers and patient's name and date of birth were entered correctly. The MOS should also review the original superbill to verify that all CPT codes, charges, and diagnoses were entered correctly. If all of those items are correct, the MOS should pull the chart to confirm that the documentation matches the procedures billed. If the facility has processed the claim correctly, a request for review of the claim must be filed with the carrier.

If a claim is denied, downcoded, or partially paid after the MOS has reviewed it and confirmed that all billing and documentation provided to the carrier were correct, an appeal must be filed with the payer for consideration of claim adjudication.

EOBs are also used as evidence of payments when another insurance company needs such information to administer **coordination of benefits (COB)**. When benefits are coordinated with another insurance carrier, the primary EOB will be copied and forwarded to the secondary payer with the claim. The secondary payer will know what amount was paid by the primary insurance carrier and what their responsibility is. The goal is to provide the necessary information primarily through an EOB to help recipients understand the claim and to make sure that proper reimbursement is received by the provider

After reviewing the EOB, the medical office specialist records EOB and payment information in the insurance log, either electronically or manually. After a payment transaction has been entered into a patient's account, an adjustment should be made if required. Each transaction entry should relate to the procedure or service billed. The MOS bills any remaining balance to the patients, if appropriate, and then files the EOBs that have been paid by that insurance carrier. This file should be available for review at any time. EOB statements are to be kept according to state retention schedule requirements, in the event questions arise as to how claims were handled and paid. A **retention schedule** dictates how long patient records are to be kept and stored. This determination is based on state regulations and federal laws, such as Medicare laws.

Adjustments to Patient Accounts

An **adjustment** is a positive or negative change to a patient's account balance. Corrections, changes, and write-offs to patients' accounts are made by means of adjustments to the existing transactions. The medical office specialist will also adjust a patient's bill as a result of any discounts given. If the provider is a PAR provider, the difference between the billed amount (the provider's UCR fee) and the allowed amount is adjusted from the amount the patient owes. After posting the payment to the specific date and procedure, the adjustment should be made in the same way. This is referred to as per line item posting.

Processing Reimbursement Information

Four steps are to be followed when an EOB is received from an insurance carrier:

1. Enter the date when the EOB and any accompanying reimbursement are received.
2. Compare the EOB with the copy of the claim filed. Check dates of services, types of services, and charges to be sure all items were included on the EOB.
3. Check the accuracy of mathematical calculations.
4. Determine the amounts of any write-offs or adjustments to the patient's account that may be required. Also note whether a balance is due from the patient, or whether a refund is due the patient or insurance carrier. For example, if a patient paid for a service in advance and it was reimbursed by the carrier or if the patient or insurance carrier overpaid on an account, then a refund is due.

Confirming Amount Paid, Making Adjustments, and Determining Amount Due from Patient

To confirm the amount paid by the payer, to determine any needed adjustments or write-offs, and to determine the amount due from the patient or to be refunded to the patient, follow the steps in Figure 14.17.

Now it is time to put all your knowledge together by completing Practice Exercises 14.14 through 14.16. Using the physician charge, allowed amount, amount insurance pays, and the deductible amount, complete the Explanation of Benefits and fill in the missing information in the blanks for each exercise. In Practice Exercises 14.17 through 14.20, review the EOB and fill in the missing information in the blanks.

STEP 1

Billed Amount	$400.00
Allowed Amount	−$200.00
	−$100.00
	$200.00
	$100.00

Write-Off
"New" Allowed Amount

STEP 2

| Allowed Amount | $200.00 |

Minus deductible or copay (if no deductible go to Step 3)

STEP 3

"New" Allowed Amount × 70%, 80%, or 90% (whichever is the correct coinsurance percentage)

For example:
$100.00
× .70
$70.00 paid by carrier to provider

STEP 4

"New" Allowed Amount × percentage of coinsurance (%) and/or copay

plus deductible = **Patient's Responsibility**

Figure 14.17

Steps for confirming what was paid by the carrier, determining any needed adjustment or write-off, and determining the amount due from the patient or to be refunded to the patient.

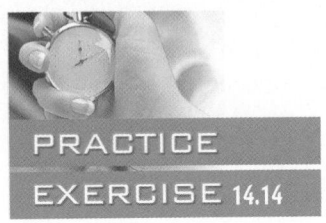

PRACTICE EXERCISE 14.14

Complete the Explanation of Benefits and fill in the blanks below.

Physician Charges	Allowed Amounts	Insurance Pays	Deductible
$200.00	$169.43	90%	0.00
25.00	23.69		

	Charge	Adjustment	Allowed	Deductible	Copay	Ins. Pays	Coinsurance
	$	$	$	$	$	$	$
	$	$	$	$	$	$	$
TOTALS	$	$	$	$	$	$	$

BALANCE DUE FROM PATIENT:

Patient's Deductible: $_____

Patient's Coinsurance: $_____

TOTAL INSURANCE PAYMENT: $_____

TOTAL PHYSICIAN WRITE-OFF: $_____

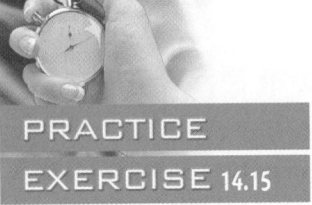

PRACTICE EXERCISE 14.15

Complete the Explanation of Benefits and fill in the blanks below.

Physician Charges	Allowed Amounts	Insurance Pays	Deductible
$1750.00	$1750.00	95%	$150.00*
925.00	925.00		
400.00	400.00		
108.00	108.00		

	Charge	Adjustment	Allowed	Deductible	Copay	Ins. Pays	Coinsurance
	$	$	$	$	$	$	$
	$	$	$	$	$	$	$
	$	$	$	$	$	$	$
	$	$	$	$	$	$	$
TOTALS	$	$	$	$	$	$	$

*Deductible not met.

BALANCE DUE FROM PATIENT:

Patient's Deductible: $_____

Patient's Coinsurance: $_____

TOTAL INSURANCE PAYMENT: $_____

TOTAL PHYSICIAN WRITE-OFF: $_____

Complete the Explanation of Benefits and fill in the blanks below.

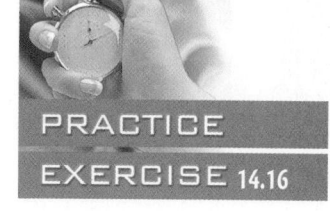

PRACTICE
EXERCISE 14.16

Physician Charges	Allowed Amounts	Insurance Pays	Deductible
$1650.00	$123.70	90%	$250.00*
1650.00	412.50		

	Charge	Adjustment	Allowed	Deductible	Copay	Ins. Pays	Coinsurance
	$	$	$	$	$	$	$
	$	$	$	$	$	$	$
TOTALS	$	$	$	$	$	$	$

*$115.00 of deductible not met.

BALANCE DUE FROM PATIENT:

Patient's Deductible: $_____

Patient's Coinsurance: $_____

TOTAL INSURANCE PAYMENT: $_____

TOTAL PHYSICIAN WRITE-OFF: $_____

On completion of this exercise, refer to Appendix J to check the accuracy of your work.

Review the Explanation of Benefits, then fill in the missing information in the blanks that follow the EOB.

PRACTICE
EXERCISE 14.17

Health Insurance Company
501 West Michigan
Milwaukee, WI 12345
800-555-7777

Explanation of Benefits   Health Insurance, Inc.

Insured Name: Betty White
Insured ID/Social Security number: 232-33-2222
Policy:
Claim Number: TI-4107081-001-1-01-13
Control Number: 204466533
Date: 02/14/09

Below is an Explanation of Benefits for your Medical Coverage

Patient: Pam White   **Patient ID/Social Security number:** 633-33-3333
Provider Name: Medical Center Subsidiary **Patient Account Number:** 96604599

Service Code	Service Description	Service Date(s)	Provider Charge	Allowed Amount	Discount Amount	Not Covered	Deductible	Copay	Pay Amt.	Remarks	Amount Paid
	Hosp Exp	12/12/08	$5363.50	$3261.10	$2102.40				100%	0054	$3261.10
			$5363.50	$3261.10	$2102.40						$3261.10
TOTALS											

(continued)

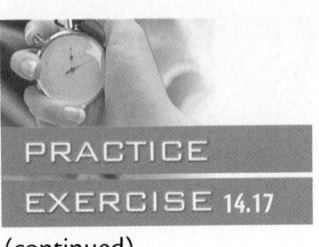

**PRACTICE
EXERCISE 14.17**

(continued)

Remarks

0054 PPO-Preferred Provider benefits applied. Your provider has agreed to the negotiated rate in accordance with the Private Healthcare Systems provider agreement. You should not be billed for this amount.

Payment Summary

Payment Sent To: Medical Center Subsidiary
Payment Amount: $3261.10
Payment Date: 02/14/09
Patient's Portion: $0.00

Total Payment Summary

Payment(s) Sent To: Medical Center Subsidiary
Total Payment Amount: $3261.10
Payment Date: 02/14/09

*TOTAL PATIENT PORTION: $0.00

Insurance company name: _____

Patient's name: _____

Patient's ID: _____

Provider's name: _____

Date of service: _____

Total charge: _____

Procedure(s): _____

Copay: _____

Deductible: _____

Coinsurance due from patient: _____

Allowed amount: _____

Discount amount: _____

Noncovered items: _____

Rate of benefit (%): _____

Amount paid: _____

Remarks: _____

Outcome: ■ Bill patient balance
            ■ Appeal
            ■ Call carrier
            ■ Claim paid in full

On completion of this exercise, refer to Appendix J to check the accuracy of your work.

Review the Explanation of Benefits, then fill in the missing information in the blanks that follow the EOB.

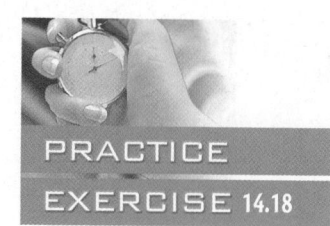

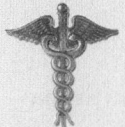

	PROVIDER CLAIM SUMMARY

Claims processed by
Medical Care
A Division of Allied Health Corp.
P.O. Box 6644
Dallas, Texas 12345
Toll Free (800) 555-0287

DATE: 01/30/03
PROVIDER NUMBER: 0000K223
CHECK NUMBER: 034324
TAX IDENTIFICATION NUMBER: 001223456

SURGICAL ASSOCIATES OF TEXAS
4001 9TH STREET
DALLAS, TX 12345

PATIENT: Joe Smith
PERF PRV: 0000000000000080430S
CLAIM NUMBER: 0000227050697800X

IDENTIFICATION NUMBER: 555-66-4444
PATIENT NUMBER: 79625C0G4   CLAIM TYPE: **MCP**

FROM / TO DATES	PROC PS* TS**	CODE	AMOUNT BILLED	CONTRACT ALLOWABLE	SERVICES NOT COVERED	DEDUCTIONS/OTHER INELIGIBLE	AMOUNT PAID
01/02–01/02/09	03 T	93880	$550.00	$190.13	$359.87 (1)	$0.00	$190.13
			$550.00	$190.13	$359.87	$0.00	$190.13

AMOUNT PAID TO PROVIDER FOR THIS CLAIM: $190.13
DEDUCTIONS/OTHER INELIGIBLE

TOTAL SERVICES NOT COVERED: $359.87
PATIENT'S SHARE: $ 0.00

Insurance company name: _____

Patient's name: _____

Patient's ID: _____

Provider's name: _____

Date of service: _____

Total charge: _____

Procedure(s): _____

Copay: _____

Deductible: _____

Coinsurance due from patient: _____

Allowed amount: _____

Discount amount: _____

Noncovered items: _____

Rate of benefit (%): _____

Amount paid: _____

Remarks: _____

(continued)

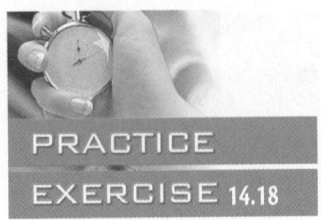

PRACTICE EXERCISE 14.18

(continued)

Outcome: ■ Bill patient balance
            ■ Appeal
            ■ Call carrier
            ■ Claim paid in full

PATIENT: **Kelly Jones**
PERF PRV: **0000000000000080430S**   IDENTIFICATION NUMBER: **444-55-6666**
CLAIM NUMBER: **0000227050697810X**   PATIENT NUMBER: **79625C0G5**   CLAIM TYPE: **MCP**

FROM / TO DATES	PROC PS* TS** CODE	AMOUNT BILLED	CONTRACT ALLOWABLE	SERVICES NOT COVERED	DEDUCTIONS/OTHER INELIGIBLE	AMOUNT PAID
01/02–01/02/09	93880	$162.00	$41.30	$120.70 (1)	$0.00	$41.30
		$162.00	$41.30	$120.70	$0.00	$41.30

AMOUNT PAID TO PROVIDER FOR THIS CLAIM: $41.30
DEDUCTIONS/OTHER INELIGIBLE

                                          TOTAL SERVICES NOT COVERED: $120.70
                                          PATIENT'S SHARE: $ 0.00

Insurance company name: _____

Patient's name: _____

Patient's ID: _____

Provider's name: _____

Date of service: _____

Total charge: _____

Procedure(s): _____

Copay: _____

Deductible: _____

Coinsurance due from patient: _____

Allowed amount: _____

Discount amount: _____

Noncovered items: _____

Rate of benefit (%): _____

Amount paid: _____

Remarks: _____

Outcome: ■ Bill patient balance
            ■ Appeal
            ■ Call carrier
            ■ Claim paid in full

PATIENT: **Mary Young**
PERF PRV: **0000000000000080430S**
CLAIM NUMBER: **0000227050697820X**

IDENTIFICATION NUMBER: **454-55-5555**
PATIENT NUMBER: **79625C0C6**　　　CLAIM TYPE: **MCP**

FROM / TO DATES 01/01–01/02/09	PROC PS* TS** CODE	AMOUNT BILLED	CONTRACT ALLOWABLE	SERVICES NOT COVERED	DEDUCTIONS/OTHER INELIGIBLE	AMOUNT PAID
	99203	$170.00	$128.00	$42.00 (1)	$10.00	$118.00
	72100	$188.00	$150.00	$38.00 (1)	$ 0.00	$150.00
		$358.00	$278.00	$80.00	$10.00	$268.00

AMOUNT PAID TO PROVIDER FOR THIS CLAIM: $268.00
DEDUCTIONS/OTHER INELIGIBLE $10.00

TOTAL SERVICES NOT COVERED: $80.00
PATIENT'S SHARE: $10.00

PROVIDER CLAIMS AMOUNT SUMMARY

NUMBER OF CLAIMS: 3
AMOUNT PAID TO PROVIDER: $499.43
RECOUPMENT AMOUNT: $0.00
NET AMOUNT PAID TO PROVIDER: $499.43

AMOUNT PAID TO SUBSCRIBER: $0.0
AMOUNT OVER MAXIMUM ALLOWANCE: $560.57
AMOUNT OF SERVICES NOT COVERED: $560.57
AMOUNT PREVIOUSLY PAID: $0.00

AMOUNT BILLED: $1070.00

(1) Contractual adjustment of billed amount

Insurance company name: _____

Patient's name: _____

Patient's ID: _____

Provider's name: _____

Date of service: _____

Total charge: _____

Procedure(s): _____

Copay: _____

Deductible: _____

Coinsurance due from patient: _____

Allowed amount: _____

Discount amount: _____

Noncovered items: _____

Rate of benefit (%): _____

Amount paid: _____

Remarks: _____

Outcome: ▪ Bill patient balance
　　　　　 ▪ Appeal
　　　　　 ▪ Call carrier
　　　　　 ▪ Claim paid in full

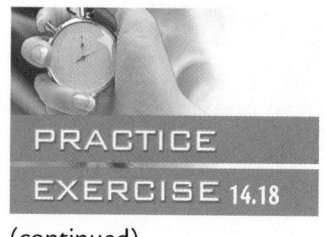

PRACTICE EXERCISE 14.18

(continued)

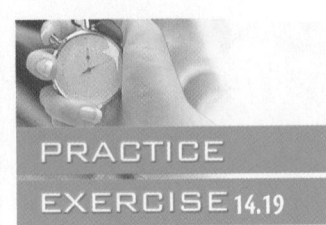

PRACTICE
EXERCISE 14.19

Review the Explanation of Benefits, then fill in the missing information in the blanks that follow the EOB. Do not treat each claim individually, instead, total the amounts from the individual claims to arrive at the correct answers.

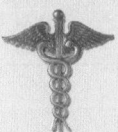

EXPLANATION OF PAYMENTS
American Insurance Company
P.O. Box 123456
Any Town, TX 12345
800-555-6543

Date: 05/10/2009 Page 1 of 3

Allied Medical Center
1933 E. Frankford Rd. Suite 110
Carrollton, TX 12345

VENDOR NUMBER: 0012CK
PROVIDER NUMBER: 85702B

PATIENT NAME: MARY DEAN   PATIENT NUMBER: DEAMA
SUBSCRIBER: MARY DEAN   GROUP NUMBER: H9852   MEMBER NUMBER: 8523697401-01

CLAIM NUMBER: 01 011905 037 04

BGDAT	ENDDAT	SVCCOD	MD	UNITS	BILLED	ALLOWED	NOT-COVD	PREPAID	COP/DED	EP1	EP2	EP3
021009	021009	99215	1		$237.00	$141.46	$0.00	$0.00	$20.00	001		
021009	021009	82270	1		$ 27.00	$ 4.54	$0.00	$0.00	$ 0.00	001		

BILLED	ALLOWED	NOT-COVD	DISCOUNT	PREPAID	WITHHOLD	COP/DED	COB	PAID
$264.00	$146.00	$0.00	$0.00	$0.00	$0.00	$20.00	$0.00	$126.00

PATIENT NAME: JOHN SMITH   PATIENT NUMBER: SMIJO
SUBSCRIBER: JOHN SMITH   GROUP NUMBER: 85230   MEMBER NUMBER: 321654753-00

CLAIM NUMBER: 01 011907 038 20

BGDAT	ENDDAT	SVCCOD	MD	UNITS	BILLED	ALLOWED	NOT-COVD	PREPAID	COP/DED	EP1	EP2	EP3
032109	032109	99213	1		$102.00	$62.78	$0.00	$0.00	$20.00	001		

BILLED	ALLOWED	NOT-COVD	DISCOUNT	PREPAID	WITHHOLD	COP/DED	COB	PAID
$102.00	$62.78	$0.00	$0.00	$0.00	$0.00	$20.00	$0.00	$42.78

PATIENT NAME: JANE DOE   PATIENT NUMBER: DOEJA
SUBSCRIBER: MARK DOE   GROUP NUMBER: 85230   MEMBER NUMBER: 741582569-03

CLAIM NUMBER: 01 012105 035 74

BGDAT	ENDDAT	SVCCOD	MD	UNITS	BILLED	ALLOWED	NOT-COVD	PREPAID	COP/DED	EP1	EP2	EP3
032109	032109	99213	1		$102.00	$62.78	$0.00	$0.00	$20.00	001		

BILLED	ALLOWED	NOT-COVD	DISCOUNT	PREPAID	WITHHOLD	COP/DED	COB	PAID
$102.00	$62.78	$0.00	$0.00	$0.00	$0.00	$25.00	$0.00	$37.78

PATIENT NAME: SHARON ALEXANDER   PATIENT NUMBER: ALESH
SUBSCRIBER: ELLEN ALEXANDER   GROUP NUMBER: 98732   MEMBER NUMBER: 654820069-04

CLAIM NUMBER: 01 011905 037 15

BGDAT	ENDDAT	SVCCOD	MD	UNITS	BILLED	ALLOWED	NOT-COVD	PREPAID	COP/DED	EP1	EP2	EP3
021009	021009	99211	1		$56.00	$25.64	$0.00	$0.00	$12.82	001		
021009	021009	36415	1		$26.00	$ 3.00	$0.00	$0.00	$ 0.00	001		

BILLED	ALLOWED	NOT-COVD	DISCOUNT	PREPAID	WITHHOLD	COP/DED	COB	PAID
$82.00	$28.64	$0.00	$0.00	$0.00	$0.00	$12.82	$0.00	$15.82

(continued)

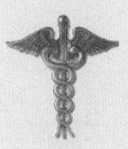

EXPLANATION OF PAYMENTS
American Insurance Company
P.O. Box 123456
Any Town, TX 12345
800-555-6543

Date: 05/10/2009 Page 2 of 3

VENDOR NUMBER: 0012CK
PROVIDER NUMBER: 85702B

PROVIDER TOTALS:

BILLED	ALLOWED	NOT-COVD	DISCOUNT	PREPAID	WITHHOLD	COP/DED	COB	PAID
$550.00	$300.20	$0.00	$0.00	$0.00	$0.00	$77.82	$0.00	$222.38

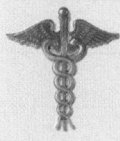

EXPLANATION OF PAYMENTS
American Insurance Company
P.O. Box 123456
Any Town, TX 12345
800-555-6543

Date: 05/10/2009 Page 3 of 3

VENDOR NUMBER: 0012CK
PROVIDER NUMBER: 85702B

PATIENT NAME: SHANNON BURG   PATIENT NUMBER: BURSH
SUBSCRIBER: SHANNON BURG   GROUP NUMBER: 63250   MEMBER NUMBER: 002586317-00

CLAIM NUMBER: 01 011210 038 60

BGDAT	ENDDAT	SVCCOD	MD	UNITS	BILLED	ALLOWED	NOT-COVD	PREPAID	COP/DED	EP1	EP2	EP3
032509	032509	99213		1	$102.00	$62.78	$0.00	$0.00	$20.00	001		

BILLED	ALLOWED	NOT-COVD	DISCOUNT	PREPAID	WITHHOLD	COP/DED	COB	PAID
$102.00	$62.78	$0.00	$0.00	$0.00	$0.00	$20.00	$0.00	$42.78

PATIENT NAME: LUCY LANGE   PATIENT NUMBER: LANLU
SUBSCRIBER: LUCY LANGE   GROUP NUMBER: 63250   MEMBER NUMBER: 54608712300

CLAIM NUMBER: 01 011907 612 14

BGDAT	ENDDAT	SVCCOD	MD	UNITS	BILLED	ALLOWED	NOT-COVD	PREPAID	COP/DED	EP1	EP2	EP3
032109	032109	99213		1	$102.00	$62.78	$0.00	$0.00	$20.00	001		

BILLED	ALLOWED	NOT-COVD	DISCOUNT	PREPAID	WITHHOLD	COP/DED	COB	PAID
$102.00	$62.78	$0.00	$0.00	$0.00	$0.00	$20.00	$0.00	$42.78

PATIENT NAME: BRUCE MONTANIO   PATIENT NUMBER: MONBR
SUBSCRIBER: TINA MONTANIO   GROUP NUMBER: 85230   MEMBER NUMBER: 098143276-05

CLAIM NUMBER: 01 012105 074 61

BGDAT	ENDDAT	SVCCOD	MD	UNITS	BILLED	ALLOWED	NOT-COVD	PREPAID	COP/DED	EP1	EP2	EP3
032109	032109	99213		1	$102.00	$62.78	$0.00	$0.00	$20.00	001		

BILLED	ALLOWED	NOT-COVD	DISCOUNT	PREPAID	WITHHOLD	COP/DED	COB	PAID
$102.00	$62.78	$0.00	$0.00	$0.00	$0.00	$20.00	$0.00	$42.78

PROVIDER TOTALS:

BILLED	ALLOWED	NOT-COVD	DISCOUNT	PREPAID	WITHHOLD	COP/DED	COB	PAID
$306.00	$188.34	$0.00	$0.00	$0.00	$0.00	$60.00	$0.00	$128.34

VENDOR TOTALS:

BILLED	ALLOWED	NOT-COVD	DISCOUNT	PREPAID	WITHHOLD	COP/DED	COB	PAID
$856.00	$488.54	$0.00	$0.00	$0.00	$0.00	$137.82	$0.00	$350.72

CHECK#—00525441284   DATE—5/10/2009   AMOUNT—$350.72

EXPLANATION OF PAYMENT CODES:

001   SERVICES PROVIDED ARE COVERED UP TO AN ALLOWED
       AMOUNT. SINCE THIS AMOUNT HAS BEEN PAID, NO
       ADDITIONAL PAYMENT CAN BE MADE

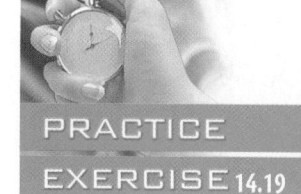

PRACTICE
EXERCISE 14.19

(continued)

(continued)

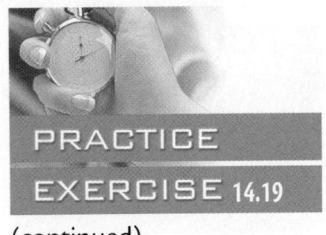

PRACTICE EXERCISE 14.19

(continued)

TOTALS ONLY

Insurance company name: _____

Patient's name: N/A _____

Patient's ID: N/A _____

Provider's name: _____

Date of services: N/A _____

Total charges: _____

Procedure(s): N/A _____

Total copay: _____

Total deductibles: _____

Total coinsurance due
from patients: _____

Total allowed amount: _____

Total discount amount: _____

Total noncovered items: _____

Rate of benefit (%): N/A _____

Total amount paid to
provider: _____

Remarks: _____

On completion of this exercise, refer to Appendix J to check the accuracy of your work.

Review the Explanation of Benefits, then fill in the missing information in the blanks that follow the EOB.

Insurance Company of America
P. O. Box 3564-1
Any Town, TX 12345
800-555-1234

CLAIM NUMBER	CHECK NUMBER
10268785-04	Nock895016

CHECK DATE	CHECK AMOUNT
05/09/2009	0.00

PRACTICE
EXERCISE 14.20

ALLIED MEDICAL CENTER
1933 E FRANKFORD RD, STE 110
CARROLLTON, TX 12345

Insurance Company of America   **EXPLANATION OF BENEFITS**

RETAIN FOR YOUR RECORDS

Date(s) of Service: 10/13/2008–10/13/2008   Check Date: 05/09/2009
Patient: Jeff Staubach   Check Number: nock895016
Insured: Jeff Staubach   Check Amount:
Patient Account #: 3265   Group: United Peoples Employer   Group # 00025
Provider: Allied Medical Center   Contract Name: American Health Network   Claim #: 10268725

Service Code	Service Description	Service Date(s)	Provider Charge	Allowed Amount	Discount Amount	Not Covered	Deductible	Copay	Pay Amt.	Remarks	Amount Paid
99214	Office visit	10/13/08	$148.00			$148.00				ab	
TOTALS			$148.00			$148.00					

Remarks
ab   This claim was previously processed.

THIS IS NOT A BILL

Insurance company name: _____

Patient's name: _____

Patient's ID: _____

Provider's name: _____

Date of service: _____

Total charge: _____

Procedure(s): _____

Copay: _____

Deductible: _____

Coinsurance due from patient: _____

Allowed amount: _____

Discount amount: _____

(continued)

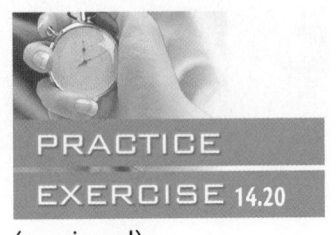

Noncovered items: _____

Rate of benefit (%): _____

Amount paid: _____

Remarks: _____

Outcome: ■ Bill patient balance
            ■ Appeal
            ■ Call carrier
            ■ Claim paid in full

On completion of this exercise, refer to Appendix J to check the accuracy of your work.

Methods of Receiving Funds

Various methods are available for carriers to remit funds to providers. These methods include check by mail, electronic funds transfer, and lockbox services.

Check by Mail

The carrier mails a check directly to the provider attached to an EOB. One or several patients can be listed on the EOB and a single check attached for all fees paid.

Electronic Funds Transfer

Electronic funds transfer (ETF) is used by participating providers and carriers. Providers can have checks that in the past would have been attached to mailed EOBs instead deposited directly into the provider's bank account. When a provider electronically files a claim, he will receive an ERA. If the provider submits a paper claim, he will receive an EOB. The ERA/EOB shows dollar amounts paid to the provider along with the amount of the patient's financial responsibility. This helps in controlling accounts receivables. The advantages of using ETFs are that funds are immediately available and the transfer is less costly than check deposits.

Lockbox Services

A lockbox service is one that is provided by a bank for accounting purposes to help control account receivables. The provider must have an account with the bank to be able to obtain this service.

A lockbox service helps control receivables by collecting and depositing customer payments faster. To remain competitive in today's environment, many practices look for opportunities to streamline their operations. A lockbox service does this by:

■ Saving time and money while improving cash flow
■ Ensuring high-quality processing of the practice's receivables
■ Employing an aggressive mail pickup schedule.

With a lockbox service, carriers and patients remit payment to a unique zip code designated only for lockbox mail. The bank's couriers pick up the payments directly from the post office. Lockbox mail is processed and deposited to the practice's account the same day. All payment information is forwarded to the practice. The bank will:

- Make copies of all checks
- Deposit checks into the practice's account
- Provide a record of all deposits and totals
- Forward receipt of all deposits with documentation.

The bank will gather all EOBs, patients' statements (that were returned with checks), and any other documentation that was attached to the check and forward it to the practice.

When the practice receives the EOBs and documentation of deposit from the lockbox, the office insurance specialist should do the following:

- Add up the copies of the checks and the deposit total to ensure they match.
- Add up the EOBs to ensure that the total equals the insurance company's check.
- If everything adds up, then begin to post the EOBs. The office insurance specialist should consider "batching" the EOBs if there are a lot of them. To "batch" means to choose a certain amount to post, for example, $1000.00 per batch (enter the amount in the Batch account), instead of posting all EOBs at once. When finished with that batch, check to see if the amount is correct. Batching makes it easier to control your posting errors because there are fewer amounts to recheck.
- When all postings have been completed, run an activities report or "day sheet" for the one day only and verify that it matches the total deposit amount reported by the bank.

If there is an error in the amount the bank deposited compared to the amount totaled by the medical office specialist, the bank should be called and the error found and corrected. Always document on the posting sheet any errors found, who was called, and how they were corrected.

Chapter Summary

- An explanation of benefits (EOB) is a notification form sent from the insurance carrier to the patient and the healthcare provider (if the provider accepted assignment) after an insurance claim has been processed.
- The EOB lists the patient, dates of services, types of service, and the charges filed on the insurance claim form. The EOB also describes the way the amount of the benefit payment was determined.
- The Medicare Fee Schedule (MFS) is based on the RBRVS fees. Therefore, the fees are based on the federal government's data of what each service costs.
- Allowed charges refer to the maximum allowed amount for a covered charge. Some payers refer to this as the maximum allowed fee, allowed amount, or allowable charge. This is the amount the payer will pay the provider for her services.

■ Depending on the medical plan, the insured may be required to make four types of payments: deductibles, copayments, coinsurance, and payments for excluded services. These are referred to as out-of-pocket expenses. The MOS will know exactly what the insured needs to pay at the time of service after verifying the insured's insurance plan benefits.

■ The MOS must be aware of and become familiar with payers' reimbursement calculations and payment method in order to review an EOB to determine if the payment amount is correct. Various methods are available for carriers to remit funds to providers. These methods include check by mail, electronic funds transfer, and lockbox services.

Chapter Review

True/False

Identify the statement as true (T) or false (F).

_____ 1. The allowed charge is the amount that a third-party payer will pay for a particular procedure when the patient has coinsurance.

_____ 2. Accounts receivable include monies owed to a practice by both payers and patients.

_____ 3. An adjustment is a negative or positive change to an account balance.

_____ 4. The claim turnaround time is the period between the patient's encounter and the transmission of the resulting claim.

_____ 5. A payer may downcode a procedure it determines was not medically necessary at the level reported.

_____ 6. A medical review is part of the provider's staff responsibilities.

_____ 7. The determination of a claim refers to the payer's decision regarding payment.

_____ 8. When a payer's ERA is received, the medical office specialist checks that the amount paid matches the expected payments.

_____ 9. When a family deductible is required, it must be met before benefits from the payer begin.

_____ 10. Under a plan with an individual deductible, the deductible amount can be met by the combination of payments from all family members.

_____ 11. Posting the payment to the specific date of service and each CPT code, and then following the same procedure for posting an adjustment is referred to as per line item posting.

_____ **12.** The provider "withhold" required by some managed care plans may be repaid to the physician.

_____ **13.** The advantages of using ETFs are that funds are immediately available and the transfer is less costly than check deposits.

Multiple Choice

Identify the letter of the choice that best completes the statement or answers the question.

_____ **1.** The three parts of an RBRVS fee are:
   a. uniform value, GPCI, and conversion factor.
   b. usual, customary, and reasonable charges.
   c. usual charges, GPCI, and conversion factor.
   d. none of the above.

_____ **2.** The purpose of the GPCI is to account for:
   a. regional differences in costs.
   b. changes in the cost of living index.
   c. differences in relative work values.
   d. none of the above.

_____ **3.** Which of the following payment methods is the newest?
   a. UCR
   b. RVS
   c. RBRVS
   d. GPCI

_____ **4.** Which of the following payment methods is the basis for Medicare's fees?
   a. UCR   c. RBRVS
   b. RVS   d. GPCI

_____ **5.** The Medicare conversion factor is set:
   a. twice a year.
   b. once each year.
   c. semiannually.
   d. each decade.

_____ **6.** Which answer correctly lists the main method(s) payers use to determine their fee structure?
   a. allowed charges
   b. allowed charges, contracted fee schedule, and capitation
   c. contracted fee schedule and capitation
   d. capitation and retrospective payments

_____ **7.** The Medicare allowed charge for a procedure is $80.00. What amount does the participating provider receive from Medicare and what amount from the patient?
   a. $64.00/$16.00   c. $40.00/$40.00
   b. $60.00/$20.00   d. $80.00/$0.00

_____ 8. The Medicare allowed charge for a procedure is $150.00, and a PAR provider's usual charge is $200.00. What amount must the provider write off?
   a. $150.00   c. $50.00
   b. $100.00   d. $30.00

_____ 9. The deductibles, coinsurance, and copayments patients pay are called their:
   a. excluded services.   c. capitation rate.
   b. out-of-pocket expenses.   d. maximum benefit limit.

_____ 10. If a non-PAR provider's usual fee is $600.00, the allowed amount is $300.00, and balance billing is permitted, what amount is written off?
   a. $150.00   c. $300.00
   b. $480.00   d. $0.00

_____ 11. A payer's automated claim edits may result in claim denial because of:
   a. lack of eligibility for a reported service.
   b. lack of medical necessity.
   c. lack of required preauthorization.
   d. all of the above.

_____ 12. A claim that is removed from a payer's automated processing system is sent for:
   a. adjudication.   c. utilization review.
   b. manual review.   d. none of the above.

_____ 13. If a provider has accepted assignment, the payer sends the ERA or EOB to:
   a. the provider.   c. the billing service.
   b. the patient.   d. the carrier.

_____ 14. The payer's decision regarding whether to pay a claim is called:
   a. determination.   c. evaluation.
   b. adjudication.   d. utilization.

_____ 15. After the claim has gone through the adjudication process and a claim has been downcoded or denied, the MOS may submit to the insurance carrier:
   a. a letter of appeal.
   b. patient's medical records.
   c. providers dictation.
   d. additional insurance information.

Completion

Complete each sentence or statement.

1. An initial review of each claim consists of _____ that screen the basic data on the claim form.

2. Although adjudication varies somewhat depending on the payer's policies, the essential steps—edits, reviews, and _____ are universal.

3. A claim examiner reviews the claim to check if the _____ and _____ are linked.

4. Downcoding is also called _____.

5. A(n) _____ is an amount that an insured must pay to the provider before the insurance benefits begin.

6. Under the formula for calculating a Medicare fee for a procedure, the sum of the adjusted totals for work, practice expense, and malpractice are multiplied by a(n) _____.

7. If a participating provider's usual charge is higher than the allowed amount, the provider must _____ the difference between the two charges.

8. Medical insurance plans require patients to pay for all _____ services.

9. Following a payment _____, the payer either pays, denies, or partially pays the claim.

10. A payer may downcode a claim if the reported procedure does not match the reported _____.

11. Corrections, changes, and write-offs to patients' account are made with _____ to the existing transactions.

12. If a carrier has continued to deny all of the practice's appeal requests, the provider can file a request to the _____ for assistance.

Resources

How to read and explain your Explanation of Benefits: *www.benplan.com*
Click on the Resources & Tools link then click on the Understanding Your Explanation of Benefits (EOB) link at the bottom of the page.

Chapter 15 Refunds and Appeals

Key Terms

administrative law judge (ALJ) hearing	insurance commissioner	redetermination
documentation	peer review	SOAP format
Employee Retirement Income Security Act (ERISA) of 1974	qualified independent contractors (QICs)	

Case Study
Refunds and Appeals

As a new accounts receivable specialist, Amy has been given a list of denied claims to work with. One of those claims was denied due to a primary diagnosis of obesity. Amy believes that the claim will be paid if the primary code of obesity is switched with the secondary code of migraine headaches. She approaches her manager with this information. Her manager explains that it is not possible to change the order of the codes, and that if they did it would be considered insurance fraud. She informs Amy that an appeal may reverse the denial with proper documentation.

Questions

1. Why would a claim be denied because of an obesity code?
2. Why can't the order of the codes be changed by the billing office if it will provide payment?
3. What kind of documentation may be needed for such an appeal?

Introduction

As discussed in Chapter 14, an *appeal* is the submission of additional clinical and other pertinent information to an insurance carrier to overturn a denied or downcoded claim by the payer.

The majority of a provider's income is generated through insurance billing. In a perfect world, the provider would be paid promptly and fully for all claims submitted. Knowing that nothing is perfect, however, the medical office specialist (MOS) will receive denial notices from the insurance carriers. What to do with the denial and balance on the patient's account is vitally important. If the practice feels that the charges should be paid by the carrier, the MOS must appeal the carrier's decision to deny all or parts of the claim. Some appeals may be conducted over the telephone, whereas others may require a written appeal. Either way, the MOS must be familiar with medical records, verification of benefits forms, precertification, preauthorization, and referral requirements, as well as the appeals process for each insurance carrier with whom the provider contracts.

Reimbursement Follow-Up

One of the critical goals of a medical office specialist is to prepare claims that will be approved and paid by insurance carriers. Another is to help ensure prompt reimbursement of charges. What steps can the MOS take to avoid claim rejection and to speed correct reimbursement from carriers and patients?

Regardless of the method of reimbursement, insurance claims must be monitored until payments are received. When payments are late or made incorrectly, the MOS must follow up. Frequently, reimbursement follow-up is as simple as calling the insurance carrier to ask for help. Most insurance carriers have staff members whose primary duty is to answer questions about the status of claims. Figure 15.1 lists some of the reasons why an MOS would inquire about an outstanding claim.

Figure 15.1

Some reasons to inquire about an insurance claim.

The following are some reasons for contacting the insurance carrier:

1. A letter from the insurance carrier states that a claim is being investigated. This might be due to preexisting conditions, workers' compensation situations, or other reasons. After a period of 30 days, however, follow-up should be done by phone or letter.
2. An unclear denial of payment is received.
3. An incorrect payment is received.
4. Reimbursement is received with no indication of the amount of the allowed charge or how much the patient is responsible for.
5. Reimbursement is received for an unknown patient. For example, a check is made out for Jamie Nussbaum, who is not a patient on record. When the carrier is called, the MOS discovers that Jamie Nussbaum's policy covers Michael Lambert, a patient recently seen by the physician.
6. A specialist has provided a service that is not listed as having a CPT® code. In response, the insurance carrier asks for a narrative description of the procedure or precise details of the service provided.

CPT is a registered trademark of the American Medical Association.

Rebilling

Some providers automatically rebill every 30 days if they have not heard from an insurance company. Before rebilling, however, the medical office specialist should be aware of the terms of his provider's managed care contract that deal with turnaround times. Some payers may think this is duplicate billing. The procedure for rebilling paper claims is to reprint the claim from the computer and write "SECOND BILLING" in black letters at the top. This lets the insurance carrier know that it is not a duplicate claim and that payment is delinquent. If the insurance carrier has already communicated with the patient, it will send the provider a record of that information in response to the second billing. For example, the notice might read "Paid to patient," "Applied to deductible," or "Not a covered benefit." Table 15.1 lists other reasons why the MOS may need to rebill a claim.

The carrier may ask for rebilling in these situations:

- The wrong diagnosis codes or procedure codes were submitted. (One wrong number can mean denial of benefits!)
- Information is incomplete or missing (for example, no policy number or no accident date).
- The charges, units, and costs do not total properly.

Occasionally, second billings are rejected as duplicates, which is why a medical office specialist must be careful with second billings. Some carriers may perceive "aggressive billing techniques" as fraudulent billing. When sending claims electronically, it is very easy to resubmit all outstanding claims. But the carrier may have just adjudicated the original claim for payment such that when a second billing is received, it may

Table 15.1	Reasons to Rebill	
	A mistake has been made in billing.	For example, during a patient's physical examination, the physician discovers an ear infection. Ear infections are covered by the patient's insurance, but physicals are not. However, the physician noted the physical but forgot to mark the ear problem on the superbill. When this error is discovered, the insurance carrier is notified. The usual procedure is for the MOS to make the correction in the computer and attach a copy of the patient's medical record for that date of service (if an authorization is on file). A cover letter is then prepared describing the billing error and mailed to the insurance representative's attention.
	Charges must be detailed to receive maximum reimbursement.	When an EOB is examined, discrepancies between the amount billed and the amount paid should be analyzed. For example, assume that, per the contract, a physician should be reimbursed for actual laboratory charges. The physician charges the patient $25.00 for a stool culture, but the actual laboratory costs for the culture were $20.00. Because the carrier's payment was for $16.00, there is probably an error. The carrier should have reimbursed the physician for the actual cost of $20.00. In this case, a copy of the bill received from the laboratory should be sent to the insurance carrier for reimbursement of $4.00, the difference between the actual charge of $20.00 and the payment of $16.00 that was received.
	A claim was overlooked by the provider's office.	This can happen when a patient undergoes a series of visits or treatments. For example, Marshall Williams gets a weekly allergy injection. He received 10 injections, but somehow claims were submitted for only 8. The 2 missing injections can still be billed. Also a corrected claim can be sent with a request for an adjustment.

also be adjudicated for payment, resulting in the carrier overpaying on the service. Third-party payers may feel that this duplication has been done deliberately and may decide to conduct an audit. An *audit* is the process of examining and verifying claims and supporting documents submitted by a physician or medical facility.

If a claim is outstanding, instead of automatically resubmitting it, the MOS can call the carrier to help resolve the problem. Another way to research an unpaid claim is via the Internet. Participating providers usually have been provided with a personal ID number (PIN) so they can access third-party websites and check the status of claims immediately.

Denied or Delayed Payments

There are many reasons the carrier might deny or delay payment. The following are some common problems and their solutions:

The claim is not for a covered contract benefit. Bill the patient, making a note of the insurance information directly on the patient's bill so that the patient knows the reason for the bill.

The patient's preexisting condition is not covered. Bill the patient, making a note of the insurance information on the patient's bill. If the physician believes the patient's condition was not preexisting, the MOS will be instructed to file an appeal (discussed in detail later in this chapter).

The patient's coverage has been canceled. Bill the patient, making a note of the insurance information directly on the patient's bill. If the MOS verified benefits prior to the visit, an appeal may be in order.

Workers' compensation (WC) is involved and the case is still under consideration. Call the employer and ask for the WC case number and the address to which the claim should be submitted. If the employer cannot give you a case number, ask if there is a "Notice of Contest." Notify the patient to follow up on the claim with an ombudsman or get a denial of the claim to attach to the health insurance claim form that will be sent to the patient's personal insurance plan.

The carrier believes that coordination of benefits should be done and has requested information about another carrier. The claim will not be processed until the patient provides the information. Call the patient. Explain to the patient what the insurance carrier is requesting and inform the patient that he will be responsible for paying the bill if the insurance carrier does not receive the requested information in a timely manner. (You may need to explain timely filing deadlines.)

The insurance company considers the physician's procedure experimental. A new procedure that requires an unlisted procedure code should always have an explanation of the procedure and proof of medical necessity attached to the original claim. Call the carrier to discuss the necessity of the procedure. If the procedure is still denied, an appeal letter explaining the procedure may need to be sent or a request made for a peer review. Ultimately, the patient may need to be billed.

The person responsible, either the physician or the patient, did not obtain preauthorization for a procedure or for hospitalization. Review the patient's contract. Some contracts impose a sanction for failure to secure preauthorization. If there are reasons why this was not done, a letter of appeal should be written. If authorization was obtained, call the carrier to give the authorization number.

The physician provided services before the patient's health insurance contract went into effect. Bill the patient. A notation such as "No insurance coverage at date of service" should be marked on the bill.

The carrier asks for additional information. Send the carrier the requested information. Follow up as needed after 15 days.

When payment is denied, the insurance carrier notifies both the provider and the patient. The medical office specialist should follow up with a letter to the patient explaining what action is being taken. In cases of preexisting conditions and canceled coverage, the patient is responsible for the bill. Any specific written correspondence received from the insurance carrier should be filed with the patient's records. If the patient has questions, the information from the insurance carrier may help to resolve them.

Answering Patients' Questions About Claims

Often, patients need a go-between, an objective third party who is not emotionally involved. A medical office specialist with expertise and objectivity can build goodwill for the provider's office by using problem-solving and communication skills to fulfill this role. The first step toward answering patients' inquiries about claims is to find out exactly what the problem is. Find out from the patient whether she has:

- Called the insurance carrier
- Talked to the company's employee representative
- Reviewed the policy.

Often, the answer is no. The patient may not understand the insurance policy or may be confused about the rules of the managed care organization (MCO).

Patients typically get upset when they receive large bills or an incorrect payment, or when there is a delayed payment. Even though their complaint is with the insurance carrier, the MOS is the patients' advocate. Helping them solve their insurance problems can soothe these angry, worried patients. Sometimes the problem is just a misunderstanding because the patient does not know the right questions to ask, does not understand the answers, or is unaware that benefits have changed. In other situations, the patient may accuse the office staff of billing incorrectly. In these cases, try to listen carefully for the facts without letting feelings interfere.

If the patient has already called the insurance carrier but is still upset or confused, the MOS should call the insurance carrier again and listen carefully to the explanation. The patient may have been too stressed to understand it. Explaining the solution again to the patient may help clear up misunderstandings.

The following are some techniques to use when explaining insurance issues to patients:

- Volunteer to explain. Speak slowly and calmly.
- Use simple language. Try to omit insurance jargon.
- Explain more than once when necessary.
- Ask the patient, "Do you understand?" or say, "Perhaps I can explain that better."
- Remember, patients are under stress. Use respect and care.

Claim Rejection Appeal

An appeal is the submission of additional clinical and other pertinent information to an insurance carrier to overturn a denied or downcoded claim by the payer. It is a formal way of asking the insurance carrier to reconsider its decision regarding a claim. An example of when a medical office specialist will submit an appeal is when an incorrect payment is received; the carrier's representative should be contacted. The carrier may have made a mistake and not entered the code that was submitted, which requires an adjustment to the Explanation of Benefits (EOB). Figures 15.2 through 15.4 are sample

Figure 15.2

Sample Explanation of Benefits showing denied claim.

Medi PPO
P.O. Box 8525
Garland, TX 12345-0000

Family Medicine Associates of Dallas
33333 Josey Lane #303
Carrollton, TX 12345

Beneficiaries: 1-800-555-2832
Providers: 1-800-555-2833
Page 1 of 1
EOB Number: 15878563214

For Participating Physicians and Facilities Only—If your practice has a change of address and/or telephone number please contact Medi online at: https://www.medi.com/providerehealthoffice/

SUMMARY OF CLAIM

Provider Number: T5478921
Patient Account Number: Tayho0
Patient Name: Hope Taylor   **Sponsor Number:** 511-64-5140
Insured Name: James Taylor   **Claim Number:** 200354 48 9144478

Provider:	Service Dates	Pos	Proc	Mod No Type	Billed	Allowed	Code
Elaine Hamm	10/15–10/15/04	11	97010	01	$ 40.00	$0.00	282
	10/15–10/15/04	11	97012	01	$100.00	$0.00	282
	10/15–10/15/04	11	97035	02	$120.00	$0.00	282
TOTAL					$260.00	$0.00	

Other Ins. Allowed	Other Ins. Paid	Reduction Days	Reduction Amount	Paid by Patient
$0.00	$00.00	0	$0.00	$0.00

Deduct	Cost-share/Co-payment	Total Payable	Interest Paid	Net Payment
$0.0	$0.00	$0.00	$0.00	$0.00

Remarks:
Code 282: Not covered; due to automobile accident, submit to auto carrier

*************************************Voucher Summary*************************************

TOTAL PAYABLE   NET PAYMENT
$0.0 $0.00

Health Care Insurance
504 Explorer Way
Milwaukee, WI 12345
800-555-7777

Explanation of Benefits

Health Care

Our Customer Service Dept. is available
Monday-Friday, between the hours of
7:30 am and 6:00 pm (CT) at 800-555-7666

Insured Name: Mike Zamora
Insured ID/Social Security number: 214-55-1711
Policy: 531AA14788
Claim Number: TI-4107081-001-1-01-13
Control Number: 204466533
Date: 06/25/09

Summary of Benefits

Patient: Maggie Zamora   **Patient ID/Social Security number:** 214-55-1711
Provider Name: Medical Center Subsidiary   **Patient Account Number:** 789624599

Service Code	Service Description	Service Date(s)	Provider Charge	Allowed Amount	Discount Amount	Not Covered	Deductible	Copay	Pay Amt.	Remarks	Amount Paid
96000	Motion analysis	06/12/09	$165.00							0023	$00.00

TOTALS

Remarks

0023   This plan does not cover services rendered that are not considered medically necessary

Figure 15.3

Sample Explanation of Benefits showing denied claims.

EOBs that list rejected or denied claims. Sometimes, instead of a routine error, the provider considers the carrier's reimbursement for services inadequate or incorrect. In either case, a claim rejection can be appealed.

An appeal is used in the following cases:

- The physician did not file for preauthorization in a timely manner due to unusual circumstances.
- The physician receives what is believed to be inadequate reimbursement for surgery or a complicated procedure.
- The physician disagrees with the carrier's preexisting condition decision.
- A patient has unusual circumstances that affect medical treatment.

For example, consider the case in which a medical office specialist filed a claim for a child who was chronically ill. When the child began choking at home, his parents called an ambulance. The ambulance took the child to his physician's hospital, which was 5 miles farther than the nearest facility. The insurance carrier denied payment, stating the ambulance was not necessary. In addition, the carrier felt that the ambulance should have gone to the nearest facility. To press payment for this claim, the physician wrote an appeal letter to the insurance carrier detailing the child's special problems that made it necessary to call an ambulance. This letter included the child's medical information from birth. The physician also explained what was done in the ambulance and why it was necessary for him to treat the child, rather than a physician in the closer emergency room.

Figure 15.4

Sample Explanation of Benefits showing denied claims.

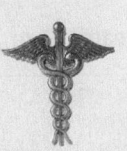

Claims processed by
Medical Care
A Division of Allied Health Corp
NUMBER: 0000K223
P.O. Box 6644
Dallas, Texas 12345
Toll Free (800) 555-0287

Date:
PROVIDER: 001223456
CHECK NUMBER: 034324
TAX IDENTIFICATION NUMBER: BV458796

SURGICAL ASSOCIATES OF TEXAS
4001 9TH STREET
DALLAS, TX 12345

PATIENT: Joe Pendergrass
PERF PRV: 0000000000000080430S
CLAIM NUMBER: 0000227050697800X

IDENTIFICATION NUMBER: 555-66-4444
PATIENT NUMBER: 79625C0G4   **CLAIM TYPE:** MCP

FROM / TO DATES	PROC PS*	CODE	AMOUNT BILLED	CONTRACT ALLOWABLE	SERVICES NOT COVERED	DEDUCTIONS/OTHER INELIGIBLE	AMOUNT PAID
01/02–01/02/09	11	99212	$50.00	$23.00	$50.00 (4)	$0.00	$0.00
			$50.00	$23.00	$50.00	$0.00	$0.00

AMOUNT PAID TO PROVIDER FOR THIS CLAIM: $0.00
DEDUCTIONS/OTHER INELIGIBLE

TOTAL SERVICES NOT COVERED: $50.00
PATIENT'S SHARE: $0.00

PATIENT: Kelly McIntire
PERF PRV: 0000000000000080430S
CLAIM NUMBER: 0000227050697810X

IDENTIFICATION NUMBER: 444-55-6666
PATIENT NUMBER: 79625C0G5   **CLAIM TYPE:** MCP

FROM / TO DATES	PROC PS*	CODE	AMOUNT BILLED	CONTRACT ALLOWABLE	SERVICES NOT COVERED	DEDUCTIONS/OTHER INELIGIBLE	AMOUNT PAID
01/02–01/02/09	11	99214	$62.00	$29.00	$62.00 (5)	$0.00	$00.00
			$62.00	$29.00	$62.00	$0.00	$00.00

AMOUNT PAID TO PROVIDER FOR THIS CLAIM: $00.00
DEDUCTIONS/OTHER INELIGIBLE

TOTAL SERVICES NOT COVERED: $62.00
PATIENT'S SHARE: $62.00

PATIENT: Ben Bates
PERF PRV: 0000000000000080430S
CLAIM NUMBER: 0000227050697820X

IDENTIFICATION NUMBER: 454-55-5555
PATIENT NUMBER: 79625C0C6   **CLAIM TYPE:** MCP

FROM / TO DATES	PROC PS*	CODE	AMOUNT BILLED	CONTRACT ALLOWABLE	SERVICES NOT COVERED	DEDUCTIONS/OTHER INELIGIBLE	AMOUNT PAID
01/01–01/02/09	11	99386	$125.00	$ 90.00	$125.00 (6)	$0.00	$00.00
		72100	$188.00	$110.00	$188.00 (6)	$0.00	$00.00
			$313.00	$200.00	$313.00	$0.00	$00.00

AMOUNT PAID TO PROVIDER FOR THIS CLAIM: $0.00
DEDUCTIONS/OTHER INELIGIBLE $0.00

TOTAL SERVICES NOT COVERED: $313.00
PATIENT'S SHARE: $313.00

PROVIDER CLAIMS AMOUNT SUMMARY

NUMBER OF CLAIMS:	3	AMOUNT PAID TO SUBSCRIBER:	$0.00
AMOUNT BILLED:	**$425.00**	**AMOUNT PAID TO PROVIDER:**	**$00.00**
AMOUNT OVER MAXIMUM ALLOWANCE:	$173.00	RECOUPMENT AMOUNT:	$0.00
AMOUNT OF SERVICES NOT COVERED:	$252.00	NET AMOUNT PAID TO PROVIDER:	$00.00
AMOUNT PREVIOUSLY PAID:	$0.00		

(4) Services rendered after termination date of coverage.
(5) This plan does not cover preexisting conditions.
(6) Only one (1) physical exam is covered for every 24-month period.

Peer Review

If, after an appeal, the insurance carrier denies what the physician considers fair compensation for services, the physician may request a peer review. (In responding to an appeal the insurance carrier sometimes sends a claim for peer review as a matter of routine.) A peer review is usually the physician's last attempt to resolve the problem after all other communications have been exhausted. In a **peer review**, an objective, unbiased group of physicians determines what payment is adequate for services provided. If the physician requests the peer review and it is determined that the procedures were not medically necessary, the physician is responsible for paying for the peer review.

State Insurance Commissioner

Each state's **insurance commissioner** is the regulatory agency for the insurance industry and serves as a liaison between the patient and the carrier, and between the physician and carrier. The MOS should contact this governmental department if multiple appeals fail. The physician, carrier, or patient may appeal to the insurance commissioner if any of the three feel unfairly treated.

For example, suppose two insurance carriers cannot determine who the primary carrier is and as a result the physician has not been paid. The physician can write to the insurance commissioner on behalf of the patient to request a resolution of the problem. First, the insurance commissioner formally notifies each party involved and asks each to present the documents that apply to the case. The commissioner then looks at all the facts and makes an impartial decision.

Carrier Audits

When a physician contracts to participate in a specific network with a particular insurance company, the company has the right to audit, or review, the physician's billing practices. Sometimes carriers audit selected providers because they provide extraordinary or very specialized services. Other audits are conducted in cases where fraud or other misrepresentation of services is suspected.

The insurance carrier will notify the provider before an audit is conducted. The dates and the types of records that will be audited are specified ahead of time. For example, the carrier may review billing practices or completeness of medical records. The role of the medical office specialist is to make sure the records are available, complete, and signed by the physician. To avoid problems, the MOS should:

- Make sure that each claim is complete and that each diagnosis matches the services provided
- Be as specific as possible when choosing diagnoses and modifiers for procedure codes
- Make sure all patients' medical records are complete; check to see if everything involved in each patient's care has been documented.

Documentation

Documentation is defined as the chronological recording of pertinent facts and observations regarding a patient's health status in a logical sequence. The structure of the medical record must be consistent, and the information must be recorded in a format that allows the physician to access it easily and quickly. Documentation helps in making a proper diagnosis and formulating a sound therapeutic plan. For those who work with a patient, it provides a means to understand quickly the patient's history and current medical status. Documentation promotes continuity of care among physicians and other healthcare providers. The medical record is also a collection of information that may be useful for research and education. It is also important to maintain a record of all the treatments received by a patient to reflect what has been reported to third-party payers. Consistently, the CPT® and ICD-9 codes reported to payers should reflect the documentation in the chart. An unwritten rule states that "If it was not documented, it was not done; if it was not done, it cannot be reported or billed." A properly documented medical record provides the legal means of verifying care. Millions of dollars are paid in malpractice cases annually because the care was good but the medical record was not.

Documentation Guidelines

Medical record documentation is required to record pertinent facts, findings, and observations about an individual's health history including past and present illnesses, examinations, tests, treatments, and outcomes. The medical record chronologically documents the care of the patient and is an important element contributing to high-quality care. An appropriately documented medical record can reduce many of the "hassles" associated with claims processing and may serve as legal documents to verify the care provided, if necessary. Because payers have a contractual obligation to enrollees, they may require reasonable documentation that services are consistent with the insurance coverage provided. They may request information to validate:

- The site of service
- The medical necessity and appropriateness of the diagnostic and/or therapeutic services provided, and/or
- That services provided have been accurately reported.

SOAP Record-Keeping Format

The method of documentation most widely used by physicians is the **SOAP format**. SOAP stands for "subjective, objective, assessment, plan." The SOAP record-keeping format is taught in medical schools and can be adapted to the evaluation and management section of the CPT-4 book. With the SOAP format, the patient's treatment is recorded in an organized and consistent sequence. Otherwise, the physician may not document important components of the Evaluation and Management (E/M) procedure codes. The SOAP format can be described as follows:

S: *Subjective* (E&M history): the chief complaint or the reason for the medical encounter. Generally includes the history of the present illness (HPI) and a review of systems. This is usually information the patient tells the doctor. The subjective format also includes past, family, and/or social history.

O: *Objective* (E&M examination): the physical examination of the patient, including vital signs, height, weight, and blood pressure.

A: *Assessment* (E&M decision making): the doctor's diagnosis at the time of the encounter or a documenting of the impression if a diagnosis cannot be made.

P: *Plan* (E&M recommended treatment): a documenting of recommended treatment, testing ordered or other workup contemplated, new medications or adjustments of medications, therapies, and planned surgical procedures.

Necessity of Appeals

There are times during the posting of the EOB/ERAs when a decision has to be made about the necessity of an appeal. Submitting an appeal is very different from submitting a new claim because an appeal involves extra time and paperwork. Additional information and paperwork must be supplied, and detailed clinical information that may involve the physician might also be requested by the carrier.

The appeals process involves a lot of administrative work by the medical office specialist and other staff members. Because the appeals process is time consuming, it is often not done properly or consistently. Rather than appeal, some facilities take the "easy road" by submitting a statement to the patient and requiring the patient to deal with the carrier, instead of doing so themselves.

Consider the example of a college student who went to her gynecologist for the insertion of an IUD. The MOS called to verify benefits and was given the information that the procedure was covered and the allowed amount. After the procedure was performed and the claim was filed, the claim was denied as a noncovered service. The verification was completed correctly, but the carrier's representative had misquoted. The patient was sent a statement to pay the full amount. The misrepresentation has placed a financial burden on the patient who is not able to pay the $700.00 now due.

It is the belief of the authors that all appeals efforts should be made by the provider prior to expecting the patient to pay for these services.

Registering a Formal Appeal

If the decision is made to go ahead with an appeal, the first step is to know and follow the appeals policy of the payer. For example, the medical office specialist must register the appeal in a timely manner, because there is often a cutoff date for doing so. Most practices learn about the appeals policies of the major plans they work with by referring to physician administrative manuals, contracts, and newsletters. Plan representatives may also be contacted to learn about specific policies. Be aware that some plans are instituting paperless review procedures, which will decrease the time spent gathering and documenting detailed information.

The next step is for the MOS to differentiate between denials of total charges and disallowances. Disallowances represent partial payment on claims because they are above the maximum allowable fee. Every practice should have a policy for determining when to appeal a disallowance. Some practices set a dollar amount limit, such as $50.00 to $200.00, depending on the specialty, beyond which an appeal will be registered with the plan. Some practices set a percentage, such as 20% of the billed charge. When a specific policy is in place regarding disallowance limits, the staff does not have to check with a supervisor before registering an appeal. Appeals are automatic and consistent. Standard form letters are used to appeal disallowances when working with a plan that does not accept verbal requests. When appealing disallowances resulting from low maximum allowable fees (MAFs), include data regarding what other plans pay for the same CPT code if the plan you are appealing to is a much lower payer than others for this code. Use phrases like "Medicare allows $1636.00, Medicaid allows $1233.00, XYZ plan allows $2100.00, and your MAF is $1088.00."

There are many other reasons why a practice may want to appeal a claim, but unfortunately some of these reasons are not easy to identify and file. This is especially true when claims are denied because the payer feels a certain procedure is excluded from coverage or feels that medical necessity was not proven. Regardless of the specific reason, a standard opening for an appeal letter can be developed. All that is left to do, then, is to insert the special explanations and attach the clinical information.

The Appeals Process

No matter how clean your claims are, there are always going to be denials or partial payments that will need to be appealed. The two types of appeals are written and telephone appeals. The circumstances of each claim will determine which appeal process is necessary. Some examples follow of simple appeals that can be handled by phone and/or fax:

- The insurance company has denied the claim because information, for example, secondary payer information, was requested from the patient and never received. Sometimes the patient will contact the insurance company and respond by phone. Once the insurance company has the correct information, the claim can be processed.
- A claim is denied because accident details are not available. An E code should be used when submitting an accident claim along with a CPT code. In the case of an auto accident, the MOS may also be requested to submit a police report. If the insurance company requests the police report, the MOS can usually fax it. The same applies to the operative report for surgery and office notes.
- An insurance company might routinely deny coverage for well-person care for a patient. This can be appealed by phone also. Simply ask the insurance representative to review the policy documentation.
- A claim might be denied because a modifier was used in a multiple procedure that the insurance company decided to bundle. Bundling occurs when multiple services are performed. The insurance companies have a list that they refer to which enables them to list procedures as inclusive to another procedure, as explained in the following example.

Example

A patient with a headache comes in for an office visit. While being examined, the patient asks the doctor to look at his toe as long as he is there. The doctor discovers an ingrown toenail and performs minor surgery. A modifier is used to establish that a distinct and separate procedure was performed. The claims examiner disregards the modifier and denies the office visit as global. The medical office specialist should try to get the claim reconsidered by phone, requesting that the claim be paid and state that the reason can be backed up with documentation. The medical office specialist should offer to fax the documentation.

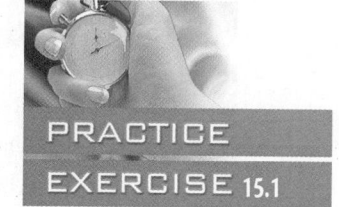

PRACTICE EXERCISE 15.1

The decision has been made to appeal the following situations. Which ones can be appealed by telephone and which would be appealed in writing? Please use a T for a telephone appeal and a W for a written appeal.

1. Diagnosis does not match procedure. _____

2. Insurance company is requesting accident details on a 3 year old. _____

3. Services not authorized. _____

4. Services not medically necessary. _____

5. Services previously paid. _____

6. Multiple surgical procedures lumped and paid under primary procedure even though modifiers were used. _____

7. Radiology charges for a precertified surgery performed by a contracted provider paid as out of network. _____

8. Lab charges for inpatient precertified stay applied toward out-of-network deductible. _____

On completion of this exercise, refer to Appendix J to check the accuracy of your work.

Appeals may be required to be in writing, for example when a claim is denied as not medically necessary or the carrier misquotes benefits.

Sometimes billed procedures are missed and even though the insurance company made the mistake it is not uncommon to be asked to submit a written appeal. One very important thing to remember is that most managed care companies set deadlines for filing an appeal, therefore, the MOS must know the contents of the contract with the carrier regarding the appeals process and deadlines.

Reason Codes That Require a Formal Appeal

In Table 15.2, reasons marked with an asterisk require a formal appeal to be initiated by the practice whenever it suspects the claim was not adjudicated properly by the insurance plan. In addition to those listed in Table 15.2, there are many other occasions that may require a special explanation when registering a formal appeal.

Employee Retirement Income Security Act of 1974

The **Employee Retirement Income Security Act (ERISA) of 1974** protects the interests of participants and their beneficiaries who depend on benefits from private employee benefit plans. ERISA sets standards for administering these plans, including a requirement that financial and other information be disclosed to plan participants and beneficiaries and requirements for the processing of claims for benefits under the plan.

Table 15.2 Reason Codes That Require a Formal Appeal

Code	Description	Code	Description
100	Services payable at 100%	DUP	*Duplicate (previously processed)
19	Dependent over age 19	ELIG	Pending eligibility
21	Dependent over age 21	ERR	Claim processing error or adjustment
1yr	*Limited to one per year	EXP	*Experimental service not covered
2ND	COB secondary payment	FUD	*Included in surgical package
3yr	*Allowed once in 3 years	INFO	Pending additional information
6MO	*Allowed once in 6 months	MAX	Maximum benefits paid
80%	Service(s) payable at 80%	MED	*Not medically necessary
ADD	Need additional information	N/C	*Noncovered services
ADM	Administrative adjustment	NER	*Noncovered emergency services
AOP	Approved out-of-plan	NOA	No answer to inquiry
AVE	*Authorized number of visits exceeded	NOD	No ordering doctor listed
BE	*Billing error	NPD	Nonparticipating doctor
BOI	Bill other insurance	NPP	Nonparticipating provider
CAP	*Capitated services	NREF	*No referral or unauthorized
CMC	*Contractual maximum charge	PCI	*Patient convenience item not covered
COB	Possible COB involved	PRE	Prior to effective date
COS	*Cosmetic service not covered	TNR	*Not related to diagnosis
DNC	*Dental service not covered	UA	*No authorization number; do not bill patient

Although some employee benefit plans are not covered by the act (such as church or government plans), the insured has certain rights if a claim is denied. Contact the plan administrator regarding filing a claim and appeal. Self-funded plans are subject to ERISA and U.S. Department of Labor regulations. Seek assistance from the U.S. Department of Labor at:

U.S. Department of Labor
Division of Technical Assistance and Inquiries
200 Constitution Ave. NW Room N-5619
Washington, DC 20210
Phone: 202-219-8776

The medical office specialist should be aware of what insurance plans fall under ERISA. ID cards for ERISA plans are marked in different ways by different payers.

Waiting Period for an ERISA Claim

Within 90 days after a claim has been filed, the insurance plan must respond as to whether it will be paid or whether additional information is needed. If additional information is requested, the plan must specify why and the day by which the plan expects to render a final decision. If no response is received within the 90-day period, the claim is considered denied. Explanation is required for a denied claim.

Appeal to ERISA

The plan administrator must inform the provider how to submit a denied claim for a fair and full review. The provider has at least 60 days to appeal. Some plans allow more time, but again this is determined according to each individual plan. If review of the appeal is going to take longer than 60 days, the insured must be notified in writing of the delay. A decision on the appeal must be made within 120 days.

The medical office specialist should separate the EOBs that are from administrators for a self-insured employer from all other carriers so their time is spent appealing in the correct format. These claims and appeals fall under federal guidelines and are not mandated by the state insurance commissioner.

Medicare Appeals

In the mid-2000s the government made significant structural and procedural changes in the existing Medicare appeals process. There are three levels of appeals as discussed next: redetermination, the second level of appeal, and the third level of appeal.

Redetermination

A provider has 120 days to file a request for a Medicare review, also known as a **redetermination**, with a Medicare carrier. A Medicare redetermination is the first level of appeal for physician claims. The law stipulates that Medicare carriers must process redeterminations within 30 days.

Second Level of Appeal

The second level of the appeals process is handled by **qualified independent contractors (QICs)** who process "reconsiderations" of carriers' initial determinations and redeterminations. As a result of the recent changes, appellants now have easier access to this second level of appeal because the $100.00 threshold for the amount in controversy was removed. Physicians can also expect a quicker turnaround on these second-level appeals than in the past, because QICs must now process their reconsiderations within 30 days. Physicians essentially have 6 months to file a second-level appeal.

Third Level of Appeal and Beyond

The third level of appeal is an **administrative law judge (ALJ) hearing**, and physicians have 60 days to file an appeal with an ALJ. With the recent changes, the minimum amount in controversy requirement is now only $100.00 and ALJs have 90 days in which to make a decision. Thus, physicians should have an easier time than in the past getting an ALJ hearing, if needed, and they should receive a quicker decision in most cases.

The levels of appeal beyond the ALJ are the Departmental Appeals Board and federal district courts. Appeals of physicians' claims rarely reach either of these levels. There have been no major changes in the process for these stages, except that there is now a 90-day time limit on decisions at the Departmental Appeals Board level; previously, there was no time limit on these decisions.

Medicare Part B has found that the number one reason an appeal is returned is for an invalid or lack of an acceptable signature. Acceptable signatures on appeals are:

- Actual signature by the provider or authorized employee
- A rubber-stamped signature of provider or authorized employee

- Signature of provider signed and initialed by an authorized employee
- The signature must be on the review request. It is not acceptable on just the operative report or claim form.

When requesting a redetermination or filing an appeal with Medicare, the Medicare redetermination request form shown in Appendix D must be used.

Appeals Letters

Many appeals letters can be standardized, with the MOS then inserting specific details and providing necessary information and documentation. Sometimes, however, the specific situation calls for an original letter. To strengthen an appeal, court rulings can and should be used in appeal letters. Returning to our earlier example of the college student whose claim was rejected, Figures 15.6 and 15.7 are examples of two appeal letters regarding the denial of payment for insertion of an IUD. The letter in Figure 15.5 does not include court rulings and is not as effective as the one in Figure 15.6, which does include court rulings. Note also that Figure 15.6 is more formal and includes more details about the patient, such as the policy number. This, too, helps its effectiveness.

Figure 15.5

Sample appeal letter regarding denial of payment for insertion of an IUD. It does not include court rulings.

Allied Medical Center
1933 E. Frankford Rd #110
Carrollton, TX 12345

Dear Claims Examiner,

I am writing to you in regards to a claim submitted for Tessa Kirk for services provided by Dr. Stewart on June 12, 2009. The charges total $700.00.

This claim was sent to ABC Insurance Company, which has since denied the charges. The reason given for the denial is that insertion of an IUD isn't covered by her health insurance plan. However, I called the customer service number listed on the back of her insurance card and was told that it would be a covered expense.

On June 9, 2009, I called and spoke with Phyllis Rose and asked about benefits for an IUD. She not only told me that it was a covered service, but she also quoted me the payment benefits and assured me that it would be paid. I feel that Dr. Stewart should not be penalized for receiving incorrect information from your insurance company. I was using the customer service number provided on the back of the insurance plan and I believe that the insurance company should be held accountable for what is quoted over the phone. Furthermore, had we known the service was not covered, we would have notified the patient in advance of that and would have given her the opportunity to make payment arrangements or not to have the procedure.

Please review this letter and reconsider the charges you have previously denied. Thank you for your time and assistance in this matter.

Sincerely,

Linda Baldwin
Medical Office Specialist

Allied Medical Center
1933 E. Frankford Rd #110
Carrollton, TX 12345

July 20, 2009
Attn: Director of Claims
ABC Insurance Company
2246 Midway Road, #110
Phoenix, AZ 12345

Re: Tessa Kirk
Policy: 455-29-2020
Insured: Tessa Kirk
Treatment Dates: June 12, 2009
Amount: $700.00

Dear Director of Claims:

The above-referenced claim was denied despite the fact that verification of benefits and/or preauthorization of care was obtained from your company on June 9, 2009. Please be advised that our facility relies on information received from your company regarding coverage. We extended treatment in good faith based on the expectation of payment. Further, state courts have held that insurers are liable for misrepresentations made during coverage verification. In *Hermann Hospital v. National Standard Insurance Company*, 776 SW 2nd 249, the Court of Appeals of Texas ruled that coverage misrepresentations could be construed as both negligent and fraudulent. In rendering this decision, the court wrote:

"Hospital and other healthcare providers must, and do, rely on the insurance carriers' representations of coverage in making their decision regarding admission of potential patients. If insurance coverage and benefits cannot be verified, or no coverage exists, the medical provider can then make alternative financial arrangements. To insulate the insurance carriers from liability leaves the medical care provider without recourse against the party causing it damage, if it acted in reliance on the representation of coverage."

Therefore, we request your review of the denial in light of the information obtained by your company at the time treatment was rendered.

Sincerely,

Dee Phillips
Medical Office Specialist

Figure 15.6

Sample appeal letter regarding the denial of payment for insertion of an IUD. It does include court rulings.

It is important for the medical office specialist to research and share information regarding the federal and state laws that affect the provider's claim submission and appeals process. We discussed earlier the importance of medical necessity and the fact that this is a reason many claims are denied. Figures 15.7 and 15.8 are examples of appeal letters that deal with denial because of medical necessity.

Figure 15.7

Sample appeal letter dealing with denial because of medical necessity.

Allied Medical Center
1933 E. Frankford Rd #110
Carrollton, TX 12345

Dear Mr. Hess,

We have received the explanation of benefits for a patient, Mr. Robert Crawford. However, we believe the charges totaling $480.00 for February 25, 2009, through March 14, 2009, have been considered incorrectly.

The EOB states that the March 15th charge of $80.00 is not a medical necessity. When I spoke to you at the claims center earlier this week, your explanation of the denial was because the patient is not homebound and the insurance company believes the visit was for patient convenience and not medically necessary.

In reviewing the nurse's notes for each skilled nursing visit, medical necessity appears to have been established. The March 15th visit should not have been denied. A new infusion therapy was started on that date and the patient required instruction on drug administration.

Skilled nursing visits are a medical necessity to follow up on how well the patient is learning and, indeed, errors in the patient's technique were discovered. Throughout the therapy the patient was fatigued, weak, and felt sick. The patient also felt overwhelmed with the therapies, requiring further instruction and reinforcement. The results of not having skilled nursing visits could lead to further complications, such as not following the drug schedule or performing inaccurate drug administration.

It appears that a review of the nurse's notes would support the medical necessity of the nursing charges. Please reconsider the denied portion of the charges and issue a payment to Value Home Care in the amount of $80.00.

Sincerely,

Bill Ingram
Collections Manager, Value Home Care

Closing Words

Note the similarities among these appeal letters. They (1) provided a specific description of the charges being appealed; (2) identified the names of people contacted at the insurance company with the dates the conversations took place; (3) gave concise explanations of what was being requested, either a re-verification of the policy requirements or asking for an exception to the rules; in either case, a strong argument defining the position of the letter writer must be stated precisely; and (4) explained clearly the anticipated result anticipated by the letter writer.

Appeals and Customer Service

Many providers view appealing denied medical claims as an unwanted, but necessary, function of back-end collections. An aggressive appeals program in a provider's office can also be a tremendous bonus to the practice's reputation for extending exemplary customer service.

Most patients recognize that a medical provider is going above the call of duty when the provider attempts to overturn an unfair claim denial for the patient. To the

Figure 15.8

Sample appeal letter for dealing with denial because of medical necessity.

Allied Medical Center
1933 E. Frankford Rd #110
Carrollton, TX 12345

April 20, 2009
Attn: Director of Claims
ABC Insurance Company
2246 Midway Road #110
Phoenix, AZ 12345

Re: Mr. Robert Crawford
Policy: 636-33-459
Insured: Robert Crawford
Treatment Dates: February 25, 2009–March 14, 2009
Amount: $80.00

Dear Director of Claims:

It is our understanding that this claim was denied pursuant to your decision that the care was not medically necessary.

The Explanation of Benefits did not give adequate information to establish the accuracy of this decision. Therefore, please provide the following information to support the denial of benefits for this treatment.

Please furnish the name and credentials of the insurance representative who reviewed the treatment records. Also, please provide an outline of the specific records reviewed and a description of any records that would be necessary in order to approve the treatment.

Further, we would appreciate copies of any expert medical opinions that have been secured by your company with regard to treatments of this nature and its efficacy so that the treating physician may respond to its applicability to this patient's condition.

Thank you for your assistance.

Sincerely,

Dee Phillips
Medical Office Specialist

patient, already beset with a medical malady, any assistance in dealing with complicated insurance issues is greatly appreciated. Further, a successful appeal letter that relieves the patient of a possible financial burden will be something the patient is sure to discuss with friends, neighbors, and mere acquaintances—all prospects for growing clientele.

Ways to reinforce this positive aspect of appealing denied claims include the following:

■ In an appeal letter, refer to the patient by name, rather than using the generic term *patient*. For example, state "Mr. Brown was treated in our office on May 5," rather than "This patient was treated. . . ."

- Send a copy of the appeal letter to the patient. Put a cc: notation at the bottom of the original so the patient will know that the carrier is being advised that the patient should be advised of all communications.
- When sending the copy of the appeal letter to the patient, include a brief cover letter explaining that the appeal was filed as a courtesy to the patient. Ask the patient to also appeal the denial, inviting him to use any information in your letter that supports the request for payment. Give the patient the name of your insurance representative who might be able to answer questions about medical appeals.
- Advise the patient of her alternatives. The provider might want to keep literature in the office from the state's Department of Insurance, Labor Department information, or business cards of companies and law firms that offer appeal assistance.
- Finally, and most importantly, give the patient a phone call when an appeal letter is sent.

Appeals Require Perseverance and Attitude

In appealing denied insurance claims, you need to have the mindset that it is the insurance carrier's burden to prove that the claim has been processed correctly and that any ambiguities in the coverage terms were construed in the insured's favor. A strong mindset will also give you the perseverance necessary to continue to appeal a claim the insurer strongly defends.

PROFESSIONAL TIP

Insurance recovery requires attitude. Perseverance is the key to a high rate of overturned denials.

"Attitude is more important than facts."

This quote is from noted psychiatrist Karl Menninger who understood the vast importance of attacking a difficult situation with a strong mind-set.

Attitude is more important than facts, because the right attitude will help you persuade the insurance carrier to look at the facts differently. The initial appeal should be addressed to the appeals department.

Many claims are overturned after a single appeal letter. However, you should persist with filing appeals until you get a satisfactory answer. When you do not receive an adequate response to your appeal from the appeals committee, it is imperative that you continue to appeal.

Persistence is often the key to overturning a denied claim. Many carriers overturn as many appeals during the second and third appeals as on the first appeal. It is crucial to keep the appeal active, even after the initial denial. In fact, statistics released from major insurance carriers indicate that about 25% of appeals are overturned on the first appeal and another 25% are overturned on the second appeal.

If you believe payment is indicated by the policy terms, continue to appeal the claim. See the next section for information on keeping your appeal alive.

Do Not Settle for "Denial Upheld"

As just mentioned, appealing denied insurance claims requires perseverance. You may find that the claims department is not reviewing your carefully researched and strongly worded appeal adequately. In such instances, you can redirect your appeal to someone in a better position to review and respond to the information you have cited. Consider sending your appeal to one of the following:

- *Carrier legal counsel.* If you have cited regulatory information, you can request a review and written response from the legal department.
- *Carrier president.* If your appeal involves a possible breach of claim processing procedures, ask the president or other senior management official to respond.
- *Department of Labor.* If the insurance is self-funded, file a complaint with the Department of Labor. Send a copy of the complaint to the insurer.
- *Employer.* The employer will have an appeals committee if the group is self-insured.
- *Department of Insurance.* File a formal complaint with your state's Department of Insurance if you are unable to get a satisfactory response. Send a copy of the complaint to the insurer.
- *State medical association.* Many medical associations now have a complaint review process and will assist you with resolving denied insurance claims.

> Additional sample appeals letters and case studies can be found at www. appealsolutions.com.

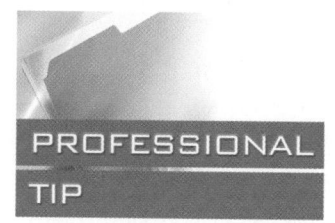

PROFESSIONAL TIP

Refund Guidelines

Credit balances and refunds are the result of overpayments by the patient or insurance company. Overpayments are not uncommon and can occur for various reasons:

- The patient pays in excess of his financial responsibility.
- The patient has both primary and secondary insurance. Both insurance companies pay as primary in error.
- The insurance company makes a duplicate payment on a previously paid claim.

A good portion of the refund process is accomplished using common sense. Do not automatically refund money to an insurance carrier just because they have requested money back. Research must first be completed. If a carrier requests a refund, it must be requested in writing. The medical office specialist must know what type of plan is involved and whether prompt payment rules apply.

Make sure the EOB or request for a refund clearly states why a refund is warranted. If the insurance carrier states coverage was canceled prior to or not in effect on the date services were performed, check to see if a verification of benefits (VOB) form is on file for that date of service. If a VOB form is on file for that date of service, appeal the refund request citing the information given on the VOB. If the insurance carrier states a refund is due because of overpayment on the patient's account, check the carrier contract and fee schedule to see if that is the case.

If the insurance carrier states other insurance should have paid first (coordination of benefits), research the other insurance coverage. If this is true, refund the money. If it is not, appeal the refund request. If the insurance carrier has paid twice for the same date of service and is requesting a refund, check the first EOB to see that is was posted to the correct date of service. If it was, refund the overpayment amount. If it was not, the first EOB needs to be posted correctly and an appeal should be sent to the insurance carrier.

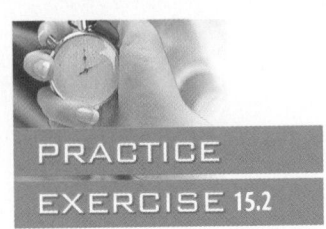

PRACTICE EXERCISE 15.2

Read the following scenarios. On a separate sheet of paper, explain what steps you would take to handle each situation. If you believe an appeal is necessary, explain why, write the appeal letter, and explain what you would attach to the appeal letter. If you believe a patient bill is necessary, type a patient bill. If you feel more research into the case is needed, explain what research should be done. Please make up an insurance address, provider address, and the patient's address, policy number, and claim number. Use your imagination with the scenarios.

1. Jane Shadrack saw Dr. Eugene A. Brady on July 8, 2009. She complained of severe headaches, blurred vision, and disorientation. Dr. Brady diagnosed her with migraine headaches. The claim was denied by her insurance carrier, Aetna, stating that her condition was preexisting. Ms. Shadrack's medical records show she has not seen Dr. Brady for these symptoms before.

2. Bobbie Montgomery, age 12, saw Dr. Eugene A. Brady on September 21, 2009. A claim was submitted to his father's insurance carrier, Great West Life, on September 24. Great West Life has sent Dr. Brady an EOB stating that coordination of benefits should be observed and is being researched.

3. Shannon Macaroni was seen by Dr. Eugene A. Brady as an emergency patient on October 5 at 9 P.M. because she had a stick in her right eye. A claim was submitted on October 8 and denied for no prior authorization number.

4. Dr. Eugene A. Brady performed surgery on Lois Buttons' index finger on August 15. The claim was submitted to Aetna and denied as an experimental procedure.

If a patient is requesting a refund due to a prepayment they made for a service, you will first need to research the patient account to ensure the patient has no other outstanding balance (i.e., from an earlier date of service). If the patient does have an outstanding balance, apply the money appropriately and refund the difference. If there is no other outstanding balance, the patient should be sent the entire refund amount.

Occasionally, a patient is lucky enough to have a secondary insurance policy that will pay her copayment amount due on the primary insurance policy. If the patient paid her copay at the time of service and both insurance companies have paid their shares—the second policy having covered the primary copay amount—then the patient may be entitled to a refund. Again, check the patient account for any outstanding balances. If there is a balance, apply the copay amount to that balance and refund the difference if any. If there is no outstanding balance, refund the entire copay amount to the patient.

Usually, the accounting department or office manager handles the actual check writing for refunds. If a refund is warranted, print out the patient's financial record for the appropriate date of service, attach a copy of the EOB/refund request and any research you completed, and give it to the accounting department or office manager.

Although there is no way to completely avoid credit balances, policies can be put in place to keep them at a minimum. Whatever the reasons for the overpayment, make sure that the reason for the credit balance is identified and do not issue a refund unless requested by the carrier.

The medical office specialist's goal should always be to keep accounts as clean as possible. To issue a refund, the MOS must first go into the computer transaction screen.

Any time financial information is entered to alter an account balance, a transaction is being performed. To issue a refund to an insurance company, the MOS makes an adjustment to the balance of patient's accounts. A negative adjustment will increase the balance, while a positive adjustment will decrease it. To issue a refund, use a positive adjustment. Entering a positive adjustment code will offset the credit. After the adjustment codes have been entered, the MOS documents the patient's account explaining the reason for the refund. After entering the notes, print a copy of the patient's ledger and attach it to the daily batch.

When an insurance company has requested a refund for an overpayment, it should be examined as soon as possible. If the carrier does not receive the refund or an appeal, the carrier has the right to automatically recoup payments from any current payment due on adjudicated claims before it is ever actually issued. The insurance company does this simply by flagging the provider's tax ID number showing that the provider owes a refund. This should be avoided at all cost. All government health plans can also do automatic recoupments without notice. Automatic recoupments can become an accounting nightmare. The insurance company will recoup money from any payment going out of their office to the provider whether this is the account where the overpayment occurred or not. Therefore, adjustments will have to be made to several accounts depending on the amount of money the insurance company has recouped.

Avoid Excessive Overpayments

Patient's copayments are to be verified with the insurance carrier at the time of service if at all possible. As companies renew their coverage each year, sometimes the deductibles and copays change. The patient may not have his new card when he comes into the office. Therefore, every effort must be made to verify copays with the carrier. If the card is asking for a $25.00 copay and the patient states that his copay has changed and it is now $10.00, take the patient's word for it. It is good customer service to do so—the patient usually knows what his copay is. A bill can be sent later if it is incorrect rather than risking losing a patient and having to issue a refund later.

The deductible should be requested up front if the services are being rendered prior to the patient meeting her deductible. Also, if the procedure is not covered by the insurance plan, the charged amount should be requested prior to the services being provided. For some services, the copays and deductibles are not applicable. For example, a routine well-person visit may not apply to the deductible. Always verify with the insurance carrier or the MCO.

Guidelines for Insurance Overpayments and Refund Requests

The American Medical Association and its staff receive questions daily from medical offices about payer requests for refunds. The following general information will help the MOS properly assess most refund requests:

Self-funded employer ERISA plans. Time limits are based on individual contractual agreements. Nothing prevents carriers from automatically recouping refunds from current or future payments, regardless of whether the physician is contracted or noncontracted.

Medicare overpayments. In general, there is no practical time limit after which Medicare cannot ask for money back. Automatic recoupments from current and/or future payments are permitted. For Medicare beneficiaries the provider who is not participating and not accepting assignment can only charge a limiting charge. A Medicare Limiting Charge form is a request for a refund to the patient by

Medicare. This form can be found in Appendix D. The form states to the patient that the provider has been informed of the overcharge.

Medicaid overpayments. In general, Medicaid may request refunds for up to 5 years. Depending on the circumstances, this time frame can be exceeded.

Civil Practice and Remedies Code §16.004. In rare situations where no contract language governs refunds, the statute of limitations is 4 years (excluding government programs).

Preauthorization. For all payer types, preauthorization pertains only to medical necessity and is never a guarantee of payment.

Wrongful retention. A physician should never retain any amount truly not owed to the practice. Wrongful retention of an overpayment is called *conversion* and is illegal. If the practice did not perform the service(s), or if the reimbursement is clearly more than the plan owes, the practice should return the overpayment.

Take the time now to complete Practice Exercises 15.3 through 15.6 to gain experience working with situations in which refunds are required.

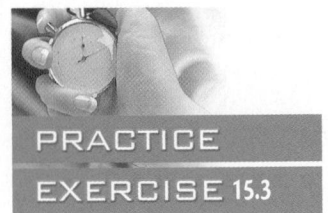

PRACTICE EXERCISE 15.3

Review the following claim information and (1) complete a CMS-1500, (2) apply refund calculations, and (3) then fill in the missing information in the blanks provided. Copy the CMS-1500 form from Appendix D or download it from the CD-ROM that accompanies this text.

Patient:	Sandra Brown	**DOB:**	09/06/1975
Address:	1658 N. Lovers Lane	**Ins Co:**	Aetna
	Dallas, TX 12345	3300 Hoppy St. Dallas, TX 12345	
Phone Number:	214-555-8288	**ID Number:**	581144448
Employer:	Central Market	**Group Number:**	1274
	Highland Park Village		
	Dallas, TX 12345		

Patient is seen for first time. Reason for visit is sore throat and fever. She is the insured and has selected your doctor, Dr. Mallard, as her PCP. Refer to Practice Exercise 11.7 for Physician Information.

DX: 487.1

Office visit	99204	$180.00
Strep Test	87081	$54.00

Sandra paid $234.00 up-front because she has a $250.00 deductible and is not sure whether or not it has been met.

You receive an EOB 30 days after submitting a paper claim. The insurance company allowed $125.00 of the visit and $20.00 of the lab charges. All allowable charges were applied to the deductible. Enter payments on account as well as any contractual write-offs.

1. Is there a credit on this account? _____

2. If so, how much? _____

3. What type of adjustment needs to be entered? _____

4. Is a refund due? _____

5. If so, how much? _____

PRACTICE

EXERCISE 15.3

(continued)

On completion of this exercise, refer to Appendix J to check the accuracy of your work.

Review the following claim information and (1) complete a CMS-1500, (2) apply refund calculations, and (3) then fill in the missing information in the blanks provided. Copy the CMS-1500 form from Appendix D or download it from the CD-ROM that accompanies this text.

PRACTICE

EXERCISE 15.4

Patient:	Elizabeth O'Connor	**DOB:** 04/08/1982	
ID Number:	625148544	**Employer:** CVS Pharmacy	
Group Number:	11158		
Address:	1900 Lemon Lane		
	Dallas, TX 12345		
Phone Number:	214-555-1589		
Ins Co:	United Health Care		
	P.O. Box 1014		
	Dallas, TX 12345		

Elizabeth was seen today for scoliosis. She is the insured and has selected Dr. Mallard as her PCP. Refer to Practice Exercise 11.7 for Physician Information.

Diagnosis code: 737.30

Office visit		
	99214	$65.00
	97260	$30.00

Elizabeth made a payment of $47.00 for her services today. Her deductible has been met for the year.

You receive an EOB 30 days after submitting a paper claim. The insurance company allowed $55.00 of the visit and $20.00 of the second charge. Rate of benefit is 80%.

1. Is there a credit on this account? _____

2. If so, how much? _____

3. What type of adjustment needs to be entered? _____

4. Is a refund due? _____

5. If so, how much? _____

On completion of this exercise, refer to Appendix J to check the accuracy of your work.

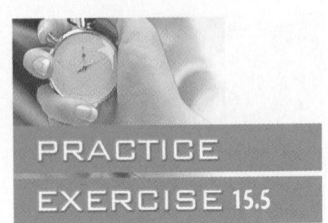

Review the following claim information and (1) complete a CMS-1500, (2) apply refund calculations, and (3) then fill in the missing information in the blanks provided. Copy the CMS-1500 form from Appendix D or download it from the CD-ROM that accompanies this text.

Patient:	Norbert Blake	**DOB:** 05/07/1984
ID Number:	514258522	**Employer:** Lizis Chicken
Group Number:	58999	
Address:	1721 Elm Street	
	Richardson, TX 12345	
Phone Number:	972-414-8544	
Ins Co:	Cigna Health Care	
	P.O. Box 99874	
	Dallas, TX 12345	

James was seen today for injury to his hand. He is the insured and has selected Dr. Mallard as his PCP. Refer to Practice Exercise 11.7 for Physician Information.

Diagnosis code: 959.4

Office visit	99213	$60.00
X-ray	73130	$45.00

James made a payment of $32.00 for his services today. His deductible has been met for the year.

You receive an EOB 30 days after submitting a paper claim. The insurance company allowed $53.00 of the visit and $33.00 of the x-ray charge. Rate of benefit is 70%.

1. Is there a credit on this account? _____

2. If so, how much? _____

3. What type of adjustment needs to be entered? _____

4. Is a refund due? _____

5. If so, how much? _____

On completion of this exercise, refer to Appendix J to check the accuracy of your work.

.Review the following claim information and (1) complete a CMS-1500, (2) apply refund calculations, and (3) then fill in the missing information in the blanks provided. Copy the CMS-1500 form from Appendix D or download it from the CD-ROM that accompanies this text.

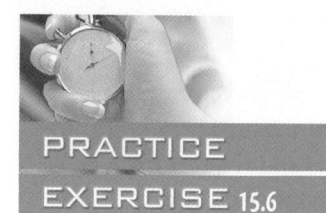

Patient:	Robert Sessions	**DOB:** 02/04/75	
ID Number:	411-65-8744	**Employer:** Tony's Tireshop	
Group Number:	15555		
Address:	1221 High Country		
	Carrollton, TX 12345		
Phone Number:	972-939-8244		
Ins Co:	All Health Care		
	P.O. Box 994		
	Dallas, TX 12345		

Robert was seen today for an upper respiratory infection. He is the insured and has selected Dr. Mallard as his PCP. Refer to Practice Exercise 11.7 for Physician Information.

Diagnosis code: 465.9

Office visit	99213	$60.00
X-ray	71040	$50.00
Lab	81000	$11.00

Robert made a payment of $35.00 for his services today. His deductible has been met for the year.

You receive an EOB 30 days after submitting a paper claim. The insurance company allowed $53.00 of the visit, $35.00 of the x-ray charge, and $9.00 on the lab. Rate of benefit is 90%.

1. Is there a credit on this account? _____

2. If so, how much? _____

3. What type of adjustment needs to be entered? _____

4. Is a refund due? _____

5. If so, how much? _____

On completion of this exercise, refer to Appendix J to check the accuracy of your work.

Figure 15.9

Example of a letter refusing a refund request from an insurance carrier.

Allied Medical Center
1933 E. Frankford Rd #110
Carrollton, TX 12345

February 10, 2009
Aetna Healthcare
OSR Department
P. O. Box 45987
Nashville, TN 12345

Re: Patient Name
Policy Number: 0000000000
Claim Number: 0000000000

Dear Sirs:

On behalf of Allied Medical Center, I am writing to notify you of our refusal to comply with your refund request on the referenced member. Attached for your review is a copy of your letter requesting a refund.

Texas courts have already decided on this issue and have ruled in favor of the providers. If 180 days have lapsed from the day payment was received, no refund is due. Your request for payment is past this deadline. Insurers are not entitled to restitution for an overpayment that resulted solely from the insurer's mistake. Instead, the courts have stated that the medical provider is an innocent party and that the party who created the situation (the insurer) leading to the loss must bear the loss. Refer to the cases of *Lincoln National Life Insurance Co v. Brown Schools, Inc.*, 787 SW 2nd 411, and *Lincoln National v. Rittman*, 79 SW 2nd 791.

Furthermore, "The Retention of Insurance Overpayments by Health Care Providers," 30 So. Tex. L. 387-395, concluded the following on the subject: "Overpayments or payments otherwise mistakenly made by an insurer may be retained by the healthcare provider who is innocent, acts in good faith without prior knowledge of the mistake, and makes no misrepresentation to the insurer, provided the amount retained relates only to the amount actually due for services rendered."

Please correct your records on this case and contact me should you have any questions.

Sincerely,

Melissa Haverty
Practice Manager
cc: Texas Medical Association

Figure 15.9 is an example of a letter refusing a refund request from an insurance carrier. Each state has its own laws and regulations regarding refunds. The medical office specialist can contact his local medical association, attorney general, or state insurance board for state and local information regarding refund guidelines.

Chapter Summary

■ Insurance claims that a third-party payer denies, downcodes, or requests more information on ultimately affect the financial status of the practice.

■ A claim appeal is a written request for a review of reimbursements. It is a formal way of asking the insurance carrier to reconsider its decision regarding a claim.

■ The structure of the medical record must be consistent, and the information must be recorded in a format that allows the physician to access it easily and quickly. Documentation helps in making a proper diagnosis and formulating a sound therapeutic plan.

■ When a physician contracts to participate in a specific network with a particular insurance company, the company has the right to audit or review the physician's billing practices or completeness of medical records.

■ The method of documentation most widely used by physicians is the SOAP (subjective, objective, assessment, plan) format for record keeping.

■ The MOS needs to differentiate between denials of total charges and disallowances. Disallowances represent partial payment on claims because they are above the maximum allowable fee. Denials are when no payment is received.

■ Self-funded plans are subject to ERISA and U.S. Department of Labor regulations. The MSO needs to contact the plan administrator regarding filing an ERISA claim and appeal.

■ The three levels of Medicare appeals include redetermination; the processing of reconsiderations of carriers' initial determinations and redeterminations by qualified independent contractors; and administrative law judge (ALJ) hearings.

■ Credit balances and refunds are a result of an overpayment by the patient or insurance company. Overpayments are not uncommon.

Chapter Review

True/False

Identify the statement as true (T) or false (F).

_____ 1. Some appeals may be conducted over the telephone, whereas others may require a written appeal.

_____ 2. If a payer has rejected all of the appeals on a claim, the claimant may take the case to the state's insurance commissioner.

_____ 3. The Medicare program provides four levels of appeals.

_____ 4. The SOAP format is used when calling insurance companies to verify benefits.

_____ 5. When a third-party payer issues a refund request in writing, the practice should issue a refund within 24 hours.

_____   6. ERISA stands for Employee Retirement Income Security Act (of 1974).

_____   7. Each state's insurance commissioner is the regulatory agency for the insurance industry and serves as a liaison between the patient and the provider.

_____   8. Regardless of the method of reimbursement, insurance claims must be monitored until payments are received.

Multiple Choice

Identify the letter of the choice that best completes the statement or answers the question.

_____   1. The governmental department you should go to if multiple appeals to an MCO fail is:
   a. the Department of Health.
   b. the CMS.
   c. the state department of insurance/insurance commissioner.
   d. HIPAA.

_____   2. What percentage of denied claims are overturned on the first appeal?
   a. 25%   c. 30%
   b. 15%   d. 45%

_____   3. If your first appeal is denied, it is appropriate to:
   a. write a second appeal.
   b. forward the denial with a bill for the unpaid portions to the patient.
   c. call the carrier and complain.
   d. all of the above.

_____   4. It is best to direct initial appeal letters to:
   a. the appeals department.
   b. the customer service representative.
   c. the claims examiner.
   d. the president of the insurance company.

_____   5. The method of documentation most widely used by physicians is the:
   a. RVU format.   c. ERA format.
   b. SOAP format.   d. HIPAA format.

_____   6. What percentage of denied claims are overturned on the second appeal?
   a. 35%   c. 20%
   b. 25%   d. 60%

_____   7. Appealing denied insurance claims requires:
   a. a college degree in mental health.
   b. perseverance.
   c. knowledge in preventative medicine.
   d. none of the above.

_____ **8.** Medicare Part B states the number one reason an appeal is returned is because:
   a. it is beyond the time limit.
   b. it is invalid or there is no acceptable signature.
   c. the benefit plan is not covered by ERISA.
   d. a modifier was not used.

Matching

Choose the best word or phrase that matches the definition.

a. audit
b. peer review
c. claim appeal
d. SOAP

e. documentation
f. administrative law judge (ALJ) hearing
g. insurance commissioner

_____ **1.** Third level of Medicare appeal

_____ **2.** An examination and verification of claims and supporting documents by a physician or medical facility

_____ **3.** A written request for a review of reimbursements

_____ **4.** An objective, unbiased group of physicians who determine what payment is adequate for services provided

_____ **5.** The regulatory agency for the insurance industry; serves as a liaison between the patient and the carrier

_____ **6.** A method of documentation most widely used by physicians for record keeping

_____ **7.** A process of examining and verifying claims and supporting documents submitted by a physician or medical facility

For Additional Practice

Review the case study and determine the necessary action to be taken.

Mary Johnson saw Dr. Nichols today for a well-woman exam. Total charges are $185.00. Mary has two insurance companies:

Primary Insurance	**Secondary Insurance**
BCBS	Cigna Health Care
Copay: $25.00	Deductible: $200.00 (already met)
100% benefit after copay	80% benefit after deductible
Allowed amount: $150.00	Allowed amount: $125.00

Both claims were submitted at the same time in error.

Money collected today from patient: $0.00

1. How much money did Dr. Nichols receive?

2. How much should BCBS have paid?

3. How much should Cigna have paid?

4. How much is this claim overpaid?

5. Who overpaid on this claim?

6. How could this situation have been avoided?

Resources

Aetna: **www.aetna.com**

Claims Resolution for Healthcare Providers: **www.appealsolutions.com**

Injured Employee Medical Claim

16 Workers' Compensation

Workers' compensation is a state-regulated insurance program that pays medical bills and some lost wages for employees who are injured on the job or who have work-related diseases or illnesses. It was developed to benefit both the injured employee and the employer. Chapter 16 presents the student with in-depth knowledge of federal and state workers' compensation programs and how to file workers' compensation insurance claims.

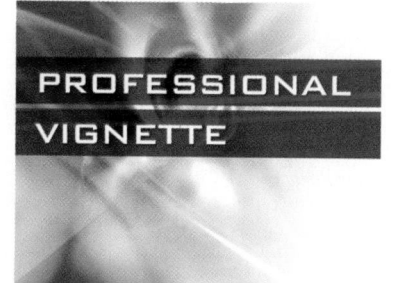

PROFESSIONAL VIGNETTE

My name is Valarie B. Clement, CMA (AAMA). I worked as a medical biller and coder for the past 18 years, before beginning my teaching career. My first introduction to medical billing and coding was when I worked for a medical laboratory. The medical coder was getting married and they needed someone to learn her position while she was on leave. I gladly volunteered as it was an opportunity to learn something new. Looking up ICD-9 and CPT codes was fascinating to me. I never realized just how many there were. While I learned a lot about medical coding from her, I recognized that I needed to go back to school to fully understand the process.

Shortly after completing my studies, I was hired by a family physician to do his billing. I was as shocked as he was to find a file cabinet full of rejected claims. These claims had been billed, but rejected for various reasons. Some were rejected for simply needing an insured's ID number. Time was of the essence in getting these claims processed, as many were close to filing time limits. I went right to work on statusing and resubmitting claims for payment. Within 45 days, 95% of the claims were paid or transferred to patients for their responsible amounts. The physician was so pleased with my results that he gave me a nice bonus for my hard work and determination. I had found a career that I fully enjoyed and that challenged me on a routine basis.

I have learned that the key to successful medical collections is to be persistent and knowledgeable. I have had a long and successful career in the medical field both as a certified medical assistant, and as a professional medical biller and coder. Today, I have the privilege of teaching medical assisting students at Everest Institute about medical billing and coding while still working part-time as a professional medical billing consultant.

Chapter 16　Workers' Compensation

Chapter Objectives

After reading this chapter, the student should be able to:

1. Understand the history of workers' compensation.
2. Distinguish between federal workers' compensation and state workers' compensation.
3. List the classifications of a work-related injury.
4. Know injured workers' responsibilities and rights.
5. Understand the responsibilities of the treating doctor.
6. Understand the role of an Ombudsman in assisting with claims.
7. Know the four types of workers' compensation benefits.
8. Be able to discuss the different types of disability.
9. Accurately complete a CMS-1500 form for a workers' compensation claim.
10. Determine the workers' compensation fee based on the Medicare Fee Schedule.

Key Terms

Admission of Liability
burial benefits
death benefits
designated doctor
disability
disability compensation
　programs
District of Columbia
　Workers' Compensation
　Act

Employer's First Report of
　Injury or Illness
Energy Employees
　Occupational Illness
　Compensation Program
　Act (EEOICP)
Federal Coal Mine Health
　and Safety Act (Black
　Lung Benefits Reform
　Act)

Federal Employees'
　Compensation Act
　(FECA)
final report
fraud indicators
impairment
impairment income
　benefits
impairment rating
income benefits

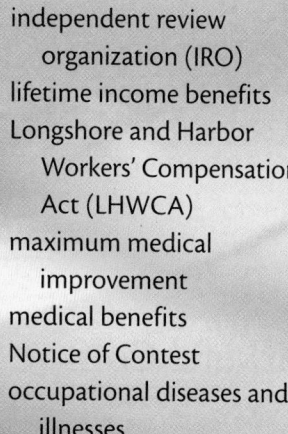

independent review
   organization (IRO)
lifetime income benefits
Longshore and Harbor
   Workers' Compensation
   Act (LHWCA)
maximum medical
   improvement
medical benefits
Notice of Contest
occupational diseases and
   illnesses

Occupational Safety and
   Health Act
Office of Workers'
   Compensation
   Programs (OWCP)
ombudsmen
physician of record
Social Security Disability
   Insurance (SSDI)
supplemental income
   benefits

temporary income
   benefits
treating doctor
Veteran's Disability
   Compensation
Veteran's Disability
   Pension Benefits
vocational rehabilitation
Work Status Report

Case Study
Workers'
Compensation

Julie, the front desk assistant, is speaking with Paula regarding a patient who just left the office. He has a worker's compensation claim involving an injury he suffered on the job. Julie feels that the patient shouldn't be allowed the claim because she thought he seemed fine when he was at the her desk. She felt that he may be faking his injury. Paula explained that it was up to the doctor to decide the type and level of injury incurred by the patient, not hers. The office manager overheard part of the conversation and told Julie that she was not to make such comments about a patient since there was no way for her to know the whole story.

Questions

1. Would you consider Julie's statements as unprofessional?

2. Do you believe that Julie's attitude toward the patient would be obvious if she felt this strongly about the issue? How could her body language be indicative of her viewpoint?

3. Do you think the office manager should take more steps to educate Julie on worker's compensation claims?

Introduction

Workers' compensation was developed to benefit both the injured employee and the employer. Prior to the availability of workers' compensation insurance, injured workers and families of workers killed on the job had to pursue legal action against the employer to attempt to receive compensation for the injury or death. In order for the court case to be successful, the injured worker had to prove that his employer was negligent. As you can imagine, the cases were difficult to prove and often took years to settle.

History of Workers' Compensation

By the late 1800s, the idea of compensating injured workers from an insurance fund to which employers would contribute had gained a foothold in the United States. A few states tried to establish such compensation programs, but organized labor successfully opposed the concept because it was not intended as a preventive measure, but more as a humanitarian measure. That is, the general level of compensation insurance premiums was so low that it didn't encourage employers to adopt safer work environments to eliminate the causes of accidents.

In 1908, Congress passed a limited workers' compensation law for federal employees. Encouraged by this example, several states tried to enact workers' compensation laws. Maryland and New York were the first. Courts later overturned both laws because they believed that mandatory, government-administered workers' compensation programs denied employer property rights without due process of law. To ease the objections, most states enacted laws that allowed employers to choose whether or not to participate in the state's workers' compensation program. In 1911, Wisconsin became the first state to successfully establish a workers' compensation program. Then, by 1947, the tide had turned and almost all states *required* employers to purchase workers' compensation insurance. Texas is the only state that currently allows private employers to choose whether or not to provide workers' compensation, although public employees and employers that enter into a building or construction contract with a governmental entity must provide workers' compensation coverage.

Helping employees receive compensation for workplace injuries was a good start. However, as stated previously, the generally small premium for the policy did not encourage employers to improve the workplace conditions that led to accidents and illnesses in the first place. Therefore, the **Occupational Safety and Health Act** was signed into law on December 29, 1970. This act gave the federal government the authority to set and enforce safety and health standards for most of the United States' employers. If covered businesses do not meet the standards set by the act, they are subject to large fines. If an employee feels that his work environment is unhealthy or unsafe, he may file a complaint directly with the Occupational Safety and Health Administration (OSHA), which was created by the act. The types of employers not regulated by that act include churches, independent contractors, and federal employees.

Federal Workers' Compensation Programs

Civilian employees of federal agencies are covered for work-related injuries and illnesses under various programs administered by the **Office of Workers' Compensation**

Programs (OWCP), which is part of the U.S. Department of Labor. The following programs are administered by the OWCP:

- The **Federal Employees' Compensation Act (FECA)**. This act provides workers' compensation benefits to millions of civilian employees of the United States, members of the Peace Corps, and AmeriCorps*VISTA volunteers.

- The **Federal Coal Mine Health and Safety Act** (also called the **Black Lung Benefits Reform Act**). This act provides benefits to current coal mine employees as well as monthly payments to surviving dependents of deceased workers.

- The **District of Columbia Workers' Compensation Act**. This act provides benefits for any employee performing work (or who did perform work—for deceased/disabled workers) on a regular (i.e., not short-term or temporary) basis in the District of Columbia. Until 1982, any job-related injuries were covered under the Longshore and Harbor Workers' Compensation Act (see next entry).

- The **Longshore and Harbor Workers' Compensation Act (LHWCA)**. This act covers maritime workers injured or killed on navigable waters of the United States, employees working on adjoining piers, docks, and terminals, plus some other special groups. Compensation under this act is paid through policies provided by private insurers or employers who are self-insured.

- The **Energy Employees Occupational Illness Compensation Program Act (EEOICP)**. The newest program administered by OWCP, this act provides benefits to eligible and former employees of the U.S Department of Energy, its contractors and subcontractors, and/or to certain survivors of such individuals.

State Workers' Compensation Plans

Each state has its own statutes that govern workers' compensation and each administers its own workers' compensation program. All states, however, provide two types of workers' compensation coverage. One pays the medical expenses that resulted from the work-related injury/illness, and the other pays the employee's lost wages while she is unable to work.

Employers can obtain workers' compensation insurance policies through a private insurance carrier or a state workers' compensation fund, or they may self-insure if they meet specific criteria. Most employers purchase policies through private insurance companies. If they use a state workers' compensation fund, the employer pays premiums into the fund and claims are paid out of it. Most states require an employer who chooses to self-insure to obtain authorization from the state. When an employer self-insures, money is set aside in a special fund that can only be used to pay workers' compensation claims. The employer pays for workers' compensation; no money is taken from an employee's pay.

Employers must file proof of their workers' compensation insurance with the state Workers' Compensation Board. The employer must also post a Notice of Workers' Compensation Coverage in a place where all employees will see it. The notice must state the name, address, and telephone number of the company's workers' compensation insurance administrator.

Overview of Covered Injuries, Illnesses, and Benefits

Workers' compensation pays medical bills and some lost wages for employees who are injured on the job or who have work-related diseases or illnesses. The injured employee is unable to earn income and consequently there will be loss of income. Injuries do not have to take place on the job site however. They may occur during the performance of duties on behalf of the company, such as driving to the store to purchase office supplies. Taking a fall in the company parking lot is also covered under workers' compensation. A **Notice of Contest** is given to the employee if the employer denies a workers' compensation claim. An **Admission of Liability** is the acknowledgment to the employee of a successful workers' compensation claim.

Each state determines the types of injuries that will be covered under workers' compensation. In general, an injury, accident, or illness is covered if:

- It occurs during the course of employment
- It arises out of employment
- It occurs by accident
- It results in personal injury or death.

Examples of compensable injuries would include:

- Falls in the company parking lot
- Injuries/accidents that occur on the employee's "personal time," such as in the restroom or lunchroom at work
- Back injuries due to required heavy lifting on the job or from a fall
- Repetitive motion/stress injuries, such as carpal tunnel syndrome.

An injured worker may not receive benefits for a generally covered injury if:

- The injury occurred while the worker was intoxicated
- The worker injured himself or herself intentionally or while unlawfully attempting to injure someone else
- The worker was injured by another person for personal reasons
- The worker was injured while voluntarily participating in an off-work activity
- The worker was injured by an act of God
- The injury occurred during horseplay
- The worker failed to use safety equipment or failed to obey safety procedures
- The worker is also receiving Social Security disability benefits
- The worker is also a recipient of unemployment insurance
- The worker receives an employer-paid pension or disability benefit.

Occupational Diseases

Occupational diseases and illnesses (also called nontraumatic injuries/illnesses) are health problems that result from exposure to a workplace health hazard, such as dust, gases, fumes, radiation, repetitive motions, and loud noises. These illnesses may come on rapidly or develop over time, such as with carpal tunnel syndrome.

Work-Related Injury Classifications

Work-related injuries are divided into the following five categories:

1. Injury without **disability**
2. Injury with temporary disability
3. Injury with permanent disability
4. Injury requiring vocational rehabilitation
5. Injury resulting in death.

Each of these categories is discussed next.

Injury without Disability

This category describes an employee who is injured on the job, requires treatment, and is able to return to work within several days. The medical expenses will be fully taken care of by workers' compensation if the injury is deemed compensable.

Injury with Temporary Disability

This category describes an employee who is injured on the job, requires treatment, but is not able to return to work within several days. Not only will all medical expenses be paid for by workers' compensation (if deemed compensable), but also, the employee will receive compensation for lost wages.

Injury with Permanent Disability

This category describes an employee who is injured on the job, requires treatment, is not able to return to work, and is not expected to be able to perform her regular job in the future. This employee usually has been on temporary disability for some time and is still unable to return to work. All medical expenses are paid by workers' compensation and the employee will receive compensation for lost wages.

Injury Requiring Vocational Rehabilitation

An employee in this category has been injured on the job, requires treatment, and is unable to return to work without vocational rehabilitation. **Vocational rehabilitation** is the retraining of the employee so he can return to the workforce. Due to the injury/illness, the employee may not be able to perform the same job duties as before and so would be trained to perform another job.

Injury Resulting in Death

In this category, the employee dies as a result of an on-the-job injury. Death benefits are paid to the worker's survivors.

Injured Worker Responsibilities and Rights

The injured worker has the right to receive medical care that is necessary to treat the work-related injury or illness. The injured worker has the right to an initial choice of doctor (called the **treating doctor** or **physician of record**) with some limitations.

■ If a covered employer contracts with an insurance carrier that establishes or contracts with a certified managed care network, the employer's employees will be required to obtain medical care for their work-related injuries through the network if the employees live within the network service area. However, the insurance carrier will be liable for approved out-of-network referred care, emergency care, and health care for an employee who does not live in the network service area.

■ An injured employee who lives in the network service area may choose a treating doctor from the list of doctors maintained by the network. If an injured employee does not make an initial choice within 14 days, the network will assign a treating doctor to the injured employee. An injured employee who does not live within the network's service area would continue to choose a treating doctor from the Approved Doctor's List (ADL). However, an injured employee may be liable for medical care that is related to the compensable injury if that employee is required to seek care within a network and that employee sees a non-network provider without network approval.

■ If an injured employee is dissatisfied with his or her initial choice of treating doctor, the injured employee is entitled to select another treating doctor from the network's list of doctors. A network cannot deny an injured employee's initial request to change treating doctors. However, any subsequent requests by an injured employee to change treating doctors are subject to network approval.

■ An injured employee may request that her primary care provider (PCP) under a group health maintenance organization (HMO) plan also serve as her treating doctor if the PCP agrees to abide by the network requirements.

■ The injured worker has the responsibility to tell his employer of a work-related injury or illness within 30 days of the injury or within 30 days of realizing the injury/illness may be the result of his employment.

The injured worker has the responsibility to tell the treating doctor/physician of record how he was injured and if he believes the injury to be work related. The worker should tell the doctor about the injury or illness and whether it may be work related before receiving medical treatment. An injured worker may not sue his employer after receiving workers' compensation benefits.

Treating Doctor's Responsibilities

If an injured worker has a managed care plan as her personal insurance and would like to see her PCP for a workers' compensation-related injury/illness, she must receive approval from the PCP in writing prior to services being rendered. The treating doctor (physician of record) is responsible for treating the injured worker's condition and determining the worker's impairment rating. **Maximum medical improvement** is the earlier of the point in time that an injured worker's injury or illness has improved as much as it is likely to improve, or 104 weeks from the date the worker became eligible to receive income benefits. At this point and time the provider determines the patient's impairment. **Impairment** is the permanent physical damage to a worker's body from a work-related injury or illness. A doctor will determine whether the worker has any permanent physical damage and will assign an impairment rating. The **impairment rating** describes the degree of permanent damage done to the worker's body as a whole. The impairment rating determines whether the worker is eligible to receive impairment income benefits and supplemental income benefits. This is described in terms of percentage, that is, 6%, 25%. It also determines the length of time the worker may receive impairment income benefits. If an injured worker disagrees with the impairment rating a doctor assigns, the worker must dispute the rating within 90 days.

The treating doctor will also determine a return-to-work date. After the initial visit with the injured worker, the treating doctor is required to file a Work Status Report. A **Work Status Report** is a state form that is used for transmission of information between the employer, employee, insurance carrier, and the treating doctor. It provides the employer and insurance carrier with information on the employee's limitations in performing her job responsibilities. The treating doctor is also required to file a new Work Status Report (sometimes referred to as a *progress report* or *supplemental report*) with the employer's workers' compensation insurance carrier if there is a substantial change to the injured worker's condition that might affect the worker's disability status or return-to-work date or when required by state rules and regulations. Anytime the injured worker is seen by the treating doctor, a Work Status Report must be sent in with the insurance claim.

The treating doctor will file a **final report** when the injured worker is released from medical care. This report affirms that the worker is fit to return to work and resume normal job responsibilities.

If an injured worker disagrees with the treating doctor's findings (i.e., the percentage of disability or maximum medical improvement), the worker may contact the insurance carrier and/or the state's workers' compensation office. The worker will be referred to a **designated doctor**. A designated doctor is an impartial doctor who helps resolve workers' compensation claim disputes about maximum medical improvement and impairment ratings. The designated doctor may be chosen by agreement between the injured worker and the insurance company. If the injured worker and the insurance company cannot agree, the designated doctor is chosen by the state's Department of Insurance for Workers' Compensation.

Selecting a Designated Doctor and Scheduling an Appointment

When the state Workers' Compensation (WC) Department receives notice about a dispute, it will select a select a designated doctor from a list of approved doctors; make an appointment with the designated doctor for the worker; and send the worker and the insurance carrier a written notice with the date, time, and location of the appointment.

The WC Department will not select a doctor who has already examined the worker; it will instead attempt to select a doctor licensed by the same medical board as the worker's treating doctor.

The worker and the insurance company may agree on a different designated doctor, however. The two sides have 10 days from the date of the notice to agree on a different doctor.

If the two sides agree on a different designated doctor, the insurance company will inform the WC Department of the agreement and the name of the doctor both sides agreed on; make an appointment with the doctor for the worker; and tell the worker and the department the date, time, and location of the appointment. If the appointment is canceled by the patient, the MOS needs to contact the WC Department.

An injured worker may reschedule the appointment with the designated doctor if necessary.

Communicating with the Designated Doctor

An injured worker may talk with the designated doctor to reschedule an appointment or to discuss the worker's medical condition. However, once the doctor has examined the worker, the worker may not contact the doctor directly. All communication with the designated doctor must go through the workers' compensation office handling the claim. No one else involved in the dispute may contact the designated doctor directly at any time. Because of this, it is suggested that the designated doctor use color-coded medical records to indicate a medical record that is strictly for an Independent Medical Examination (IME). That way, if a patient calls with questions after the appointment, the medical office specialist (MOS) will know not to release information to anyone.

What the Designated Doctor Will Do

The designated doctor will:

- Review medical information from the treating doctor and other doctors who have treated the worker for the work-related injury or illness
- Examine, test, and evaluate the parts of the worker's body affected by the injury or illness
- Determine if the worker has reached maximum medical improvement and, if so, when
- Give the worker an impairment rating if the worker has reached maximum medical improvement
- Submit an IME report, including a narrative report and documentation of the impairment rating, to the WC Department within 7 days of the date the worker was examined. The designated doctor also must send a copy of the report to the worker and the insurance company. The doctor will determine the impairment rating using the American Medical Association's *Guides to the Evaluation of Permanent Impairment* (fifth edition, second printing, dated February 1989). If the worker has not reached maximum medical improvement, the designated doctor cannot assign an impairment rating.

Disputing the Designated Doctor's Findings

The injured worker or the insurance company may dispute the designated doctor's findings. To dispute the designated doctor's findings, call the WC Department office handling the claim. Both sides may have to attend a dispute resolution proceeding to resolve the dispute.

If the worker and the insurance company agreed on the designated doctor, the WC Department is required by law to accept the impairment rating the designated doctor assigned. Otherwise, the WC Department must accept the maximum medical improvement date and the impairment rating the designated doctor assigned unless stronger medical evidence clearly indicates that another date or rating is more appropriate.

Disputing Maximum Medical Improvement or Impairment Rating

The injured worker or insurance company may dispute the maximum medical improvement date or the impairment rating a doctor assigned the worker. The worker will be required to see a designated doctor to resolve the dispute.

Either side has 90 days from the date the notice of the rating was received to dispute the rating and notify the WC Department of the dispute. The worker or the insurance carrier must call the workers' compensation office handling the claim if one disagrees with the maximum medical improvement date or impairment rating. The WC Department will tell the other side that there is a dispute.

Ombudsmen

If the injured worker needs assistance with her workers' compensation claim, a Worker's Compensation Department of Insurance Ombudsmen can help. **Ombudsmen** are division employees that can help the worker with her claim, at no charge, once a proceeding has been scheduled. The injured worker may ask for help from an ombudsman if she has not hired an attorney to represent her and does not have any other type of representation.

Ombudsmen can:

- Give the injured worker information to help make decisions
- Communicate with employers, insurance companies, and healthcare providers on the worker's behalf
- Show how to gather and prepare facts and evidence for dispute resolution proceedings
- Help present facts and evidence at dispute resolution proceedings
- Help the injured worker ask questions of witnesses and raise questions about evidence at dispute resolution proceedings
- Give information about how to appeal a dispute resolution decision.

Note, however, that ombudsmen are not attorneys and so they may not give legal advice, make any decisions for the injured worker, or sign agreements or forms on the worker's behalf.

Indicate which of the following scenarios would qualify for workers' compensation benefits and which would not by circling the appropriate answer.

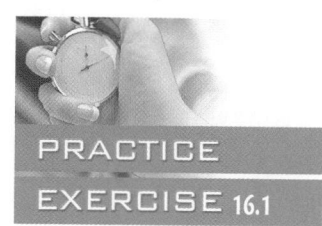

PRACTICE

EXERCISE 16.1

1. Mary drove to the office supply store to buy supplies for the office as instructed by her boss. On her way back to the office she stopped at the post office to mail her tax return. While exiting her car at the post office, her skirt got caught in her car door. As a result, Mary fell down and landed on her left knee, which immediately became swollen and painful. Mary found it quite difficult to walk.

   WC covered   Not WC covered

2. Theo slipped and bruised his tailbone in the employee lunchroom because of a mess a coworker left on the floor.

   WC covered   Not WC covered

3. Louis and Robert work in a warehouse. When the supervisor isn't around, they often goof around on skateboards or roller skates. One day Robert and Louis were racing each other on skateboards from one end of the warehouse

(continued)

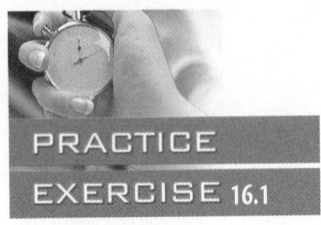

to the other. Louis wasn't paying close attention to where he was going and slammed into a hand cart filled with empty wooden pallets. The hand cart was not supposed to be in that part of the warehouse; another employee left it there before going on break. Louis takes a fall, spills all the pallets, and breaks his arm.

WC covered   Not WC covered

4. Nicholas was encouraged by his fellow employees to play on the softball team sponsored by their employer. Participation on the team is voluntary, but his coworkers pressured him to play. He joined the team and enjoyed the camaraderie and spirit of his coworkers. All was going well until one day he slid into second base and sprained his ankle.

WC covered   Not WC covered

5. Cynthia and her coworker, Monica, play practical jokes on each other all the time. One day while Cynthia was sneaking away from Monica's cubicle after smearing everything in sight with petroleum jelly, she tripped on a rip in the carpet that all of the employees had been complaining about for the past month. Because the rip in the carpet has not been fixed, Cynthia fell down and landed on her wrist, spraining it.

WC covered   Not WC covered

6. On a day when the wind was gusting up to 50 miles per hour, Norma Jean was blown into a light pole in the company parking lot while trying to get to her car to leave for the day. She bruised her left hip and sprained vertebrae in her neck.

WC covered   Not WC covered

7. Scott has a data entry position and has served his company well for the past 3 years. One day he told his supervisor that his hands and wrists ached and that sometimes he felt pain that radiated up his arm to his shoulder.

WC covered   Not WC covered

8. Betty returned to work after a doctor's appointment. She stated to her supervisor that she had to have back surgery for a slipped disk. She told her supervisor that she probably wouldn't have had this problem if she hadn't fallen off the ladder 2 years ago while replacing light bulbs in the employee lounge. That was the first time Betty's supervisor had heard about the fall from the ladder and there was no mention of it in Betty's employee file.

WC covered   Not WC covered

On completion of this exercise, refer to Appendix J to check the accuracy of your work.

Types of Workers' Compensation Benefits

The four types of workers' compensation benefits—medical, income, death, and burial—are discussed next.

Medical Benefits

Medical benefits pay for any medical care that is reasonable and necessary to treat a work-related injury or illness. The employer's workers' compensation insurance company pays medical benefits directly to the doctor or healthcare provider who treated the injured worker.

Amount of Medical Benefits

Medical benefits pay only for the treatment of work-related injuries and illnesses. They do not pay for the treatment of other injuries or illnesses, even if the treatment was provided at the same time as the treatment for the work-related injury. A doctor or healthcare provider may not bill an injured worker for treating a work-related injury or illness, but may bill the worker for treating other injuries or illnesses.

When Medical Benefits Begin and End

Injured workers may receive reasonable and necessary medical care immediately after the injury or illness. The worker may choose a doctor, but the doctor must be on a list of doctors approved by the Worker's Compensation Department. Except in an emergency, the injured worker's treating doctor must approve all medical care for an injury or illness.

An injured worker may receive medical care that is reasonable and necessary to treat a work-related injury or illness without any specific time limit.

Income Benefits

Income benefits replace a portion of any wages a worker loses because of a work-related injury or illness. The four types of income benefits are:

1. Temporary income benefits
2. Impairment income benefits
3. Supplemental income benefits
4. Lifetime income benefits.

Income benefits may not exceed a maximum weekly amount. Temporary income benefits, impairment income benefits, and lifetime income benefits also are subject to a minimum amount.

Temporary Income Benefits

An injured worker may get **temporary income benefits** if the injury or illness causes the worker to lose some or all income for more than 7 days.

When Temporary Income Benefits Begin and End   An injured worker becomes eligible for temporary income benefits on the eighth day of disability. Benefits are not paid for the first week of lost wages unless disability lasts for 4 weeks or more.

Temporary income benefits end at the earlier of:

- The date the worker reaches maximum medical improvement (MMI), which is the earlier of the point in time when the work-related injury or illness has improved as much as it is going to improve or 104 weeks from the date the worker became eligible to receive temporary income benefits
- The date the worker is again physically able to earn the average weekly wage.

Impairment Income Benefits

An injured worker may get **impairment income benefits** if the worker has a permanent impairment from a work-related injury or illness.

When Impairment Income Benefits Begin and End   An injured worker becomes eligible for impairment income benefits the day after the worker reaches MMI. Impairment income benefits end after the worker has received 3 weeks of payments for each percentage point of impairment rating. For example, if an injured worker has an impairment rating of 6%, the worker would receive 18 weeks of impairment income benefits.

Supplemental Income Benefits

An injured worker may get **supplemental income benefits** if:

- The worker has an impairment rating of 15% or more and
- The worker has not returned to work because of the impairment, or has returned to work but is earning less than 80% of the state weekly wage because of the impairment and
- The worker did not take a lump sum payment of impairment income benefits and
- The worker has tried to find a job that matches his or her ability to work.

When Supplemental Income Benefits Begin and End   An injured worker becomes eligible for supplemental income benefits the day after impairment income benefits end. Each quarter, the worker must send a form to the insurance company showing that the worker is eligible to receive supplemental income benefits. If the worker is eligible, she will receive benefits the next quarter.

Eligibility to receive supplemental income benefits ends 401 weeks from the date of injury. If the worker has an occupational illness, eligibility ends 401 weeks from the date the worker first became eligible to receive income benefits.

Lifetime Income Benefits

Certain work-related injuries may result in a condition for which you are entitled to income benefits for your lifetime. **Lifetime income benefits** are paid if the worker incurs:

- Total and permanent loss of sight in both eyes
- Loss of both feet at or above the ankle
- Loss of both hands at or above the wrist
- Loss of one foot at or above the ankle and the loss of one hand, at or above the wrist
- An injury to the spine that results in permanent and complete paralysis of both arms
- Both legs, or one arm and one leg

- A physically traumatic injury to the brain resulting in incurable insanity or imbecility
- Third-degree burns that cover at least 40% of the body and require grafting, or
- Third-degree burns covering the majority of either both hands or one hand and the face.

When Lifetime Income Benefits Begin and End   The injured worker becomes eligible for lifetime income benefits from his date of disability if the injury is the loss of both feet at or above the ankle; the loss of both hands at or above the wrist; or the loss of one foot at or above the ankle and the loss of one hand, at or above the wrist.

All other listed qualifying injuries become eligible for lifetime income benefits from the date the worker is certified to have reached maximum medical improvement.

Death and Burial Benefits

Death benefits can replace a portion of lost family income for the eligible family members of workers killed on the job and pay for some of the deceased worker's funeral expenses. **Burial benefits** are paid to the person who paid the deceased worker's burial expenses. The maximum burial benefit allowed is $6,000.00.

When Death Benefits Begin and End

A beneficiary becomes eligible for death benefits the day after the worker's death. Death benefits end at different times depending on the beneficiary's qualifications to be entitled.

Death benefits are paid if there is a surviving spouse, dependent child, dependent grandchild, or other eligible dependent family member of an employee killed on the job. Except for the spouse and minor children, other family members must have been at least 20% dependent on the deceased worker's income to receive death benefits.

Eligible Beneficiaries

A spouse is eligible to receive death benefits for life unless she remarries. Upon remarriage, the insurance carrier will pay a 2-year (104 weeks) lump sum payment. If there are minor children, the benefit is divided between the spouse and the minor children. One-half is paid to the spouse and the other half is divided equally among the children. If the spouse remarries and the insurance carrier pays the lump sum, at the end of the 104 weeks, if there are still minor children who are eligible for benefits, the entire benefit will be divided equally among the minor children.

Eligible children can receive death benefits until age 18 or 25 if enrolled as a full-time student in an accredited college. If there is more than one minor child, as a child loses eligibility the benefits are redistributed among the other eligible children.

A dependent child, such as a stepchild or dependent child, over the age of 18 is only entitled to benefits for 364 weeks unless the child has a physical or mental disability. In this instance, benefits are paid until the child no longer has a disability.

If the grandchild is a minor at the time of death, benefits are paid until the child is no longer a minor. If the grandchild is not a minor but a dependent of the deceased at the time of death, the benefits are limited to 364 weeks.

Dependent Child, Grandchild, and Other Eligible Parties

These benefits are limited to 364 weeks and the beneficiaries must show at least 20% dependency on the deceased worker. This includes the parents or stepparents of the deceased, a brother, sister, or grandparent. If at any time there are no eligible beneficiaries, or the eligible beneficiaries are no longer eligible and at least 364 weeks have not been paid by the insurance carrier, the remaining benefits are paid to the Subsequent Injury Fund administered by the Worker's Compensation Department.

Benefits and Compensation Termination

Temporary partial and temporary permanent disability benefits are terminated when one of the following things occurs:

- The injured worker is released from treatment by his treating doctor and is authorized to return to his regular job.
- The injured worker has returned to work.
- The injured worker has been offered a different job by her employer and has either accepted (returning to work) or has rejected the job offer.
- The injured worker has exhausted the maximum workers' compensation benefits for the injury or illness.
- The injured worker does not cooperate with requests for a medical examination that will determine the type and duration of the disability and the relationship of the injury to the patient's condition.
- The worker has died. However, death benefits will be paid to the worker's survivors.

Disability Compensation Programs

Disability compensation programs reimburse a covered individual for lost wages that occur due to a disability that prevents the individual from working. Disability programs do not pay for medical treatment. Unlike with workers' compensation benefits, the injury is not required to be work related to qualify for lost wages benefits. Some employers offer disability insurance to employees, but they are not required to do so. Individuals may purchase their own disability policy.

State and federal employees are eligible for a public disability program. Many individuals who are covered by employer disability programs or private policies are also eligible for government-sponsored programs, such as Social Security Disability Insurance or the veterans compensation programs (discussed next). If the individual is eligible for benefits under a government program, the employer-sponsored or private disability policy would supplement the government program's coverage. This means that the government program would pay first, followed by the other policy if applicable.

Types of Government Disability Policies

Various types of government disability policies are available:

- **Veteran's Disability Compensation** is a benefit paid to a veteran because of injuries or diseases that happened while on active duty, or were made worse by active military service.

- **Veteran's Disability Pension Benefits** is a benefit paid to wartime veterans with limited income who are no longer able to work.
- **Social Security Disability Insurance (SSDI)** pays benefits to people who cannot work because they have a medical condition that is expected to last at least 1 year (12 months) or result in death. Federal law requires this very strict definition of disability. While some programs give money to people with partial disability or short-term disability, SSDI does not. SSDI is funded by workers' payroll deductions—as a result of the Federal Insurance Contribution Act (FICA)—and matching employer contributions.

In general, to receive disability benefits, a person must meet certain requirements. General requirements include the following:

- Employed or self-employed individuals with disabilities who are under age 65 and have paid Social Security taxes for a minimum number of calendar year quarters. The number of quarters worked varies depending on the age of the individual.
- Persons disabled before the age of 22 who have a parent receiving Social Security benefits who retires, becomes disabled, or dies.
- Employees who are blind or whose vision cannot be corrected to better than 20/200 in their better eye, or if their visual field is 20 degrees or less in their better eye. The blind employee also must have worked long enough in a job that she paid Social Security taxes.

Certain family members of a worker with a disability may qualify for benefits based on the worker's work history:

- Workers' spouse, if he or she is 62 or older
- Workers' spouse, at any age if he or she is caring for a child of the worker with a disability who is younger than age 16 or has a disability
- The worker's unmarried child, including an adopted child, or, in some cases, a stepchild or grandchild. The child must be under age 18 or under age 19 if in elementary or secondary school full time
- The worker's unmarried child, age 18 or older, if he or she has a disability that started before age 22. (The child's disability also must meet the definition of disability for adults.)

After submitting an application for SSDI, the approval process can take from 3 to 5 months. If the application is approved, the first Social Security disability benefits will be paid for the sixth full month after the date the disability began. (Meaning there is a 5-month waiting period).

Example

If the state agency decides the disability began on January 15, the first disability benefit will be paid for the month of July. Social Security benefits are paid in the month following the month for which they are due, so the worker with the disability will receive her July benefit in August. The amount of the monthly disability benefit is based on the worker's average lifetime earnings.

Supplemental Security Income (SSI) is another type of federal income supplement program funded by general tax revenues (not Social Security taxes).It is designed to help the elderly, people who are blind or have disabilities, and those who have little or no income (i.e., are eligible for welfare). It provides cash to meet basic needs for food, clothing, and shelter.

Whether a person is eligible to receive SSI depends on his income and resources (the things he owns). Also, to receive SSI, the individual must live in the United States or the Northern Mariana Islands and be a U.S. citizen or national. In some cases, noncitizen residents can qualify for SSI.

Verifying Insurance Benefits

As with any patient, prior to treating a patient with a workers' compensation injury (except in emergency cases), it is necessary to verify insurance information. The MOS should obtain the injured worker's employer information prior to the appointment. A call to the employer will confirm whether or not the employer carries workers' compensation insurance and whether or not the employer has filed an **Employer's First Report of Injury or Illness** form. The MOS should also ask for a workers' compensation case number at this time if it's available.

As soon as the employer has completed and sent the Employer's First Report of Injury or Illness form to its insurance carrier, the carrier will assign a case number for the injured worker. If, however, the employer has not filed an Employer's First Report of Injury or Illness form, the MOS will not be able to obtain a case number. This is the first indication that there may be some trouble regarding insurance payment. A workers' compensation claim will not be paid by the carrier if there is no case number. If the form hasn't been filed or the employer doesn't carry workers' compensation insurance, you must request the patient's personal health insurance information because this is the insurance company to whom you will end up submitting claims.

Preauthorization

Preauthorization is prospective approval of health care based solely on medical necessity. Preauthorization is obtained from an insurance carrier by the requester or injured worker before the health care is provided.

Requirements for the Preauthorization Request

The requester (the healthcare provider or designated representative, including office staff or a referral healthcare provider/facility, who requests preauthorization, concurrent review, or voluntary certification) or injured worker must request preauthorization from the insurance carrier via the carrier's designated phone line, fax line, or e-mail address. Preauthorization must be obtained before the health care is rendered. Health care for an emergency does not require preauthorization.

Filing Insurance Claims

Universal claim forms CMS-1500 and UB-04 are used to file workers' compensation insurance claims. The completion of the forms for a workers' compensation claim, however, differs from submitting a standard medical insurance claim. For example, the patient's (injured worker) signature is not required on the form and payment will automatically be sent directly to the medical provider. The billed amount for services rendered is calculated using the Medicare Fee Schedule (MFS) for the procedure and multiplying that amount by a certain amount designated by the state insurance commissioner. If the employer is contracted though a managed care organization, the physician's usual fee is billed and the carrier indicates the monetary contractual adjustments (write-offs) on the Explanation of Benefits (EOB) or Electronic Remittance Advice (ERA). The MOS makes the adjustments to the patient's account after the EOB/ERA is received. Additional information for calculating the fees for service is covered later in this chapter.

A healthcare provider waives any right to payment unless a medical bill is submitted to the insurance carrier on or before the 95th day after the date of service. The insurance carrier, in turn, must pay, reduce, deny, or determine to audit the claim not later than the 45th day after receipt of the claim.

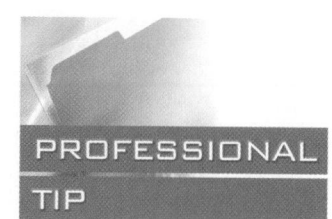

An updated treating doctor's Work Status Report is sent in with every claim that is submitted. If this is not done, the carrier will assume the injured worker has reached maximum medical improvement and will cease paying for future claims.

PROFESSIONAL TIP

Completing the CMS-1500 for Workers' Compensation Claims

Detailed instructions for completing the CMS-1500 claim form are given in Chapter 9; details about the UB-04 claim form are given in Chapter 10. Here, we discuss the specific form locators on the CMS-1500 that are different when submitting a workers' compensation claim. Note that workers compensation claims procedures vary from state to state.

Form Locator 1: Type of Insurance   Check the "Other" or FECA Black Lung box.

Form Locator 1a: Insured's ID Number   Enter the WC case number and the injured employee's Social Security number (SSN). If the SSN is not available, enter the injured employee's driver's license number and jurisdiction, green card number and "ZY", visa number and "TA", or passport number and "ZZ."

Form Locator 4: Insured's Name   Enter the insured employer's local name. This is the employer at the time of the injury.

Form Locator 7: Insured's Address   Enter the insured employer's current business address, including city, state, zip code, and phone number.

Form Locator 10: Is Patient's Condition Related To?   Check the YES box in part a to indicate this is an employment-related condition.

Form Locator 11: Insured's Policy Group or FECA Number   Leave blank or check with state-specific guidelines.

Form Locator 11c: Insurance Plan Name or Program Name   Enter "Workers' Compensation Insurance Plan."

Form Locators 12 and 13: Patient's/Insured's or Authorized Person's Signature   Leave blank. No signature is required for workers' compensation claims.

Form Locator 14: Date of Current: Illness, Injury, Pregnancy   Enter date of injury or occupational illness.

Form Locator 16: Dates Patient Unable to Work in Current Occupation   Enter date patient was first unable to work in his or her present position.

Form Locator 18: Hospitalization Dates Related to Current Services   Enter the dates of hospitalization related to injury or the occupational illness.

Form Locator 33: Billing Provider Information and Phone Number   Enter the billing name of the provider/supplier, including complete address, city, state, zip code, and telephone number. The PIN number for a workers' compensation claim is the provider's license number with the state in front of it or a specific identification number from the Workers' Compensation Department.

Independent Review Organizations

If a health insurer or HMO refuses to pay for a treatment because it considers the treatment medically unnecessary or inappropriate, the injured worker/treating doctor may be able to have an **independent review organization (IRO)** review the decision. An IRO review is a system for final administrative review of the medical necessity and appropriateness of healthcare services provided or proposed to patients. The IRO's decision is binding on the healthcare plan, which pays for the review. An independent review is available if:

- The employer's plan or its utilization review agent (URA) determines that a treatment recommended, but not yet performed, is medically unnecessary or inappropriate
- The employer's plan or its URA determines that an ongoing treatment is medically unnecessary or inappropriate.

A healthcare plan must base its denial on written screening criteria established and updated with involvement by practicing physicians and other providers. The injured worker, the worker's representative, or the injured worker's treating doctor may request an independent review. Only the injured worker or the worker's legal guardian, however, may sign a medical records release form.

In most cases, the injured worker must use the healthcare plan's internal appeal process before requesting an IRO review. The injured worker can bypass the appeal process, however, if the worker or treating doctor believes the injured worker's condition is life threatening.

An independent review is not available if:

- The employer's WC healthcare plan refuses to pay for a service the plan doesn't cover, such as cosmetic surgery
- The injured worker has already received treatment and the plan then determines that the treatment was not medically necessary or appropriate
- The employer's healthcare plan is not subject to the law related to the IRO process. For example, Medicaid and Medicare, including Medicare HMO healthcare plans, are not required to participate in the IRO process. Other healthcare plans may not be subject to the IRO process and you should contact your health plan to find out if it participates in the IRO process.

If the IRO process is not available, the injured worker, the worker's treating doctor, or another provider may file a complaint or appeal regarding the denial of health care or the denial of payment for health care already performed.

How to Obtain an Independent Review

If the employer's WC healthcare plan participates in the IRO process and denies a treatment because it regards the treatment as medically unnecessary or inappropriate, the plan must provide the injured worker with the necessary form for requesting an appeal and an independent review.

> The healthcare plan or the URA must give the injured worker the independent review request form again after denying an appeal.

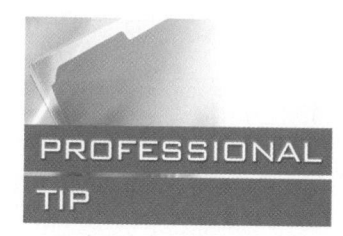

PROFESSIONAL
TIP

If the injured worker wants an independent review, she must complete the form and return it to the health plan or URA.

The IRO Decision

The WC insurer or HMO must pay for a treatment if the IRO decides the care is medically necessary or appropriate. The IRO will provide the injured worker and treating doctor with a notice of its decision that includes the clinical basis for the decision, the screening criteria used to make the decision, a list of qualifications of the IRO staff who reviewed the case, and a statement certifying that the IRO has no conflict of interests involving the insurer, HMO, or the URA.

Medical Records

Workers' compensation medical records are to be kept separate from a patient's regular medical records. If a previously established patient is being seen for a workers' compensation–related case, make sure not to mix the two medical records. A worker's compensation chart is made for the specific injury only. It is suggested that the medical office use color-coded charts for workers' compensation cases. Color-coded charts are an immediate indication that the case is for workers' compensation and that specific information needs to be collected from the patient, including a copy of the patient's state driver's license or state identification card and Social Security card. Another reason to keep workers' compensation files separate from a patient's regular medical records is because workers' compensation claim information is not subject to the same confidentiality rules or laws as private medical records. In most states, carriers, claim adjusters, and employers are allowed unrestricted access to workers' compensation medical records but not private/regular medical records. The financial information (transactions) relating to a workers' compensation case should be kept separate as well.

Fraud

Workers' compensation fraud costs millions of dollars each year. Employers, employees, insurance carriers, and consumers pay the cost of fraud in lost jobs and profit, lower wages and benefits, and higher costs for services and premiums.

The Workers' Compensation Commission's Office of Investigations works with numerous special investigation units to deter fraud by assisting in the prosecution of those who commit fraud. These units include state and federal law enforcement, other regulatory agencies, and insurance carrier special investigation units.

Investigations often lead to prosecution and recovery of money gained through fraudulent schemes. Fraud can be committed by employers, employees, healthcare providers, attorneys, insurance agents, and others.

Fraud occurs when a person knowingly or intentionally conceals, misrepresents, or makes a false statement to either deny or obtain workers' compensation benefits or insurance coverage, or otherwise profit from the deceit. The key to conviction is proving in court that the misrepresentation or concealment occurred knowingly or intentionally. Premium fraud and benefit fraud are the most common types of workers' compensation fraud. Premium fraud is usually committed by an employer who misrepresents the amount of payroll or classification of employees, or who attempts to avoid a higher insurance risk modifier by transferring employees to a new business entity rated as a lower risk category.

Benefit fraud is usually committed by:

- A worker who works full time at an unreported job and draws benefits when he or she is supposed to be unable to work, or when a worker fakes an injury
- A healthcare provider or attorney who assists the worker in fraudulent schemes, or participates in double billing or billing for services not provided.

Fraud indicators do not mean fraud has occurred, but they may require a closer review of the claim or application. Employer fraud indicators include but are not limited to:

- Classification codes not consistent with duties normally associated with the employer's type of business, for example, a construction company that reports mainly clerical classifications
- Much larger premium paid for the previous year's policy
- Small payroll reported by a large company or employee leasing company
- Frequent addition and cancellation of coverage, especially if several business entities appear to be owned or controlled by the same person or group.

Employee fraud indicators include but are not limited to:

- Injuries that have no witness other than the worker
- Injuries occurring late Friday or early Monday
- Injuries not reported until a week or more after they occur
- Injuries occurring before a strike or holiday, or in anticipation of a layoff or termination
- Injuries occurring where the worker would not usually work
- Injuries not usually occurring in the particular job description, for example, a secretary injured while lifting a heavy object
- Worker observed in activities inconsistent with the reported injury
- Worker history of workers' compensation claims
- Conflicting diagnoses from subsequent treating doctors
- Any evidence of working elsewhere while drawing benefits.

Attorney and healthcare provider fraud indicators include:

- Submission of bills or Explanation of Benefits forms for services that seem unnecessary or fictitious
- Submission of "boilerplate" medical reports, or reports that are merely copies of previously submitted reports

- Treatment dates on holidays for nonemergency situations
- Bills from a healthcare provider or attorney that present an unreasonable amount or hours per day
- Complaints from the worker that the attorney is "never" available although the attorney files fee affidavits for services
- Attorney relationship with a healthcare provider that appears to be a partnership in handling workers' compensation claims.

Penalties

If an investigation establishes criminal fraud, the local district attorney may begin prosecution. Workers' compensation fraud involving amounts of $1500.00 or more in benefits or premiums is a felony punishable by fines, orders for restitution, and imprisonment. If the amount is below $1500.00, the action is a Class A misdemeanor punishable by fines, orders for restitution, and imprisonment.

Medical Provider Fraud

Fraud by medical providers can evolve as the nature of medical care changes over time. Outright fraud occurs when providers bill for treatments that never occur or were blatantly unnecessary. Some of the newer forms of medical provider fraud include specialists and other treatment providers giving kickbacks to referring physicians and provider upcoding, in which the provider's charges exceed the scheduled amount. Fraud also occurs when providers shift from the less expensive, all-inclusive patient report to supplemental reports, which add evaluations as a charge and thus incur separate charges.

Medical provider fraud schemes include:

- *Creative billing*: billing for services not performed
- *Self-referrals*: occurs when medical providers inappropriately refer a patient to a clinic or laboratory in which the provider has an interest
- *Upcoding*: billing for a more expensive treatment than the one performed
- *Unbundling*: performing a single service but billing it as a series of separate procedures
- *Product switching*: occurs when a pharmacy or other provider bills for one type of product but dispenses a cheaper version, such as a generic drug.

According to the National Council on Compensation, "The increased use of managed care for workers' compensation, as well as for other insurance lines, is bringing new twists to old schemes." Managed care creates more opportunities for fraud because of the financial relationships and incentives between players. Newer forms of fraud and abuse occurring under managed care arrangements include:

- *Underutilization*: doctors receiving a fixed fee per patient may not provide a sufficient level of treatment
- *Overutilization*: unnecessary treatments or tests are ordered to justify higher patient fees in a new contract year
- *Kickbacks*: incentives for patient referrals
- *Internal fraud*: providers collude with the medical plan or insurance company to defraud the employer through a number of schemes.

Calculating Reimbursements

When the insured employer's insurance policy is not a managed care plan, the fees for services will need to be calculated using the Medicare Fee Schedule (MFS) and multiplying the MFS fees by a certain percentage that is determined by each individual state. Conveniently, the MFS can be found on the Internet. Each state contracts with a carrier to administrate Medicare and Medicaid claims. For example, Trailblazer Health contracts with the states of Colorado, New Mexico, Delaware, Maryland, Texas, and Virginia and the District of Columbia metropolitan area. Each carrier may have a website to provide information on workers' compensation claims. The Trailblazer Health website (http://trailblazerhealth.com) has each CPT® code listed along with its MFS amount. Instructions for the use of the Trailblazer site follow:

1. Go to the Internet website for Trailblazer Health Enterprises, LLC, at http://trailblazerhealth.com.
2. On the homepage, click on the "payment link".
3. On the payment page, you will see a navigation link on the left of the page. Click on "fee schedule".
4. On the fee schedule page, click on "Medicare Fee Schedule", found in the middle of the page.
5. Select the year of the fee schedule you want and your state and locality in the appropriate windows.
6. Fill in the CPT code and modifier for which you are seeking information.
7. Refer to the column that applies to the service provided (facility or nonfacility) and find the "participating amount". "Facility" refers to a hospital or ambulatory surgery center. "Nonfacility" refers to a medical provider such as a physician.
8. Multiply this amount by 125%.

CPT is a registered trademark of the American Medical Association.

As an example to determine the fee, use the Trailblazer Health website for the state of Texas and a multiple of 125%. Fill in each box in the following grid. Specifics about each procedure code are listed below the grid.

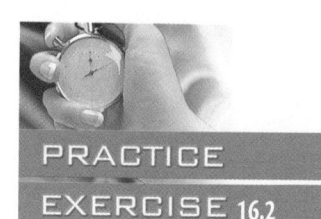

| | Dallas County 2005 | | Dallas County 2006 | | Dallas County 2007 | |
CPT Code	MFS	WC	MFS	WC	MFS	WC
95861						
95900						
95904						
99201						
99202						
99203						
99204						

Workers' Compensation Fees

95861 Needle Electromyography: 2 extremities with or without paraspinal areas
95900 Nerve conduction, amplitude, latency, velocity study (each nerve); motor without F wave
95904 Sensory
99201 New Patient Outpatient O.V. problem-focused history, problem-focused exam, and straightforward medical decision making
99202 New Patient Outpatient O.V. expanded problem-focused history, expanded problem-focused examination, and straightforward medical decision making
99203 New Patient detailed history, detailed examination, and medical decision making of low complexity
99204 New Patient comprehensive history, comprehensive examination, and medical decision making of moderate complexity

On completion of this exercise, refer to Appendix J to check the accuracy of your work.

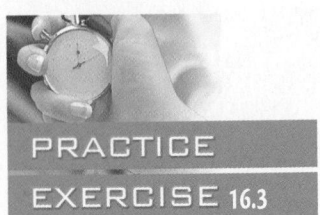

PRACTICE EXERCISE 16.3

Use the information provided to prepare a workers' compensation claim. To complete this exercise, copy the CMS-1500 form provided in Appendix D or download it from the CD-ROM that accompanies this text.

Physician Information:

Name:	Dennis J. Bonner, M.D.
Address:	980 Frederick Road
	Dallas, TX 12345
Phone:	800-555-5000
Employer ID Number:	57-5562147
License Number:	TX 5529
UPIN Number:	224861
NPI:	7536982100

Patient Information Form:

Name:	Kennedy Moore
Birth Date:	April 25, 1944
Phone:	972-555-0087
Address:	346 Austin Boulevard
	Dallas, TX 12345
Sex:	Female
Status:	Married
Social Security number:	968-44-9876
Insurance Carrier:	Aetna TX
Insurance Carrier Address:	20 Forester Avenue
	San Antonio, TX 12345
	555-443-3987
Insurance Group Number:	AR 187267-T
Insurance ID/Policy Number:	66543
Employer:	Datamatic Inc.
	644 San Juan Street
	Dallas, TX 12345
Phone:	214-555-8674
WC Case Number:	0856

Please note that the employer is self-insured.

Patient's Encounter Form:

Date:	Use today's date

Patient Encounter Information:

CC: Patient presents complaining of numbness and tingling in the left hand. She states her job description is data entry.
Patient presents for evaluation of left hand numbness intermittently for the past 3 weeks.

(continued)

| Dx: | Carpal tunnel syndrome. (354.0) |
| Service and Charges: | 99203—Office visit; for the evaluation and management of a new patient, which includes a detailed history, detailed examination, and medical decision of low complexity. |

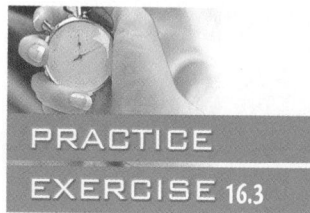

PRACTICE EXERCISE 16.3

(continued)

Check the accuracy of your work by comparing your claim form to the completed claim form in Appendix J.

Use the information provided to prepare a workers' compensation claim. To complete this exercise, copy the CMS-1500 form provided in Appendix D or download it from the CD-ROM that accompanies this text.

PRACTICE EXERCISE 16.4

Physician Information:	Charles H. Hess, M.D.
	980 Frederick Road
	Dallas, TX 12345
Phone:	899-555-2276
EIN:	22-9872767
Professional License:	TX2056
UPIN:	3468923
NPI:	1471236545
Patient Information:	Catherine Daley
	346 Highpoint Drive
	Dallas, TX 12345
	999-555-0756
DOB:	04/25/1969
Social Security number:	968-34-0025
Status:	Married
Sex:	Female
Patient's Insurance Information:	BC/BS
	ID/Policy Number 2543097
	Gr Number 08632
	1123 High Point
	Dallas, TX 12345
	800-555-1123
Employer's Information:	Coca-Cola Corp.
	6345 Harvey Drive
	Dallas, TX 12345
	998-555-6785

(continued)

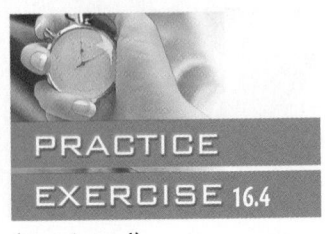

Employer Insurance Carrier: Aetna TX
ID/Policy Number 0231
Gr Number 55111
20 Forest Drive
Plano, TX 12345
972-555-0050

Reason for Visit: Injured at work
Workers' Compensation Case Number: 81526

Use today's date.

Patient Encounter Information:

CC: Patient presents with low back pain.
"Patient states that she slipped
on a wet floor two days ago,
which had recently been cleaned,
and landed on her back and has
been unable to go to work."
Anterior and posterior x-rays of
lumbar spine

DX: Lumbar Sprain 847.2

List of fees for services for Catherine Daley:
Listed below are our UCR fees:

- 99202 NP Office Visit Problem focused-history and examination, straightforward decision making $100.00
- 95861 Needle Electromyography 2 extremities $250.00
- 95900 Nerve Conduction (each nerve) motor (6x) $75.00 each nerve
- 95904 Nerve Conduction (each nerve) sensory (3x) $60.00 each nerve

Check the accuracy of your work by comparing your claim form to the completed claim form in Appendix J.

Chapter Summary

- All states provide two types of workers' compensation coverage. One pays the medical expenses that resulted from the work-related injury/illness and the other pays the employee's lost wages while he or she is unable to work.
- Civilian employees of federal agencies are covered for work-related injuries and illnesses under various programs administered by the Office of Workers' Compensation Programs.
- Worker's Compensation benefits pay only for the treatment of work-related injuries and illnesses. They do not pay for the treatment of other injuries or illnesses, even if the treatment was provided at the same time as the treatment for the work-related injury.

■ The medical office specialist must have knowledge of covered and non-covered workers compensation services.

■ Work-related injuries are divided into the following five categories:
  ● Injury without disability
  ● Injury with temporary disability
  ● Injury with permanent disability
  ● Injury requiring vocational rehabilitation
  ● Injury resulting in death

■ The injured worker has the right to receive medical care that is necessary to treat the work-related injury or illness. The injured worker has the right to an initial choice of doctor (called the treating doctor or physician of record) with some limitations.

■ The injured worker has the responsibility to his tell his employer of a work-related injury or illness within 30 days of the injury or within 30 days of realizing the illness/nontraumatic injury may be the result of his employment.

  ● The treating doctor (physician of record) is responsible for treating the injured worker's condition, determining whether the worker has any permanent physical damage, and determining the worker's impairment rating. The treating doctor will also determine a return-to-work date and is required to file a Work Status Report.

  ● The four types of workers' compensation benefits are medical, income, death, and burial.

  ● Medical providers send their insurance claims directly to the employer's workers' compensation insurance carrier and the carrier pays them directly. The fees for services are limited to the established state fees or the managed care network's fees.

  ● Universal claim forms CMS-1500 and UB-04 are used to file workers' compensation insurance claims. The completion of the forms for a workers' compensation claim, however, differs from submitting a standard medical insurance claim.

  ● A provider waives any right to payment unless a medical bill is submitted to the insurance carrier on or before the 95th day after the date of service. The insurance carrier, in turn, must pay, reduce, deny, or determine to audit the claim not later than the 45th day after receipt of the claim.

  ● If a health insurer or HMO refuses to pay for a treatment because it considers the treatment medically unnecessary or inappropriate, the injured worker/treating doctor may be able to have an independent review organization (IRO) review the decision.

  ● Fraud can be committed by the employee, employer, and provider. The medical office specialist should be aware of all the ways a provider and patient can conduct fraud.

Chapter Review

True/False

Identify the statement as true (T) or false (F).

_____ 1. MMI stands for major medical income.

_____ 2. Disability compensation programs reimburse the insured only when a work-related injury causes the person to lose income.

_____ **3.** The Admission of Liability and the Notice of Contest determinations both find the employer liable in a workers' compensation case.

_____ **4.** An occupational disease or illness is caused by some factor in the work environment that exists over a period of time.

_____ **5.** Under workers' compensation regulations, the treating doctor is the provider who prepares the final report.

_____ **6.** FECA is the abbreviation for Federal Employees' Compensation Act.

_____ **7.** Disability means loss of income.

_____ **8.** Disability compensation programs do not pay medical benefits.

_____ **9.** OSHA is the abbreviation for Occupational Safety and Hazard Administration.

_____ **10.** Vocational rehabilitation is not covered by workers' compensation plans.

_____ **11.** The employer sends in the First Report of Injury or Illness in a workers' compensation case.

_____ **12.** The fee for workers' compensation cases are based on the UCR fee.

_____ **13.** Any employee can purchase a disability plan.

_____ **14.** IME is an abbreviation for Individual Medical Examination.

Multiple Choice

Identify the letter of the choice that best completes the statement or answers the question.

_____ **1.** After discharging a workers' compensation patient, the provider must file a(n):
   a. First Report of Injury.   c. Admission of Liability.
   b. First Report of Illness.   d. final report.

_____ **2.** When a provider initially examines a workers' compensation patient, what document must be filed with the state?
   a. final report
   b. Admission of Liability
   c. Work Status Report
   d. vocational report

_____ **3.** Social Security Disability Insurance provides compensation for lost wages to individuals who:
   a. are qualified for welfare programs.
   b. have contributed to Social Security.
   c. either a or b.
   d. neither a nor b.

_____ **4.** Supplemental Security Income provides financial assistance to individuals who:

a. are qualified for welfare programs.

b. have contributed to Social Security.

c. either a or b.

d. neither a nor b.

_____ **5.** What information is required in form locator 1a when preparing a workers' compensation claim?

a. patient's name

b. patient's Social Security number

c. employer's name

d. insured's ID number

_____ **6.** Workers' compensation fees are based on what fee schedule and a percentage?

a. Aetna   c. Medicare

b. state insurance fees   d. Medicaid

_____ **7.** What form locators are left blank on a CMS-1500 claim form for a workers' compensation claim?

a. Form locators 4 and 5

b. Form locators 12 and 13

c. Form locators 32 and 33

d. Form locators 25 and 26

Completion

Complete each sentence or statement.

1. _____ is the permanent physical damage to a worker's body from a work-related injury or illness.

2. The Federal Employees' Compensation Act provides _____ insurance for civilian employees of the federal government.

3. In the workers' compensation classification of injuries, _____ injury occurs when a worker is injured on the job and cannot resume work within a few days of receiving treatment.

4. In the workers' compensation classification of injuries, _____ injury occurs when a worker is injured on the job, is unable to resume work, and is not expected to be able to return to the regular job in the future.

5. In the workers' compensation classification of injuries, an injury requiring _____ occurs when a worker is injured on the job and cannot resume work without retraining.

6. When a person knowingly or intentionally conceals, misrepresents, or makes a false statement to either deny or obtain workers' compensation benefits or insurance coverage, or otherwise profit from the deceit, this action is called _____.

7. Carpal tunnel syndrome is an example of a(n) _____ illness.

8. _____ describes the degree of permanent damage done to a worker's body as a whole.

9. An injured worker may not receive benefits if _____.

10. MMI is the abbreviation for _____.

11. Workers' compensation bills need to be submitted with a(n) _____.

Resources

U.S. Department of Labor—Federal workers' compensation: **www.dol.gov/dol/topic/workcomp**
U.S. Department of Labor—OSHA: **www.osha.gov**
U.S. Department of Labor—State Workers' Compensation: **www.dol.gov/esa/regs/compliance**

Use of Medical Practice Management Software

17 Electronic Medical Claims Processing

The process of posting payments includes posting of charges, insurance payments, patient payments, and contractual adjustments. Payment posting is an accounts receivable position that may also require the medical office specialist to collect payments, follow up on accounts, and review aging reports. Chapter 17 allows the student to practice entering patient demographic information and posting charges, payments, and adjustments using medical practice management software.

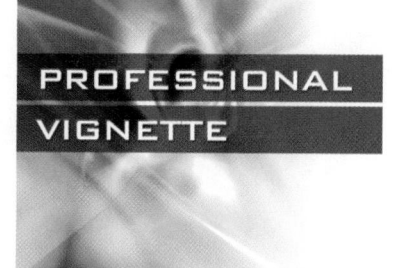

PROFESSIONAL VIGNETTE

My name is Shanna Eaquinta and I'm a certified coding professional (CPC). My first job out of school was as a call center operator for a 20-physician orthopedic clinic, but within a few months, I was offered the position of coding support specialist!

I prepared operative reports for the coder. I printed the fee ticket and gathered all the reports related to the patient's stay, such as emergency department, consultations, hospital visits, pathology, and the operative report. Soon, I was promoted to coder and performed what was considered "straightforward" coding such as carpal tunnel and spinal injections.

When the position of Coding Coordinator opened up I was asked to obtain my CPC certification and apply for the position. This was less than one year after I started! Now I oversee the coding for all three locations and enter all the surgery charges into the computer. I am the "go to" person when we receive an insurance denial. I review the case and determine how we can appeal it. Every insurance provider has unique coding rules, especially for modifiers, which we use often. We keep a master list of how each insurance company wants codes and modifiers reported. One thing is for sure, the job is never boring!

My advice to others entering the field is the same advice my instructor gave me, "Don't be afraid to take something that isn't exactly what you dreamed of because it could open doors to even better opportunities." I'm so glad I did!

Chapter 17 · Electronic Medical Claims Processing

Chapter Objectives

After reading this chapter, the student should be able to:

1. Enter all patient demographic information and post charges, payments, and adjustments using medical practice management software.

2. Print a walkout receipt for each patient who has charges posted to his or her account.

3. Balance the batch at the end of each day.

4. Print insurance claim forms for patients who are covered by insurance.

Key Terms

batch out	payments	walkout receipt
charges	transactions	

Case Study
Medical
Claims
Processing

The office of Dr. Patrick has decided to change to a different medical practice management software system. Since the new software cannot download information from the existing software, Jackie has been hired to enter the patient demographics, insurance information and accounts into the new system. The new system has a list of the insurance carriers and their addresses in place.

Questions

1. What type of information will Jackie be responsible for entering?
2. Where will she obtain patient demographic information?
3. How will she enter this information into the medical practice management software?

Introduction

Payment posting is a position in a medical office or hospital that handles accounts receivables. The payment posting process includes entering patient demographic information and posting (entering into a computer) of **charges** (the physician fee for a service), insurance **payments** (money received for services rendered), patient payments, contractual adjustments, and other **transactions** (records of charges, payments, and adjustments) into a medical software program. This position may also require the medical office specialist (MOS) to collect payments, follow up on accounts, and review aging reports. To successfully post payments, the MOS must have knowledge of insurance companies and contract payers. The MOS must also be able to recognize and understand an Explanation of Benefits (EOB) form.

Nowadays, most entering of patient information and posting of transactions is done using medical practice management software. There are many medical software programs for providers to choose from. Examples of medical practice management software packages are Medisoft, MedicsElite, Mysis Healthcare Systems, Centricity Practice Solutions, and AdvanceMD. Appendix I provides an introduction to Medisoft Advanced.

This chapter will familiarize the student with some of the generic tasks involved in the use of such software. Each medical software program will have its own commands and formats unique to that software, but the steps are generally the same. Review Appendix I prior to begining the office simulation to familiaize yourself with some of the basic tasks the MOS should be able to perform with medical practice management software.

Simulation Instructions

For this medical practice management office simulation, you are the medical office specialist for your medical practice. It is your job to enter all patient demographic information and post charges, payments, and adjustments using computer software.

New patients will need to be entered into the patient list database. The patient's name, address, telephone number, insurance information, employer name and address, and any other pertinent information from the Patient Information Form needs to be entered. Insurance information should match exactly what is printed on the patient insurance identification card.

When posting transactions, it may be necessary to enter the ICD-9 and CPT® codes and charges exactly as they appear on the superbills. This may require you to enter the codes into the database (as a new code) as well as the specific patient's account. The medical practice management (MPM) software you are using may already have all codes entered into the database. Your instructor will provide you with the directions for either entering or searching for the correct code(s).

You are responsible for printing a **walkout receipt** (a record of the patient's financial transactions for the encounter) for each patient account to which you post charges. It is your responsibility to balance your batch at the end of each day and to print insurance claim forms for the patients who are covered by insurance.

Before class ends each day, you may be instructed to stop posting transactions and **"batch out"**. Batching out is when you calculate all monies received, tally all cash on

CPT is a registered trademark of the American Medical Association.

hand and compare your totals with the Patient Day Sheet report totals. Access the **Reports** menu and run the **Patient Day Sheet** report for today's date. After printing your report, you will use it to make sure you "balance." To do this, you must separately add up all of the charges, payments, and adjustments from all of the superbills (or EOBs) you posted during the day. Your charges should add up to the amount on the **Total Charges** line on the Patient Day Sheet report. Your payments should equal the negative amount on the **Total Receipts** line of the report, and your adjustments should match the **Total Adjustments** line. If the amounts you totaled from your super-bills/EOBs do not match the report totals, you will need to go over the report patient by patient as you look at each patient superbill/EOB to find the discrepancy. After you have balanced your totals, your instructor may require you to batch your super-bills/EOBs and correct Patient Day Sheet report together and turn them in before you leave each day. If this is the case, it means you will have to remove or copy the super-bills/EOBs you posted from your textbook. The Patient Day Sheet report is to be placed on top of your superbills/EOBs, followed by your walkout receipts, and stapled together.

Once your batch is complete, it is time to create insurance claims for the patients for whom you entered transaction information. All medical software programs allow you to view your insurance claims on screen prior to printing them or sending them electronically. You must look over the claims on the computer screen to make sure there are no errors. If you find any errors, close the claims window and go back to the specific patient's account in the computer and correct it. The claim will automatically be updated with the corrected information. Check your electronic claim batch again to make sure all claims are correct. When you are sure there are no errors, print the claims.

Paper clip your CMS-1500 forms to the bottom of your batch material and turn it in to your instructor.

Before beginning the simulation, you will need to enter the physician's information if it has not been preprogrammed into the MPM software. Open the **Provider List** and click **New**.

Enter the following information in the **Provider List** window:

Enter your own name as the provider's name.		
1933 E. Frankford Rd., #110	Office Phone: 972-555-5482	Home Phone: 214-555-8888
Carrollton, TX 12345	Cell Phone: 469-555-3657	Fax: 972-555-5416
Medicare Participating, Signature on File		License No.: B1740
Specialty: General Practice		
In the **Default PINs** folder enter 75-1234567 for Federal Tax ID Indicator.		
Medicare PIN: B94765	Medicaid: K89J2	UPIN: B94765

Be sure to save any data entered. All of the patients you enter during the simulation will be seeing you.

You are ready to begin the simulation. Please use the following cases (patient registration, encounter, and EOB forms) to complete the simulation.

If at any time you have a question, do not hesitate to ask your instructor. Do not worry if the person seated next to you is farther in the textbook than you are. Concentrate on being accurate.

Allied Medical Center
REGISTRATION FORM
(Please Print)

Today's date: _____   PCP: _____

PATIENT INFORMATION

Patient's last name: DUPONT	First: MARGARET	Middle: B	☐ Mr. ☒ Mrs.	☐ Miss ☐ Ms.	Marital status (circle one) Single / (Mar) / Div / Sep / Wid

Is this your legal name? ☒ Yes ☐ No	If not, what is your legal name?	(Former name):	Birth date: 09/21/1946	Age:	Sex: ☐ M ☒ F

Street address: 12 BRIAR LANE	Social Security no.: 717-87-0054	Home phone no.: (214) 555-9871

P.O. box:	City: DALLAS	State: TX	ZIP Code: 12345

Occupation: MANAGER	Employer: SHARON'S BRIDAL SHOPPE	Employer phone no.: (214) 555-8878

Chose clinic because/Referred to clinic by (please check one box):	☐ Dr.	☒ Insurance Plan	☐ Hospital

☐ Family	☐ Friend	☐ Close to home/work	☐ Yellow Pages	Other

Other family members seen here:
LISA DUPONT   **REASON FOR THIS VISIT:** Persistent cough

INSURANCE INFORMATION

(Please give your insurance card to the receptionist.)

Person responsible for bill: SELF	Birth date: / /	Address (if different):	Home phone no.: ( )

Is this person a patient here? ☒ Yes ☐ No			

Occupation:	Employer:	Employer address:	Employer phone no.: ( )

Is this patient covered by insurance? ☒ Yes ☐ No			

Please indicate primary insurance:	PHYSICIAN ALLIANCE PPO	Claims Mailing Address:	P O BOX 1256	Philadelphia, PA	12345
		PHONE: 800-555-5522			

Subscriber's name: SELF	Subscriber's S.S. no.:	Birth date: / /	☐ M ☒ F	Group no.: A435	Policy no.: 621382	Co-payment: $10.00

Patient's relationship to subscriber: ☒ Self ☐ Spouse ☐ Child ☐ Other

Name of secondary insurance (if applicable): BLUE CROSS BLUE SHIELD TX PPO	Subscriber's name and DOB: FRANK DUPONT 07/21/1941	☒ M ☐ F	Group no.: 126	Policy no.: BHR716830061

Patient's relationship to subscriber: ☐ Self ☒ Spouse ☐ Child ☐ Other Claims Mailing Address: P O BOX 660044 DALLAS 12345

IN CASE OF EMERGENCY

Name of local friend or relative (not living at same address): SHARON THELANER	Relationship to patient: SISTER	Home phone no.: (469) 555-3259	Work phone no.: (817) 555-8114

The above information is true to the best of my knowledge. I authorize my insurance benefits to be paid directly to the physician. I understand that I am financially responsible for any balance. I also authorize ALLIED MEDICAL CENTER or insurance company to release any information required to process my claims.

Maggie Dupont

_____   _____
Patient/Guardian signature   Date

ENCOUNTER FORM

Patient Information		Payment Method		Visit Information	
Patient ID number		**Primary**	Physician's Alliance	Visit date	
Patient name	Margaret Dupont	Primary ID number	621382	Visit number	
Address	12 Briar Lane	Primary group number	A435	Rendering physician	
City/State	Dallas, TX 12345	**Secondary**	BCBS TX	Referring physician	
Phone number	214-555-9871	Secondary ID number	BHR716830061	Reason for visit	Cough
Date of birth	09/21/1946	Secondary group no.	126		
Age		Cash/credit card			
		Other billing			

E/M Modifiers	Procedure Modifiers	DIAGNOSIS:
21 — Prolonged E&M Service	22 — Unusual, excessive procedure	
24 — Unrelated E/M service during postop.	50 — Bilateral procedure	ACUTE SINUSITIS 461.9
25 — Significant, separately identifiable E/M	51 — Multiple surgical procedures in same day	
32 — Mandated Service	52 — Reduced/incomplete procedure	
57 — Decision for surgery	55 — Postop. management only	
	59 — Distinct multiple procedures	

CATEGORY	CODE	MOD	FEE	CATEGORY	CODE	MOD	FEE
Office Visit — New Patient				**Wound Care**			
Minimal office visit	99201			Debride partial thickness burn	11040		
20 minutes	99202			Debride full thickness burn	11041		
30 minutes	99203			Debride wound, not a burn	11000		
45 minutes	99204	X	135.00	Unna boot application	29580		
60 minutes	99205			Unna boot removal	29700		
Other				Other			
Office Visit — Established				**Supplies**			
Minimal office visit	99211			Ace bandage, 2"	A6448		
10 minutes	99212			Ace bandage, 3"-4"	A6449		
15 minutes	99213			Ace bandage, 6"	A6450		
25 minutes	99214			Cast, fiberglass	A4590		
40 minutes	99215			Coban wrap	A6454		
Other				Foley catheter	A4338		
General Procedures				Immobilizer	L3670		
Anoscopy	46600			Kerlix roll	A6220		
Audiometry	92551			Oxygen mask/cannula	A4620		
Breast aspiration	19000			Sleeve, elbow	E0191		
Cerumen removal	69210			Sling	A4565		
Circumcision	54150			Splint, ready-made	A4570		
DDST	96110			Splint, wrist	S8451		
Flex sigmoidoscopy	45330			Sterile packing	A6407		
Flex sig. w/ biopsy	45331			Surgical tray	A4550		
Foreign body removal—foot	28190			Other			
Nail removal	11730			OB Care			
Nail removal/phenol	11750			Routine OB care	59400		
Trigger point injection	20552			Postpartum care only (separate procedure)	59430		
Tympanometry	92567			Ante partum 4–6 visits	59425		
Visual acuity	99173			Ante partum 7 or more visits	59426		
Other				Other			
Other				Other			

Other Visit Information: _____

Lab Work to Order: _____

Referral to: _____

Provider Signature: _____

Next Appointment: _____ RETURN IN A FEW DAYS IF NOT BETTER _____

Fees:

Total Charges: $ 135.00
Copay Received: $ 10.00
Other Payment: $_____
Total Due: **$125.00**

Allied Medical Center 1933 E. Frankford Rd. Carrollton, TX 12345 **972-555-5482**

Allied Medical Center
REGISTRATION FORM
(Please Print)

Today's date: _____   PCP: _____

PATIENT INFORMATION

Patient's last name:	First:	Middle:	☐ Mr.	☒ Miss	Marital status (circle one)
DUPONT	LISA	M	☐ Mrs.	☐ Ms.	(Single) / Mar / Div / Sep / Wid

Is this your legal name?	If not, what is your legal name?	(Former name):	Birth date:	Age:	Sex:
☒ Yes ☐ No			06/03/1996		☐ M ☒ F

Street address:	Social Security no.:	Home phone no.:
12 BRIAR LANE	212-55-3311	(214) 555-9871

P.O. box:	City:	State:	ZIP Code:
	DALLAS	TX	12345

Occupation:	Employer:	Employer phone no.:
STUDENT		( )

Chose clinic because/Referred to clinic by (please check one box):	☐ Dr.	☒ Insurance Plan	☐ Hospital
☐ Family ☐ Friend ☐ Close to home/work ☐ Yellow Pages Other			

Other family members seen here:	
MARGARET DUPONT	**REASON FOR THIS VISIT:** School physical

INSURANCE INFORMATION

(Please give your insurance card to the receptionist.)

Person responsible for bill:	Birth date:	Address (if different):	Home phone no.:
FRANK DUPONT	07/21/1941	SAME	( ) SAME

Is this person a patient here?	☐ Yes	☒ No

Occupation:	Employer:	Employer address:	Employer phone no.:
ACCOUNTANT	MASTERLOCK	1902 CROSBY RD CARROLLTON TX 12345	(972) 555-3211

Is this patient covered by insurance?	☒ Yes	☐ No

Please indicate primary insurance:	BLUE CROSS BLUE SHIELD TX PPO	Claims Mailing Address:	P O BOX 660044	DALLAS, TX	12345
		PHONE: 800-555-4563			

Subscriber's name:	Subscriber's S.S. no.:	Birth date:	☒ M ☐ F	Group no.:	Policy no.:	Co-payment:
FRANK DUPONT	716-83-0061	07/21/1941		126	BHR716830061	$12.00

Patient's relationship to subscriber:	☐ Self	☐ Spouse	☒ Child	☐ Other

Name of secondary insurance (if applicable):	Subscriber's name and DOB:	☐ M ☒ F	Group no.:	Policy no.:
PHYSICIAN ALLIANCE PPO	MARGARET DUPONT 09/21/1946		A435	621382

Patient's relationship to subscriber:	☐ Self	☐ Spouse	☒ Child	☐ Other Claims Mailing Address: P O BOX 1256 PHILA PA 12345

IN CASE OF EMERGENCY

Name of local friend or relative (not living at same address):	Relationship to patient:	Home phone no.:	Work phone no.:
SHARON THELANER	AUNT	(469) 555-3259	(817) 555-8114

The above information is true to the best of my knowledge. I authorize my insurance benefits to be paid directly to the physician. I understand that I am financially responsible for any balance. I also authorize ALLIED MEDICAL CENTER or insurance company to release any information required to process my claims.

Frank Dupont

Patient/Guardian signature   _Date_

ENCOUNTER FORM

Patient Information		Payment Method		Visit Information	
Patient ID number		**Primary**	BCBS TX	Visit date	
Patient name	Lisa Dupont	Primary ID number	BHR716830061	Visit number	
Address	12 Briar Lane	Primary group number	126	Rendering physician	
City/State	Dallas, TX 12345	**Secondary**	Physician's Alliance	Referring physician	
Phone number	214-555-9871	Secondary ID number	621382	Reason for visit	Well-child exam
Date of birth	06/03/1993	Secondary group no.	A435		
Age		Cash/credit card			
		Other billing			

E/M Modifiers	Procedure Modifiers	DIAGNOSIS:
21 — Prolonged E&M Service	22 — Unusual, excessive procedure	Normal state — V65.5
24 — Unrelated E/M service during postop.	50 — Bilateral procedure	Immunization — V05.9
25 — Significant, separately identifiable E/M	51 — Multiple surgical procedures in same day	
32 — Mandated Service	52 — Reduced/incomplete procedure	
57 — Decision for surgery	55 — Postop. management only	
	59 — Distinct multiple procedures	

CATEGORY	CODE	MOD	FEE	CATEGORY	CODE	MOD	FEE
Office Visit — New Patient				**Wound Care**			
Minimal office visit	99201			Debride partial thickness burn	11040		
20 minutes	99202			Debride full thickness burn	11041		
30 minutes	99203	X	120.00	Debride wound, not a burn	11000		
45 minutes	99204			Unna boot application	29580		
60 minutes	99205			Unna boot removal	29700		
Other				Other			
Office Visit — Established				**Supplies**			
Minimal office visit	99211			Ace bandage, 2"	A6448		
10 minutes	99212			Ace bandage, 3"-4"	A6449		
15 minutes	99213			Ace bandage, 6"	A6450		
25 minutes	99214			Cast, fiberglass	A4590		
40 minutes	99215			Coban wrap	A6454		
Other				Foley catheter	A4338		
General Procedures				Immobilizer	L3670		
Anoscopy	46600			Kerlix roll	A6220		
Audiometry	92551			Oxygen mask/cannula	A4620		
Breast aspiration	19000			Sleeve, elbow	E0191		
Cerumen removal	69210			Sling	A4565		
Circumcision	54150			Splint, ready-made	A4570		
DDST	96110			Splint, wrist	S8451		
Flex sigmoidoscopy	45330			Sterile packing	A6407		
Flex sig. w/ biopsy	45331			Surgical tray	A4550		
Foreign body removal—foot	28190			Other			
Nail removal	11730			**OB Care**			
Nail removal/phenol	11750			Routine OB care	59400		
Trigger point injection	20552			Postpartum care only (separate procedure)	59430		
Tympanometry	92567			Ante partum 4–6 visits	59425		
Visual acuity	99173			Ante partum 7 or more visits	59426		
Other	90707	X	30.00	Other			
Other				Other			

Other Visit Information:

Lab Work to Order: _____

Referral to: _____

Provider Signature: _____

Next Appointment: _____

Fees:

Total Charges: $150.00

Copay Received: $ 12.00

Other Payment: $_____

Total Due: **$138.00**

Allied Medical Center 1933 E. Frankford Rd. Carrollton, TX 12345 **972-555-5482**

Allied Medical Center
REGISTRATION FORM
(Please Print)

Today's date: _____   PCP: _____

PATIENT INFORMATION

Patient's last name:	First:	Middle:	☐ Mr.	☒ Miss	Marital status (circle one)
SMYTH	SAMANTHA	M	☐ Mrs.	☐ Ms.	(Single) / Mar / Div / Sep / Wid

Is this your legal name?	If not, what is your legal name?	(Former name):	Birth date:	Age:	Sex:
☒ Yes ☐ No			03/17/1968		☐ M ☒ F

Street address:		Social Security no.:	Home phone no.:
9401 Winding Valley		455-94-8204	(972) 555-9871

P.O. box:	City:	State:	ZIP Code:
	PLANO	TX	12345

Occupation:	Employer:	Employer phone no.:
FOOD SERVER	WENDY'S HAMBURGERS	(972) 555-8936

Chose clinic because/Referred to clinic by (please check one box):	☐ Dr.	☐ Insurance Plan	☐ Hospital
☐ Family ☒ Friend ☐ Close to home/work	☐ Yellow Pages	Other	

Other family members seen here: _____   **REASON FOR THIS VISIT:** Cholesterol check

INSURANCE INFORMATION

(Please give your insurance card to the receptionist.)

Person responsible for bill:	Birth date:	Address (if different):	Home phone no.:
SAMANTHA SMYTH	03/17/1968	same	( )

Is this person a patient here?   ☒ Yes   ☐ No

Occupation:	Employer:	Employer address:	Employer phone no.:
			( )

Is this patient covered by insurance?   ☐ Yes   ☒ No

Please indicate primary insurance:	NONE	Claims Mailing Address:		
		PHONE:		

Subscriber's name:	Subscriber's S.S. no.:	Birth date:	☐ M ☐ F	Group no.:	Policy no.:	Co-payment:
		/ /				$

Patient's relationship to subscriber: ☐ Self   ☐ Spouse   ☐ Child   ☐ Other

Name of secondary insurance (if applicable):	Subscriber's name and DOB:	☐ M ☐ F	Group no.:	Policy no.:

Patient's relationship to subscriber: ☐ Self   ☐ Spouse   ☐ Child   ☐ Other   Claims Mailing Address:

IN CASE OF EMERGENCY

Name of local friend or relative (not living at same address):	Relationship to patient:	Home phone no.:	Work phone no.:
CARRIE TINKHAM	FRIEND	(972) 555-1502	(972) 555-0074

The above information is true to the best of my knowledge. I authorize my insurance benefits to be paid directly to the physician. I understand that I am financially responsible for any balance. I also authorize ALLIED MEDICAL CENTER or insurance company to release any information required to process my claims.

Samantha Smyth
_____   _____
Patient/Guardian signature   Date

ENCOUNTER FORM

Patient Information		Payment Method		Visit Information	
Patient ID number		**Primary**		Visit date	
Patient name	Samantha Smyth	Primary ID number		Visit number	
Address	9401 Winding Valley	Primary group number		Rendering physician	
City/State	Plano, TX 12345	**Secondary**		Referring physician	
Phone number	972-555-9871	Secondary ID number		Reason for visit	Cholesterol Check
Date of birth	03/17/1968	Secondary group no.			
Age		Cash/credit card	CHECK		
		Other billing			

E/M Modifiers	Procedure Modifiers	DIAGNOSIS:
21 — Prolonged E&M Service	22 — Unusual, excessive procedure	Hypercholesteremia 272.00
24 — Unrelated E/M service during postop.	50 — Bilateral procedure	
25 — Significant, separately identifiable E/M	51 — Multiple surgical procedures in same day	
32 — Mandated Service	52 — Reduced/incomplete procedure	
57 — Decision for surgery	55 — Postop. management only	
	59 — Distinct multiple procedures	

CATEGORY	CODE	MOD	FEE	CATEGORY	CODE	MOD	FEE
Office Visit — New Patient				**Wound Care**			
Minimal office visit	99201			Debride partial thickness burn	11040		
20 minutes	99202			Debride full thickness burn	11041		
30 minutes	99203			Debride wound, not a burn	11000		
45 minutes	99204			Unna boot application	29580		
60 minutes	99205			Unna boot removal	29700		
Other				Other			
Office Visit — Established				**Supplies**			
Minimal office visit	99211			Ace bandage, 2"	A6448		
10 minutes	99212	X	35.00	Ace bandage, 3"-4"	A6449		
15 minutes	99213			Ace bandage, 6"	A6450		
25 minutes	99214			Cast, fiberglass	A4590		
40 minutes	99215			Coban wrap	A6454		
Other				Foley catheter	A4338		
General Procedures				Immobilizer	L3670		
Anoscopy	46600			Kerlix roll	A6220		
Audiometry	92551			Oxygen mask/cannula	A4620		
Breast aspiration	19000			Sleeve, elbow	E0191		
Cerumen removal	69210			Sling	A4565		
Circumcision	54150			Splint, ready-made	A4570		
DDST	96110			Splint, wrist	S8451		
Flex sigmoidoscopy	45330			Sterile packing	A6407		
Flex sig. w/ biopsy	45331			Surgical tray	A4550		
Foreign body removal—foot	28190			Other			
Nail removal	11730			OB Care			
Nail removal/phenol	11750			Routine OB care	59400		
Trigger point injection	20552			Postpartum care only (separate procedure)	59430		
Tympanometry	92567			Ante partum 4–6 visits	59425		
Visual acuity	99173			Ante partum 7 or more visits	59426		
Other	82465	X	30.00	Other			
Other				Other			

Other Visit Information: _____

Lab Work to Order: _____
Referral to: _____
Provider Signature: _____
Next Appointment: _____ RETURN IN A FEW DAYS IF NOT BETTER _____

Fees:
Total Charges: $65.00
Copay Received: $____
Other Payment: $65.00 CK #1235
Total Due: $0

Allied Medical Center 1933 E. Frankford Rd. Carrollton, TX 12345 **972-555-5482**

Allied Medical Center
REGISTRATION FORM
(Please Print)

Today's date: _____   PCP: _____

PATIENT INFORMATION

Patient's last name: BAILEY	First: EILEEN	Middle: B	☐ Mr. ☐ Mrs.	☐ Miss ☒ Ms.	Marital status (circle one) Single / Mar / Div / Sep /(Wid)

Is this your legal name? ☒ Yes ☐ No	If not, what is your legal name?	(Former name): EILEEN STANFORD	Birth date: 04/26/1961	Age:	Sex: ☐ M ☒ F

Street address: 2531 BENT TREE COURT		Social Security no.: 555-63-2112	Home phone no.: (972) 555-6058

P.O. box:	City: DALLAS	State: TX	ZIP Code: 12345

Occupation: SUPERVISOR	Employer: DISCOUNT COMPUTER WAREHOUSE	Employer phone no.: (972) 555-6577

Chose clinic because/Referred to clinic by (please check one box):	☐ Dr.	☒ Insurance Plan	☐ Hospital
☐ Family ☐ Friend ☐ Close to home/work	☐ Yellow Pages	Other	

Other family members seen here: _____   **REASON FOR THIS VISIT:** Yearly Physical

INSURANCE INFORMATION
(Please give your insurance card to the receptionist.)

Person responsible for bill: EILEEN BAILEY	Birth date: / /	Address (if different): Same	Home phone no.: ( )

Is this person a patient here?   ☒ Yes   ☐ No

Occupation:	Employer:	Employer address:	Employer phone no.: ( )

Is this patient covered by insurance?   ☒ Yes   ☐ No

Please indicate primary insurance:	PHYSICIAN'S CHOICE EPO	Claims Mailing Address:	P O BOX 9873	Dover, OH	12345
		PHONE: 800-555-8637			

Subscriber's name: EILEEN BAILEY	Subscriber's S.S. no.: 555-63-2112	Birth date: 04/26/1961	☐ M ☐ F	Group no.: K1047	Policy no.: 13056	Co-payment: $

Patient's relationship to subscriber: ☒ Self   ☐ Spouse   ☐ Child   ☐ Other

Name of secondary insurance (if applicable):	Subscriber's name and DOB:	☐ M ☐ F	Group no.:	Policy no.:

Patient's relationship to subscriber: ☐ Self   ☐ Spouse   ☐ Child   ☐ Other Claims Address:

IN CASE OF EMERGENCY

Name of local friend or relative (not living at same address): MALCOLM JOHNSON	Relationship to patient: FRIEND	Home phone no.: (214) 555-5277	Work phone no.: (214) 555-8788

The above information is true to the best of my knowledge. I authorize my insurance benefits to be paid directly to the physician. I understand that I am financially responsible for any balance. I also authorize ALLIED MEDICAL CENTER or insurance company to release any information required to process my claims.

Eileen Bailey

_____   _____
Patient/Guardian signature   *Date*

ENCOUNTER FORM

Patient Information		Payment Method		Visit Information	
Patient ID number		**Primary**		Visit date	
Patient name	Eileen Bailey	Primary ID number	Physician's Choice EPO	Visit number	
Address	2531 Bent Tree Ct	Primary group number	13056	Rendering physician	
City/State	Dallas, TX 12345	**Secondary**	K1047	Referring physician	
Phone number	972-555-6058	Secondary ID number		Reason for visit	Yearly Physical
Date of birth	04/26/1961	Secondary group no.			
Age		Cash/credit card	CHECK		
		Other billing			

E/M Modifiers	Procedure Modifiers	DIAGNOSIS:
21 — Prolonged E&M Service	22 — Unusual, excessive procedure	Routine Exam V70.0
24 — Unrelated E/M service during postop.	50 — Bilateral procedure	
25 — Significant, separately identifiable E/M	51 — Multiple surgical procedures in same day	
32 — Mandated Service	52 — Reduced/incomplete procedure	
57 — Decision for surgery	55 — Postop. management only	
	59 — Distinct multiple procedures	

CATEGORY	CODE	MOD	FEE	CATEGORY	CODE	MOD	FEE
Office Visit — New Patient				**Wound Care**			
Minimal office visit	99201			Debride partial thickness burn	11040		
20 minutes	99202			Debride full thickness burn	11041		
30 minutes	99203			Debride wound, not a burn	11000		
45 minutes	99204			Unna boot application	29580		
60 minutes	99205	X	160.00	Unna boot removal	29700		
Other				Other			
Office Visit — Established				**Supplies**			
Minimal office visit	99211			Ace bandage, 2"	A6448		
10 minutes	99212			Ace bandage, 3"-4"	A6449		
15 minutes	99213			Ace bandage, 6"	A6450		
25 minutes	99214			Cast, fiberglass	A4590		
40 minutes	99215			Coban wrap	A6454		
Other				Foley catheter	A4338		
General Procedures				Immobilizer	L3670		
Anoscopy	46600			Kerlix roll	A6220		
Audiometry	92551			Oxygen mask/cannula	A4620		
Breast aspiration	19000			Sleeve, elbow	E0191		
Cerumen removal	69210			Sling	A4565		
Circumcision	54150			Splint, ready-made	A4570		
DDST	96110			Splint, wrist	S8451		
Flex sigmoidoscopy	45330			Sterile packing	A6407		
Flex sig. w/ biopsy	45331			Surgical tray	A4550		
Foreign body removal—foot	28190			Other			
Nail removal	11730			OB Care			
Nail removal/phenol	11750			Routine OB care	59400		
Trigger point injection	20552			Postpartum care only (separate procedure)	59430		
Tympanometry	92567			Ante partum 4–6 visits	59425		
Visual acuity	99173			Ante partum 7 or more visits	59426		
Other	82465			Other			
Other				Other			

Other Visit Information: _____

Lab Work to Order: _____

Referral to: _____

Provider Signature: _____

Next Appointment: _____ AS NEEDED _____

Fees:

Total Charges: $160.00

Copay Received: $ 32.00

Other Payment: $_____

Total Due: $128.00

Allied Medical Center 1933 E. Frankford Rd. Carrollton, TX 12345 **972-555-5482**

Allied Medical Center
REGISTRATION FORM
(Please Print)

Today's date:	PCP:

PATIENT INFORMATION

Patient's last name: CATHER	First: JIM	Middle: S	☒ Mr. ❑ Mrs.	❑ Miss ❑ Ms.	Marital status (circle one) Single / (Mar) / Div / Sep / Wid

Is this your legal name? ☒ Yes ❑ No	If not, what is your legal name? JAMES CATHER	(Former name):	Birth date: 10/01/1953	Age:	Sex: ☒ M ❑ F

Street address: 425 LAVENDER STREET	Social Security no.: 188-38-3833	Home phone no.: (972) 555-3394

P.O. box:	City: GARLAND	State: TX	ZIP Code: 12345

Occupation: SALESPERSON	Employer: MERRY MILER VANS	Employer phone no.: (972) 555-3337

Chose clinic because/Referred to clinic by (please check one box):	☒ Dr. LESLIE MCNEICE	❑ Insurance Plan	❑ Hospital

❑ Family	❑ Friend	❑ Close to home/work	❑ Yellow Pages	Other **AUTH # A569874, 30 DAYS, 3 VISITS**

Other family members seen here: **REASON FOR THIS VISIT:** Hyperglycemia check up

INSURANCE INFORMATION
(Please give your insurance card to the receptionist.)

Person responsible for bill: JIM CATHER	Birth date: / /	Address (if different): SAME	Home phone no.: ( )

Is this person a patient here?	☒ Yes	❑ No	

Occupation:	Employer:	Employer address:	Employer phone no.: ( )

Is this patient covered by insurance?	☒ Yes	❑ No

Please indicate primary insurance:	PHYSICIAN'S ALLIANCE HMO	Claims Mailing Address:	P O BOX 65	TOLEDO, OH	12345

			PHONE: 800-555-9865		

Subscriber's name: SAME AS PATIENT	Subscriber's S.S. no.: 188-38-3833	Birth date: / /	❑ M ❑ F	Group no.: 145	Policy no.: 188383833	Co-payment: $25.00

Patient's relationship to subscriber:	☒ Self	❑ Spouse	❑ Child	❑ Other

Name of secondary insurance (if applicable):	Subscriber's name and DOB:	❑ M ❑ F	Group no.:	Policy no.:

Patient's relationship to subscriber:	❑ Self	❑ Spouse	❑ Child	❑ Other Claims Address:

IN CASE OF EMERGENCY

Name of local friend or relative (not living at same address): MARILYN CATHER	Relationship to patient: SIBLING	Home phone no.: (214) 555-3329	Work phone no.: (469) 555-8200

The above information is true to the best of my knowledge. I authorize my insurance benefits to be paid directly to the physician. I understand that I am financially responsible for any balance. I also authorize ALLIED MEDICAL CENTER or insurance company to release any information required to process my claims.

Jim Cather

Patient/Guardian signature   Date

ENCOUNTER FORM

Patient Information		Payment Method		Visit Information	
Patient ID number		**Primary**	Physician's Alliance HMO	Visit date	
Patient name	Jim Cather	Primary ID number	188383833	Visit number	
Address	425 Lavender St	Primary group number	145	Rendering physician	
City/State	Garland, TX 12345	**Secondary**		Referring physician	Leslie McNeice
Phone number	972-555-3394	Secondary ID number		Reason for visit	Hyperglyce-mia CK
Date of birth	10/01/1953	Secondary group no.			
Age		Cash/credit card			
		Other billing			

E/M Modifiers	Procedure Modifiers	DIAGNOSIS:
21 — Prolonged E&M Service	22 — Unusual, excessive procedure	Hyperglycemia 790.6
24 — Unrelated E/M service during postop.	50 — Bilateral procedure	
25 — Significant, separately identifiable E/M	51 — Multiple surgical procedures in same day	
32 — Mandated Service	52 — Reduced/incomplete procedure	
57 — Decision for surgery	55 — Postop. management only	
	59 — Distinct multiple procedures	

CATEGORY	CODE	MOD	FEE	CATEGORY	CODE	MOD	FEE
Office Visit — New Patient				**Wound Care**			
Minimal office visit	99201			Debride partial thickness burn	11040		
20 minutes	99202			Debride full thickness burn	11041		
30 minutes	99203			Debride wound, not a burn	11000		
45 minutes	99204			Unna boot application	29580		
60 minutes	99205			Unna boot removal	29700		
Other				Other			
Office Visit — Established				**Supplies**			
Minimal office visit	99211			Ace bandage, 2"	A6448		
10 minutes	99212			Ace bandage, 3"-4"	A6449		
15 minutes	99213			Ace bandage, 6"	A6450		
25 minutes	99214	X	65.00	Cast, fiberglass	A4590		
40 minutes	99215			Coban wrap	A6454		
Other				Foley catheter	A4338		
General Procedures				Immobilizer	L3670		
Anoscopy	46600			Kerlix roll	A6220		
Audiometry	92551			Oxygen mask/cannula	A4620		
Breast aspiration	19000			Sleeve, elbow	E0191		
Cerumen removal	69210			Sling	A4565		
Circumcision	54150			Splint, ready-made	A4570		
DDST	96110			Splint, wrist	S8451		
Flex sigmoidoscopy	45330			Sterile packing	A6407		
Flex sig. w/ biopsy	45331			Surgical tray	A4550		
Foreign body removal—foot	28190			Other			
Nail removal	11730			**OB Care**			
Nail removal/phenol	11750			Routine OB care	59400		
Trigger point injection	20552			Postpartum care only (separate procedure)	59430		
Tympanometry	92567			Ante partum 4–6 visits	59425		
Visual acuity	99173			Ante partum 7 or more visits	59426		
Other	93000	X	45.00	Other			
Other	82954	X	12.00	Other			

Other Visit Information: _____

Lab Work to Order: _____

Referral to: _____

Provider Signature: _____

Next Appointment: _____

Fees:

Total Charges: $122.00

Copay Received: $ 25.00

Other Payment: $_____

Total Due: **$97.00**

Allied Medical Center 1933 E. Frankford Rd. Carrollton, TX 12345 **972-555-5482**

Allied Medical Center
REGISTRATION FORM
(Please Print)

| Today's date: | | | PCP: | | |

PATIENT INFORMATION

Patient's last name: BAE	First: YONG	Middle: JOON	☒ Mr. ❑ Mrs.	❑ Miss ❑ Ms.	Marital status (circle one) Single / (Mar) / Div / Sep / Wid

Is this your legal name? ☒ Yes ❑ No	If not, what is your legal name?	(Former name):	Birth date: 02/23/1972	Age:	Sex: ☒ M ❑ F

Street address: 4549 EXPLORER DRIVE #110		Social Security no.: 661-39-2520	Home phone no.: (469) 555-0719

P.O. box:	City: FRISCO	State: TX	ZIP Code: 12345

Occupation: SUPERVISOR	Employer: SUGARLAND DAIRY FARM	Employer phone no.: (903) 555-8663

Chose clinic because/Referred to clinic by (please check one box):	☒ Dr. MALCOLM MAZOW	❑ Insurance Plan	❑ Hospital
❑ Family	❑ Friend	❑ Close to home/work	❑ Yellow Pages	❑ Other REFERRAL # FOR TODAY–1644401

Other family members seen here:	REASON FOR THIS VISIT: Shoulder Pain

INSURANCE INFORMATION

(Please give your insurance card to the receptionist.)

Person responsible for bill: PATIENT	Birth date: / /	Address (if different): SAME	Home phone no.: ( )

Is this person a patient here?	☒ Yes	❑ No

Occupation:	Employer:	Employer address:	Employer phone no.: ( )

Is this patient covered by insurance?	☒ Yes	❑ No

Please indicate primary insurance:	METLIFE HMO	Claims Mailing Address:	P O BOX 6983	NEWARK, DE	12345
		PHONE: 800-555-6897			

Subscriber's name: SELF	Subscriber's S.S. no.: 661-39-2520	Birth date: / /	❑ M ❑ F	Group no.: 62440	Policy no.: 661392520-01	Co-payment: $10.00

Patient's relationship to subscriber:	☒ Self	❑ Spouse	❑ Child	❑ Other

Name of secondary insurance (if applicable):	Subscriber's name and DOB:	❑ M ❑ F	Group no.:	Policy no.:

Patient's relationship to subscriber:	❑ Self	❑ Spouse	❑ Child	❑ Other Claims Address:

IN CASE OF EMERGENCY

Name of local friend or relative (not living at same address): YUJIN JEONG	Relationship to patient: MOTHER	Home phone no.: (214) 650-9801	Work phone no.: ( )

The above information is true to the best of my knowledge. I authorize my insurance benefits to be paid directly to the physician. I understand that I am financially responsible for any balance. I also authorize ALLIED MEDICAL CENTER or insurance company to release any information required to process my claims.

Yong Joon Bae

Patient/Guardian signature	Date

ENCOUNTER FORM

Patient Information		Payment Method		Visit Information	
Patient ID number		**Primary**	MetLife HMO	Visit date	
Patient name	Yong Joon Bae	Primary ID number	661392520-01	Visit number	
Address	4549 Explorer Dr	Primary group number	62440	Rendering physician	
City/State	Frisco, TX 12345	**Secondary**		Referring physician	Malcolm Mazow
Phone number	469-555-0719	Secondary ID number		Reason for visit	Shoulder Pain
Date of birth	02/23/1972	Secondary group no.			**Auth # for today: 1644401**
Age		Cash/credit card			
		Other billing			

E/M Modifiers	Procedure Modifiers	DIAGNOSIS:
21 — Prolonged E&M Service	22 — Unusual, excessive procedure	Bursitis, Shoulder 726.10
24 — Unrelated E/M service during postop.	50 — Bilateral procedure	
25 — Significant, separately identifiable E/M	51 — Multiple surgical procedures in same day	
32 — Mandated Service	52 — Reduced/incomplete procedure	
57 — Decision for surgery	55 — Postop. management only	
	59 — Distinct multiple procedures	

CATEGORY	CODE	MOD	FEE	CATEGORY	CODE	MOD	FEE
Office Visit — New Patient				**Wound Care**			
Minimal office visit	99201			Debride partial thickness burn	11040		
20 minutes	99202			Debride full thickness burn	11041		
30 minutes	99203			Debride wound, not a burn	11000		
45 minutes	99204			Unna boot application	29580		
60 minutes	99205			Unna boot removal	29700		
Other				Other			
Office Visit — Established				**Supplies**			
Minimal office visit	99211			Ace bandage, 2"	A6448		
10 minutes	99212			Ace bandage, 3"-4"	A6449		
15 minutes	99213	X	45.00	Ace bandage, 6"	A6450		
25 minutes	99214			Cast, fiberglass	A4590		
40 minutes	99215			Coban wrap	A6454		
Other				Foley catheter	A4338		
General Procedures				Immobilizer	L3670		
Anoscopy	46600			Kerlix roll	A6220		
Audiometry	92551			Oxygen mask/cannula	A4620		
Breast aspiration	19000			Sleeve, elbow	E0191		
Cerumen removal	69210			Sling	A4565		
Circumcision	54150			Splint, ready-made	A4570		
DDST	96110			Splint, wrist	S8451		
Flex sigmoidoscopy	45330			Sterile packing	A6407		
Flex sig. w/ biopsy	45331			Surgical tray	A4550		
Foreign body removal—foot	28190			Other			
Nail removal	11730			**OB Care**			
Nail removal/phenol	11750			Routine OB care	59400		
Trigger point injection	20552			Postpartum care only (separate procedure)	59430		
Tympanometry	92567			Ante partum 4–6 visits	59425		
Visual acuity	99173			Ante partum 7 or more visits	59426		
Other				Other			
Other				Other			

Other Visit Information: _____

Lab Work to Order: _____

Referral to: _____

Provider Signature: _____

Next Appointment: _____

Fees:

Total Charges: $45.00

Copay Received: $10.00

Other Payment: $_____

Total Due: **$35.00**

Allied Medical Center 1933 E. Frankford Rd. Carrollton, TX 12345 **972-555-5482**

Allied Medical Center
REGISTRATION FORM
(Please Print)

Today's date:	PCP:

PATIENT INFORMATION

Patient's last name: BAE	First: JOANNE	Middle:	☐ Mr. ☒ Mrs.	☐ Miss ☐ Ms.	Marital status (circle one) Single / (Mar) / Div / Sep / Wid		
Is this your legal name? ☒ Yes ☐ No	If not, what is your legal name?		(Former name):		Birth date: 01/16/1974	Age:	Sex: ☐ M ☒ F
Street address: 4549 EXPLORER DRIVE			Social Security no.: 401-63-4272			Home phone no.: (469) 555-0719	
P.O. box:	City: FRISCO			State: TX		ZIP Code: 12345	
Occupation: HOMEMAKER	Employer:				Employer phone no.: ( )		

Chose clinic because/Referred to clinic by (please check one box):	☒ Dr. MALCOLM MAZOW	☐ Insurance Plan	☐ Hospital
☐ Family ☐ Friend ☐ Close to home/work	☐ Yellow Pages	Other **REFERRAL # FOR TODAY: 1644404**	

Other family members seen here: YONG JOON BAE	**REASON FOR THIS VISIT:** Coughing, fever

INSURANCE INFORMATION

(Please give your insurance card to the receptionist.)

Person responsible for bill: JOANNE BAE	Birth date: / /	Address (if different): SAME	Home phone no.: ( )
Is this person a patient here? ☒ Yes ☐ No			
Occupation:	Employer:	Employer address:	Employer phone no.: ( )
Is this patient covered by insurance? ☒ Yes ☐ No			

Please indicate primary insurance:	METLIFE HMO	Claims Mailing Address:	P O BOX 6983	NEWARK, DE	12345
		PHONE: 800-555-6897			

Subscriber's name: YONG JOON BAE	Subscriber's S.S. no.: 661-39-2520	Birth date: 02/23/1972	☐ M ☐ F	Group no.: 62440	Policy no.: 661392520-02	Co-payment: $10.00
Patient's relationship to subscriber: ☐ Self ☒ Spouse ☐ Child ☐ Other						
Name of secondary insurance (if applicable):		Subscriber's name and DOB:	☐ M ☐ F	Group no.:	Policy no.:	
Patient's relationship to subscriber: ☐ Self ☐ Spouse ☐ Child ☐ Other Claims Address:						

IN CASE OF EMERGENCY

Name of local friend or relative (not living at same address): YUJIN JEONG	Relationship to patient: MOTHER IN LAW	Home phone no.: (214) 555-9801	Work phone no.: ( )

The above information is true to the best of my knowledge. I authorize my insurance benefits to be paid directly to the physician. I understand that I am financially responsible for any balance. I also authorize ALLIED MEDICAL CENTER or insurance company to release any information required to process my claims.

Joanne Bae

Patient/Guardian signature   _Date_

ENCOUNTER FORM

Patient Information		Payment Method		Visit Information	
Patient ID number		**Primary**	MetLife HMO	Visit date	
Patient name	Joanne Bae	Primary ID number	661392520-02	Visit number	
Address	4549 Explorer Dr	Primary group number	62440	Rendering physician	
City/State	Frisco, TX 12345	**Secondary**		Referring physician	
Phone number	469-555-0719	Secondary ID number		Reason for visit	Coughing, fever
Date of birth	01/16/1974	Secondary group no.			**Auth # for today: 164404**
Age		Cash/credit card			
		Other billing			

E/M Modifiers	Procedure Modifiers	DIAGNOSIS:
21 — Prolonged E&M Service	22 — Unusual, excessive procedure	URI 465.9
24 — Unrelated E/M service during postop.	50 — Bilateral procedure	
25 — Significant, separately identifiable E/M	51 — Multiple surgical procedures in same day	
32 — Mandated Service	52 — Reduced/incomplete procedure	
57 — Decision for surgery	55 — Postop. management only	
	59 — Distinct multiple procedures	

CATEGORY	CODE	MOD	FEE	CATEGORY	CODE	MOD	FEE
Office Visit — New Patient				**Wound Care**			
Minimal office visit	99201			Debride partial thickness burn	11040		
20 minutes	99202			Debride full thickness burn	11041		
30 minutes	99203			Debride wound, not a burn	11000		
45 minutes	99204			Unna boot application	29580		
60 minutes	99205			Unna boot removal	29700		
Other				Other			
Office Visit — Established				**Supplies**			
Minimal office visit	99211			Ace bandage, 2"	A6448		
10 minutes	99212	X	35.00	Ace bandage, 3"-4"	A6449		
15 minutes	99213			Ace bandage, 6"	A6450		
25 minutes	99214			Cast, fiberglass	A4590		
40 minutes	99215			Coban wrap	A6454		
Other				Foley catheter	A4338		
General Procedures				Immobilizer	L3670		
Anoscopy	46600			Kerlix roll	A6220		
Audiometry	92551			Oxygen mask/cannula	A4620		
Breast aspiration	19000			Sleeve, elbow	E0191		
Cerumen removal	69210			Sling	A4565		
Circumcision	54150			Splint, ready-made	A4570		
DDST	96110			Splint, wrist	S8451		
Flex sigmoidoscopy	45330			Sterile packing	A6407		
Flex sig. w/ biopsy	45331			Surgical tray	A4550		
Foreign body removal—foot	28190			Other			
Nail removal	11730			**OB Care**			
Nail removal/phenol	11750			Routine OB care	59400		
Trigger point injection	20552			Postpartum care only (separate procedure)	59430		
Tympanometry	92567			Ante partum 4–6 visits	59425		
Visual acuity	99173			Ante partum 7 or more visits	59426		
Other	82465 CBC	X	18.00	Other			
Other				Other			

Other Visit Information:
Lab Work to Order: _____
Referral to: _____
Provider Signature: _____
Next Appointment: _____

Fees:
Total Charges: $53.00
Copay Received: $10.00
Other Payment: $_____
Total Due: $43.00

Allied Medical Center
REGISTRATION FORM
(Please Print)

Today's date:	PCP:

PATIENT INFORMATION

Patient's last name: WALVOORD	First: JENNY	Middle:	☐ Mr. ☒ Mrs.	☐ Miss ☐ Ms.	Marital status (circle one) Single / (Mar)/ Div / Sep / Wid

Is this your legal name? ☒ Yes ☐ No	If not, what is your legal name?	(Former name):	Birth date: 04/26/1969	Age:	Sex: ☐ M ☒ F

Street address: 1650 YALE BLVD	Social Security no.: 658-91-4736	Home phone no.: (214) 555-6542

P.O. box:	City: DALLAS	State: TX	ZIP Code: 12345

Occupation: ADMIN ASSISTANT	Employer: GRUBB-ELLIS REALTORS	Employer phone no.: (972) 555-7591

Chose clinic because/Referred to clinic by (please choose one):	☒ Dr.	☐ Insurance Plan	☐ Hospital

☐ Family	☒ Friend	☐ Close to home/work	☐ Yellow Pages	Other

Other family members seen here: **REASON FOR THIS VISIT:** Diabetes check up

INSURANCE INFORMATION
(Please give your insurance card to the receptionist.)

Person responsible for bill: JENNY WALVOORD	Birth date: 04/26/1969	Address (if different): SAME	Home phone no.: ( )

Is this person a patient here? ☒ Yes ☐ No

Occupation:	Employer:	Employer address:	Employer phone no.: ( )

Is this patient covered by insurance? ☒ Yes ☐ No

Please indicate primary insurance:	Pro-Net PPO	Claims Mailing Address:	P O BOX 98621	DARIEN, CT	12345
		PHONE: 800-555-6555			

Subscriber's name: CARL WALVOORD	Subscriber's S.S. no.: 456-00-2531	Birth date: 09/21/1971	☐ M ☐ F	Group no.: 6209	Policy no.: 50632	Co-payment: $15.00

Patient's relationship to subscriber:	☐ Self	☒ Spouse	☐ Child	☐ Other

Name of secondary insurance (if applicable):	Subscriber's name and DOB:	☐ M ☐ F	Group no.:	Policy no.:

Patient's relationship to subscriber:	☐ Self	☐ Spouse	☐ Child	☐ Other	Claims Address:

IN CASE OF EMERGENCY

Name of local friend or relative (not living at same address): VALERIE PENNINGTON	Relationship to patient: FRIEND	Home phone no.: (972) 555-6102	Work phone no.: ( )

The above information is true to the best of my knowledge. I authorize my insurance benefits to be paid directly to the physician. I understand that I am financially responsible for any balance. I also authorize ALLIED MEDICAL CENTER or insurance company to release any information required to process my claims.

Jenny Walvoord

Patient/Guardian signature	Date

ENCOUNTER FORM

Patient Information		Payment Method		Visit Information	
Patient ID number		**Primary**	Pro-Net PPO	Visit date	
Patient name	Jenny Walvoord	Primary ID number	50632	Visit number	
Address	1650 Yale Blvd	Primary group number	6209	Rendering physician	
City/State	Dallas, TX 12345	**Secondary**		Referring physician	
Phone number	214-555-6542	Secondary ID number		Reason for visit	Diabetes check up
Date of birth	04/26/1969	Secondary group no.			
Age		Cash/credit card			
		Other billing			

E/M Modifiers	Procedure Modifiers	DIAGNOSIS:
21 — Prolonged E&M Service	22 — Unusual, excessive procedure	DIABETES MELLITUS 250.00
24 — Unrelated E/M service during postop.	50 — Bilateral procedure	
25 — Significant, separately identifiable E/M	51 — Multiple surgical procedures in same day	
32 — Mandated Service	52 — Reduced/incomplete procedure	
57 — Decision for surgery	55 — Postop. management only	
	59 — Distinct multiple procedures	

CATEGORY	CODE	MOD	FEE	CATEGORY	CODE	MOD	FEE
Office Visit — New Patient				**Wound Care**			
Minimal office visit	99201			Debride partial thickness burn	11040		
20 minutes	99202			Debride full thickness burn	11041		
30 minutes	99203			Debride wound, not a burn	11000		
45 minutes	99204			Unna boot application	29580		
60 minutes	99205			Unna boot removal	29700		
Other				Other			
Office Visit — Established				**Supplies**			
Minimal office visit	99211	X	25.00	Ace bandage, 2"	A6448		
10 minutes	99212			Ace bandage, 3"-4"	A6449		
15 minutes	99213			Ace bandage, 6"	A6450		
25 minutes	99214			Cast, fiberglass	A4590		
40 minutes	99215			Coban wrap	A6454		
Other				Foley catheter	A4338		
General Procedures				Immobilizer	L3670		
Anoscopy	46600			Kerlix roll	A6220		
Audiometry	92551			Oxygen mask/cannula	A4620		
Breast aspiration	19000			Sleeve, elbow	E0191		
Cerumen removal	69210			Sling	A4565		
Circumcision	54150			Splint, ready-made	A4570		
DDST	96110			Splint, wrist	S8451		
Flex sigmoidoscopy	45330			Sterile packing	A6407		
Flex sig. w/ biopsy	45331			Surgical tray	A4550		
Foreign body removal—foot	28190			Other			
Nail removal	11730			**OB Care**			
Nail removal/phenol	11750			Routine OB care	59400		
Trigger point injection	20552			Postpartum care only (separate procedure)	59430		
Tympanometry	92567			Ante partum 4–6 visits	59425		
Visual acuity	99173			Ante partum 7 or more visits	59426		
Other				Other			
Other				Other			

Other Visit Information: _____

Lab Work to Order: _____

Referral to: _____

Provider Signature: _____

Next Appointment: _____

Fees:

Total Charges: $25.00

Copay Received: $15.00

Other Payment: $_____

Total Due: $10.00

Allied Medical Center
REGISTRATION FORM
(Please Print)

Today's date: _____   PCP: _____

PATIENT INFORMATION

Patient's last name:	First:	Middle:	☒ Mr.	☐ Miss	Marital status (circle one)
SUAREZ	MARCO	R.	☐ Mrs.	☐ Ms.	(Single) / Mar / Div / Sep / Wid

Is this your legal name?	If not, what is your legal name?	(Former name):		Birth date:	Age:	Sex:
☒ Yes ☐ No				05/29/1971		☒ M ☐ F

Street address:	Social Security no.:	Home phone no.:
45 SOUTHERN OAKS	310-10-3101	(214) 555-5564

P.O. box:	City:	State:	ZIP Code:
	DESOTO	TX	12345

Occupation:	Employer:	Employer phone no.:
SALESPERSON	MONKEY BUSINESS PET STORE	(972) 555-8200

Chose clinic because/Referred to clinic by (please choose one):	☒ Dr. REYNALDO SANCHEZ	☐ Insurance Plan	☐ Hospital
☐ Family ☐ Friend ☐ Close to home/work	☐ Yellow Pages	Other **AUTH #3 OVS, 30 DAYS: 650125400**	

Other family members seen here: _____   **REASON FOR THIS VISIT:** Hemorrhoids

INSURANCE INFORMATION

(Please give your insurance card to the receptionist.)

Person responsible for bill:	Birth date:	Address (if different):	Home phone no.:
MARCO SUAREZ	/ /	SAME	( )

Is this person a patient here?   ☒ Yes   ☐ No

Occupation:	Employer:	Employer address:	Employer phone no.:
			( )

Is this patient covered by insurance?   ☒ Yes   ☐ No

Please indicate primary insurance:	Physician Alliance HMO	Claims Mailing Address:	P O BOX 65	TOLEDO, OH	12345
		PHONE: 800-555-9866			

Subscriber's name:	Subscriber's S.S. no.:	Birth date:	☐ M	Group no.:	Policy no.:	Co-payment:
MARCO SUAREZ	310-10-3101	/ /	☐ F	MB456	310103101	$12.00

Patient's relationship to subscriber: ☒ Self   ☐ Spouse   ☐ Child   ☐ Other

Name of secondary insurance (if applicable):	Subscriber's name and DOB:	☐ M ☐ F	Group no.:	Policy no.:

Patient's relationship to subscriber: ☐ Self   ☐ Spouse   ☐ Child   ☐ Other   Claims Address:

IN CASE OF EMERGENCY

Name of local friend or relative (not living at same address):	Relationship to patient:	Home phone no.:	Work phone no.:
LOUISE PEREZ	FRIEND	(214) 555-9014	(972) 555-6630

The above information is true to the best of my knowledge. I authorize my insurance benefits to be paid directly to the physician. I understand that I am financially responsible for any balance. I also authorize ALLIED MEDICAL CENTER or insurance company to release any information required to process my claims.

Marco Suarez

_____   _____
Patient/Guardian signature   *Date*

ENCOUNTER FORM

Patient Information		Payment Method		Visit Information	
Patient ID number		**Primary**	Physician Alliance HMO	Visit date	
Patient name	Marco Suarez	Primary ID number	310103101	Visit number	
Address	45 Southern Oaks	Primary group number	MB456	Rendering physician	
City/State	Desoto, TX 12345	**Secondary**		Referring physician	Reynaldo Sanchez
Phone number	214-555-5564	Secondary ID number		Reason for visit	Hemorrhoids
Date of birth	05/29/1971	Secondary group no.			**Auth # for today: 650125400**
Age		Cash/credit card			
		Other billing			

E/M Modifiers	Procedure Modifiers	DIAGNOSIS:
21 — Prolonged E&M Service	22 — Unusual, excessive procedure	EXTERNAL HEMORRHOIDS 455.3
24 — Unrelated E/M service during postop.	50 — Bilateral procedure	
25 — Significant, separately identifiable E/M	51 — Multiple surgical procedures in same day	
32 — Mandated Service	52 — Reduced/incomplete procedure	
57 — Decision for surgery	55 — Postop. management only	
	59 — Distinct multiple procedures	

CATEGORY	CODE	MOD	FEE	CATEGORY	CODE	MOD	FEE
Office Visit — New Patient				**Wound Care**			
Minimal office visit	99201			Debride partial thickness burn	11040		
20 minutes	99202			Debride full thickness burn	11041		
30 minutes	99203			Debride wound, not a burn	11000		
45 minutes	99204			Unna boot application	29580		
60 minutes	99205			Unna boot removal	29700		
Other				Other			
Office Visit — Established				**Supplies**			
Minimal office visit	99211			Ace bandage, 2"	A6448		
10 minutes	99212			Ace bandage, 3"-4"	A6449		
15 minutes	99213	X	45.00	Ace bandage, 6"	A6450		
25 minutes	99214			Cast, fiberglass	A4590		
40 minutes	99215			Coban wrap	A6454		
Other				Foley catheter	A4338		
General Procedures				Immobilizer	L3670		
Anoscopy	46600			Kerlix roll	A6220		
Audiometry	92551			Oxygen mask/cannula	A4620		
Breast aspiration	19000			Sleeve, elbow	E0191		
Cerumen removal	69210			Sling	A4565		
Circumcision	54150			Splint, ready-made	A4570		
DDST	96110			Splint, wrist	S8451		
Flex sigmoidoscopy	45330			Sterile packing	A6407		
Flex sig. w/ biopsy	45331			Surgical tray	A4550		
Foreign body removal—foot	28190			Other			
Nail removal	11730			**OB Care**			
Nail removal/phenol	11750			Routine OB care	59400		
Trigger point injection	20552			Postpartum care only (separate procedure)	59430		
Tympanometry	92567			Ante partum 4–6 visits	59425		
Visual acuity	99173			Ante partum 7 or more visits	59426		
Other				Other			
Other				Other			

Other Visit Information: _____

Lab Work to Order: _____

Referral to: _____

Provider Signature: _____

Next Appointment: _____

Fees:

Total Charges: $45.00

Copay Received: $

Other Payment: $_____

Total Due: **$45.00**

Allied Medical Center 1933 E. Frankford Rd. Carrollton, TX 12345 **972-555-5482**

Allied Medical Center
REGISTRATION FORM
(Please Print)

Today's date: _____   PCP: _____

PATIENT INFORMATION

Patient's last name: FITZGERALD	First: SHANNON	Middle: M	☐ Mr. ☒ Miss ☐ Mrs. ☐ Ms.	Marital status (circle one) (Single) / Mar / Div / Sep / Wid

Is this your legal name? ☒ Yes ☐ No	If not, what is your legal name?	(Former name):	Birth date: 12/19/1994	Age:	Sex: ☐ M ☒ F

Street address: 2601 Mint Leaf Drive #56B	Social Security no.: 698-73-6581	Home phone no.: (214) 555-8000

P.O. box:	City: DALLAS	State: TX	ZIP Code: 12345

Occupation: STUDENT	Employer:	Employer phone no.: ( )

Chose clinic because/Referred to clinic by (please choose one):   ☐ Dr.   ☐ Insurance Plan   ☐ Hospital

☐ Family   ☐ Friend   ☐ Close to home/work   ☐ Yellow Pages   ☒ Other

Other family members seen here: _____   **REASON FOR THIS VISIT:** Dizziness

INSURANCE INFORMATION
(Please give your insurance card to the receptionist.)

Person responsible for bill: MICHAEL FITZGERALD	Birth date: 11/27/1955	Address (if different): SAME	Home phone no.: ( )

Is this person a patient here?   ☐ Yes   ☒ No

Occupation: RETIRED	Employer:	Employer address:	Employer phone no.: ( )

Is this patient covered by insurance?   ☒ Yes   ☐ No

Please indicate primary insurance:	CHAMPVA	Claims Mailing Address:	P O BOX 8993	MADISON, WI	12345
		PHONE: 800-555-1230			

Subscriber's name: MIKE FITZGERALD	Subscriber's S.S. no.: 455836914	Birth date: 11/27/1955 ☒ M ☐ F	Group no.:	Policy no.: 455836914	Co-payment: $12.00

Patient's relationship to subscriber: ☐ Self   ☐ Spouse   ☒ Child   ☐ Other

Name of secondary insurance (if applicable):	Subscriber's name and DOB:	☐ M ☐ F	Group no.:	Policy no.:

Patient's relationship to subscriber: ☐ Self   ☐ Spouse   ☐ Child   ☐ Other   Claims Address:

IN CASE OF EMERGENCY

Name of local friend or relative (not living at same address): MATTHEW BUCHANAN	Relationship to patient: FRIEND	Home phone no.: (469) 555-3259	Work phone no.: (972) 555-3722

The above information is true to the best of my knowledge. I authorize my insurance benefits to be paid directly to the physician. I understand that I am financially responsible for any balance. I also authorize ALLIED MEDICAL CENTER or insurance company to release any information required to process my claims.

Shannon Fitzgerald
_____
Patient/Guardian signature   *Date*

ENCOUNTER FORM

Patient Information		Payment Method		Visit Information	
Patient ID number		**Primary**	CHAMPVA	Visit date	
Patient name	Shannon Fitzgerald	Primary ID number	455836914	Visit number	
Address	2601 Mint Leaf Dr #56B	Primary group number		Rendering physician	
City/State	Dallas, TX 12345	**Secondary**		Referring physician	
Phone number	214-555-8000	Secondary ID number		Reason for visit	Dizziness
Date of birth	12/19/1994	Secondary group no.			
Age		Cash/credit card			
		Other billing			

E/M Modifiers	Procedure Modifiers	DIAGNOSIS:
21 — Prolonged E&M Service	22 — Unusual, excessive procedure	ESSENTIAL HYPERTENSION 401.1
24 — Unrelated E/M service during postop.	50 — Bilateral procedure	
25 — Significant, separately identifiable E/M	51 — Multiple surgical procedures in same day	
32 — Mandated Service	52 — Reduced/incomplete procedure	
57 — Decision for surgery	55 — Postop. management only	
	59 — Distinct multiple procedures	

CATEGORY	CODE	MOD	FEE	CATEGORY	CODE	MOD	FEE
Office Visit — New Patient				**Wound Care**			
Minimal office visit	99201			Debride partial thickness burn	11040		
20 minutes	99202			Debride full thickness burn	11041		
30 minutes	99203			Debride wound, not a burn	11000		
45 minutes	99204			Unna boot application	29580		
60 minutes	99205			Unna boot removal	29700		
Other				Other			
Office Visit — Established				**Supplies**			
Minimal office visit	99211	X	25.00	Ace bandage, 2"	A6448		
10 minutes	99212			Ace bandage, 3"-4"	A6449		
15 minutes	99213			Ace bandage, 6"	A6450		
25 minutes	99214			Cast, fiberglass	A4590		
40 minutes	99215			Coban wrap	A6454		
Other				Foley catheter	A4338		
General Procedures				Immobilizer	L3670		
Anoscopy	46600			Kerlix roll	A6220		
Audiometry	92551			Oxygen mask/cannula	A4620		
Breast aspiration	19000			Sleeve, elbow	E0191		
Cerumen removal	69210			Sling	A4565		
Circumcision	54150			Splint, ready-made	A4570		
DDST	96110			Splint, wrist	S8451		
Flex sigmoidoscopy	45330			Sterile packing	A6407		
Flex sig. w/ biopsy	45331			Surgical tray	A4550		
Foreign body removal—foot	28190			Other			
Nail removal	11730			**OB Care**			
Nail removal/phenol	11750			Routine OB care	59400		
Trigger point injection	20552			Postpartum care only (separate procedure)	59430		
Tympanometry	92567			Ante partum 4–6 visits	59425		
Visual acuity	99173			Ante partum 7 or more visits	59426		
Other	**82465**	X	10.00	Other			
Other				Other			

Other Visit Information: _____

Lab Work to Order: _____

Referral to: _____

Provider Signature: _____

Next Appointment: _____

Fees:

Total Charges: $35.00

Copay Received: $12.00

Other Payment: $_____

Total Due: **$23.00**

Allied Medical Center
REGISTRATION FORM
(Please Print)

Today's date: _____   PCP: _____

PATIENT INFORMATION

Patient's last name:	First:	Middle:	☒ Mr.	☐ Miss	Marital status (circle one)
ABERNATHY	STEPHEN	J.	☐ Mrs.	☐ Ms.	Single / Mar / Div / Sep / (Wid)

Is this your legal name?	If not, what is your legal name?	(Former name):	Birth date:	Age:	Sex:
☒ Yes ☐ No			07/07/1939		☒ M ☐ F

Street address:	Social Security no.:	Home phone no.:
175 MEANDERING WAY	888-91-4637	(214) 555-6488

P.O. box:	City:	State:	ZIP Code:
	DALLAS	TX	12345

Occupation:	Employer:	Employer phone no.:
OWNER	GAMESTOP	(214) 555-8741

Chose clinic because/Referred to clinic by (please choose one): ☐ Dr. ____ ☐ Insurance Plan ☐ Hospital

☐ Family   ☐ Friend   ☐ Close to home/work   ☒ Yellow Pages   ☐ Other

Other family members seen here: _____   **REASON FOR THIS VISIT:** Coughing Chest Pain

INSURANCE INFORMATION

(Please give your insurance card to the receptionist.)

Person responsible for bill:	Birth date:	Address (if different):	Home phone no.:
SELF	/ /		( )

Is this person a patient here?   ☒ Yes   ☐ No

Occupation:	Employer:	Employer address:	Employer phone no.:
			( )

Is this patient covered by insurance?   ☐ Yes   ☒ No

Please indicate primary insurance:		Claims Mailing Address:		
		PHONE:		

Subscriber's name:	Subscriber's S.S. no.:	Birth date:	☐ M ☐ F	Group no.:	Policy no.:	Co-payment: $
		/ /				

Patient's relationship to subscriber: ☐ Self   ☐ Spouse   ☐ Child   ☐ Other

Name of secondary insurance (if applicable):	Subscriber's name and DOB:	☐ M ☐ F	Group no.:	Policy no.:

Patient's relationship to subscriber: ☐ Self   ☐ Spouse   ☐ Child   ☐ Other   Claims Address: .

IN CASE OF EMERGENCY

Name of local friend or relative (not living at same address):	Relationship to patient:	Home phone no.:	Work phone no.:
MAGGIE SCOFIELD	SISTER	(972) 555-8775	(214) 555-3774

The above information is true to the best of my knowledge. I authorize my insurance benefits to be paid directly to the physician. I understand that I am financially responsible for any balance. I also authorize ALLIED MEDICAL CENTER or insurance company to release any information required to process my claims.

Stephen Abernathy

_____   _____
Patient/Guardian signature   Date

ENCOUNTER FORM

Patient Information		Payment Method		Visit Information	
Patient ID number		**Primary**	NONE	Visit date	
Patient name	Stephen Abernathy	Primary ID number		Visit number	
Address	175 Meandering Way	Primary group number		Rendering physician	
City/State	Dallas, TX 12345	**Secondary**		Referring physician	
Phone number	214-555-6488	Secondary ID number		Reason for visit	Coughing, Chest Pain
Date of birth	07/07/1939	Secondary group no.			
Age		Cash/credit card	CHECK		
		Other billing			

E/M Modifiers	Procedure Modifiers	DIAGNOSIS:
21 — Prolonged E&M Service	22 — Unusual, excessive procedure	Acute Bronchitis 466.0
24 — Unrelated E/M service during postop.	50 — Bilateral procedure	
25 — Significant, separately identifiable E/M	51 — Multiple surgical procedures in same day	
32 — Mandated Service	52 — Reduced/incomplete procedure	
57 — Decision for surgery	55 — Postop. management only	
	59 — Distinct multiple procedures	

CATEGORY	CODE	MOD	FEE	CATEGORY	CODE	MOD	FEE
Office Visit — New Patient				**Wound Care**			
Minimal office visit	99201			Debride partial thickness burn	11040		
20 minutes	99202			Debride full thickness burn	11041		
30 minutes	99203			Debride wound, not a burn	11000		
45 minutes	99204			Unna boot application	29580		
60 minutes	99205			Unna boot removal	29700		
Other				Other			
Office Visit — Established				**Supplies**			
Minimal office visit	99211			Ace bandage, 2"	A6448		
10 minutes	99212			Ace bandage, 3"-4"	A6449		
15 minutes	99213	X	35.00	Ace bandage, 6"	A6450		
25 minutes	99214			Cast, fiberglass	A4590		
40 minutes	99215			Coban wrap	A6454		
Other				Foley catheter	A4338		
General Procedures				Immobilizer	L3670		
Anoscopy	46600			Kerlix roll	A6220		
Audiometry	92551			Oxygen mask/cannula	A4620		
Breast aspiration	19000			Sleeve, elbow	E0191		
Cerumen removal	69210			Sling	A4565		
Circumcision	54150			Splint, ready-made	A4570		
DDST	96110			Splint, wrist	S8451		
Flex sigmoidoscopy	45330			Sterile packing	A6407		
Flex sig. w/ biopsy	45331			Surgical tray	A4550		
Foreign body removal—foot	28190			Other			
Nail removal	11730			OB Care			
Nail removal/phenol	11750			Routine OB care	59400		
Trigger point injection	20552			Postpartum care only (separate procedure)	59430		
Tympanometry	92567			Ante partum 4–6 visits	59425		
Visual acuity	99173			Ante partum 7 or more visits	59426		
Other	**71020**	X	53.00	Other			
Other				Other			

Other Visit Information: _____

Lab Work to Order: _____

Referral to: _____

Provider Signature: _____

Next Appointment: _____

Fees:

Total Charges: $88.00

Copay Received: $_____

Other Payment: $88.00 CK# 5316

Total Due: **$0.00**

Allied Medical Center
REGISTRATION FORM
(Please Print)

Today's date:	PCP:

PATIENT INFORMATION

Patient's last name: ANDREWS	First: THERESA	Middle: L	☐ Mr. ☒ Mrs.	☐ Miss ☐ Ms.	Marital status (circle one) Single / (Mar) / Div / Sep / Wid

Is this your legal name? ☒ Yes ☐ No	If not, what is your legal name?	(Former name):	Birth date: 06/08/1967	Age:	Sex: ☐ M ☒ F

Street address: 4569 Avenue K, APT. 120	Social Security no.: 332-49-0432	Home phone no.: (972) 555-4448

P.O. box:	City: PLANO	State: TX	ZIP Code: 12345

Occupation: CLERK	Employer: TOWN DRUG STORE	Employer phone no.: (972) 555-5593

Chose clinic because/Referred to clinic by (please choose one):	☐ Dr.	☒ Insurance Plan	☐ Hospital

☐ Family	☐ Friend	☐ Close to home/work	☐ Yellow Pages	☐ Other

Other family members seen here: **REASON FOR THIS VISIT:** Chest Pain

INSURANCE INFORMATION
(Please give your insurance card to the receptionist.)

Person responsible for bill: THERESA ANDREWS	Birth date: / /	Address (if different): SAME	Home phone no.: ( )

Is this person a patient here?	☒ Yes ☐ No

Occupation:	Employer:	Employer address:	Employer phone no.: ( )

Is this patient covered by insurance?	☒ Yes ☐ No

Please indicate primary insurance:	TRUSTMARK PPO	Claims Mailing Address:	P O BOX 12345	Green Bay, WI	12345
		PHONE: 800-555-9863			

Subscriber's name: SAME AS PATIENT	Subscriber's S.S. no.: 332-49-0432	Birth date: / /	☐ M ☐ F	Group no.: 2038831	Policy no.: 332490432	Co-payment: $20.00

Patient's relationship to subscriber:	☒ Self ☐ Spouse ☐ Child ☐ Other

Name of secondary insurance (if applicable): Guardian PPO	Subscriber's name and DOB: BOB Andrews 12/01/1964	☒ M ☐ F	Group no.: 1122191	Policy no.: 341599392

Patient's relationship to subscriber:	☐ Self ☒ Spouse ☐ Child ☐ Other	Claims Address: PO BOX 40328

ST LOUIS, MO 12345 800-555-1212

IN CASE OF EMERGENCY

Name of local friend or relative (not living at same address): LUCILLE MCGOWEN	Relationship to patient: FRIEND	Home phone no.: (469) 555-2001	Work phone no.: (972) 555-9648

The above information is true to the best of my knowledge. I authorize my insurance benefits to be paid directly to the physician. I understand that I am financially responsible for any balance. I also authorize ALLIED MEDICAL CENTER or insurance company to release any information required to process my claims.

Theresa Andrews

Patient/Guardian signature   _Date_

ENCOUNTER FORM

Patient Information		Payment Method		Visit Information	
Patient ID number		**Primary**	TRUSTMARK PPO	Visit date	
Patient name	Theresa Andrews	Primary ID number	332490432	Visit number	
Address	4569 Ave. K #120	Primary group number	2038831	Rendering physician	
City/State	Plano, TX 12345	**Secondary**	Guardian PPO	Referring physician	
Phone number	972-555-4448	Secondary ID number	341599392	Reason for visit	Chest Pain
Date of birth	06/08/1967	Secondary group no.	1122191		
Age		Cash/credit card			
		Other billing			

E/M Modifiers	Procedure Modifiers	DIAGNOSIS:
21 — Prolonged E&M Service	22 — Unusual, excessive procedure	BRONCHOPNEUMONIA WITH FLU
24 — Unrelated E/M service during postop.	50 — Bilateral procedure	487.0
25 — Significant, separately identifiable E/M	51 — Multiple surgical procedures in same day	
32 — Mandated Service	52 — Reduced/incomplete procedure	
57 — Decision for surgery	55 — Postop. management only	
	59 — Distinct multiple procedures	

CATEGORY	CODE	MOD	FEE	CATEGORY	CODE	MOD	FEE
Office Visit — New Patient				**Wound Care**			
Minimal office visit	99201			Debride partial thickness burn	11040		
20 minutes	99202			Debride full thickness burn	11041		
30 minutes	99203			Debride wound, not a burn	11000		
45 minutes	99204			Unna boot application	29580		
60 minutes	99205			Unna boot removal	29700		
Other				Other			
Office Visit — Established				**Supplies**			
Minimal office visit	99211			Ace bandage, 2"	A6448		
10 minutes	99212	X	35.00	Ace bandage, 3"-4"	A6449		
15 minutes	99213			Ace bandage, 6"	A6450		
25 minutes	99214			Cast, fiberglass	A4590		
40 minutes	99215			Coban wrap	A6454		
Other				Foley catheter	A4338		
General Procedures				Immobilizer	L3670		
Anoscopy	46600			Kerlix roll	A6220		
Audiometry	92551			Oxygen mask/cannula	A4620		
Breast aspiration	19000			Sleeve, elbow	E0191		
Cerumen removal	69210			Sling	A4565		
Circumcision	54150			Splint, ready-made	A4570		
DDST	96110			Splint, wrist	S8451		
Flex sigmoidoscopy	45330			Sterile packing	A6407		
Flex sig. w/ biopsy	45331			Surgical tray	A4550		
Foreign body removal—foot	28190			Other			
Nail removal	11730			OB Care			
Nail removal/phenol	11750			Routine OB care	59400		
Trigger point injection	20552			Postpartum care only (separate procedure)	59430		
Tympanometry	92567			Ante partum 4–6 visits	59425		
Visual acuity	99173			Ante partum 7 or more visits	59426		
Other	**71020**		53.00	Other			
Other				Other			

Other Visit Information: _____

Lab Work to Order: _____

Referral to: _____

Provider Signature: _____

Next Appointment: _____

Fees:

Total Charges: $88.00

Copay Received: $20.00

Other Payment: $_____

Total Due: **$68.00**

Allied Medical Center
REGISTRATION FORM
(Please Print)

Today's date:	PCP:

PATIENT INFORMATION

Patient's last name: ANDREWS	First: ROBERT "BOB"	Middle: C	☒ Mr. ❑ Mrs.	❑ Miss ❑ Ms.	Marital status (circle one) Single / (Mar) / Div / Sep / Wid

Is this your legal name? ☒ Yes ❑ No	If not, what is your legal name?	(Former name):	Birth date: 12/01/1964	Age:	Sex: ☒ M ❑ F

Street address: 4569 Avenue K, APT. 120	Social Security no.: 341-59-9392	Home phone no.: (972) 555-4448

P.O. box:	City: PLANO	State: TX	ZIP Code: 12345

Occupation: MECHANIC	Employer: DISCOUNT TIRE COMPANY	Employer phone no.: (972) 555-8256

Chose clinic because/Referred to clinic by (please choose one):   ❑ Dr.   ☒ Insurance Plan   ❑ Hospital

❑ Family   ❑ Friend   ❑ Close to home/work   ❑ Yellow Pages   ❑ Other

Other family members seen here: **REASON FOR THIS VISIT:** ROUTINE YEARLY PHYSICAL

INSURANCE INFORMATION
(Please give your insurance card to the receptionist.)

Person responsible for bill: ROBERT ANDREWS	Birth date: / /	Address (if different): SAME	Home phone no.: ( )

Is this person a patient here?   ☒ Yes   ❑ No

Occupation:	Employer:	Employer address:	Employer phone no.: ( )

Is this patient covered by insurance?   ☒ Yes   ❑ No

Please indicate primary insurance:	GUARDIAN PPO	Claims Mailing Address:	P O BOX 40328	St Louis, Mo	12345
		PHONE: 800-555-1212			

Subscriber's name: SAME AS PATIENT	Subscriber's S.S. no.:	Birth date: / /	❑ M ❑ F	Group no.: 1122191	Policy no.: 341599392	Co-payment: $30.00

Patient's relationship to subscriber: ☒ Self   ❑ Spouse   ❑ Child   ❑ Other

Name of secondary insurance (if applicable): TRUSTMARK PPO	Subscriber's name and DOB: THERESA ANDREWS 06/08/1967	❑ M ☒ F	Group no.: 2038831	Policy no.: 332490432

Patient's relationship to subscriber: ❑ Self ☒ Spouse ❑ Child ❑ Other Claims Address: PO BOX 12459 Green Bay, WI 12345

800-555-9863

IN CASE OF EMERGENCY

Name of local friend or relative (not living at same address): TED LATHAM	Relationship to patient: FRIEND	Home phone no.: (214) 555-4197	Work phone no.: (214) 555-4197

The above information is true to the best of my knowledge. I authorize my insurance benefits to be paid directly to the physician. I understand that I am financially responsible for any balance. I also authorize ALLIED MEDICAL CENTER or insurance company to release any information required to process my claims.

Robert Andrews

Patient/Guardian signature   _Date_

ENCOUNTER FORM

Patient Information		Payment Method		Visit Information	
Patient ID number		**Primary**	GUARDIAN PPO	Visit date	
Patient name	Robert Andrews	Primary ID number	341599392	Visit number	
Address	4569 Ave. K #120	Primary group number	1122191	Rendering physician	
City/State	Plano, TX 12345	**Secondary**	Trustmark PPO	Referring physician	
Phone number	972-555-4448	Secondary ID number	332490432	Reason for visit	ROUTINE PHYSICAL
Date of birth	12/01/1964	Secondary group no.	2038831		
Age		Cash/credit card			
		Other billing			

E/M Modifiers	Procedure Modifiers	DIAGNOSIS:
21 — Prolonged E&M Service	22 — Unusual, excessive procedure	ROUTINE EXAM V70.0
24 — Unrelated E/M service during postop.	50 — Bilateral procedure	
25 — Significant, separately identifiable E/M	51 — Multiple surgical procedures in same day	
32 — Mandated Service	52 — Reduced/incomplete procedure	
57 — Decision for surgery	55 — Postop. management only	
	59 — Distinct multiple procedures	

CATEGORY	CODE	MOD	FEE	CATEGORY	CODE	MOD	FEE
Office Visit — New Patient				**Wound Care**			
Minimal office visit	99201			Debride partial thickness burn	11040		
20 minutes	99202			Debride full thickness burn	11041		
30 minutes	99203			Debride wound, not a burn	11000		
45 minutes	99204			Unna boot application	29580		
60 minutes	99205			Unna boot removal	29700		
Other				Other			
Office Visit — Established				**Supplies**			
Minimal office visit	99211			Ace bandage, 2"	A6448		
10 minutes	99212			Ace bandage, 3"-4"	A6449		
15 minutes	99213			Ace bandage, 6"	A6450		
25 minutes	99214			Cast, fiberglass	A4590		
40 minutes	99215	X	80.00	Coban wrap	A6454		
Other				Foley catheter	A4338		
General Procedures				Immobilizer	L3670		
Anoscopy	46600			Kerlix roll	A6220		
Audiometry	92551			Oxygen mask/cannula	A4620		
Breast aspiration	19000			Sleeve, elbow	E0191		
Cerumen removal	69210			Sling	A4565		
Circumcision	54150			Splint, ready-made	A4570		
DDST	96110			Splint, wrist	S8451		
Flex sigmoidoscopy	45330			Sterile packing	A6407		
Flex sig. w/ biopsy	45331			Surgical tray	A4550		
Foreign body removal—foot	28190			Other			
Nail removal	11730			OB Care			
Nail removal/phenol	11750			Routine OB care	59400		
Trigger point injection	20552			Postpartum care only (separate procedure)	59430		
Tympanometry	92567			Ante partum 4–6 visits	59425		
Visual acuity	99173			Ante partum 7 or more visits	59426		
Other				Other			
Other				Other			

Other Visit Information: _____

Lab Work to Order: _____

Referral to: _____

Provider Signature: _____

Next Appointment: _____

Fees:

Total Charges:	$80.00
Copay Received:	$30.00
Other Payment:	$_____
Total Due:	**$50.00**

Allied Medical Center 1933 E. Frankford Rd. Carrollton, TX 12345 **972-555-5482**

ENCOUNTER FORM

Patient Information		Payment Method			Visit Information	
Patient ID number		**Primary**		Physician's Alliance	Visit date	
Patient name	Margaret Dupont	Primary ID number		621382	Visit number	
Address	12 Briar Lane	Primary group number		A435	Rendering physician	
City/State	Dallas, TX 12345	**Secondary**		BCBS TX	Referring physician	
Phone number	214-555-9871	Secondary ID number		BHR716830061	Reason for visit	SINUSITIS
Date of birth	09/21/1946	Secondary group no.		126		
Age		Cash/credit card				
		Other billing				

E/M Modifiers	Procedure Modifiers	DIAGNOSIS:
21 — Prolonged E&M Service	22 — Unusual, excessive procedure	SINUSITIS, ACUTE 461.9
24 — Unrelated E/M service during postop.	50 — Bilateral procedure	
25 — Significant, separately identifiable E/M	51 — Multiple surgical procedures in same day	
32 — Mandated Service	52 — Reduced/incomplete procedure	
57 — Decision for surgery	55 — Postop. management only	
	59 — Distinct multiple procedures	

CATEGORY	CODE	MOD	FEE	CATEGORY	CODE	MOD	FEE
Office Visit — New Patient				**Wound Care**			
Minimal office visit	99201			Debride partial thickness burn	11040		
20 minutes	99202			Debride full thickness burn	11041		
30 minutes	99203			Debride wound, not a burn	11000		
45 minutes	99204			Unna boot application	29580		
60 minutes	99205			Unna boot removal	29700		
Other				Other			
Office Visit — Established				**Supplies**			
Minimal office visit	99211			Ace bandage, 2"	A6448		
10 minutes	99212	X	35.00	Ace bandage, 3"-4"	A6449		
15 minutes	99213			Ace bandage, 6"	A6450		
25 minutes	99214			Cast, fiberglass	A4590		
40 minutes	99215			Coban wrap	A6454		
Other				Foley catheter	A4338		
General Procedures				Immobilizer	L3670		
Anoscopy	46600			Kerlix roll	A6220		
Audiometry	92551			Oxygen mask/cannula	A4620		
Breast aspiration	19000			Sleeve, elbow	E0191		
Cerumen removal	69210			Sling	A4565		
Circumcision	54150			Splint, ready-made	A4570		
DDST	96110			Splint, wrist	S8451		
Flex sigmoidoscopy	45330			Sterile packing	A6407		
Flex sig. w/ biopsy	45331			Surgical tray	A4550		
Foreign body removal—foot	28190			Other			
Nail removal	11730			OB Care			
Nail removal/phenol	11750			Routine OB care	59400		
Trigger point injection	20552			Postpartum care only (separate procedure)	59430		
Tympanometry	92567			Ante partum 4–6 visits	59425		
Visual acuity	99173			Ante partum 7 or more visits	59426		
Other				Other			
Other				Other			

Other Visit Information: _____

Lab Work to Order: _____

Referral to: _____

Provider Signature: _____

Next Appointment: _____

Fees:

Total Charges:	$35.00
Copay Received:	$10.00
Other Payment:	$_____
Total Due:	**$25.00**

Allied Medical Center 1933 E. Frankford Rd. Carrollton, TX 12345 **972-555-5482**

Allied Medical Center
REGISTRATION FORM
(Please Print)

Today's date: _____   PCP: _____

PATIENT INFORMATION

Patient's last name: MONROE	First: KEVIN	Middle: L	☒ Mr. ❏ Mrs.	❏ Miss ❏ Ms.	Marital status (circle one) Single / Mar / Div / Sep / Wid

Is this your legal name? ☒ Yes ❏ No	If not, what is your legal name?	(Former name):	Birth date: 05/21/1946	Age:	Sex: ☒ M ❏ F

Street address: 1609 KILKIRK AVE	Social Security no.: 645-28-9631	Home phone no.: (972) 555-3219

P.O. box:	City: DALLAS	State: TX	ZIP Code: 12345

Occupation: SALESPERSON	Employer: THE HOME IMPROVEMENT STORE	Employer phone no.: (972) 555-9516

Chose clinic because/Referred to clinic by (please choose one):   ❏ Dr.   ❏ Insurance Plan   ❏ Hospital

❏ Family   ☒ Friend   ❏ Close to home/work   ❏ Yellow Pages   ❏ Other

Other family members seen here:

REASON FOR THIS VISIT:

INSURANCE INFORMATION

(Please give your insurance card to the receptionist.)

Person responsible for bill: PATIENT	Birth date: / /	Address (if different): SAME AS ABOVE	Home phone no.: ( )

Is this person a patient here?   ☒ Yes   ❏ No

Occupation:	Employer:	Employer address:	Employer phone no.: ( )

Is this patient covered by insurance?   ❏ Yes   ☒ No

Please indicate primary insurance:	NONE	Claims Mailing Address:		
		PHONE:		

Subscriber's name:	Subscriber's S.S. no.:	Birth date: / /	❏ M ❏ F	Group no.:	Policy no.:	Co-payment: $

Patient's relationship to subscriber: ❏ Self   ❏ Spouse   ❏ Child   ❏ Other

Name of secondary insurance (if applicable):	Subscriber's name and DOB:	❏ M ❏ F	Group no.:	Policy no.:

Patient's relationship to subscriber: ❏ Self   ❏ Spouse   ❏ Child   ❏ Other   Claims Address: PO BOX 12459 Green Bay, WI 12345

IN CASE OF EMERGENCY

Name of local friend or relative (not living at same address): MARK WILLIAMS	Relationship to patient: FRIEND/NEIGHBOR	Home phone no.: (972) 555-8809	Work phone no.: (903) 555-1764

The above information is true to the best of my knowledge. I authorize my insurance benefits to be paid directly to the physician. I understand that I am financially responsible for any balance. I also authorize ALLIED MEDICAL CENTER or insurance company to release any information required to process my claims.

Kevin Monroe

Patient/Guardian signature   _Date_

ENCOUNTER FORM

Patient Information		Payment Method		Visit Information	
Patient ID number		**Primary**		Visit date	
Patient name	Kevin Monroe	Primary ID number		Visit number	
Address	1609 Kilkirk Ave.	Primary group number		Rendering physician	
City/State	Dallas, TX 12345	**Secondary**		Referring physician	
Phone number	972-555-3219	Secondary ID number		Reason for visit	Cholesterol CK
Date of birth	05/21/1946	Secondary group no.			
Age		Cash/credit card	VISA		
		Other billing			

E/M Modifiers	Procedure Modifiers	DIAGNOSIS:
21 — Prolonged E&M Service	22 — Unusual, excessive procedure	HYPERCHOLESTEROLEMIA –272.0
24 — Unrelated E/M service during postop.	50 — Bilateral procedure	
25 — Significant, separately identifiable E/M	51 — Multiple surgical procedures in same day	
32 — Mandated Service	52 — Reduced/incomplete procedure	
57 — Decision for surgery	55 — Postop. management only	
	59 — Distinct multiple procedures	

CATEGORY	CODE	MOD	FEE	CATEGORY	CODE	MOD	FEE
Office Visit — New Patient				**Wound Care**			
Minimal office visit	99201			Debride partial thickness burn	11040		
20 minutes	99202			Debride full thickness burn	11041		
30 minutes	99203			Debride wound, not a burn	11000		
45 minutes	99204			Unna boot application	29580		
60 minutes	99205			Unna boot removal	29700		
Other				Other			
Office Visit — Established				**Supplies**			
Minimal office visit	99211			Ace bandage, 2"	A6448		
10 minutes	99212	X	35.00	Ace bandage, 3"-4"	A6449		
15 minutes	99213			Ace bandage, 6"	A6450		
25 minutes	99214			Cast, fiberglass	A4590		
40 minutes	99215			Coban wrap	A6454		
Other				Foley catheter	A4338		
General Procedures				Immobilizer	L3670		
Anoscopy	46600			Kerlix roll	A6220		
Audiometry	92551			Oxygen mask/cannula	A4620		
Breast aspiration	19000			Sleeve, elbow	E0191		
Cerumen removal	69210			Sling	A4565		
Circumcision	54150			Splint, ready-made	A4570		
DDST	96110			Splint, wrist	S8451		
Flex sigmoidoscopy	45330			Sterile packing	A6407		
Flex sig. w/ biopsy	45331			Surgical tray	A4550		
Foreign body removal—foot	28190			Other			
Nail removal	11730			**OB Care**			
Nail removal/phenol	11750			Routine OB care	59400		
Trigger point injection	20552			Postpartum care only (separate procedure)	59430		
Tympanometry	92567			Ante partum 4–6 visits	59425		
Visual acuity	99173			Ante partum 7 or more visits	59426		
Other	80061	X	20.00	Other			
Other				Other			

Other Visit Information: _____

Lab Work to Order: _____

Referral to: _____

Provider Signature: _____

Next Appointment: _____

Fees:

Total Charges: $55.00

Copay Received: $_____

Other Payment: $55.00 VISA

Total Due: **$0.00**

Allied Medical Center
REGISTRATION FORM
(Please Print)

Today's date:	PCP:

PATIENT INFORMATION

Patient's last name: SAMPSON	First: DEAN	Middle:	☒ Mr. ❑ Mrs.	❑ Miss ❑ Ms.	Marital status (circle one) (Single) / Mar / Div / Sep / Wid

Is this your legal name? ☒ Yes ❑ No	If not, what is your legal name?	(Former name):	Birth date: 11/16/1993	Age:	Sex: ☒ M ❑ F

Street address: 1940 Frankford RD. Apt 132	Social Security no.: 999-87-5624	Home phone no.: (972) 555-8666

P.O. box:	City: CARROLLTON	State: TX	ZIP Code: 12345

Occupation:	Employer:	Employer phone no.: ( )

Chose clinic because/Referred to clinic by (please choose one):	❑ Dr.	☒ Insurance Plan	❑ Hospital

❑ Family	❑ Friend	❑ Close to home/work	❑ Yellow Pages	❑ Other

Other family members seen here:

REASON FOR THIS VISIT: ELBOW PAIN

INSURANCE INFORMATION

(Please give your insurance card to the receptionist.)

Person responsible for bill: ANNETTE SAMPSON	Birth date: 08/25/1963	Address (if different): SAME	Home phone no.: ( )

Is this person a patient here?	❑ Yes	☒ No

Occupation: IT SPECIALIST	Employer: COMPUTER GEEKS	Employer address: 2306 W. Beltline RD. #210 Carrollton TX 12345	Employer phone no.: (972) 555-6530

Is this patient covered by insurance?	☒ Yes	❑ No

Please indicate primary insurance:	PHCS EPO	Claims Mailing Address:	PO BOX 4658	IRVING, TX	12345
		PHONE: 800-555-2569			

Subscriber's name: ANNETTE SAMPSON	Subscriber's S.S. no.: 655-88-9520	Birth date: 08/25/1963	❑ M ☒ F	Group no.: 365280	Policy no.: 655889520	Co-payment: $25.00

Patient's relationship to subscriber:	❑ Self	❑ Spouse	☒ Child	❑ Other

Name of secondary insurance (if applicable):	Subscriber's name and DOB:	❑ M ❑ F	Group no.:	Policy no.:

Patient's relationship to subscriber:	❑ Self	❑ Spouse	❑ Child	❑ Other Claims Address:

IN CASE OF EMERGENCY

Name of local friend or relative (not living at same address): LELAND SAMPSON	Relationship to patient: SIBLING	Home phone no.: (469) 555-8716	Work phone no.: (972) 555-8500

The above information is true to the best of my knowledge. I authorize my insurance benefits to be paid directly to the physician. I understand that I am financially responsible for any balance. I also authorize ALLIED MEDICAL CENTER or insurance company to release any information required to process my claims.

Annette Sampson

Patient/Guardian signature	_Date_

ENCOUNTER FORM

Patient Information		Payment Method		Visit Information	
Patient ID number		**Primary**	PHCS EPO	Visit date	
Patient name	Dean Sampson	Primary ID number	655885520	Visit number	
Address	1940 Frankford Rd #132	Primary group number	365280	Rendering physician	
City/State	Carrollton, TX 12345	**Secondary**		Referring physician	
Phone number	972-555-8666	Secondary ID number		Reason for visit	ELBOW PAIN
Date of birth	11/16/1993	Secondary group no.			
Age		Cash/credit card			
		Other billing			

E/M Modifiers	Procedure Modifiers	DIAGNOSIS:
21 — Prolonged E&M Service	22 — Unusual, excessive procedure	SPRAIN ULNOHUMERAL JOINT 841.3
24 — Unrelated E/M service during postop.	50 — Bilateral procedure	
25 — Significant, separately identifiable E/M	51 — Multiple surgical procedures in same day	
32 — Mandated Service	52 — Reduced/incomplete procedure	
57 — Decision for surgery	55 — Postop. management only	
	59 — Distinct multiple procedures	

CATEGORY	CODE	MOD	FEE	CATEGORY	CODE	MOD	FEE
Office Visit — New Patient				**Wound Care**			
Minimal office visit	99201			Debride partial thickness burn	11040		
20 minutes	99202			Debride full thickness burn	11041		
30 minutes	99203			Debride wound, not a burn	11000		
45 minutes	99204			Unna boot application	29580		
60 minutes	99205			Unna boot removal	29700		
Other				Other			
Office Visit — Established				**Supplies**			
Minimal office visit	99211			Ace bandage, 2"	A6448		
10 minutes	99212			Ace bandage, 3"-4"	A6449		
15 minutes	99213			Ace bandage, 6"	A6450		
25 minutes	99214	X	65.00	Cast, fiberglass	A4590		
40 minutes	99215			Coban wrap	A6454		
Other				Foley catheter	A4338		
General Procedures				Immobilizer	L3670		
Anoscopy	46600			Kerlix roll	A6220		
Audiometry	92551			Oxygen mask/cannula	A4620		
Breast aspiration	19000			Sleeve, elbow	E0191		
Cerumen removal	69210			Sling	A4565		
Circumcision	54150			Splint, ready-made	A4570		
DDST	96110			Splint, wrist	S8451		
Flex sigmoidoscopy	45330			Sterile packing	A6407		
Flex sig. w/ biopsy	45331			Surgical tray	A4550		
Foreign body removal—foot	28190			Other			
Nail removal	11730			OB Care			
Nail removal/phenol	11750			Routine OB care	59400		
Trigger point injection	20552			Postpartum care only (separate procedure)	59430		
Tympanometry	92567			Ante partum 4–6 visits	59425		
Visual acuity	99173			Ante partum 7 or more visits	59426		
Other	73090	X	45.00	Other			
Other				Other			

Other Visit Information: _____

Lab Work to Order: _____

Referral to: _____

Provider Signature: _____

Next Appointment: _____

Fees:

Total Charges: $110.00

Copay Received: $ 25.00 CASH

Other Payment: $_____

Total Due: **$85.00**

Allied Medical Center 1933 E. Frankford Rd. Carrollton, TX 12345 **972-555-5482**

Allied Medical Center
REGISTRATION FORM
(Please Print)

Today's date:	PCP:

PATIENT INFORMATION

Patient's last name: BLACK	First: DIANNE	Middle: E	☐ Mr. ☒ Mrs.	☐ Miss ☐ Ms.	Marital status (circle one) Single / (Mar) / Div / Sep / Wid

Is this your legal name? ☒ Yes ☐ No	If not, what is your legal name?	(Former name):	Birth date: 01/06/1947	Age:	Sex: ☐ M ☒ F

Street address: 1222 ELDER RD	Social Security no.: 321-22-8787	Home phone no.: (972) 555-5277

P.O. box:	City: CARROLLTON	State: TX	ZIP Code: 12345

Occupation: MEDICAL SPECIALIST	Employer: DR. WALTER WEISS	Employer phone no.: (972) 555-8759

Chose clinic because/Referred to clinic by (please choose one):	☒ Dr. WALTER WEISS	☐ Insurance Plan	☐ Hospital

☐ Family	☐ Friend	☐ Close to home/work	☐ Yellow Pages	☐ Other **AUTH# R85946100016, 60 DAYS**

Other family members seen here:

REASON FOR THIS VISIT: SHORTNESS OF BREATH

INSURANCE INFORMATION

(Please give your insurance card to the receptionist.)

Person responsible for bill: PATIENT	Birth date: / /	Address (if different): SAME	Home phone no.: ( )

Is this person a patient here? ☒ Yes ☐ No

Occupation: SAME AS ABOVE	Employer:	Employer address:	Employer phone no.: ( )

Is this patient covered by insurance? ☒ Yes ☐ No

Please indicate primary insurance:	BCBS TX HMO	Claims Mailing Address:	PO BOX 550066	DALLAS, TX	12345

		PHONE: 800-555-6582	

Subscriber's name: DIANNE BLACK	Subscriber's S.S. no.: 321-22-8787	Birth date: 01/06/1947	☐ M ☒ F	Group no.: 65981	Policy no.: ABC321228787	Co-payment: $5.00

Patient's relationship to subscriber: ☒ Self ☐ Spouse ☐ Child ☐ Other

Name of secondary insurance (if applicable): AETNA PPO	Subscriber's name and DOB: Sean Black 12/13/1948	☒ M ☐ F	Group no.: 65002	Policy no.: 129874

Patient's relationship to subscriber: ☐ Self ☒ Spouse ☐ Child ☐ Other	Claims Address: P O BOX 915 Arlington, TX 12345 800-555-7462

IN CASE OF EMERGENCY

Name of local friend or relative (not living at same address): LISA ADAMS	Relationship to patient: NEIGHBOR/FRIEND	Home phone no.: (972) 555-2681	Work phone no.: (214) 555-7016

The above information is true to the best of my knowledge. I authorize my insurance benefits to be paid directly to the physician. I understand that I am financially responsible for any balance. I also authorize ALLIED MEDICAL CENTER or insurance company to release any information required to process my claims.

Dianne Black

Patient/Guardian signature   _Date_

ENCOUNTER FORM

Patient Information		Payment Method		Visit Information	
Patient ID number		**Primary**	BCBS TX HMO	Visit date	
Patient name	Dianne Black	Primary ID number	ABC321228787	Visit number	
Address	1222 Elder Rd	Primary group number	65981	Rendering physician	
City/State	Carrollton, TX 12345	**Secondary**	Aetna PPO	Referring physician	
Phone number	972-555-5277	Secondary ID number	129874	Reason for visit	SHORTNESS OF BREATH
Date of birth	01/06/1947	Secondary group no.	65002		
Age		Cash/credit card			
		Other billing			

E/M Modifiers	Procedure Modifiers	DIAGNOSIS:
21 — Prolonged E&M Service	22 — Unusual, excessive procedure	PERSISTENT SINUS BRADYCARDIA
24 — Unrelated E/M service during postop.	50 — Bilateral procedure	427.81
25 — Significant, separately identifiable E/M	51 — Multiple surgical procedures in same day	
32 — Mandated Service	52 — Reduced/incomplete procedure	
57 — Decision for surgery	55 — Postop. management only	
	59 — Distinct multiple procedures	

CATEGORY	CODE	MOD	FEE	CATEGORY	CODE	MOD	FEE
Office Visit — New Patient				**Wound Care**			
Minimal office visit	99201			Debride partial thickness burn	11040		
20 minutes	99202			Debride full thickness burn	11041		
30 minutes	99203	X	120.00	Debride wound, not a burn	11000		
45 minutes	99204			Unna boot application	29580		
60 minutes	99205			Unna boot removal	29700		
Other				Other			
Office Visit — Established				**Supplies**			
Minimal office visit	99211			Ace bandage, 2"	A6448		
10 minutes	99212			Ace bandage, 3"-4"	A6449		
15 minutes	99213			Ace bandage, 6"	A6450		
25 minutes	99214			Cast, fiberglass	A4590		
40 minutes	99215			Coban wrap	A6454		
Other				Foley catheter	A4338		
General Procedures				Immobilizer	L3670		
Anoscopy	46600			Kerlix roll	A6220		
Audiometry	92551			Oxygen mask/cannula	A4620		
Breast aspiration	19000			Sleeve, elbow	E0191		
Cerumen removal	69210			Sling	A4565		
Circumcision	54150			Splint, ready-made	A4570		
DDST	96110			Splint, wrist	S8451		
Flex sigmoidoscopy	45330			Sterile packing	A6407		
Flex sig. w/ biopsy	45331			Surgical tray	A4550		
Foreign body removal—foot	28190			Other			
Nail removal	11730			**OB Care**			
Nail removal/phenol	11750			Routine OB care	59400		
Trigger point injection	20552			Postpartum care only (separate procedure)	59430		
Tympanometry	92567			Ante partum 4–6 visits	59425		
Visual acuity	99173			Ante partum 7 or more visits	59426		
Other				Other			
Other				Other			

Other Visit Information: _____

Lab Work to Order: _____
Referral to: _____
Provider Signature: _____
Next Appointment: _____

Fees:
Total Charges: $120.00
Copay Received: $ 5.00 CK # 6548
Other Payment: $_____
Total Due: **$115.00**

Allied Medical Center
REGISTRATION FORM
(Please Print)

Today's date: _____   PCP: _____

PATIENT INFORMATION

Patient's last name: BONNER	First: ALICE	Middle: C	☐ Mr. ☐ Mrs.	☒ Miss ☐ Ms.	Marital status (circle one) (Single) / Mar / Div / Sep / Wid

Is this your legal name? ☒ Yes ☐ No	If not, what is your legal name?	(Former name):	Birth date: 02/13/1994	Age:	Sex: ☐ M ☒ F

Street address: 10362 Marsh Lane, APT 208	Social Security no.: 655-47-2111	Home phone no.: (972) 555-8526

P.O. box:	City: DALLAS	State: TX	ZIP Code: 12345

Occupation: STUDENT	Employer:	Employer phone no.: ( )

Chose clinic because/Referred to clinic by (please choose one): ☐ Dr. ☒ Insurance Plan ☐ Hospital

☐ Family ☐ Friend ☐ Close to home/work ☐ Yellow Pages ☐ Other

Other family members seen here:

REASON FOR THIS VISIT: SORE THROAT

INSURANCE INFORMATION

(Please give your insurance card to the receptionist.)

Person responsible for bill: HERB BONNER	Birth date: 03/01/1995	Address (if different): SAME AS PATIENT	Home phone no.: ( )

Is this person a patient here? ☐ Yes ☒ No

Occupation: INSTRUCTOR	Employer: ST MARK'S SCHOOL	Employer address: 15201 PRESTON RD. DALLAS, TX 12345	Employer phone no.: (214) 555-1470

Is this patient covered by insurance? ☒ Yes ☐ No

Please indicate primary insurance:	OXFORD HEALTH EPO	Claims Mailing Address:	PO BOX 9998	ARLINGTON, TX	12345
		PHONE: 800-555-8693			

Subscriber's name: HERBERT BONNER	Subscriber's S.S. no.: 369-58-9514	Birth date: 03/01/1965 ☒ M ☐ F	Group no.: 500	Policy no.: 369589514-03	Co-payment: $40.00

Patient's relationship to subscriber: ☐ Self ☐ Spouse ☒ Child ☐ Other

Name of secondary insurance (if applicable):	Subscriber's name and DOB:	☐ M ☐ F	Group no.:	Policy no.:

Patient's relationship to subscriber: ☐ Self ☐ Spouse ☐ Child ☐ Other Claims Address:

IN CASE OF EMERGENCY

Name of local friend or relative (not living at same address): JOSEPH BROWN	Relationship to patient: FRIEND	Home phone no.: (972) 555-4957	Work phone no.: (972) 555-0062

The above information is true to the best of my knowledge. I authorize my insurance benefits to be paid directly to the physician. I understand that I am financially responsible for any balance. I also authorize ALLIED MEDICAL CENTER or insurance company to release any information required to process my claims.

Herb Bonner

Patient/Guardian signature   _Date_

ENCOUNTER FORM

Patient Information		Payment Method			Visit Information	
Patient ID number		**Primary**		Oxford Health EPO	Visit date	
Patient name	Alice Bonner	Primary ID number		369589514-03	Visit number	
Address	10362 Marsh Ln #208	Primary group number		500	Rendering physician	
City/State	Carrollton, TX 12345	**Secondary**			Referring physician	
Phone number	972-555-8526	Secondary ID number			Reason for visit	SORE THROAT
Date of birth	02/13/1994	Secondary group no.				
Age		Cash/credit card	•			
		Other billing				

E/M Modifiers	Procedure Modifiers	DIAGNOSIS:
21 — Prolonged E&M Service	22 — Unusual, excessive procedure	STREP THROAT 034.0
24 — Unrelated E/M service during postop.	50 — Bilateral procedure	
25 — Significant, separately identifiable E/M	51 — Multiple surgical procedures in same day	
32 — Mandated Service	52 — Reduced/incomplete procedure	
57 — Decision for surgery	55 — Postop. management only	
	59 — Distinct multiple procedures	

CATEGORY	CODE	MOD	FEE	CATEGORY	CODE	MOD	FEE
Office Visit — New Patient				**Wound Care**			
Minimal office visit	99201			Debride partial thickness burn	11040		
20 minutes	99202			Debride full thickness burn	11041		
30 minutes	99203			Debride wound, not a burn	11000		
45 minutes	99204			Unna boot application	29580		
60 minutes	99205			Unna boot removal	29700		
Other				Other			
Office Visit — Established				**Supplies**			
Minimal office visit	99211	X	25.00	Ace bandage, 2"	A6448		
10 minutes	99212			Ace bandage, 3"-4"	A6449		
15 minutes	99213			Ace bandage, 6"	A6450		
25 minutes	99214			Cast, fiberglass	A4590		
40 minutes	99215			Coban wrap	A6454		
Other				Foley catheter	A4338		
General Procedures				Immobilizer	L3670		
Anoscopy	46600			Kerlix roll	A6220		
Audiometry	92551			Oxygen mask/cannula	A4620		
Breast aspiration	19000			Sleeve, elbow	E0191		
Cerumen removal	69210			Sling	A4565		
Circumcision	54150			Splint, ready-made	A4570		
DDST	96110			Splint, wrist	S8451		
Flex sigmoidoscopy	45330			Sterile packing	A6407		
Flex sig. w/ biopsy	45331			Surgical tray	A4550		
Foreign body removal—foot	28190			Other			
Nail removal	11730			**OB Care**			
Nail removal/phenol	11750			Routine OB care	59400		
Trigger point injection	20552			Postpartum care only (separate procedure)	59430		
Tympanometry	92567			Ante partum 4–6 visits	59425		
Visual acuity	99173			Ante partum 7 or more visits	59426		
Other	86403	X	20.00	Other			
Other				Other			

Other Visit Information: _____

Lab Work to Order: _____

Referral to: _____

Provider Signature: _____

Next Appointment: _____

Fees:

Total Charges: $45.00

Copay Received: $40.00 CK # 582

Other Payment: $_____

Total Due: $5.00

Allied Medical Center 1933 E. Frankford Rd. Carrollton, TX 12345 **972-555-5482**

Allied Medical Center
REGISTRATION FORM
(Please Print)

Today's date:		PCP:

PATIENT INFORMATION

Patient's last name: TINKHAM	First: ROSE	Middle:	☐ Mr. ☐ Mrs.	☒ Miss ☐ Ms.	Marital status (circle one) Single / Mar / Div / Sep / Wid

Is this your legal name? ☒ Yes ☐ No	If not, what is your legal name?	(Former name):	Birth date: 04/07/1978	Age:	Sex: ☐ M ☒ F

Street address: 1249 DAVENPORT CIRCLE	Social Security no.: 614-55-9229	Home phone no.: (972) 555-7419

P.O. box:	City: FARMERS BRANCH	State: TX	ZIP Code: 12345

Occupation: SERVICE PERSON	Employer: ABC AIR CONDITIONING	Employer phone no.: (972) 555-6543

Chose clinic because/Referred to clinic by (please choose one): ☒ Dr. MICKEY ROONEY   ☐ Insurance Plan   ☐ Hospital

☐ Family   ☐ Friend   ☐ Close to home/work   ☐ Yellow Pages   ☐ Other **REFERRAL#: 2584–TODAY ONLY**

Other family members seen here:

REASON FOR THIS VISIT: FLU

INSURANCE INFORMATION

(Please give your insurance card to the receptionist.)

Person responsible for bill: SAME	Birth date: / /	Address (if different):	Home phone no.: ( )

Is this person a patient here? ☒ Yes ☐ No

Occupation:	Employer:	Employer address:	Employer phone no.: ( )

Is this patient covered by insurance? ☒ Yes ☐ No

Please indicate primary insurance:	BCBS TX HMO	Claims Mailing Address:	P O BOX 55006	DALLAS, TX	12345
		PHONE: 800-555-6582			

Subscriber's name: SAME	Subscriber's S.S. no.:	Birth date: / /	☐ M ☐ F	Group no.: 95214	Policy no.: BLM614559229	Co-payment: $15.00

Patient's relationship to subscriber: ☒ Self   ☐ Spouse   ☐ Child   ☐ Other

Name of secondary insurance (if applicable):	Subscriber's name and DOB:	☒ M ☐ F	Group no.:	Policy no.:

Patient's relationship to subscriber: ☐ Self   ☐ Spouse   ☐ Child   ☐ Other   Claims Address:

IN CASE OF EMERGENCY

Name of local friend or relative (not living at same address): KIM BOSEMAN	Relationship to patient: AUNT	Home phone no.: (972) 555-5670	Work phone no.: (214) 555-8777

The above information is true to the best of my knowledge. I authorize my insurance benefits to be paid directly to the physician. I understand that I am financially responsible for any balance. I also authorize ALLIED MEDICAL CENTER or insurance company to release any information required to process my claims.

Rose Tinkham

Patient/Guardian signature   _Date_

ENCOUNTER FORM

Patient Information		Payment Method		Visit Information	
Patient ID number		**Primary**		Visit date	
Patient name	Rose Tinkham	Primary ID number	BCBS TX HMO	Visit number	
Address	1249 Davenport Cir	Primary group number	BLM614559229	Rendering physician	
City/State	Farmers Branch, TX 12345	**Secondary**	95214	Referring physician	Mickey Rooney, M.D.
Phone number	972-555-7419	Secondary ID number		Reason for visit	FLU
Date of birth	04/07/1978	Secondary group no.			
Age		Cash/credit card			
		Other billing			

E/M Modifiers	Procedure Modifiers	DIAGNOSIS:
21 — Prolonged E&M Service	22 — Unusual, excessive procedure	INFLUENZA WITH URI 487.1
24 — Unrelated E/M service during postop.	50 — Bilateral procedure	
25 — Significant, separately identifiable E/M	51 — Multiple surgical procedures in same day	
32 — Mandated Service	52 — Reduced/incomplete procedure	
57 — Decision for surgery	55 — Postop. management only	
	59 — Distinct multiple procedures	

CATEGORY	CODE	MOD	FEE	CATEGORY	CODE	MOD	FEE
Office Visit — New Patient				**Wound Care**			
Minimal office visit	99201			Debride partial thickness burn	11040		
20 minutes	99202			Debride full thickness burn	11041		
30 minutes	99203			Debride wound, not a burn	11000		
45 minutes	99204			Unna boot application	29580		
60 minutes	99205			Unna boot removal	29700		
Other				Other			
Office Visit — Established				**Supplies**			
Minimal office visit	99211	X	25.00	Ace bandage, 2"	A6448		
10 minutes	99212			Ace bandage, 3"-4"	A6449		
15 minutes	99213			Ace bandage, 6"	A6450		
25 minutes	99214			Cast, fiberglass	A4590		
40 minutes	99215			Coban wrap	A6454		
Other				Foley catheter	A4338		
General Procedures				Immobilizer	L3670		
Anoscopy	46600			Kerlix roll	A6220		
Audiometry	92551			Oxygen mask/cannula	A4620		
Breast aspiration	19000			Sleeve, elbow	E0191		
Cerumen removal	69210			Sling	A4565		
Circumcision	54150			Splint, ready-made	A4570		
DDST	96110			Splint, wrist	S8451		
Flex sigmoidoscopy	45330			Sterile packing	A6407		
Flex sig. w/ biopsy	45331			Surgical tray	A4550		
Foreign body removal—foot	28190			Other			
Nail removal	11730			OB Care			
Nail removal/phenol	11750			Routine OB care	59400		
Trigger point injection	20552			Postpartum care only (separate procedure)	59430		
Tympanometry	92567			Ante partum 4–6 visits	59425		
Visual acuity	99173			Ante partum 7 or more visits	59426		
Other				Other	·		
Other				Other			

Other Visit Information: _____

Lab Work to Order: _____

Referral to: _____

Provider Signature: _____

Next Appointment: _____

Fees:

Total Charges:	$25.00
Copay Received:	$15.00
Other Payment:	$_____
Total Due:	**$10.00**

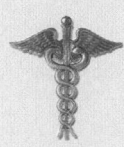

Claims processed by	**PROVIDER CLAIM**
Medi Health Insurance	
A Division of Health Care Corp.	DATE:
P.O. Box 5554	PROVIDER NUMBER: 0000K223
Dallas, Texas 12345	CHECK NUMBER: 034324
Toll Free (800) 555-5563	TAX IDENTIFICATION NUMBER: 75-1234567

1933 E. Frankford Rd. Suite 110
Carrollton, TX 12345

PATIENT: **Lisa Dupont**
PERF PRV: **0000000000000080430S**
CLAIM Number: **0000227050697800X**

IDENTIFICATION Number: **BHR716830061**
PATIENT Number: CLAIM TYPE: **MCP**

FROM / TO DATES	PROC CODE	AMOUNT BILLED	CONTRACT ALLOWABLE	SERVICES NOT COVERED	DEDUCTIONS/OTHER INELIGIBLE	AMOUNT PAID
TODAY	99203	$120.00	$86.29	$33.71 (1)	$0.00	$74.29
	90707	$ 30.00	$19.25	$10.75 (1)	$0.00	$19.25

AMOUNT PAID TO PROVIDER FOR THIS CLAIM: $93.54
DEDUCTIONS/OTHER INELIGIBLE

TOTAL SERVICES NOT COVERED:
PATIENT'S SHARE: $12.00

PATIENT: **Dianne Black**
PERF PRV: **0000000000000080430S**
CLAIM Number: **0000227050697800X**

IDENTIFICATION Number: **ABC321228787**
PATIENT Number: CLAIM TYPE: **MCP**

FROM / TO DATES	CODE	AMOUNT BILLED	CONTRACT ALLOWABLE	SERVICES NOT COVERED	DEDUCTIONS/OTHER INELIGIBLE	AMOUNT PAID
TODAY	99203	$120.00	$86.29	$33.71 (1)	$0.00	$81.29

AMOUNT PAID TO PROVIDER FOR THIS CLAIM: $81.29
DEDUCTIONS/OTHER INELIGIBLE

TOTAL SERVICES NOT COVERED: $33.71
PATIENT'S SHARE: $ 5.00

PROVIDER CLAIMS AMOUNT SUMMARY

NUMBER OF CLAIMS: 2	AMOUNT PAID TO SUBSCRIBER: $0.00	AMOUNT BILLED: $270.00
AMOUNT PAID TO PROVIDER: $174.83	AMOUNT OVER MAXIMUM ALLOWANCE: $78.17	
RECOUPMENT AMOUNT: $0.00	AMOUNT OF SERVICES NOT COVERED: $78.17	
NET AMOUNT PAID TO PROVIDER: $174.83	AMOUNT PREVIOUSLY PAID: $0.00	

(1) Contractual adjustment of billed amount

Explanation of Benefits

If you have any questions contact:

PHYSICIAN ALLIANCE INSURANCE GROUP
CENTRAL PROCESSING CENTER
Telephone: (800) 555-9901

Date:
Provider Name:
Provider TIN: **75-1234567**
Telephone Number: **972-555-5482**
Suffix (internal use): **015**
Check Number: **244183696**

1933 E FRANKFORD RD #110
CARROLLTON TX 12345

Page 1 of 2

CLAIM DETAIL SECTION (if there are numbers in the "SEE REMARKS" column, see the Remarks Section for explanation.)

Patient Name: **Margaret Dupont**   Patient Account Number:
Patient ID: **621382**   Insured's Name: **Margaret Dupont**   GROUP Number: **A435**
Provider Name: Inventory Number: **0036070010900-569**   Claim Control Number: **0101031742047-74**

SERVICE DATE(S)	PROCEDURE	TOTAL CHARGES	CONTRACT ADJUSTMENT	CONTRACT AMOUNT	PT'S COPAY	PT'SDED/ NOT COV	PAID AMT.	PT'S COINS	TOTAL PAYMENT	SEE REMARKS
	99204	$135.00	$38.47	$121.53	$10.00	$0.00	100%	$0.00	$111.53	PA
	99212	$ 35.00	$ 0.00	$ 30.00	$10.00	$0.00	100%	$0.00	$ 20.00	PA
TOTALS		$170.00	$38.47	$151.53	$20.00	$0.00		$0.00	$ 131.53	

TOTAL PAID $131.53

BALANCE DUE FROM PATIENT: PT'S DED/NOT COV: $0.00 PLUS
PT'S COINS. $0.00 = $0.00

Patient Name: **James Cather**   Patient Account Number:
Patient ID: **188383833**   Insured's Name: **James Cather**   GROUP Number: **145**
Provider Name: Inventory Number: **0036070010900-570**   Claim Control Number: **0101031742047-75**

SERVICE DATE(S)	PROCEDURE	TOTAL CHARGES	CONTRACT ADJUSTMENT	CONTRACT AMOUNT	PT'S COPAY	PT'SDED/ NOT COV	PAID AMT.	PT'S COINS	TOTAL PAYMENT	SEE REMARKS
	99214	$65.00	$27.35	$37.65	$25.00	$0.00	100%	$0.00	$12.65	PA
	93000	$45.00	$ 3.00	$42.00	$ 0.00	$0.00	100%	$0.00	$42.00	
	82954	$12.00		$12.00	$ 0.00	$0.00	100%	$0.00	$12.00	
TOTALS		$122.00	$30.35	$91.65	$25.00	$0.00		$0.00	$ 66.65	

TOTAL PAID $66.65

BALANCE DUE FROM PATIENT: PT'S DED/NOT COV: $0.00 PLUS
PT'S COINS. $0.00 = $0.00

Patient Name: **Marco Suarez**   Patient Account Number:
Patient ID: **310103101**   Insured's Name: **Marco Suarez**   GROUP Number: **MB456**
Provider Name: Inventory Number: **0036070010900-571**   Claim Control Number: **0101031742047-75**

SERVICE DATE(S)	PROCEDURE	TOTAL CHARGES	CONTRACT ADJUSTMENT	CONTRACT AMOUNT	PT'S COPAY	PT'SDED/ NOT COV	PAID AMT.	PT'S COINS	TOTAL PAYMENT	SEE REMARKS
	99213	$45.00	$2.00	$43.00	$12.00	$0.00	100%	$0.00	$31.00	PA
TOTALS		$45.00	$2.00	$43.00	$12.00	$0.00		$0.00	$31.00	

TOTAL PAID 31.00

(continued)

Explanation of Benefits

If you have any questions contact:

PHYSICIAN ALLIANCE INSURANCE GROUP
CENTRAL PROCESSING CENTER
Telephone: (800) 555-9901

Date:
Provider Name:
Provider TIN: **75-1234567**
Telephone Number: **972-555-5482**
Suffix (internal use): **015**
Check Number: **244183696**

1933 E FRANKFORD RD #110
CARROLLTON TX 12345

Page 2 of 2

CLAIM DETAIL SECTION (if there are numbers in the "SEE REMARKS" column, see the Remarks Section for explanation.)

BALANCE DUE FROM PATIENT: PT'S DED/NOT COV: $0.00 PLUS
PT'S COINS. $0.00 = $0.00

Payment Summary Section

TOTAL CHARGES	TOTAL CONTRACT ADJUSTMENT	TOTAL CONTRACT AMOUNT	TOTAL PT'S COPAY	TOTAL PT'S DED/ NOT COV	TOTAL PT'S COINS.	TOTAL PAID	CHECK #
$337.00	$70.82	$286.18	57.00	$0.00	$0.00	$229.18	244163696

Remarks Section

PA—PPO Provisions have been applied

Chapter Summary

- The responsibility of entering patient demographics requires accuracy of all data entered.
- To successfully post payments, the MOS must have knowledge of insurance companies and contract payers and must also be able to recognize and understand an Explanation of Benefits (EOB).
- Reports are generated daily to total receipts and adjustments.

Chapter Review

Complete each sentence or statement.

1. _____ is when the medical office specialist calculates all monies received, tallies all cash on hand, and compares the totals with the Patient Day Sheet report totals.

2. An amount a practice charges for medical services rendered is a(n) _____.

3. Money received in the practice is referred to as _____.

4. A(n) _____ is a record of charges, payments, and adjustments.

5. A(n) _____ is a printed report that reflects the patient's charges for a specific day.

For Additional Practice

Enter the following cases and charges into MPM software. Follow the directions provided for the office simulation and enter your own name as the provider's name.

- ▪ Print a primary claim form.
- ▪ Post the payment(s) from the EOB.
- ▪ Print the Day Sheet.
- ▪ Staple everything together and turn in to your instructor.

CASE 1

Patient Information:

Amanda L. Swanson
13956 Ohio Dr. Apt. 2011
Plano, TX 12345
972-555-3599

DOB: March 21, 1994
Single, Full-time Student
Social Security number: 456-11-7171
Account Number: Swaam

Reason for Visit: Fatigue, blurred vision, weight loss

Guarantor Information:

Louis R. Swanson (father)
13956 Ohio Dr. Apt. 2011
Plano, TX 12345
972-555-3599
Cellular: 469-555-6811

DOB: February 23, 1973
Married
Employed full time
Social Security number: 455-30-8741

Employer:
Sara Lee Foods
3905 Josey Lane
Carrollton, TX 12345
972-555-3254

Primary Insurance Information:
United HealthCare HMO
P. O. Box 36547
Darien, CT 12345
800-555-3369
Subscriber: Louis R. Swanson
ID: W54189 12242
Group: 893754-20-000
Copay: $15.00

PCP: Milam Pharo, M.D.
8226 Douglas Ave. #555
Dallas, TX 12345
NPI: 0927199510
United Healthcase PIN: 12122

Referral/Authorization Number: A56874100009

Charges:
99205 $75.00
85023 $18.00
81000 $11.00
82954 $10.00
Diagnosis: Juvenile Diabetes—IDDM—250.01
Patient paid $15.00 copay at time of service (cash)

Explanation of Benefits

For Student Use Only

Payer Name, and Address

United Healthcare
P.O. Box 36547
Darien, CT 12345

Provider's Name and Address   **Today's Date**

1933 East Frankford Rd. #110
Carrollton, TX 12345

This statement covers payments for the following patient(s): Swanson, Amanda

CLAIM DETAIL SECTION

Patient Name: Amanda Swanson   **Patient Account Number:**
Patient ID Number: W5418912242   **Insured's Name:** Louis R. Swanson
Group Number: 893754-20-000
Provider Name: **Inventory Number:**   **Claim Control Number:**

Service Date(s)	Procedure	Charges	Adjustment	Allowed	Copay	Deduct/Not Covered	Coins	Paid Amt.	Provider Paid/Remarks
	99205	$ 75.00	$11.46	$ 63.54	$15.00			100%	$48.54
	85023	$ 18.00		$ 18.00				100%	$18.00
	81000	$ 11.00	$ 2.00	$ 9.00				100%	$ 9.00
	82954	$ 10.00		$ 10.00				100%	$10.00
TOTALS		$114.00	$13.46	$100.54	$15.00				$85.54

CASE 2

Patient Information:

Mortimer "Morty" B. Rollins
1729 Frankford Rd.
Dallas, TX 12345
972-555-4111

DOB: September 21, 1971
Married
Employed full time
Social Security number: 657-20-6683

Reason for Visit: Low back pain

Employer:
VIYU Network Solutions
1701 N. Greenville Ave. #205
Richardson, TX 12345
972-555-1900

Primary Insurance Information:
United HealthCare PPO
P. O. Box 5687
Darien, CT 12345
800-555-5699

Subscriber: Self
ID: 657-20-6683
Group: 20050-45-365
Copay: $10.00

Charges:
99202 $40.00
97010 $10.00
Diagnosis: Low back pain 724.2

Explanation of Benefits

For Student Use Only

Payer Name, and Address

United Healthcare
P.O. Box 36547
Darien, CT 12345

Provider's Name and Address   **Today's Date**

Carlas Acosta, M.D.
1933 East Frankford Rd. #110
Carrollton, TX 12345

This statement covers payments for the following patient(s): Rollins, Mortimer

CLAIM DETAIL SECTION

Patient Name: Mortimer Rollins   **Patient Account Number:**
Patient ID Number: 657-20-6683   **Insured's Name:** Mortimer Rollins
Group Number: 20050-45-365
Provider Name: **Inventory Number:**   **Claim Control Number:**

Service Date(s)	Procedure	Charges	Adjustment	Allowed	Copay	Deduct/Not Covered	Coins	Paid At.	Provider Paid/Remarks
	99202	$40.00	$1.25	$38.75	$10.00			100%	$28.75
	97010	$10.00		$ 0.00		$10.00		100%	$ 0.00
TOTALS		$50.00	$1.25	$38.75	$10.00	$10.00			$28.75

PAYMENT SUMMARY SECTION (TOTALS)

Charges	Adjustment	Allowed	Copay	Deduct/Not Covered	Coins	Total Paid
$164.00	$14.71	$139.29	$25.00	$10.00		$114.29

Check Number.: 6547821100

Completing the CMS-1500 Form for Physician Outpatient Billing

The case studies in this appendix are provided for additional practice in coding and in completing the CMS-1500 claim form for physician outpatient billing. By applying what you have learned in this text, your objective is to accurately code and complete each case study. In addition to completing the CMS-1500 form, you will be required to insert the correct diagnostic and procedure codes on the SOAP forms for each patient, for which you will need both the ICD and CPT® manuals. Patient demographics and a brief case history are provided. Complete the cases based on the following criteria. All patients have release of information and assignment of benefit signatures on file. All providers are participating and accept assignment. The group practice is the billing entity. The national transition to NPI numbers is complete and legacy PINs of individual payers are no longer used. 2007 ICD-9-CM and CPT codes are used. Use 8 digit dates for birthdates. Use 6 digit dates for all other dates. All street names should be entered using standard postal abbreviations, even if they are spelled out on the source documents. To complete each case study, copy the CMS-1500 form provided in Appendix D or download it from the CD-ROM that accompanies this text. Refer to the Capital City Medical Fee Schedule on page 638 to determine the correct fees. For a list of abbreviations used in these case studies and their meanings, please refer to the CD-ROM that accompanies this text.

CASE STUDIES

Primary

Case	Patient	Primary Payer
A-1	Dennis Hurst	Medicaid
A-2	Tamara Jackson	Blue Cross Blue Shield
A-3	Zeb Nickles	Medicaid
A-4	Connie Aven	Health America
A-5	Celeste Donegan	Aetna
A-6	Carlos Clemenza	Blue Cross Blue Shield
A-7	Guy Colich	Aetna
A-8	Klaus Davies	Blue Cross Blue Shield
A-9	Matilda Vogel	TRICARE
A-10	Isaac Houston	Advantage Compensation Insurance (workers' comp)

Primary/Secondary

Case	Patient	Primary Payer/Secondary Payer
A-11	Kenneth Sung	Medicare/Medicaid
A-12	Viola Harrison	Medicare/Medicaid
A-13	Quaylord Quigley	Medicare/Medicaid
A-14	Winifred Myers	Medicare/Aetna (Retiree)
A-15	Stella Jaworski	Medicare/Medicaid
A-16	Murphy Bromley	Medicare/Blue Cross Blue Shield (Medigap)
A-17	Gus Powers	Medicare/Aetna (Retiree)
A-18	Kimber Acosta	Aetna/Medicare (MSP)
A-19	Chester Fields	Medicare/Blue Cross Blue Shield (Medigap)
A-20	Gertrude Huckle	Medicare/Health America (Retiree)

CASE A-1

Patient Information:

Name: (Last, First) <u>Hurst, Dennis</u>   ☒ Male   ☐ Female   Birth Date: <u>10/21/1992</u>

Address: <u>347 Fern St, Capital City, NY 12345</u>   Phone: <u>(555) 555-6337</u>

Social Security Number: <u>723-58-3742</u>   Full-Time Student: ☐ Yes   ☒ No

Marital Status: ☒ Single   ☐ Married   ☐ Divorced   ☐ Other

Employment:

Employer: _____ Phone: ( ) _____

Address: _____

Condition Related to: ☐ Auto Accident   ☐ Employment   ☐ Other Accident

Date of Accident: _____ State _____

Emergency Contact: _____ Phone: ( ) _____

Primary Insurance: <u>Medicaid</u>   Phone: ( ) _____

Address: <u>4875 Capital Blvd, Capital City, NY 12345</u>

Insurance Policyholder's Name: <u>Same</u>   ☐ M   ☐ F   DOB: _____

Address: <u>Same</u>

Phone: _____ Relationship to Insured: ☒ Self   ☐ Spouse   ☐ Child   ☐ Other

Employer: <u>McDinkles</u>   Phone: <u>(555) 555-1597</u>

Employer's Address: <u>7563 W. Washington St, Capital City, NY 12345</u>

Policy/ID No: <u>0000652381139</u>   Group No: _____ Percent Covered: ___%, Copay Amt: $<u>5.00</u>

Secondary Insurance: _____ Phone: ( ) _____

Address: _____

Insurance Policyholder's Name: _____ ☐ M   ☐ F   DOB: _____

Address: _____

Phone: _____ Relationship to Insured: ☐ Self   ☐ Spouse   ☐ Child   ☐ Other

Employer: _____ Phone: ( ) _____

Employer's Address: _____

Policy/ID No: _____ Group No: _____ Percent Covered: ___%, Copay Amt: $_____

Reason for Visit: <u>Stitches infected from recent surgery for the removal of a ganglion cyst</u>

Known Allergies: _____

Were you referred here? If so, by whom?: <u>Dr. Eva N. Good, Internal Medicine, NPI: 8976453201</u>

**CASE A-1
SOAP**

06/27/20XX
Assignment of Benefits: Y
Signature on File: Y
Referring Physician: Y

S: Dennis Hurst presents for complications of infected sutures.
O: Pt. had a ganglion cyst removed from his left hand on 6/25/XX. Mother concerned that the sutures are infected. On exam, there is noted infection at the site. This infection is localized. T: 99.9°F.
A: 1. Infected sutures—998.59
   2. Status postsurgery—V45.89
   3. Ganglion cyst—727.43
P: 1. Start on oral antibiotic for 10 days.
   2. Keep area clean and dry.
   3. Call office if condition worsens.
   4. Return in one week for suture removal.

Mannie Mends, MD
General Surgeon
NPI: 0123456789
Medicaid PIN: 5324896

CASE A-1 ENCOUNTER FORM

Patient Name Dennis Hurst

Capital City Medical
123 Unknown Boulevard, Capital City, NY 12345-2222

Date of Service
06-27-20XX

New Patient			Other Invasive/Noninvasive			Laboratory	
Problem Focused	99201		Arthrocentesis/Aspiration/Injection			Amylase	82150
Expanded Problem, Focused	99202		Small Joint		20600	B12	82607
Detailed	99203		Interm Joint		20605	CBC & Diff	85025
Comprehensive	99204		Major Joint		20610	Comp Metabolic Panel	80053
Comprehensive/High Complex	99205		**Other Invasive/Noninvasive**			Chlamydia Screen	87110
Well Exam Infant (up to 12 mos.)	99381		Audiometry		92552	Cholesterol	82465
Well Exam 1–4 yrs.	99382		Cast Application			Digoxin	80162
Well Exam 5–11 yrs.	99383		Location Long Short			Electrolytes	80051
Well Exam 12–17 yrs.	99384		Catheterization		51701	Ferritin	82728
Well Exam 18–39 yrs.	99385		Circumcision		54150	Folate	82746
Well Exam 40–64 yrs.	99386		Colposcopy		57452	GC Screen	87070
			Colposcopy w/Biopsy		57454	Glucose	82947
			Cryosurgery Premalignant Lesion			Glucose 1 HR	82950
			Location (s):			Glycosylated HGB A1C	83036
Established Patient			Cryosurgery Warts			HCT	85014
Post-Op Follow Up Visit	99024		Location (s):			HDL	83718
Minimum	99211		Curettement Lesion			Hep BSAG	87340
Problem Focused	99212	X	Single		11055	Hepatitis panel, acute	80074
Expanded Problem Focused	99213		2–4		11056	HGB	85018
Detailed	99214		>4		11057	HIV	86703
Comprehensive/High Complex	99215		Diaphragm Fitting		57170	Iron & TIBC	83550
Well Exam Infant (up to 12 mos.)	99391		Ear Irrigation		69210	Kidney Profile	80069
Well exam 1–4 yrs.	99392		ECG		93000	Lead	83655
Well Exam 5–11 yrs.	99393		Endometrial Biopsy		58100	Liver Profile	80076
Well Exam 12–17 yrs.	99394		Exc. Lesion Malignant			Mono Test	86308
Well Exam 18–39 yrs.	99395		Benign			Pap Smear	88155
Well Exam 40–64 yrs.	99396		Location			Pregnancy Test	84703
Obstetrics			Exc. Skin Tags (1–15)		11200	Obstetric Panel	80055
Total OB Care	59400		Each Additional 10		11201	Pro Time	85610
Injections			Fracture Treatment			PSA	84153
Administration Sub. / IM	90772		Loc			RPR	86592
Drug			w/Reduc w/o Reduc			Sed. Rate	85651
Dosage			I & D Abscess Single/Simple		10060	Stool Culture	87045
Allergy	95115		Multiple or Comp		10061	Stool O & P	87177
Cocci Skin Test	86490		I & D Pilonidal Cyst Simple		10080	Strep Screen	87880
DPT	90701		Pilonidal Cyst Complex		10081	Theophylline	80198
Hemophilus	90646		IV Therapy—To One Hour		90760	Thyroid Uptake	84479
Influenza	90658		Each Additional Hour		90761	TSH	84443
MMR	90707		Laceration Repair			Urinalysis	81000
OPV	90712		Location Size Simp/Comp			Urine Culture	87088
Pneumovax	90732		Laryngoscopy		31505	Drawing Fee	36415
TB Skin Test	86580		Oximetry		94760	Specimen Collection	99000
TD	90718		Punch Biopsy			**Other:**	
Unlisted Immun	90749		Rhythm Strip		93040		
Tetanus Toxoid	90703		Treadmill		93015		
Vaccine/Toxoid Admin <8 Yr Old w/ Counseling	90465		Trigger Point or Tendon Sheath Inj.		20550		
Vaccine/Toxoid Administration for Adult	90471		Tympanometry		92567		

Diagnosis/ICD-9: **998.59, V45.89, 727.43**

I acknowledge receipt of medical services and authorize the release of any medical information necessary to process this claim for healthcare payment only. I do authorize payment to the provider.

Patient Signature Dennis Hurst

Total Estimated Charges: _____

Payment Amount: _____

Next Appointment: _____

Capital City Medical—123 Unknown Boulevard, Capital City, NY 12345-2222 (555)555-1234

Phil Wells, MD, Mannie Mends, MD, Bette R. Soone, MD

Patient Information Form

Tax ID: 75-0246810

Group NPI: 1513171216

Patient Information:

Name: (Last, First) Jackson, Tamara   ☐ Male ☒ Female   Birth Date: 07/16/1988

Address: 41 Acorn Dr, Capital City, NY 12345   Phone: (555) 555-7650

Social Security Number: 201-19-4399   Full-Time Student: ☐ Yes ☒ No

Marital Status: ☐ Single ☒ Married ☐ Divorced ☐ Other

Employment:

Employer: Capital City Hospital   Phone: (555) 555-1516

Address: One Quality Care Way, Capital City, NY 12345

Condition Related to: ☐ Auto Accident ☐ Employment ☐ Other Accident

Date of Accident: _____ State _____

Emergency Contact: _____ Phone: ( ) _____

Primary Insurance: Blue Cross Blue Shield   Phone: ( ) _____

Address: 379 Blue Plaza, Capital City, NY 12345

Insurance Policyholder's Name: Same   ☐ M ☐ F DOB: _____

Address: _____

Phone: _____ Relationship to Insured: ☒ Self ☐ Spouse ☐ Child ☐ Other

Employer: _____ Phone: _____

Employer's Address: _____

Policy/ID No: YYZ401528821   Group No: 20639 Percent Covered: ____%, Copay Amt: $ 25.00

Secondary Insurance: _____   Phone: ( ) _____

Address: _____

Insurance Policyholder's Name: _____   ☐ M ☐ F DOB: _____

Address: _____

Phone: _____ Relationship to Insured: ☐ Self ☐ Spouse ☐ Child ☐ Other

Employer: _____ Phone: ( ) _____

Employer's Address: _____

Policy/ID No: _____ Group No: ____ Percent Covered: ____%, Copay Amt: $____

Reason for Visit: My period is about 2 weeks late

Known Allergies: _____

Were you referred here? If so, by whom?: _____

CASE A-2
SOAP

07/19/20XX
Assignment of Benefits: Y
Signature on File: Y
Referring Physician: N

S: Tamara Jackson is a new patient who complains of a missed menses x2 weeks. She has an irregular cycle. She also says that an OTC urine pregnancy test was positive yesterday.

O: Pt. denies any birth control methods. She is married and has a zero pregnancy history. Nausea is present. Denies vomiting. Says she has lost 12 lbs. in the past 2 weeks. Menses began at age 14. Pregnancy test today.

A: 1. Irregular menstrual cycle—626.4
2. Abnormal weight loss—783.21

P: 1. Serum pregnancy test today.
2. Will call pt. with results.

_____

Bette R. Soone, MD
Obstetrics/Gynecology
NPI: 0987654321
PIN: 654321

Patient Name <u>Tamara Jackson</u>

Capital City Medical
123 Unknown Boulevard, Capital City, NY 12345-2222

Date of Service
07-19-20XX

CASE A–2 ENCOUNTER FORM

New Patient			Arthrocentesis/Aspiration/Injection		Laboratory	
Problem Focused	99201		Arthrocentesis/Aspiration/Injection		Amylase	82150
Expanded Problem, Focused	99202	X	Small Joint	20600	B12	82607
Detailed	99203		Interm Joint	20605	CBC & Diff	85025
Comprehensive	99204		Major Joint	20610	Comp Metabolic Panel	80053
Comprehensive/High Complex	99205		**Other Invasive/Noninvasive**		Chlamydia Screen	87110
Well Exam Infant (up to 12 mos.)	99381		Audiometry	92552	Cholesterol	82465
Well Exam 1–4 yrs.	99382		Cast Application		Digoxin	80162
Well Exam 5–11 yrs.	99383		Location Long Short		Electrolytes	80051
Well Exam 12–17 yrs.	99384		Catheterization	51701	Ferritin	82728
Well Exam 18–39 yrs.	99385		Circumcision	54150	Folate	82746
Well Exam 40–64 yrs.	99386		Colposcopy	57452	GC Screen	87070
			Colposcopy w/Biopsy	57454	Glucose	82947
			Cryosurgery Premalignant Lesion		Glucose 1 HR	82950
			Location (s):		Glycosylated HGB A1C	83036
Established Patient			Cryosurgery Warts		HCT	85014
Post-Op Follow Up Visit	99024		Location (s):		HDL	83718
Minimum	99211		Curettement Lesion		Hep BSAG	87340
Problem Focused	99212		Single	11055	Hepatitis panel, acute	80074
Expanded Problem Focused	99213		2–4	11056	HGB	85018
Detailed	99214		>4	11057	HIV	86703
Comprehensive/High Complex	99215		Diaphragm Fitting	57170	Iron & TIBC	83550
Well Exam Infant (up to 12 mos.)	99391		Ear Irrigation	69210	Kidney Profile	80069
Well exam 1–4 yrs.	99392		ECG	93000	Lead	83655
Well Exam 5–11 yrs.	99393		Endometrial Biopsy	58100	Liver Profile	80076
Well Exam 12–17 yrs.	99394		Exc. Lesion Malignant		Mono Test	86308
Well Exam 18–39 yrs.	99395		Benign		Pap Smear	88155
Well Exam 40–64 yrs.	99396		Location		Pregnancy Test	84703	X
Obstetrics			Exc. Skin Tags (1–15)	11200	Obstetric Panel	80055
Total OB Care	59400		Each Additional 10	11201	Pro Time	85610
Injections			Fracture Treatment		PSA	84153
Administration Sub. / IM	90772		Loc		RPR	86592
Drug			w/Reduc w/o Reduc		Sed. Rate	85651
Dosage			I & D Abscess Single/Simple	10060	Stool Culture	87045
Allergy	95115		Multiple or Comp	10061	Stool O & P	87177
Cocci Skin Test	86490		I & D Pilonidal Cyst Simple	10080	Strep Screen	87880
DPT	90701		Pilonidal Cyst Complex	10081	Theophylline	80198
Hemophilus	90646		IV Therapy—To One Hour	90760	Thyroid Uptake	84479
Influenza	90658		Each Additional Hour	90761	TSH	84443
MMR	90707		Laceration Repair		Urinalysis	81000
OPV	90712		Location Size Simp/Comp		Urine Culture	87088
Pneumovax	90732		Laryngoscopy	31505	Drawing Fee	36415	X
TB Skin Test	86580		Oximetry	94760	Specimen Collection	99000
TD	90718		Punch Biopsy		**Other:**	
Unlisted Immun	90749		Rhythm Strip	93040		
Tetanus Toxoid	90703		Treadmill	93015		
Vaccine/Toxoid Admin <8 Yr Old w/ Counseling	90465		Trigger Point or Tendon Sheath Inj.	20550		
Vaccine/Toxoid Administration for Adult	90471		Tympanometry	92567		

Diagnosis/ICD-9: **626.4, 783.21**

I acknowledge receipt of medical services and authorize the release of any medical information necessary to process this claim for healthcare payment only. I do authorize payment to the provider.

Patient Signature <u>Tamara Jackson</u>

Total Estimated Charges: _____

Payment Amount: _____

Next Appointment: _____

CASE A-3

Capital City Medical—123 Unknown Boulevard, Capital City, NY 12345-2222 (555)555-1234

Phil Wells, MD, Mannie Mends, MD, Bette R. Soone, MD

Patient Information Form

Tax ID: 75-0246810

Group NPI: 1513171216

Patient Information:

Name: (Last, First) Nickles, Zeb   ☒ Male   ☐ Female   Birth Date: 01/14/1966

Address: 409 Elm St., Township, NY 12345   Phone: (555) 555-0123

Social Security Number: 251-89-3485   Full-Time Student: ☐ Yes   ☒ No

Marital Status: ☐ Single   ☒ Married   ☐ Divorced   ☐ Other

Employment:

Employer: Calver and Associates, Esq.   Phone: (555) 555-0123

Address: 4702 Hillman Ave., Suite 201, Township, NY 12345

Condition Related to: ☐ Auto Accident   ☐ Employment   ☐ Other Accident

Date of Accident: _____ State _____

Emergency Contact: _____ Phone: ( ) _____

Primary Insurance: Medicaid   Phone: ( ) _____

Address: 4875 Capital City Blvd, Capital City, NY 12345

Insurance Policyholder's Name: Same   ☐ M   ☐ F DOB: _____

Address: _____

Phone: _____ Relationship to Insured: ☒ Self   ☐ Spouse   ☐ Child   ☐ Other

Employer: _____ Phone: _____

Employer's Address: _____

Policy/ID No: 94099483171   Group No: _____ Percent Covered: ____%, Copay Amt: $20.00

Secondary Insurance: _____ Phone: ( ) _____

Address: _____

Insurance Policyholder's Name: _____   ☐ M   ☐ F DOB: _____

Address: _____

Phone: _____ Relationship to Insured: ☐ Self   ☐ Spouse   ☐ Child   ☐ Other

Employer: _____ Phone: ( ) _____

Employer's Address: _____

Policy/ID No: _____ Group No: _____ Percent Covered: ____%, Copay Amt: $____

Reason for Visit: My face hurts, my nose is draining, and I have been sneezing

Known Allergies: _____

Were you referred here? If so, by whom?: _____

07/16/20XX
Assignment of Benefits: Y
Signature on File: Y
Referring Physician: N

**CASE A-3
SOAP**

S: Zeb Nickles presents today with complaints of facial pressure, nasal drainage, and sneezing.

O: Respiratory tract reveals postnasal drip, edema, and yellowish-green mucus.

A: 1. Acute sinusitis—461.9
  2. Acute rhinitis—460

P: 1. Z-Pak.
  2. Nasonex one spray each nostril once daily.
  3. Return p.r.n.

Phil Wells, MD
Family Practice
NPI: 1234567890
Medicaid PIN: 5324896

CASE A-3 ENCOUNTER FORM

Patient Name Zeb Nickles

Capital City Medical
123 Unknown Boulevard, Capital City, NY 12345-2222

Date of Service
07-16-20XX

New Patient			Other Invasive/Noninvasive			Laboratory	
Problem Focused	99201		Arthrocentesis/Aspiration/Injection			Amylase	82150
Expanded Problem, Focused	99202		Small Joint	20600		B12	82607
Detailed	99203		Interm Joint	20605		CBC & Diff	85025
Comprehensive	99204		Major Joint	20610		Comp Metabolic Panel	80053
Comprehensive/High Complex	99205		Other Invasive/Noninvasive			Chlamydia Screen	87110
Well Exam Infant (up to 12 mos.)	99381		Audiometry	92552		Cholesterol	82465
Well Exam 1–4 yrs.	99382		Cast Application			Digoxin	80162
Well Exam 5–11 yrs.	99383		Location Long Short			Electrolytes	80051
Well Exam 12–17 yrs.	99384		Catheterization	51701		Ferritin	82728
Well Exam 18–39 yrs.	99385		Circumcision	54150		Folate	82746
Well Exam 40–64 yrs.	99386		Colposcopy	57452		GC Screen	87070
			Colposcopy w/Biopsy	57454		Glucose	82947
			Cryosurgery Premalignant Lesion			Glucose 1 HR	82950
			Location (s):			Glycosylated HGB A1C	83036
Established Patient			Cryosurgery Warts			HCT	85014
Post-Op Follow Up Visit	99024		Location (s):			HDL	83718
Minimum	99211		Curettement Lesion			Hep BSAG	87340
Problem Focused	99212	X	Single	11055		Hepatitis panel, acute	80074
Expanded Problem Focused	99213		2–4	11056		HGB	85018
Detailed	99214		>4	11057		HIV	86703
Comprehensive/High Complex	99215		Diaphragm Fitting	57170		Iron & TIBC	83550
Well Exam Infant (up to 12 mos.)	99391		Ear Irrigation	69210		Kidney Profile	80069
Well exam 1–4 yrs.	99392		ECG	93000		Lead	83655
Well Exam 5–11 yrs.	99393		Endometrial Biopsy	58100		Liver Profile	80076
Well Exam 12–17 yrs.	99394		Exc. Lesion Malignant			Mono Test	86308
Well Exam 18–39 yrs.	99395		Benign			Pap Smear	88155
Well Exam 40–64 yrs.	99396		Location			Pregnancy Test	84703
Obstetrics			Exc. Skin Taqs (1–15)	11200		Obstetric Panel	80055
Total OB Care	59400		Each Additional 10	11201		Pro Time	85610
Injections			Fracture Treatment			PSA	84153
Administration Sub. / IM	90772		Loc			RPR	86592
Drug			w/Reduc w/o Reduc			Sed. Rate	85651
Dosage			I & D Abscess Single/Simple	10060		Stool Culture	87045
Allergy	95115		Multiple or Comp	10061		Stool O & P	87177
Cocci Skin Test	86490		I & D Pilonidal Cyst Simple	10080		Strep Screen	87880
DPT	90701		Pilonidal Cyst Complex	10081		Theophylline	80198
Hemophilus	90646		IV Therapy—To One Hour	90760		Thyroid Uptake	84479
Influenza	90658		Each Additional Hour	90761		TSH	84443
MMR	90707		Laceration Repair			Urinalysis	81000
OPV	90712		Location Size Simp/Comp			Urine Culture	87088
Pneumovax	90732		Laryngoscopy	31505		Drawing Fee	36415
TB Skin Test	86580		Oximetry	94760		Specimen Collection	99000
TD	90718		Punch Biopsy			Other:	
Unlisted Immun	90749		Rhythm Strip	93040			
Tetanus Toxoid	90703		Treadmill	93015			
Vaccine/Toxoid Admin <8 Yr Old w/ Counseling	90465		Trigger Point or Tendon Sheath Inj.	20550			
Vaccine/Toxoid Administration for Adult	90471		Tympanometry	92567			

Diagnosis/ICD-9: **461.9, 460**

I acknowledge receipt of medical services and authorize the release of any medical information necessary to process this claim for healthcare payment only. I do authorize payment to the provider.

Patient Signature Zeb Nickles

Total Estimated Charges: _____

Payment Amount: _____

Next Appointment: _____

Capital City Medical—123 Unknown Boulevard, Capital City,
NY 12345-2222 (555)555-1234
Phil Wells, MD, Mannie Mends, MD, Bette R. Soone, MD

Patient Information Form
Tax ID: 75-0246810
Group NPI: 1513171216

Patient Information:

Name: (Last, First) Aven, Connie   ☐ Male   ☒ Female   Birth Date: 01/28/1984

Address: 55 Buckeye Dr, Capital City, NY 12345   Phone: (555) 555-3165

Social Security Number: 309-14-7286   Full-Time Student: ☐ Yes   ☒ No

Marital Status: ☐ Single   ☒ Married   ☐ Divorced   ☐ Other

Employment:

Employer: Swellsville Fireworks International   Phone: (555) 555-2200

Address: 1019 Kaboom Rd, Township, NY 12345

Condition Related to: ☐ Auto Accident   ☐ Employment   ☐ Other Accident

Date of Accident: _____ State _____

Emergency Contact: _____   **Phone: ( )** _____

Primary Insurance: Health America   Phone: ( ) _____

Address: 2031 Healthica Center, Capital City, NY 12345

Insurance Policyholder's Name: Marc Aven   ☒ M ☐ F DOB: 08/18/1983

Address: Same

Phone: _____ Relationship to Insured: ☐ Self ☒ Spouse ☐ Child ☐ Other

Employer: Computer Training Academy   Phone: (555) 555-8852

Employer's Address: 10 Parkway Center, Capital City, NY 12345

Policy/ID No: 7325185   Group No: 01429 Percent Covered: ___%, Copay Amt: $15.00

Secondary Insurance: _____   Phone: ( ) _____

Address: _____

Insurance Policyholder's Name: _____   ☐ M ☐ F DOB: _____

Address: _____

Phone: _____ Relationship to Insured: ☐ Self ☐ Spouse ☐ Child ☐ Other

Employer: _____   Phone: ( ) _____

Employer's Address: _____

Policy/ID No: _____ Group No: _____ Percent Covered: ___%, Copay Amt: $_____

Reason for Visit: I am having pain in my right eye and it is swollen

Known Allergies: _____

Were you referred here? If so, by whom?: _____

CASE A-4
SOAP

12/01/20XX
Assignment of Benefits: Y
Signature on File: Y
Referring Physician: N

S: Connie Aven presents in the office for a painful and swollen right eye.
O: Pt. denies any injury to the eye. She doesn't have any seasonal allergies. On exam, the right eye is infected. She can barely open it.
A: 1. Conjunctivitis, right eye—372.00
P: 1. Ophthalmic ointment 1 drop q 6 h.
     2. Return as needed.

_____

Phil Wells, MD
Family Practice
NPI: 1234567890
PIN: 822093

Patient Name _Connie Aven_

Capital City Medical
123 Unknown Boulevard, Capital City, NY 12345-2222

Date of Service
12-01-20XX

**CASE A-4
ENCOUNTER
FORM**

New Patient					Laboratory	
Problem Focused	99201	Arthrocentesis/Aspiration/Injection			Amylase	82150
Expanded Problem, Focused	99202	Small Joint		20600	B12	82607
Detailed	99203	Interm Joint		20605	CBC & Diff	85025
Comprehensive	99204	Major Joint		20610	Comp Metabolic Panel	80053
Comprehensive/High Complex	99205	**Other Invasive/Noninvasive**			Chlamydia Screen	87110
Well Exam Infant (up to 12 mos.)	99381	Audiometry		92552	Cholesterol	82465
Well Exam 1–4 yrs.	99382	Cast Application			Digoxin	80162
Well Exam 5–11 yrs.	99383	Location Long Short			Electrolytes	80051
Well Exam 12–17 yrs.	99384	Catheterization		51701	Ferritin	82728
Well Exam 18–39 yrs.	99385	Circumcision		54150	Folate	82746
Well Exam 40–64 yrs.	99386	Colposcopy		57452	GC Screen	87070
		Colposcopy w/Biopsy		57454	Glucose	82947
		Cryosurgery Premalignant Lesion			Glucose 1 HR	82950
		Location (s):			Glycosylated HGB A1C	83036
Established Patient		Cryosurgery Warts			HCT	85014
Post-Op Follow Up Visit	99024	Location (s):			HDL	83718
Minimum	99211	Curettement Lesion			Hep BSAG	87340
Problem Focused	99212 X	Single		11055	Hepatitis panel, acute	80074
Expanded Problem Focused	99213	2–4		11056	HGB	85018
Detailed	99214	>4		11057	HIV	86703
Comprehensive/High Complex	99215	Diaphragm Fitting		57170	Iron & TIBC	83550
Well Exam Infant (up to 12 mos.)	99391	Ear Irrigation		69210	Kidney Profile	80069
Well exam 1–4 yrs.	99392	ECG		93000	Lead	83655
Well Exam 5–11 yrs.	99393	Endometrial Biopsy		58100	Liver Profile	80076
Well Exam 12–17 yrs.	99394	Exc. Lesion Malignant			Mono Test	86308
Well Exam 18–39 yrs.	99395	Benign			Pap Smear	88155
Well Exam 40–64 yrs.	99396	Location			Pregnancy Test	84703
Obstetrics		Exc. Skin Taqs (1–15)		11200	Obstetric Panel	80055
Total OB Care	59400	Each Additional 10		11201	Pro Time	85610
Injections		Fracture Treatment			PSA	84153
Administration Sub. / IM	90772	Loc			RPR	86592
Drug		w/Reduc		w/o Reduc	Sed. Rate	85651
Dosage		I & D Abscess Single/Simple		10060	Stool Culture	87045
Allergy	95115	Multiple or Comp		10061	Stool O & P	87177
Cocci Skin Test	86490	I & D Pilonidal Cyst Simple		10080	Strep Screen	87880
DPT	90701	Pilonidal Cyst Complex		10081	Theophylline	80198
Hemophilus	90646	IV Therapy—To One Hour		90760	Thyroid Uptake	84479
Influenza	90658	Each Additional Hour		90761	TSH	84443
MMR	90707	Laceration Repair			Urinalysis	81000
OPV	90712	Location Size Simp/Comp			Urine Culture	87088
Pneumovax	90732	Laryngoscopy		31505	Drawing Fee	36415
TB Skin Test	86580	Oximetry		94760	Specimen Collection	99000
TD	90718	Punch Biopsy			**Other:**	
Unlisted Immun	90749	Rhythm Strip		93040		
Tetanus Toxoid	90703	Treadmill		93015		
Vaccine/Toxoid Admin <8 Yr Old w/ Counseling	90465	Trigger Point or Tendon Sheath Inj.		20550		
Vaccine/Toxoid Administration for Adult	90471	Tympanometry		92567		

Diagnosis/ICD-9: **372.00**

I acknowledge receipt of medical services and authorize the release of any medical information necessary to process this claim for healthcare payment only. I do authorize payment to the provider.

Patient Signature _Connie Aven_

Total Estimated Charges: _____

Payment Amount: _____

Next Appointment: _____

CASE A-5

Capital City Medical—123 Unknown Boulevard, Capital City,
NY 12345-2222 (555)555-1234
Phil Wells, MD, Mannie Mends, MD, Bette R. Soone, MD

Patient Information Form
Tax ID: 75-0246810
Group NPI: 1513171216

Patient Information:

Name: (Last, First) Donegan, Celeste _____ ☐ Male ☒ Female Birth Date: 12/20/1981

Address: 2829 Pine Ln, Township, NY 12345 _____ Phone: (555) 555-6789

Social Security Number: 453-80-0147 _____ Full-Time Student: ☐ Yes ☒ No

Marital Status: ☐ Single ☒ Married ☐ Divorced ☐ Other

Employment:

Employer: Drexell Business College _____ Phone: (555) 555-1500

Address: 2426 Clark Bldg, Township, NY 12345

Condition Related to: ☐ Auto Accident ☐ Employment ☐ Other Accident

Date of Accident: _____ State _____

Emergency Contact: _____ **Phone: ( )** _____

Primary Insurance: Aetna _____ Phone: ( ) _____

Address: 1625 Healthcare Bldg, Capital City, NY 12345

Insurance Policyholder's Name: Douglas Donegan _____ ☒ M ☐ F DOB: 09/20/1981

Address: Same

Phone: _____ Relationship to Insured: ☐ Self ☒ Spouse ☐ Child ☐ Other

Employer: Number One Construction, Inc. _____ Phone: (555) 555-1063

Employer's Address: 1700 King Ave, Township, NY 12345

Policy/ID No: 4983282 _____ Group No: 60531 Percent Covered: 90 %, Copay Amt: $___

Secondary Insurance: _____ Phone: ( ) _____

Address: _____

Insurance Policyholder's Name: _____ ☐ M ☐ F DOB: _____

Address: _____

Phone: _____ Relationship to Insured: ☐ Self ☐ Spouse ☐ Child ☐ Other

Employer: _____ Phone: ( ) _____

Employer's Address: _____

Policy/ID No: _____ Group No: ___ Percent Covered: ___%, Copay Amt: $___

Reason for Visit: Yearly gynecological exam _____

Known Allergies: _____

Were you referred here? If so, by whom?: _____

01/23/20XX
Assignment of Benefits: Y
Signature on File: Y
Referring Physician: N

S: Celeste Donegan is in office today for a gynecological exam. She presents without complaints.
O: Pelvic and abdominal exam negative. Breasts: No masses felt.
A: 1. Routine gynecological exam with pap—V72.31
P: 1. Healthy female gynecological examination.
      2. Chlamydia screen today.
      3. Return p.r.n.

_____

Bette R. Soone, MD
Obstetrics/Gynecology
NPI: 0987654321
UPIN: 654321

CASE A-5
SOAP

CASE A-5 ENCOUNTER FORM

Patient Name *Celeste Donegan*

Capital City Medical
123 Unknown Boulevard, Capital City, NY 12345-2222

Date of Service
01-23-20XX

New Patient		Other Invasive/Noninvasive			Laboratory		
Problem Focused	99201	Arthrocentesis/Aspiration/Injection			Amylase	82150	
Expanded Problem, Focused	99202	Small Joint	20600		B12	82607	
Detailed	99203	Interm Joint	20605		CBC & Diff	85025	
Comprehensive	99204	Major Joint	20610		Comp Metabolic Panel	80053	
Comprehensive/High Complex	99205	**Other Invasive/Noninvasive**			Chlamydia Screen	87110	X
Well Exam Infant (up to 12 mos.)	99381	Audiometry	92552		Cholesterol	82465	
Well Exam 1–4 yrs.	99382	Cast Application			Digoxin	80162	
Well Exam 5–11 yrs.	99383	Location Long Short			Electrolytes	80051	
Well Exam 12–17 yrs.	99384	Catheterization	51701		Ferritin	82728	
Well Exam 18–39 yrs.	99385	Circumcision	54150		Folate	82746	
Well Exam 40–64 yrs.	99386	Colposcopy	57452		GC Screen	87070	
		Colposcopy w/Biopsy	57454		Glucose	82947	
		Cryosurgery Premalignant Lesion			Glucose 1 HR	82950	
		Location (s):			Glycosylated HGB A1C	83036	
Established Patient		Cryosurgery Warts			HCT	85014	
Post-Op Follow Up Visit	99024	Location (s):			HDL	83718	
Minimum	99211	Curettement Lesion			Hep BSAG	87340	
Problem Focused	99212	Single	11055		Hepatitis panel, acute	80074	
Expanded Problem Focused	99213	2–4	11056		HGB	85018	
Detailed	99214	>4	11057		HIV	86703	
Comprehensive/High Complex	99215	Diaphragm Fitting	57170		Iron & TIBC	83550	
Well Exam Infant (up to 12 mos.)	99391	Ear Irrigation	69210		Kidney Profile	80069	
Well exam 1–4 yrs.	99392	ECG	93000		Lead	83655	
Well Exam 5–11 yrs.	99393	Endometrial Biopsy	58100		Liver Profile	80076	
Well Exam 12–17 yrs.	99394	Exc. Lesion Malignant			Mono Test	86308	
Well Exam 18–39 yrs.	99395 X	Benign			Pap Smear	88155	X
Well Exam 40–64 yrs.	99396	Location			Pregnancy Test	84703	
Obstetrics		Exc. Skin Taqs (1–15)	11200		Obstetric Panel	80055	
Total OB Care	59400	Each Additional 10	11201		Pro Time	85610	
Injections		Fracture Treatment			PSA	84153	
Administration Sub. / IM	90772	Loc			RPR	86592	
Drug		w/Reduc w/o Reduc			Sed. Rate	85651	
Dosage		I & D Abscess Single/Simple	10060		Stool Culture	87045	
Allergy	95115	Multiple or Comp	10061		Stool O & P	87177	
Cocci Skin Test	86490	I & D Pilonidal Cyst Simple	10080		Strep Screen	87880	
DPT	90701	Pilonidal Cyst Complex	10081		Theophylline	80198	
Hemophilus	90646	IV Therapy—To One Hour	90760		Thyroid Uptake	84479	
Influenza	90658	Each Additional Hour	90761		TSH	84443	
MMR	90707	Laceration Repair			Urinalysis	81000	X
OPV	90712	Location Size Simp/Comp			Urine Culture	87088	
Pneumovax	90732	Laryngoscopy	31505		Drawing Fee	36415	X
TB Skin Test	86580	Oximetry	94760		Specimen Collection	99000	
TD	90718	Punch Biopsy			**Other:**		
Unlisted Immun	90749	Rhythm Strip	93040				
Tetanus Toxoid	90703	Treadmill	93015				
Vaccine/Toxoid Admin <8 Yr Old w/ Counseling	90465	Trigger Point or Tendon Sheath Inj.	20550				
Vaccine/Toxoid Administration for Adult	90471	Tympanometry	92567				
					Pap Smear Procedure	88142	X

Diagnosis/ICD-9: **V72.31**

I acknowledge receipt of medical services and authorize the release of any medical information necessary to process this claim for healthcare payment only. I do authorize payment to the provider.

Patient Signature *Celeste Donegan*

Total Estimated Charges: _____

Payment Amount: _____

Next Appointment: _____

CASE A-6

Capital City Medical—123 Unknown Boulevard, Capital City,
NY 12345-2222 (555)555-1234
Phil Wells, MD, Mannie Mends, MD, Bette R. Soone, MD

Patient Information Form
Tax ID: 75-0246810
Group NPI: 1513171216

Patient Information:

Name: (Last, First) Clemenza, Carlos   ☒ Male   ☐ Female   Birth Date: 02/27/2003
Address: 33 Oak St, Capital City, NY 12345   Phone: (555) 555-4577
Social Security Number: 313-80-7422   Full-Time Student: ☐ Yes   ☒ No
Marital Status: ☒ Single   ☐ Married   ☐ Divorced   ☐ Other

Employment:

Employer: _____   Phone: ( ) _____
Address: _____
Condition Related to: ☐ Auto Accident   ☐ Employment   ☐ Other Accident
Date of Accident: _____   State _____
Emergency Contact: _____   **Phone: ( )** _____

Primary Insurance: Blue Cross Blue Shield HMO   Phone: ( ) _____
Address: 379 Blue Plaza, Capital City, NY 12345
Insurance Policyholder's Name: Maria Clemenza   ☐ M ☒ F DOB: 06/25/1985
Address: Same
Phone: _____ Relationship to Insured: ☐ Self ☐ Spouse ☒ Child ☐ Other
Employer: Carrollton Wing Shack   Phone: (555) 555-1717
Employer's Address: 1604 State St, Capital City, NY 12345
Policy/ID No: YYJ885631259   Group No: 162878 Percent Covered: ____%, Copay Amt: $10.00

Secondary Insurance: _____   Phone: ( ) _____
Address: _____
Insurance Policyholder's Name: _____   ☐ M ☐ F DOB: _____
Address: _____
Phone: _____ Relationship to Insured: ☐ Self ☐ Spouse ☐ Child ☐ Other
Employer: _____   Phone: ( ) _____
Employer's Address: _____
Policy/ID No: _____   Group No: _____ Percent Covered: ____%, Copay Amt: $_____

Reason for Visit: Right ear pain

Known Allergies: _____

Were you referred here? If so, by whom?: _____

CASE A-6
SOAP

07/16/20XX
Assignment of Benefits: Y
Signature on File: Y
Referring Physician: N

S: Carlos Clemenza presents for his well exam. His mother says he has been complaining of pain in his right ear since yesterday evening.

O: Pt. is 5 years old. His right ear is swollen and there is minimal drainage. His left ear is unremarkable.

A: 1. Otitis media—382.9
    2. Well child exam—V20.2

P: 1. Start Amox one b.i.d. x10 days.

_____

Phil Wells, MD
Family Practice
NPI: 1234567890
UPIN: 123456

Patient Name *Carlos Clemenza*

Capital City Medical
123 Unknown Boulevard, Capital City, NY 12345-2222

Date of Service
07-16-20XX

New Patient			Other Invasive/Noninvasive			Laboratory	
Problem Focused	99201		Arthrocentesis/Aspiration/Injection			Amylase	82150
Expanded Problem, Focused	99202		Small Joint		20600	B12	82607
Detailed	99203		Interm Joint		20605	CBC & Diff	85025
Comprehensive	99204		Major Joint		20610	Comp Metabolic Panel	80053
Comprehensive/High Complex	99205		**Other Invasive/Noninvasive**			Chlamydia Screen	87110
Well Exam Infant (up to 12 mos.)	99381		Audiometry		92552	Cholesterol	82465
Well Exam 1–4 yrs.	99382		Cast Application			Digoxin	80162
Well Exam 5–11 yrs.	99383		Location Long Short			Electrolytes	80051
Well Exam 12–17 yrs.	99384		Catheterization		51701	Ferritin	82728
Well Exam 18–39 yrs.	99385		Circumcision		54150	Folate	82746
Well Exam 40–64 yrs.	99386		Colposcopy		57452	GC Screen	87070
			Colposcopy w/Biopsy		57454	Glucose	82947
			Cryosurgery Premalignant Lesion			Glucose 1 HR	82950
			Location (s):			Glycosylated HGB A1C	83036
Established Patient			Cryosurgery Warts			HCT	85014
Post-Op Follow Up Visit	99024		Location (s):			HDL	83718
Minimum	99211		Curettement Lesion			Hep BSAG	87340
Problem Focused	99212	X	Single		11055	Hepatitis panel, acute	80074
Expanded Problem Focused	99213		2–4		11056	HGB	85018
Detailed	99214		>4		11057	HIV	86703
Comprehensive/High Complex	99215		Diaphragm Fitting		57170	Iron & TIBC	83550
Well Exam Infant (up to 12 mos.)	99391		Ear Irrigation		69210	Kidney Profile	80069
Well exam 1–4 yrs.	99392		ECG		93000	Lead	83655
Well Exam 5–11 yrs.	99393	X	Endometrial Biopsy		58100	Liver Profile	80076
Well Exam 12–17 yrs.	99394		Exc. Lesion Malignant			Mono Test	86308
Well Exam 18–39 yrs.	99395		Benign			Pap Smear	88155
Well Exam 40–64 yrs.	99396		Location			Pregnancy Test	84703
Obstetrics			Exc. Skin Tags (1–15)		11200	Obstetric Panel	80055
Total OB Care	59400		Each Additional 10		11201	Pro Time	85610
Injections			Fracture Treatment			PSA	84153
Administration Sub. / IM	90772		Loc			RPR	86592
Drug			w/Reduc w/o Reduc			Sed. Rate	85651
Dosage			I & D Abscess Single/Simple		10060	Stool Culture	87045
Allergy	95115		Multiple or Comp		10061	Stool O & P	87177
Cocci Skin Test	86490		I & D Pilonidal Cyst Simple		10080	Strep Screen	87880
DPT	90701		Pilonidal Cyst Complex		10081	Theophylline	80198
Hemophilus	90646		IV Therapy—To One Hour		90760	Thyroid Uptake	84479
Influenza	90658		Each Additional Hour		90761	TSH	84443
MMR	90707		Laceration Repair			Urinalysis	81000
OPV	90712		Location Size Simp/Comp			Urine Culture	87088
Pneumovax	90732		Laryngoscopy		31505	Drawing Fee	36415
TB Skin Test	86580		Oximetry		94760	Specimen Collection	99000
TD	90718		Punch Biopsy			**Other:**	
Unlisted Immun	90749		Rhythm Strip		93040	Modifier 99212-25	X
Tetanus Toxoid	90703		Treadmill		93015		
Vaccine/Toxoid Admin <8 Yr Old w/ Counseling	90465		Trigger Point or Tendon Sheath Inj.		20550		
Vaccine/Toxoid Administration for Adult	90471		Tympanometry		92567		

Diagnosis/ICD-9: **382.90, V20.2**

I acknowledge receipt of medical services and authorize the release of any medical information necessary to process this claim for healthcare payment only. I do authorize payment to the provider.

Patient Signature *Maria Clemenza*

Total Estimated Charges: _____

Payment Amount: _____

Next Appointment: _____

CASE A-7

Capital City Medical—123 Unknown Boulevard, Capital City,
NY 12345-2222 (555)555-1234

Phil Wells, MD, Mannie Mends, MD, Bette R. Soone, MD

Patient Information Form
Tax ID: 75-0246810
Group NPI: 1513171216

Patient Information:

Name: (Last, First) Colich, Guy   ☒ Male   ☐ Female   Birth Date: 04/23/1958

Address: 872 Hickory Pl, Capital City, NY 12345   Phone: (555) 555-9069

Social Security Number: 142-86-2078   Full-Time Student: ☐ Yes   ☒ No

Marital Status: ☐ Single   ☒ Married   ☐ Divorced   ☐ Other

Employment:

Employer: None   Phone: ( )

Address:

Condition Related to: ☐ Auto Accident   ☐ Employment   ☐ Other Accident

Date of Accident: State

Emergency Contact: **Phone: ( )**

Primary Insurance: Aetna   Phone: ( )

Address: 1625 Healthcare Bldg, Capital City, NY 12345

Insurance Policyholder's Name: Same   ☐ M ☐ F DOB:

Address:

Phone: Relationship to Insured: ☒ Self ☐ Spouse ☐ Child ☐ Other

Employer: Phone:

Employer's Address:

Policy/ID No: 9567305   Group No: 511669 Percent Covered: ___%, Copay Amt: $35.00

Secondary Insurance: Phone: ( )

Address:

Insurance Policyholder's Name: ☐ M ☐ F DOB:

Address:

Phone: Relationship to Insured: ☐ Self ☐ Spouse ☐ Child ☐ Other

Employer: Phone: ( )

Employer's Address:

Policy/ID No: Group No: ____ Percent Covered: ___%, Copay Amt: $____

Reason for Visit: I am here for a recheck on my manic depression

Known Allergies:

Were you referred here? If so, by whom?:

10/07/20XX
Assignment of Benefits: Y
Signature on File: Y
Referring Physician: N

CASE A-7
SOAP

S: Guy Colich presents today for a checkup on his manic depression.
O: Pt. says that he has been taking his medicine faithfully since the last visit. Lab displays good value. Mental status is normal, alert, and oriented x3. He has no complaints today.
A: 1. Bipolar disorder—296.80
P: 1. Pt. is to keep psychotherapy appointment for this month.
2. Return in one month for recheck on lithium level.

_____

Phil Wells, MD
Family Practice
NPI: 1234567890
UPIN: 123456

CASE A-7 ENCOUNTER FORM

Patient Name Guy Colich

Capital City Medical
123 Unknown Boulevard, Capital City, NY 12345-2222

Date of Service
10-07-20XX

New Patient			Arthrocentesis/Aspiration/Injection			Laboratory	
Problem Focused	99201		Arthrocentesis/Aspiration/Injection			Amylase	82150
Expanded Problem, Focused	99202		Small Joint		20600	B12	82607
Detailed	99203		Interm Joint		20605	CBC & Diff	85025
Comprehensive	99204		Major Joint		20610	Comp Metabolic Panel	80053
Comprehensive/High Complex	99205		**Other Invasive/Noninvasive**			Chlamydia Screen	87110
Well Exam Infant (up to 12 mos.)	99381		Audiometry		92552	Cholesterol	82465
Well Exam 1–4 yrs.	99382		Cast Application			Digoxin	80162
Well Exam 5–11 yrs.	99383		Location Long Short			Electrolytes	80051
Well Exam 12–17 yrs.	99384		Catheterization		51701	Ferritin	82728
Well Exam 18–39 yrs.	99385		Circumcision		54150	Folate	82746
Well Exam 40–64 yrs.	99386		Colposcopy		57452	GC Screen	87070
			Colposcopy w/Biopsy		57454	Glucose	82947
			Cryosurgery Premalignant Lesion			Glucose 1 HR	82950
			Location (s):			Glycosylated HGB A1C	83036
Established Patient			Cryosurgery Warts			HCT	85014
Post-Op Follow Up Visit	99024		Location (s):			HDL	83718
Minimum	99211		Curettement Lesion			Hep BSAG	87340
Problem Focused	99212		Single		11055	Hepatitis panel, acute	80074
Expanded Problem Focused	99213	X	2–4		11056	HGB	85018
Detailed	99214		>4		11057	HIV	86703
Comprehensive/High Complex	99215		Diaphragm Fitting		57170	Iron & TIBC	83550
Well Exam Infant (up to 12 mos.)	99391		Ear Irrigation		69210	Kidney Profile	80069
Well exam 1–4 yrs.	99392		ECG		93000	Lead	83655
Well Exam 5–11 yrs.	99393		Endometrial Biopsy		58100	Liver Profile	80076
Well Exam 12–17 yrs.	99394		Exc. Lesion Malignant			Mono Test	86308
Well Exam 18–39 yrs.	99395		Benign			Pap Smear	88155
Well Exam 40–64 yrs.	99396		Location			Pregnancy Test	84703
Obstetrics			Exc. Skin Tags (1–15)		11200	Obstetric Panel	80055
Total OB Care	59400		Each Additional 10		11201	Pro Time	85610
Injections			Fracture Treatment			PSA	84153
Administration Sub. / IM	90772		Loc			RPR	86592
Drug			w/Reduc	w/o Reduc		Sed. Rate	85651
Dosage			I & D Abscess Single/Simple		10060	Stool Culture	87045
Allergy	95115		Multiple or Comp		10061	Stool O & P	87177
Cocci Skin Test	86490		I & D Pilonidal Cyst Simple		10080	Strep Screen	87880
DPT	90701		Pilonidal Cyst Complex		10081	Theophylline	80198
Hemophilus	90646		IV Therapy—To One Hour		90760	Thyroid Uptake	84479
Influenza	90658		Each Additional Hour		90761	TSH	84443
MMR	90707		Laceration Repair			Urinalysis	81000
OPV	90712		Location Size Simp/Comp			Urine Culture	87088
Pneumovax	90732		Laryngoscopy		31505	Drawing Fee	36415
TB Skin Test	86580		Oximetry		94760	Specimen Collection	99000
TD	90718		Punch Biopsy			**Other:**	
Unlisted Immun	90749		Rhythm Strip		93040		
Tetanus Toxoid	90703		Treadmill		93015		
Vaccine/Toxoid Admin <8 Yr Old w/ Counseling	90465		Trigger Point or Tendon Sheath Inj.		20550		
Vaccine/Toxoid Administration for Adult	90471		Tympanometry		92567		

Diagnosis/ICD-9: **296.80**

I acknowledge receipt of medical services and authorize the release of any medical information necessary to process this claim for healthcare payment only. I do authorize payment to the provider.

Patient Signature Guy Colich

Total Estimated Charges: _____

Payment Amount: _____

Next Appointment: _____

CASE A-8

Capital City Medical—123 Unknown Boulevard, Capital City, NY 12345-2222 (555)555-1234

Phil Wells, MD, Mannie Mends, MD, Bette R. Soone, MD

Patient Information Form

Tax ID: 75-0246810

Group NPI: 1513171216

Patient Information:

Name: (Last, First) Davies, Klaus   ☒ Male   ☐ Female   Birth Date: 10/24/1965

Address: 19 Willow Rd, Capital City, NY 12345   Phone: (555) 555-1276

Social Security Number: 631-03-4305   Full-Time Student: ☐ Yes   ☒ No

Marital Status: ☐ Single   ☒ Married   ☐ Divorced   ☐ Other

Employment:

Employer: Organic Food Mart   Phone: (555) 555-5619

Address: 13 Mile Blvd, Township, NY 12345

Condition Related to: ☐ Auto Accident   ☐ Employment   ☐ Other Accident

Date of Accident: _____ State _____

Emergency Contact: _____ Phone: ( ) _____

Primary Insurance: Blue Cross Blue Shield PPO   Phone: ( ) _____

Address: 379 Blue Plaza, Capital City, NY 12345

Insurance Policyholder's Name: Same   ☐ M ☐ F DOB: _____

Address: _____

Phone: _____ Relationship to Insured: ☒ Self ☐ Spouse ☐ Child ☐ Other

Employer: _____ Phone: ( ) _____

Employer's Address: _____

Policy/ID No: YYZ8436489   Group No: 326463 Percent Covered: ____%, Copay Amt: $35.00

Secondary Insurance: _____ Phone: ( ) _____

Address: _____

Insurance Policyholder's Name: _____ ☐ M ☐ F DOB: _____

Address: _____

Phone: _____ Relationship to Insured: ☐ Self ☐ Spouse ☐ Child ☐ Other

Employer: _____ Phone: ( ) _____

Employer's Address: _____

Policy/ID No: _____ Group No: _____ Percent Covered: ____%, Copay Amt: $____

Reason for Visit: Need my blood pressure and cholesterol checked today

Known Allergies: _____

Were you referred here? If so, by whom?: _____

CASE A-8
SOAP

10/26/20XX
Assignment of Benefits: Y
Signature on File: Y
Referring Physician: N

S: Klaus Davies is in the office for a checkup on HTN and hypercholesterolemia.
O: Pt. denies any headaches, dizziness, or CP. Says he feels good. Vitals: P: 88, R: 16, BP: 142/72. Review of lab shows stable numbers with total cholesterol at 222.
A: 1. HTN—401.9
  2. Hypercholesterolemia—272.0
P: 1. Refill Lipitor 20 mg one daily, 30 x 3.
  2. Repeat fasting lab in 3 months.
  3. Schedule checkup in 3 months.

Phil Wells, MD
Family Practice
NPI: 1234567890
UPIN: 123456

Patient Name Klaus Davies

Capital City Medical
123 Unknown Boulevard, Capital City, NY 12345-2222

Date of Service
10-26-20XX

New Patient			Other Invasive/Noninvasive			Laboratory		
Problem Focused	99201		Arthrocentesis/Aspiration/Injection			Amylase	82150	
Expanded Problem, Focused	99202		Small Joint	20600		B12	82607	
Detailed	99203		Interm Joint	20605		CBC & Diff	85025	X
Comprehensive	99204		Major Joint	20610		Comp Metabolic Panel	80053	
Comprehensive/High Complex	99205		**Other Invasive/Noninvasive**			Chlamydia Screen	87110	
Well Exam Infant (up to 12 mos.)	99381		Audiometry	92552		Cholesterol	82465	
Well Exam 1–4 yrs.	99382		Cast Application			Digoxin	80162	
Well Exam 5–11 yrs.	99383		Location Long Short			Electrolytes	80051	
Well Exam 12–17 yrs.	99384		Catheterization	51701		Ferritin	82728	
Well Exam 18–39 yrs.	99385		Circumcision	54150		Folate	82746	
Well Exam 40–64 yrs.	99386		Colposcopy	57452		GC Screen	87070	
			Colposcopy w/Biopsy	57454		Glucose	82947	
			Cryosurgery Premalignant Lesion			Glucose 1 HR	82950	
			Location (s):			Glycosylated HGB A1C	83036	
Established Patient			Cryosurgery Warts			HCT	85014	
Post-Op Follow Up Visit	99024		Location (s):			HDL	83718	
Minimum	99211		Curettement Lesion			Hep BSAG	87340	
Problem Focused	99212		Single	11055		Hepatitis panel, acute	80074	
Expanded Problem Focused	99213	X	2–4	11056		HGB	85018	
Detailed	99214		>4	11057		HIV	86703	
Comprehensive/High Complex	99215		Diaphragm Fitting	57170		Iron & TIBC	83550	
Well Exam Infant (up to 12 mos.)	99391		Ear Irrigation	69210		Kidney Profile	80069	
Well exam 1–4 yrs.	99392		ECG	93000		Lead	83655	
Well Exam 5–11 yrs.	99393		Endometrial Biopsy	58100		Liver Profile	80076	X
Well Exam 12–17 yrs.	99394		Exc. Lesion Malignant			Mono Test	86308	
Well Exam 18–39 yrs.	99395		Benign			Pap Smear	88155	
Well Exam 40–64 yrs.	99396		Location			Pregnancy Test	84703	
Obstetrics			Exc. Skin Tags (1–15)	11200		Obstetric Panel	80055	
Total OB Care	59400		Each Additional 10	11201		Pro Time	85610	
Injections			Fracture Treatment			PSA	84153	
Administration Sub. / IM	90772		Loc			RPR	86592	
Drug			w/Reduc w/o Reduc			Sed. Rate	85651	
Dosage			I & D Abscess Single/Simple	10060		Stool Culture	87045	
Allergy	95115		Multiple or Comp	10061		Stool O & P	87177	
Cocci Skin Test	86490		I & D Pilonidal Cyst Simple	10080		Strep Screen	87880	
DPT	90701		Pilonidal Cyst Complex	10081		Theophylline	80198	
Hemophilus	90646		IV Therapy—To One Hour	90760		Thyroid Uptake	84479	
Influenza	90658		Each Additional Hour	90761		TSH	84443	
MMR	90707		Laceration Repair			Urinalysis	81000	
OPV	90712		Location Size Simp/Comp			Urine Culture	87088	
Pneumovax	90732		Laryngoscopy	31505		Drawing Fee	36415	X
TB Skin Test	86580		Oximetry	94760		Specimen Collection	99000	
TD	90718		Punch Biopsy			**Other:**		
Unlisted Immun	90749		Rhythm Strip	93040				
Tetanus Toxoid	90703		Treadmill	93015				
Vaccine/Toxoid Admin <8 Yr Old w/ Counseling	90465		Trigger Point or Tendon Sheath Inj.	20550				
Vaccine/Toxoid Administration for Adult	90471		Tympanometry	92567				
						Lipid Panel	80061	X

Diagnosis/ICD-9: **401.9, 272.0**

I acknowledge receipt of medical services and authorize the release of any medical information necessary to process this claim for healthcare payment only. I do authorize payment to the provider.

Total Estimated Charges: _____

Payment Amount: _____

Patient Signature Klaus Davies _____

Next Appointment: _____

CASE A-9

Capital City Medical—123 Unknown Boulevard, Capital City, NY 12345-2222 (555)555-1234

Phil Wells, MD, Mannie Mends, MD, Bette R. Soone, MD

Patient Information Form

Tax ID: 75-0246810

Group NPI: 1513171216

Patient Information:

Name: (Last, First) Vogel, Matilda   ☐ Male   ☒ Female   Birth Date: 05/19/1974

Address: 431 Forrest Ave, Capital City, NY 12345   Phone: (555) 555-5634

Social Security Number: 601–51–7806   Full-Time Student: ☐ Yes   ☒ No

Marital Status: ☐ Single   ☒ Married   ☐ Divorced   ☐ Other

Employment:

Employer: Roxie's Record Den   Phone: (555) 555-9873

Address: 6446 Lockhurst Ave, Capital City, NY 12345

Condition Related to: ☐ Auto Accident   ☐ Employment   ☐ Other Accident

Date of Accident: _____ State _____

Emergency Contact: _____   **Phone: ( )** _____

Primary Insurance: Tricare   Phone: ( ) _____

Address: 7594 Forces-Run Rd, Millitaryville, NY 12345

Insurance Policyholder's Name: Edward Vogel   ☒ M   ☐ F   DOB: 02/17/1979

Address: Same

Phone: _____ Relationship to Insured: ☐ Self ☒ Spouse ☐ Child ☐ Other

Employer: United States Army Reserves   Phone: ( ) _____

Employer's Address: 43 S. Army Blvd, Millitaryville, NY 12345

Policy/ID No: 333 22 9867   Group No: _____   Percent Covered: ____%, Copay Amt: $35.00

Secondary Insurance: _____   Phone: ( ) _____

Address: _____

Insurance Policyholder's Name: _____   ☐ M   ☐ F   DOB: _____

Address: _____

Phone: _____ Relationship to Insured: ☐ Self ☐ Spouse ☐ Child ☐ Other

Employer: _____   Phone: ( ) _____

Employer's Address: _____

Policy/ID No: _____ Group No: _____ Percent Covered: ____%, Copay Amt: $_____

Reason for Visit: I have burning when I urinate

Known Allergies: _____

Were you referred here? If so, by whom?: _____

12/30/20XX
Assignment of Benefits: Y
Signature on File: Y
Referring Physician: N

CASE A-9
SOAP

S: New patient, Matilda Vogel, is in the office for a burning sensation upon urination. She thinks it may be a vaginal yeast infection.

O: Social history negative for any promiscuity. Vulva negative for yeast. U/A with C&S ordered. Positive for WBCs.

A: 1. UTI—559.0, due to *E. coli* infection—041.4

P: 1. Septra DS one q.i.d. for seven days.
2. Recommended cranberry juice.

_____

Bette R. Soone, MD
Obstetrics/Gynecology
NPI: 9876543210
UPIN: 654321

CASE A-9 ENCOUNTER FORM

Patient Name Matilda Vogel

Capital City Medical
123 Unknown Boulevard, Capital City, NY 12345-2222

Date of Service
12-30-20XX

New Patient			Arthrocentesis/Aspiration/Injection			Laboratory		
Problem Focused	99201		Arthrocentesis/Aspiration/Injection			Amylase	82150	
Expanded Problem, Focused	99202		Small Joint	20600		B12	82607	
Detailed	99203	X	Interm Joint	20605		CBC & Diff	85025	
Comprehensive	99204		Major Joint	20610		Comp Metabolic Panel	80053	
Comprehensive/High Complex	99205		**Other Invasive/Noninvasive**			Chlamydia Screen	87110	
Well Exam Infant (up to 12 mos.)	99381		Audiometry	92552		Cholesterol	82465	
Well Exam 1–4 yrs.	99382		Cast Application			Digoxin	80162	
Well Exam 5–11 yrs.	99383		Location Long Short			Electrolytes	80051	
Well Exam 12–17 yrs.	99384		Catheterization	51701		Ferritin	82728	
Well Exam 18–39 yrs.	99385		Circumcision	54150		Folate	82746	
Well Exam 40–64 yrs.	99386		Colposcopy	57452		GC Screen	87070	
			Colposcopy w/Biopsy	57454		Glucose	82947	
			Cryosurgery Premalignant Lesion			Glucose 1 HR	82950	
			Location (s):			Glycosylated HGB A1C	83036	
Established Patient			Cryosurgery Warts			HCT	85014	
Post-Op Follow Up Visit	99024		Location (s):			HDL	83718	
Minimum	99211		Curettement Lesion			Hep BSAG	87340	
Problem Focused	99212		Single	11055		Hepatitis panel, acute	80074	
Expanded Problem Focused	99213		2–4	11056		HGB	85018	
Detailed	99214		>4	11057		HIV	86703	
Comprehensive/High Complex	99215		Diaphragm Fitting	57170		Iron & TIBC	83550	
Well Exam Infant (up to 12 mos.)	99391		Ear Irrigation	69210		Kidney Profile	80069	
Well exam 1–4 yrs.	99392		ECG	93000		Lead	83655	
Well Exam 5–11 yrs.	99393		Endometrial Biopsy	58100		Liver Profile	80076	
Well Exam 12–17 yrs.	99394		Exc. Lesion Malignant			Mono Test	86308	
Well Exam 18–39 yrs.	99395		Benign			Pap Smear	88155	
Well Exam 40–64 yrs.	99396		Location			Pregnancy Test	84703	
Obstetrics			Exc. Skin Tags (1–15)	11200		Obstetric Panel	80055	
Total OB Care	59400		Each Additional 10	11201		Pro Time	85610	
Injections			Fracture Treatment			PSA	84153	
Administration Sub. / IM	90772		Loc			RPR	86592	
Drug			w/Reduc w/o Reduc			Sed. Rate	85651	
Dosage			I & D Abscess Single/Simple	10060		Stool Culture	87045	
Allergy	95115		Multiple or Comp	10061		Stool O & P	87177	
Cocci Skin Test	86490		I & D Pilonidal Cyst Simple	10080		Strep Screen	87880	
DPT	90701		Pilonidal Cyst Complex	10081		Theophylline	80198	
Hemophilus	90646		IV Therapy—To One Hour	90760		Thyroid Uptake	84479	
Influenza	90658		Each Additional Hour	90761		TSH	84443	
MMR	90707		Laceration Repair			Urinalysis	81000	X
OPV	90712		Location Size Simp/Comp			Urine Culture	87088	X
Pneumovax	90732		Laryngoscopy	31505		Drawing Fee	36415	
TB Skin Test	86580		Oximetry	94760		Specimen Collection	99000	
TD	90718		Punch Biopsy			**Other:**		
Unlisted Immun	90749		Rhythm Strip	93040				
Tetanus Toxoid	90703		Treadmill	93015				
Vaccine/Toxoid Admin <8 Yr Old w/ Counseling	90465		Trigger Point or Tendon Sheath Inj.	20550				
Vaccine/Toxoid Administration for Adult	90471		Tympanometry	92567				

Diagnosis/ICD-9: **559.0, 041.4**

I acknowledge receipt of medical services and authorize the release of any medical information necessary to process this claim for healthcare payment only. I do authorize payment to the provider.

Total Estimated Charges: _____

Payment Amount: _____

Patient Signature Matilda Vogel _____

Next Appointment: _____

CASE A-10

Capital City Medical—123 Unknown Boulevard, Capital City, NY 12345-2222 (555)555-1234

Phil Wells, MD, Mannie Mends, MD, Bette R. Soone, MD

Patient Information Form

Tax ID: 75-0246810

Group NPI: 1513171216

Patient Information:

Name: (Last, First) Houston, Isaac ☒ Male ☐ Female Birth Date: 09/02/1961

Address: 71 Fern St, Capital City, NY 12345 Phone: (555) 555-2021

Social Security Number: 542-78-1236 Full-Time Student: ☐ Yes ☐ No

Marital Status: ☒ Single ☐ Married ☐ Divorced ☐ Other

Employment:

Employer: Mr. Construction Co. Phone: (555) 555-6211

Address: 44 Builder's Dr, Capital City, NY 12345

Condition Related to: ☐ Auto Accident ☒ Employment ☐ Other Accident

Date of Accident: 05/18/20XX State NY

Emergency Contact: Phone: ( )

Primary Insurance: Advantage Compensation Ins. Phone: ( )

Address: 1629 Accident Ave, Sickville NY 12345

Insurance Policyholder's Name: Mr. Construction Co. ☐ M ☐ F DOB:

Address: See employer

Phone: Relationship to Insured: ☐ Self ☐ Spouse ☐ Child ☒ Other

Employer: Mr. Construction Co. Phone: ( )

Employer's Address: See employer

Policy/ID No: Claim # H135246901 Group No: Percent Covered: %, Copay Amt: $

Secondary Insurance: Health America (if denied by WC) Phone: ( )

Address: 2031 Healthica Ctr, Capital City, NY 12345

Insurance Policyholder's Name: Same ☐ M ☐ F DOB:

Address:

Phone: Relationship to Insured: ☒ Self ☐ Spouse ☐ Child ☐ Other

Employer: Phone: ( )

Employer's Address:

Policy/ID No: 35643166 Group No: MRC753 Percent Covered: %, Copay Amt: $ 35.00

Reason for Visit: I fell off a ladder at work and hurt my chest

Known Allergies:

Were you referred here? If so, by whom?:

CASE A-10
SOAP

05/18/20XX
Assignment of Benefits: Y
Signature on File: Y
Referring Physician: N

S: Isaac Houston presents today with pain in the right thoracic area. He fell off of a ladder at work today; almost 2 hours ago.

O: Pt. denies any trauma to any other body area. He does have pain during inspiration and expiration. Pt. was on a ladder putting up a shutter on a house when suddenly he lost his balance and fell to the ground. CXR shows three cracked ribs on the right side.

A: 1. Fracture; ribs—807.03
2. Fall off of ladder—E881.0

P: 1. Ibuprofen one b.i.d. for 15 days.
2. Vicodin one q6h p.r.n. # 20.
3. Off work 3 days, then light duty
4. Please bill his workers' compensation. Info is as follows:
   Advantage Compensation Ins.
   1629 Accident Avenue
   Sickville, NY 12345
   Claim # H135246901

_____

Phil Wells, MD
Family Practice
NIP: 1234567890
PIN: 123456

Patient Name <u>Isaac Houston</u>

Capital City Medical
123 Unknown Boulevard, Capital City, NY 12345-2222

Date of Service
05-18-20XX

CASE A-10 ENCOUNTER FORM

New Patient			Other Invasive/Noninvasive		Laboratory	
Problem Focused	99201	Arthrocentesis/Aspiration/Injection		Amylase	82150
Expanded Problem, Focused	99202	Small Joint	20600	B12	82607
Detailed	99203	Interm Joint	20605	CBC & Diff	85025
Comprehensive	99204	Major Joint	20610	Comp Metabolic Panel	80053
Comprehensive/High Complex	99205	**Other Invasive/Noninvasive**		Chlamydia Screen	87110
Well Exam Infant (up to 12 mos.)	99381	Audiometry	92552	Cholesterol	82465
Well Exam 1–4 yrs.	99382	Cast Application		Digoxin	80162
Well Exam 5–11 yrs.	99383	Location Long Short		Electrolytes	80051
Well Exam 12–17 yrs.	99384	Catheterization	51701	Ferritin	82728
Well Exam 18–39 yrs.	99385	Circumcision	54150	Folate	82746
Well Exam 40–64 yrs.	99386	Colposcopy	57452	GC Screen	87070
		Colposcopy w/Biopsy	57454	Glucose	82947
		Cryosurgery Premalignant Lesion		Glucose 1 HR	82950
		Location (s):		Glycosylated HGB A1C	83036
Established Patient		Cryosurgery Warts		HCT	85014
Post-Op Follow Up Visit	99024	Location (s):		HDL	83718
Minimum	99211	Curettement Lesion		Hep BSAG	87340
Problem Focused	99212	Single	11055	Hepatitis panel, acute	80074
Expanded Problem Focused	99213 X	2–4	11056	HGB	85018
Detailed	99214	>4	11057	HIV	86703
Comprehensive/High Complex	99215	Diaphragm Fitting	57170	Iron & TIBC	83550
Well Exam Infant (up to 12 mos.)	99391	Ear Irrigation	69210	Kidney Profile	80069
Well exam 1–4 yrs.	99392	ECG	93000	Lead	83655
Well Exam 5–11 yrs.	99393	Endometrial Biopsy	58100	Liver Profile	80076
Well Exam 12–17 yrs.	99394	Exc. Lesion Malignant		Mono Test	86308
Well Exam 18–39 yrs.	99395	Benign		Pap Smear	88155
Well Exam 40–64 yrs.	99396	Location		Pregnancy Test	84703
Obstetrics		Exc. Skin Tags (1–15)	11200	Obstetric Panel	80055
Total OB Care	59400	Each Additional 10	11201	Pro Time	85610
Injections		Fracture Treatment		PSA	84153
Administration Sub. / IM	90772	Loc		RPR	86592
Drug		w/Reduc w/o Reduc		Sed. Rate	85651
Dosage		I & D Abscess Single/Simple	10060	Stool Culture	87045
Allergy	95115	Multiple or Comp	10061	Stool O & P	87177
Cocci Skin Test	86490	I & D Pilonidal Cyst Simple	10080	Strep Screen	87880
DPT	90701	Pilonidal Cyst Complex	10081	Theophylline	80198
Hemophilus	90646	IV Therapy—To One Hour	90760	Thyroid Uptake	84479
Influenza	90658	Each Additional Hour	90761	TSH	84443
MMR	90707	Laceration Repair		Urinalysis	81000
OPV	90712	Location Size Simp/Comp		Urine Culture	87088
Pneumovax	90732	Laryngoscopy	31505	Drawing Fee	36415
TB Skin Test	86580	Oximetry	94760	Specimen Collection	99000
TD	90718	Punch Biopsy		**Other:**	
Unlisted Immun	90749	Rhythm Strip	93040		
Tetanus Toxoid	90703	Treadmill	93015		
Vaccine/Toxoid Admin <8 Yr Old w/ Counseling	90465	Trigger Point or Tendon Sheath Inj.	20550		
Vaccine/Toxoid Administration for Adult	90471	Tympanometry	92567		
				CXR	71030 X

Diagnosis/ICD-9: **807.03, E881.0**

I acknowledge receipt of medical services and authorize the release of any medical information necessary to process this claim for healthcare payment only. I do authorize payment to the provider.

Patient Signature <u>Isaac Houston</u>

Total Estimated Charges: _____

Payment Amount: _____

Next Appointment: _____

CASE A-11

Patient Information:

Name: (Last, First) Sung, Kenneth   ☒ Male   ☐ Female   Birth Date: 10/03/1930

Address: 501 Locust St, Capital City, NY 12345   Phone: (555) 555-1718

Social Security Number: 189-42-9163   Full-Time Student: ☐ Yes   ☒ No

Marital Status: ☐ Single   ☒ Married   ☐ Divorced   ☐ Other

Employment:

Employer: Retired   Phone: ( )

Address:

Condition Related to: ☐ Auto Accident   ☐ Employment   ☐ Other Accident

Date of Accident: _____ State _____

Emergency Contact: _____ Phone: ( ) _____

Primary Insurance: Medicare   Phone: ( )

Address: P.O. Box 9834, Capital City, NY 12345

Insurance Policyholder's Name: Same   ☐ M ☐ F DOB: _____

Address:

Phone: _____ Relationship to Insured: ☒ Self ☐ Spouse ☐ Child ☐ Other

Employer: _____ Phone: ( ) _____

Employer's Address:

Policy/ID No: 894362514A   Group No: _____ Percent Covered: 80 %, Copay Amt: $_____

Secondary Insurance: Medicaid   Phone: ( )

Address: 4875 Capital Blvd, Capital City, NY 12345

Insurance Policyholder's Name: Same   ☐ M ☐ F DOB: _____

Address:

Phone: _____ Relationship to Insured: ☒ Self ☐ Spouse ☐ Child ☐ Other

Employer: _____ Phone: ( ) _____

Employer's Address:

Policy/ID No: 000684493216   Group No: _____ Percent Covered: ___%, Copay Amt: $5.00

Reason for Visit: High blood pressure and my past stroke

Known Allergies: _____

Were you referred here? If so, by whom?: _____

08/11/20XX
Assignment of Benefits: Y
Signature on File: Y
Referring Physician: N

S: Kenneth Sung is seen in the office for a follow-up on HTN and an old CVA.
O: Pt. denies any complaints. ROS unremarkable. BP: 136/88. EKG normal.
A: 1. HTN, malignant—401.0
    2. Old CVA—V12.59
P: 1. Refill medicine.
    2. PT and INR today.
    3. Return in six months.

_____

Phil Wells, MD
Family Practice
NPI: 1234567890
UPIN: 123456
Medicaid: 53248961

CASE A-11 ENCOUNTER FORM

Patient Name Kenneth Sung

Capital City Medical
123 Unknown Boulevard, Capital City, NY 12345-2222

Date of Service
08-11-20XX

New Patient					Laboratory		
Problem Focused	99201	Arthrocentesis/Aspiration/Injection			Amylase	82150	
Expanded Problem, Focused	99202	Small Joint	20600		B12	82607	
Detailed	99203	Interm Joint	20605		CBC & Diff	85025	X
Comprehensive	99204	Major Joint	20610		Comp Metabolic Panel	80053	X
Comprehensive/High Complex	99205	**Other Invasive/Noninvasive**			Chlamydia Screen	87110	
Well Exam Infant (up to 12 mos.)	99381	Audiometry	92552		Cholesterol	82465	
Well Exam 1–4 yrs.	99382	Cast Application			Digoxin	80162	
Well Exam 5–11 yrs.	99383	Location Long Short			Electrolytes	80051	
Well Exam 12–17 yrs.	99384	Catheterization	51701		Ferritin	82728	
Well Exam 18–39 yrs.	99385	Circumcision	54150		Folate	82746	
Well Exam 40–64 yrs.	99386	Colposcopy	57452		GC Screen	87070	
		Colposcopy w/Biopsy	57454		Glucose	82947	
		Cryosurgery Premalignant Lesion			Glucose 1 HR	82950	
		Location (s):			Glycosylated HGB A1C	83036	
		Cryosurgery Warts			HCT	85014	
Established Patient		Location (s):			HDL	83718	
Post-Op Follow Up Visit	99024	Curettement Lesion			Hep BSAG	87340	
Minimum	99211	Single	11055		Hepatitis panel, acute	80074	
Problem Focused	99212	2–4	11056		HGB	85018	
Expanded Problem Focused	99213	X	>4	11057	HIV	86703	
Detailed	99214	Diaphragm Fitting	57170		Iron & TIBC	83550	
Comprehensive/High Complex	99215	Ear Irrigation	69210		Kidney Profile	80069	
Well Exam Infant (up to 12 mos.)	99391	ECG	93000	X	Lead	83655	
Well exam 1–4 yrs.	99392	Endometrial Biopsy	58100		Liver Profile	80076	
Well Exam 5–11 yrs.	99393	Exc. Lesion Malignant			Mono Test	86308	
Well Exam 12–17 yrs.	99394	Benign			Pap Smear	88155	
Well Exam 18–39 yrs.	99395	Location			Pregnancy Test	84703	
Well Exam 40–64 yrs.	99396	Exc. Skin Tags (1–15)	11200		Obstetric Panel	80055	
Obstetrics		Each Additional 10	11201		Pro Time	85610	X
Total OB Care	59400	Fracture Treatment			PSA	84153	
Injections		Loc			RPR	86592	
Administration Sub. / IM	90772	w/Reduc w/o Reduc			Sed. Rate	85651	
Drug		I & D Abscess Single/Simple	10060		Stool Culture	87045	
Dosage		Multiple or Comp	10061		Stool O & P	87177	
Allergy	95115	I & D Pilonidal Cyst Simple	10080		Strep Screen	87880	
Cocci Skin Test	86490	Pilonidal Cyst Complex	10081		Theophylline	80198	
DPT	90701	IV Therapy—To One Hour	90760		Thyroid Uptake	84479	
Hemophilus	90646	Each Additional Hour	90761		TSH	84443	
Influenza	90658	Laceration Repair			Urinalysis	81000	
MMR	90707	Location Size Simp/Comp			Urine Culture	87088	
OPV	90712	Laryngoscopy	31505		Drawing Fee	36415	X
Pneumovax	90732	Oximetry	94760		Specimen Collection	99000	
TB Skin Test	86580	Punch Biopsy			**Other:**		
TD	90718	Rhythm Strip	93040				
Unlisted Immun	90749	Treadmill	93015				
Tetanus Toxoid	90703	Trigger Point or Tendon Sheath Inj.	20550				
Vaccine/Toxoid Admin <8 Yr Old w/ Counseling	90465						
Vaccine/Toxoid Administration for Adult	90471	Tympanometry	92567				
					EKG	93000	

Diagnosis/ICD-9: **401.0, V12.59**

I acknowledge receipt of medical services and authorize the release of any medical information necessary to process this claim for healthcare payment only. I do authorize payment to the provider.

Patient Signature Kenneth Sung

Total Estimated Charges: _____

Payment Amount: _____

Next Appointment: _____

CASE A-12

Capital City Medical—123 Unknown Boulevard, Capital City, NY 12345-2222 (555)555-1234	Patient Information Form
Phil Wells, MD, Mannie Mends, MD, Bette R. Soone, MD	Tax ID: 75-0246810
	Group NPI: 1513171216

Patient Information:

Name: (Last, First) Harrison, Viola   ☐ Male   ☒ Female   Birth Date: 01/31/1935

Address: 567 Walnut St, Capital City, NY 12345   Phone: (555) 555-8641

Social Security Number: 918-49-1978   Full-Time Student: ☐ Yes   ☒ No

Marital Status: ☒ Single   ☐ Married   ☐ Divorced   ☐ Other

Employment:

Employer: Retired   Phone: ( )

Address:

Condition Related to: ☐ Auto Accident   ☐ Employment   ☐ Other Accident

Date of Accident: _____ State _____

Emergency Contact: _____ **Phone: ( )** _____

Primary Insurance: Medicare   Phone: ( )

Address: P.O. Box 9834, Capital City, NY 12345

Insurance Policyholder's Name: Same   ☐ M ☐ F DOB:

Address:

Phone: _____ Relationship to Insured: ☒ Self ☐ Spouse ☐ Child ☐ Other

Employer: _____ Phone: ( ) _____

Employer's Address:

Policy/ID No: 881536935A   Group No: _____ Percent Covered: 80 %, Copay Amt: $_____

Secondary Insurance: Medicaid   Phone: ( )

Address: 4875 Capital Blvd, Capital City, NY 12345

Insurance Policyholder's Name: Same   ☐ M ☐ F DOB:

Address:

Phone: _____ Relationship to Insured: ☒ Self ☐ Spouse ☐ Child ☐ Other

Employer: _____ Phone: ( ) _____

Employer's Address:

Policy/ID No: 00009916596   Group No: _____ Percent Covered: ___%, Copay Amt: $5.00

Reason for Visit: My rheumatoid arthritis

Known Allergies:

Were you referred here? If so, by whom?:

CASE A-12
SOAP

05/05/20XX
Assignment of Benefits: Y
Signature on File: Y
Referring Physician: N

S: Viola Harrison is being seen today for a check on her rheumatoid arthritis.

O: ROS is unremarkable, otherwise than what is noted in the CC. Pt. has no new progression of this disease. Lab work reviewed.

A: 1. Rheumatoid arthritis—714.0
2. Polyarthralgia—719.49

P: 1. Recheck in three months.
2. Gold injection at next visit.
3. Continue Celebrex.

_____

Phil Wells, MD
Family Practice
UPIN: 123456
NPI: 1234567890
Medicaid: 53248961

Patient Name Viola Harrison

Capital City Medical
123 Unknown Boulevard, Capital City, NY 12345-2222

Date of Service
05-05-20XX

CASE A-12 ENCOUNTER FORM

New Patient		
Problem Focused	99201	
Expanded Problem, Focused	99202	
Detailed	99203	
Comprehensive	99204	
Comprehensive/High Complex	99205	
Well Exam Infant (up to 12 mos.)	99381	
Well Exam 1–4 yrs.	99382	
Well Exam 5–11 yrs.	99383	
Well Exam 12–17 yrs.	99384	
Well Exam 18–39 yrs.	99385	
Well Exam 40–64 yrs.	99386	

Established Patient		
Post-Op Follow Up Visit	99024	
Minimum	99211	
Problem Focused	99212	
Expanded Problem Focused	99213	
Detailed	99214	X
Comprehensive/High Complex	99215	
Well Exam Infant (up to 12 mos.)	99391	
Well exam 1–4 yrs.	99392	
Well Exam 5–11 yrs.	99393	
Well Exam 12–17 yrs.	99394	
Well Exam 18–39 yrs.	99395	
Well Exam 40–64 yrs.	99396	

Obstetrics		
Total OB Care	59400	

Injections		
Administration Sub. / IM	90772	
Drug		
Dosage		
Allergy	95115	
Cocci Skin Test	86490	
DPT	90701	
Hemophilus	90646	
Influenza	90658	
MMR	90707	
OPV	90712	
Pneumovax	90732	
TB Skin Test	86580	
TD	90718	
Unlisted Immun	90749	
Tetanus Toxoid	90703	
Vaccine/Toxoid Admin <8 Yr Old w/ Counseling	90465	
Vaccine/Toxoid Administration for Adult	90471	

Diagnosis/ICD-9: **714.0, 719.49**

Arthrocentesis/Aspiration/Injection		
Small Joint	20600	
Interm Joint	20605	
Major Joint	20610	

Other Invasive/Noninvasive		
Audiometry	92552	
Cast Application		
Location Long Short		
Catheterization	51701	
Circumcision	54150	
Colposcopy	57452	
Colposcopy w/Biopsy	57454	
Cryosurgery Premalignant Lesion		
Location (s):		
Cryosurgery Warts		
Location (s):		
Curettement Lesion		
Single	11055	
2–4	11056	
>4	11057	
Diaphragm Fitting	57170	
Ear Irrigation	69210	
ECG	93000	
Endometrial Biopsy	58100	
Exc. Lesion Malignant		
Benign		
Location		
Exc. Skin Taqs (1–15)	11200	
Each Additional 10	11201	
Fracture Treatment		
Loc		
w/Reduc w/o Reduc		
I & D Abscess Single/Simple	10060	
Multiple or Comp	10061	
I & D Pilonidal Cyst Simple	10080	
Pilonidal Cyst Complex	10081	
IV Therapy—To One Hour	90760	
Each Additional Hour	90761	
Laceration Repair		
Location Size Simp/Comp		
Laryngoscopy	31505	
Oximetry	94760	
Punch Biopsy		
Rhythm Strip	93040	
Treadmill	93015	
Trigger Point or Tendon Sheath Inj.	20550	
Tympanometry	92567	

Laboratory		
Amylase	82150	
B12	82607	
CBC & Diff	85025	X
Comp Metabolic Panel	80053	X
Chlamydia Screen	87110	
Cholesterol	82465	
Digoxin	80162	
Electrolytes	80051	
Ferritin	82728	
Folate	82746	
GC Screen	87070	
Glucose	82947	
Glucose 1 HR	82950	
Glycosylated HGB A1C	83036	
HCT	85014	
HDL	83718	
Hep BSAG	87340	
Hepatitis panel, acute	80074	
HGB	85018	
HIV	86703	
Iron & TIBC	83550	
Kidney Profile	80069	
Lead	83655	
Liver Profile	80076	
Mono Test	86308	
Pap Smear	88155	
Pregnancy Test	84703	
Obstetric Panel	80055	
Pro Time	85610	
PSA	84153	
RPR	86592	
Sed. Rate	85651	X
Stool Culture	87045	
Stool O & P	87177	
Strep Screen	87880	
Theophylline	80198	
Thyroid Uptake	84479	
TSH	84443	
Urinalysis	81000	
Urine Culture	87088	
Drawing Fee	36415	X
Specimen Collection	99000	
Other:		
Pap Smear	88142	

I acknowledge receipt of medical services and authorize the release of any medical information necessary to process this claim for healthcare payment only. I do authorize payment to the provider.

Total Estimated Charges: _____

Payment Amount: _____

Patient Signature Viola Harrison _____

Next Appointment: _____

CASE A-13

Patient Information:

Name: (Last, First) Quigley, Quaylord   ☒ Male   ☐ Female   Birth Date: 06/02/1943

Address: 54 Chesnut Ave, Capital City, NY 12345   Phone: (555) 555-9123

Social Security Number: 767-40-7981   Full-Time Student: ☐ Yes   ☒ No

Marital Status: ☐ Single   ☒ Married   ☐ Divorced   ☐ Other

Employment:

Employer: Retired   Phone: ( )

Address:

Condition Related to: ☐ Auto Accident   ☐ Employment   ☒ Other Accident

Date of Accident: _____ State _____

Emergency Contact: _____ **Phone: ( )** _____

Primary Insurance: Medicare   Phone: ( )

Address: P.O. Box 9834, Capital City, NY 12345

Insurance Policyholder's Name: Same   ☐ M ☐ F DOB: _____

Address:

Phone: _____ Relationship to Insured: ☒ Self ☐ Spouse ☐ Child ☐ Other

Employer: _____ Phone: ( ) _____

Employer's Address:

Policy/ID No: 645800022A   Group No: _____ Percent Covered: 80 %, Copay Amt: $_____

Secondary Insurance: Medicaid   Phone: ( )

Address: 4875 Capital Blvd, Capital City, NY 12345

Insurance Policyholder's Name: Same   ☐ M ☐ F DOB: _____

Address:

Phone: _____ Relationship to Insured: ☒ Self ☐ Spouse ☐ Child ☐ Other

Employer: _____ Phone: ( ) _____

Employer's Address:

Policy/ID No: 0005486598735   Group No: _____ Percent Covered: ___%, Copay Amt: $5.00

Reason for Visit: I fell off of my bike and now my back hurts

Known Allergies:

Were you referred here? If so, by whom?:

11/09/20XX
Assignment of Benefits: Y
Signature on File: Y
Referring Physician: N

CASE A-13
SOAP

S: Quaylord Quigley presents today for a fall off of his bike earlier today causing him LBP.
O: On exam, there are a few scratches. No noted bruising or bleeding. Patient has pain with movement. ROM unremarkable. Pt. does have a history of HTN.
A: 1. LBP—724.2
   2. Fall off bicycle—E826.1
P: 1. X-ray of lumbar spine reveals no evidence of fracture or sprain.
   2. Ibuprofen 800 mg one b.id. p.r.n.
   3. Patient to return to office if no improvement.

_____

Phil Wells, MD
Family Practice
NPI: 1234567890
UPIN: 123456
Medicaid: 53248961

CASE A-13 ENCOUNTER FORM

Patient Name Quaylord Quigley

Capital City Medical
123 Unknown Boulevard, Capital City, NY 12345-2222

Date of Service
11-09-20XX

New Patient					Laboratory	
Problem Focused	99201		Arthrocentesis/Aspiration/Injection		Amylase	82150
Expanded Problem, Focused	99202		Small Joint	20600	B12	82607
Detailed	99203		Interm Joint	20605	CBC & Diff	85025
Comprehensive	99204		Major Joint	20610	Comp Metabolic Panel	80053
Comprehensive/High Complex	99205		**Other Invasive/Noninvasive**		Chlamydia Screen	87110
Well Exam Infant (up to 12 mos.)	99381		Audiometry	92552	Cholesterol	82465
Well Exam 1–4 yrs.	99382		Cast Application		Digoxin	80162
Well Exam 5–11 yrs.	99383		Location　Long　Short		Electrolytes	80051
Well Exam 12–17 yrs.	99384		Catheterization	51701	Ferritin	82728
Well Exam 18–39 yrs.	99385		Circumcision	54150	Folate	82746
Well Exam 40–64 yrs.	99386		Colposcopy	57452	GC Screen	87070
			Colposcopy w/Biopsy	57454	Glucose	82947
			Cryosurgery Premalignant Lesion		Glucose 1 HR	82950
			Location (s):		Glycosylated HGB A1C	83036
Established Patient			Cryosurgery Warts		HCT	85014
Post-Op Follow Up Visit	99024		Location (s):		HDL	83718
Minimum	99211		Curettement Lesion		Hep BSAG	87340
Problem Focused	99212		Single	11055	Hepatitis panel, acute	80074
Expanded Problem Focused	99213	X	2–4	11056	HGB	85018
Detailed	99214		>4	11057	HIV	86703
Comprehensive/High Complex	99215		Diaphragm Fitting	57170	Iron & TIBC	83550
Well Exam Infant (up to 12 mos.)	99391		Ear Irrigation	69210	Kidney Profile	80069
Well exam 1–4 yrs.	99392		ECG	93000	Lead	83655
Well Exam 5–11 yrs.	99393		Endometrial Biopsy	58100	Liver Profile	80076
Well Exam 12–17 yrs.	99394		Exc. Lesion Malignant		Mono Test	86308
Well Exam 18–39 yrs.	99395		Benign		Pap Smear	88155
Well Exam 40–64 yrs.	99396		Location		Pregnancy Test	84703
Obstetrics			Exc. Skin Tags (1–15)	11200	Obstetric Panel	80055
Total OB Care	59400		Each Additional 10	11201	Pro Time	85610
Injections			Fracture Treatment		PSA	84153
Administration Sub. / IM	90772		Loc		RPR	86592
Drug			w/Reduc　w/o Reduc		Sed. Rate	85651
Dosage			I & D Abscess Single/Simple	10060	Stool Culture	87045
Allergy	95115		Multiple or Comp	10061	Stool O & P	87177
Cocci Skin Test	86490		I & D Pilonidal Cyst Simple	10080	Strep Screen	87880
DPT	90701		Pilonidal Cyst Complex	10081	Theophylline	80198
Hemophilus	90646		IV Therapy—To One Hour	90760	Thyroid Uptake	84479
Influenza	90658		Each Additional Hour	90761	TSH	84443
MMR	90707		Laceration Repair		Urinalysis	81000
OPV	90712		Location　Size　Simp/Comp		Urine Culture	87088
Pneumovax	90732		Laryngoscopy	31505	Drawing Fee	36415
TB Skin Test	86580		Oximetry	94760	Specimen Collection	99000
TD	90718		Punch Biopsy		**Other:**	
Unlisted Immun	90749		Rhythm Strip	93040		
Tetanus Toxoid	90703		Treadmill	93015		
Vaccine/Toxoid Admin <8 Yr Old w/ Counseling	90465		Trigger Point or Tendon Sheath Inj.	20550		
Vaccine/Toxoid Administration for Adult	90471		Tympanometry	92567		
					X-Ray Lumbar Spine	72100 X

Diagnosis/ICD-9: **724.2, E826.1**

I acknowledge receipt of medical services and authorize the release of any medical information necessary to process this claim for healthcare payment only. I do authorize payment to the provider.

Patient Signature Quaylord Quigley

Total Estimated Charges: _____

Payment Amount: _____

Next Appointment: _____

CASE A-14

Capital City Medical—123 Unknown Boulevard, Capital City, NY 12345-2222 (555)555-1234
Phil Wells, MD, Mannie Mends, MD, Bette R. Soone, MD

Patient Information Form
Tax ID: 75-0246810
Group NPI: 1513171216

Patient Information:

Name: (Last, First) Myers, Winifred   ❑ Male   ☒ Female   Birth Date: 08/10/1936
Address: 80 Wintergreen Ave, Capital City, NY 12345   Phone: (555) 555-1984
Social Security Number: 143-22-6433   Full-Time Student: ❑ Yes   ☒ No
Marital Status: ❑ Single   ☒ Married   ❑ Divorced   ❑ Other

Employment:

Employer: Retired   Phone: ( )
Address:
Condition Related to: ❑ Auto Accident   ❑ Employment   ❑ Other Accident
Date of Accident: _____ State _____
Emergency Contact: _____ **Phone: ( )** _____

Primary Insurance: Medicare   Phone: ( )
Address: P.O. Box 9834, Capital City, NY 12345
Insurance Policyholder's Name: Same   ❑ M   ❑ F   DOB:
Address:
Phone: _____ Relationship to Insured: ☒ Self   ❑ Spouse   ❑ Child   ❑ Other
Employer: _____ Phone: ( ) _____
Employer's Address:
Policy/ID No: 115272728A   Group No: ____ Percent Covered: 80 %, Copay Amt: $____

Secondary Insurance: Aetna   Phone: ( )
Address: 1625 Healthcare Bldg, Capital City, NY 12345
Insurance Policyholder's Name: Same   ❑ M   ❑ F   DOB:
Address:
Phone: _____ Relationship to Insured: ☒ Self   ❑ Spouse   ❑ Child   ❑ Other
Employer: Retired   Phone: ( ) _____
Employer's Address:
Policy/ID No: 12656489   Group No: 6896 Percent Covered: ___%, Copay Amt: $10.00

Reason for Visit: I'm having skin tags removed

Known Allergies:

Were you referred here? If so, by whom?:

CASE A-14
SOAP

03/24/20XX
Assignment of Benefits: Y
Signature on File: Y
Referring Physician: N

S: Winifred Myers (established patient) comes in today for the removal of 18 skin tags.
O: Pt. was prepped and draped in the usual fashion. Skin tags were removed successfully without any complications.
A: 1. Skin tags; congenital—757.39
P: 1. Keep area clean and dry.
    2. Follow up in one week.

_____

Mannie Mends, MD
General Surgeon
NPI: 0123456789
UPIN: 012345
PIN: 654321

Patient Name <u>Winifred Myers</u>

Capital City Medical
123 Unknown Boulevard, Capital City, NY 12345-2222

Date of Service
03-24-20XX

CASE A-14 ENCOUNTER FORM

New Patient			Laboratory		
Problem Focused	99201	Arthrocentesis/Aspiration/Injection	Amylase	82150	
Expanded Problem, Focused	99202	Small Joint	20600	B12	82607	
Detailed	99203	Interm Joint	20605	CBC & Diff	85025	X
Comprehensive	99204	Major Joint	20610	Comp Metabolic Panel	80053	X
Comprehensive/High Complex	99205	**Other Invasive/Noninvasive**	Chlamydia Screen	87110	
Well Exam Infant (up to 12 mos.)	99381	Audiometry	92552	Cholesterol	82465	
Well Exam 1–4 yrs.	99382	Cast Application	Digoxin	80162	
Well Exam 5–11 yrs.	99383	Location	Long	Short	Electrolytes	80051	
Well Exam 12–17 yrs.	99384	Catheterization	51701	Ferritin	82728	
Well Exam 18–39 yrs.	99385	Circumcision	54150	Folate	82746	
Well Exam 40–64 yrs.	99386	Colposcopy	57452	GC Screen	87070	
		Colposcopy w/Biopsy	57454	Glucose	82947	
		Cryosurgery Premalignant Lesion	Glucose 1 HR	82950	
		Location (s):	Glycosylated HGB A1C	83036	
Established Patient		Cryosurgery Warts	HCT	85014	
Post-Op Follow Up Visit	99024	Location (s):	HDL	83718	
Minimum	99211	Curettement Lesion	Hep BSAG	87340	
Problem Focused	99212	Single	11055	Hepatitis panel, acute	80074	
Expanded Problem Focused	99213	2–4	11056	HGB	85018	
Detailed	99214	>4	11057	HIV	86703	
Comprehensive/High Complex	99215	Diaphragm Fitting	57170	Iron & TIBC	83550	
Well Exam Infant (up to 12 mos.)	99391	Ear Irrigation	69210	Kidney Profile	80069	
Well exam 1–4 yrs.	99392	ECG	93000	Lead	83655	
Well Exam 5–11 yrs.	99393	Endometrial Biopsy	58100	Liver Profile	80076	
Well Exam 12–17 yrs.	99394	Exc. Lesion Malignant	Mono Test	86308	
Well Exam 18–39 yrs.	99395	Benign	Pap Smear	88155	
Well Exam 40–64 yrs.	99396	Location	Pregnancy Test	84703	
Obstetrics		Exc. Skin Tags (1–15)	11200	X Obstetric Panel	80055	
Total OB Care	59400	Each Additional 10	11201	X Pro Time	85610	
Injections		Fracture Treatment	PSA	84153	
Administration Sub. / IM	90772	Loc	RPR	86592	
Drug		w/Reduc	w/o Reduc	Sed. Rate	85651	
Dosage		I & D Abscess Single/Simple	10060	Stool Culture	87045	
Allergy	95115	Multiple or Comp	10061	Stool O & P	87177	
Cocci Skin Test	86490	I & D Pilonidal Cyst Simple	10080	Strep Screen	87880	
DPT	90701	Pilonidal Cyst Complex	10081	Theophylline	80198	
Hemophilus	90646	IV Therapy—To One Hour	90760	Thyroid Uptake	84479	
Influenza	90658	Each Additional Hour	90761	TSH	84443	
MMR	90707	Laceration Repair	Urinalysis	81000	
OPV	90712	Location	Size	Simp/Comp	Urine Culture	87088	
Pneumovax	90732	Laryngoscopy	31505	Drawing Fee	36415	
TB Skin Test	86580	Oximetry	94760	Specimen Collection	99000	
TD	90718	Punch Biopsy	**Other:**		
Unlisted Immun	90749	Rhythm Strip	93040		
Tetanus Toxoid	90703	Treadmill	93015		
Vaccine/Toxoid Admin <8 Yr Old w/ Counseling	90465	Trigger Point or Tendon Sheath Inj.	20550		
Vaccine/Toxoid Administration for Adult	90471	Tympanometry	92567		

Diagnosis/ICD-9: **757.39**

I acknowledge receipt of medical services and authorize the release of any medical information necessary to process this claim for healthcare payment only. I do authorize payment to the provider.

Total Estimated Charges: _____

Payment Amount: _____

Patient Signature <u>Winifred Myers</u>

Next Appointment: _____

CASE A-15

Capital City Medical—123 Unknown Boulevard, Capital City,
NY 12345-2222 (555)555-1234

Phil Wells, MD, Mannie Mends, MD, Bette R. Soone, MD

Patient Information Form

Tax ID: 75-0246810

Group NPI: 1513171216

Patient Information:

Name: (Last, First) Jaworski, Stella   ☐ Male ☒ Female Birth Date: 04/04/1936

Address: 13 Evergreen Ave, Capital City, NY 12345   Phone: (555) 555-3456

Social Security Number: 954-24-9835   Full-Time Student: ☐ Yes ☒ No

Marital Status: ☐ Single ☒ Married ☐ Divorced ☐ Other

Employment:

Employer: Retired   Phone: ( )

Address:

Condition Related to: ☐ Auto Accident ☐ Employment ☐ Other Accident

Date of Accident: State

Emergency Contact: **Phone: ( )**

Primary Insurance: Medicare   Phone: ( )

Address: P.O. Box 9834, Capital City, NY 12345

Insurance Policyholder's Name: Joseph Jaworski   ☒ M ☐ F DOB: 08/18/1935

Address: Same

Phone: Relationship to Insured: ☐ Self ☒ Spouse ☐ Child ☐ Other

Employer: Retired   Phone: ( )

Employer's Address:

Policy/ID No: 843648901A   Group No: Percent Covered: 80 %, Copay Amt: $

Secondary Insurance: Medicaid   Phone: ( )

Address: 4875 Capital Blvd, Capital City, NY 12345

Insurance Policyholder's Name: Same   ☐ M ☐ F DOB:

Address:

Phone: Relationship to Insured: ☒ Self ☐ Spouse ☐ Child ☐ Other

Employer: Phone: ( )

Employer's Address:

Policy/ID No: 0015358763896   Group No: Percent Covered: ___%, Copay Amt: $5.00

Reason for Visit: I have chills, a sick stomach, body aches, and I have been vomiting

Known Allergies:

Were you referred here? If so, by whom?:

09/09/20XX
Assignment of Benefits: Y
Signature on File: Y
Referring Physician: N

CASE A-15
SOAP

S: Stella Jaworski presents today with complaints of N&V, chills, and her body aches.
O: On exam, pt. has fever; T: 100.6°F. No diarrhea. Other systems unremarkable.
A: 1. Influenza—487.1
P: 1. Clear liquids for the next 24 hours.
    2. Bed rest.
    3. If symptoms worsen, she is to call the office.

_____

Phil Wells, MD
Family Practice
NPI: 1234567890
UPIN: 123456
Medicaid: 53248961

CASE A-15 ENCOUNTER FORM

Patient Name Stella Jaworski

Capital City Medical
123 Unknown Boulevard, Capital City, NY 12345-2222

Date of Service
09-09-20XX

New Patient						Laboratory		
Problem Focused	99201	Arthrocentesis/Aspiration/Injection				Amylase	82150	
Expanded Problem, Focused	99202	Small Joint			20600	B12	82607	
Detailed	99203	Interm Joint			20605	CBC & Diff	85025	X
Comprehensive	99204	Major Joint			20610	Comp Metabolic Panel	80053	
Comprehensive/High Complex	99205	**Other Invasive/Noninvasive**				Chlamydia Screen	87110	
Well Exam Infant (up to 12 mos.)	99381	Audiometry			92552	Cholesterol	82465	
Well Exam 1–4 yrs.	99382	Cast Application				Digoxin	80162	
Well Exam 5–11 yrs.	99383	Location	Long	Short		Electrolytes	80051	X
Well Exam 12–17 yrs.	99384	Catheterization			51701	Ferritin	82728	
Well Exam 18–39 yrs.	99385	Circumcision			54150	Folate	82746	
Well Exam 40–64 yrs.	99386	Colposcopy			57452	GC Screen	87070	
		Colposcopy w/Biopsy			57454	Glucose	82947	
		Cryosurgery Premalignant Lesion				Glucose 1 HR	82950	
		Location (s):				Glycosylated HGB A1C	83036	
Established Patient		Cryosurgery Warts				HCT	85014	
Post-Op Follow Up Visit	99024	Location (s):				HDL	83718	
Minimum	99211	Curettement Lesion				Hep BSAG	87340	
Problem Focused	99212	Single			11055	Hepatitis panel, acute	80074	
Expanded Problem Focused	99213 X	2–4			11056	HGB	85018	
Detailed	99214	>4			11057	HIV	86703	
Comprehensive/High Complex	99215	Diaphragm Fitting			57170	Iron & TIBC	83550	
Well Exam Infant (up to 12 mos.)	99391	Ear Irrigation			69210	Kidney Profile	80069	
Well exam 1–4 yrs.	99392	ECG			93000	Lead	83655	
Well Exam 5–11 yrs.	99393	Endometrial Biopsy			58100	Liver Profile	80076	
Well Exam 12–17 yrs.	99394	Exc. Lesion Malignant				Mono Test	86308	
Well Exam 18–39 yrs.	99395	Benign				Pap Smear	88155	
Well Exam 40–64 yrs.	99396	Location				Pregnancy Test	84703	
Obstetrics		Exc. Skin Tags (1–15)			11200	Obstetric Panel	80055	
Total OB Care	59400	Each Additional 10			11201	Pro Time	85610	
Injections		Fracture Treatment				PSA	84153	
Administration Sub. / IM	90772	Loc				RPR	86592	
Drug		w/Reduc		w/o Reduc		Sed. Rate	85651	
Dosage		I & D Abscess Single/Simple			10060	Stool Culture	87045	
Allergy	95115	Multiple or Comp			10061	Stool O & P	87177	
Cocci Skin Test	86490	I & D Pilonidal Cyst Simple			10080	Strep Screen	87880	
DPT	90701	Pilonidal Cyst Complex			10081	Theophylline	80198	
Hemophilus	90646	IV Therapy—To One Hour			90760	Thyroid Uptake	84479	
Influenza	90658	Each Additional Hour			90761	TSH	84443	
MMR	90707	Laceration Repair				Urinalysis	81000	
OPV	90712	Location	Size	Simp/Comp		Urine Culture	87088	
Pneumovax	90732	Laryngoscopy			31505	Drawing Fee	36415	X
TB Skin Test	86580	Oximetry			94760	Specimen Collection	99000	
TD	90718	Punch Biopsy				**Other:**		
Unlisted Immun	90749	Rhythm Strip			93040			
Tetanus Toxoid	90703	Treadmill			93015			
Vaccine/Toxoid Admin <8 Yr Old w/ Counseling	90465	Trigger Point or Tendon Sheath Inj.			20550			
Vaccine/Toxoid Administration for Adult	90471	Tympanometry			92567			

Diagnosis/ICD-9: **487.1**

I acknowledge receipt of medical services and authorize the release of any medical information necessary to process this claim for healthcare payment only. I do authorize payment to the provider.

Total Estimated Charges: _____

Payment Amount: _____

Patient Signature Stella Jaworski

Next Appointment: _____

CASE A-16

Capital City Medical—123 Unknown Boulevard, Capital City, NY 12345-2222 (555)555-1234

Phil Wells, MD, Mannie Mends, MD, Bette R. Soone, MD

Patient Information Form

Tax ID: 75-0246810

Group NPI: 1513171216

Patient Information:

Name: (Last, First) Bromley, Murphy   ☒ Male   ❑ Female   Birth Date: 09/13/1956

Address: 9 Redwood Dr, Township, NY 12345   Phone: (555) 555-4972

Social Security Number: 785-10-8339   Full-Time Student: ❑ Yes   ☒ No

Marital Status: ❑ Single   ☒ Married   ❑ Divorced   ❑ Other

Employment:

Employer: Retired   Phone: ( )

Address:

Condition Related to: ❑ Auto Accident   ❑ Employment   ❑ Other Accident

Date of Accident: State

Emergency Contact: **Phone: ( )**

Primary Insurance: Medicare   Phone: ( )

Address: P.O. Box 9834, Capital City, NY 12345

Insurance Policyholder's Name: Same   ❑ M ❑ F DOB:

Address:

Phone: Relationship to Insured: ☒ Self   ❑ Spouse   ❑ Child   ❑ Other

Employer: Phone: ( )

Employer's Address:

Policy/ID No: 481654563A   Group No: Percent Covered: 80 %, Copay Amt: $

Secondary Insurance: Blue Cross Blue Shield Medigap   Phone: ( )

Address: 379 Blue Plaza, Capital City, NY 12345

Insurance Policyholder's Name: Same   ❑ M ❑ F DOB:

Address:

Phone: Relationship to Insured: ☒ Self   ❑ Spouse   ❑ Child   ❑ Other

Employer: Phone: ( )

Employer's Address:

Policy/ID No: YYJ0472009   Group No: Percent Covered: %, Copay Amt: $

Reason for Visit: My three-month check up on high blood pressure, migraines, and diabetes

Known Allergies:

Were you referred here? If so, by whom?:

CASE A-16
SOAP

03/17/20XX
Assignment of Benefits: Y
Signature on File: Y
Referring Physician: N

S: Murphy Bromley is in the office today for a checkup on HTN, DM I, and migraine disorder.

O: Pt. is in no acute distress. BP: 152/90. He says that his diastolic pressure has been running higher than normal for the past couple of weeks. He denies any stress or increased salt intake. Migraines have been under control with medicine. Wt. is stable at 174 lbs.

A: 1. HTN—401.9
2. Atypical migraines—346.10
3. DM I—250.01

P: 1. DC Norvasc.
2. Start Diazide one b.i.d.
3. Return to office for BP check around the same time everyday x4 days.
4. Refill insulin.
5. Schedule appointment for 2 months.

_____

Phil Wells, MD
Family Practice
NPI: 1234567890
UPIN: 123456
PIN: 358612

Patient Name Murphy Bromley

Capital City Medical
123 Unknown Boulevard, Capital City, NY 12345-2222

Date of Service
03-17-20XX

New Patient			Other Invasive/Noninvasive			Laboratory		
Problem Focused	99201		Arthrocentesis/Aspiration/Injection			Amylase	82150	
Expanded Problem, Focused	99202		Small Joint		20600	B12	82607	
Detailed	99203		Interm Joint		20605	CBC & Diff	85025	X
Comprehensive	99204		Major Joint		20610	Comp Metabolic Panel	80053	X
Comprehensive/High Complex	99205		**Other Invasive/Noninvasive**			Chlamydia Screen	87110	
Well Exam Infant (up to 12 mos.)	99381		Audiometry		92552	Cholesterol	82465	
Well Exam 1–4 yrs.	99382		Cast Application			Digoxin	80162	
Well Exam 5–11 yrs.	99383		Location Long Short			Electrolytes	80051	
Well Exam 12–17 yrs.	99384		Catheterization		51701	Ferritin	82728	
Well Exam 18–39 yrs.	99385		Circumcision		54150	Folate	82746	
Well Exam 40–64 yrs.	99386		Colposcopy		57452	GC Screen	87070	
			Colposcopy w/Biopsy		57454	Glucose	82947	
			Cryosurgery Premalignant Lesion			Glucose 1 HR	82950	
			Location (s):			Glycosylated HGB A1C	83036	
Established Patient			Cryosurgery Warts			HCT	85014	
Post-Op Follow Up Visit	99024		Location (s):			HDL	83718	
Minimum	99211		Curettement Lesion			Hep BSAG	87340	
Problem Focused	99212		Single		11055	Hepatitis panel, acute	80074	
Expanded Problem Focused	99213	X	2–4		11056	HGB	85018	
Detailed	99214		>4		11057	HIV	86703	
Comprehensive/High Complex	99215		Diaphragm Fitting		57170	Iron & TIBC	83550	
Well Exam Infant (up to 12 mos.)	99391		Ear Irrigation		69210	Kidney Profile	80069	
Well exam 1–4 yrs.	99392		ECG		93000	Lead	83655	
Well Exam 5–11 yrs.	99393		Endometrial Biopsy		58100	Liver Profile	80076	
Well Exam 12–17 yrs.	99394		Exc. Lesion Malignant			Mono Test	86308	
Well Exam 18–39 yrs.	99395		Benign			Pap Smear	88155	
Well Exam 40–64 yrs.	99396		Location			Pregnancy Test	84703	
Obstetrics			Exc. Skin Tags (1–15)		11200	Obstetric Panel	80055	
Total OB Care	59400		Each Additional 10		11201	Pro Time	85610	
Injections			Fracture Treatment			PSA	84153	
Administration Sub. / IM	90772		Loc			RPR	86592	
Drug			w/Reduc	w/o Reduc		Sed. Rate	85651	
Dosage			I & D Abscess Single/Simple		10060	Stool Culture	87045	
Allergy	95115		Multiple or Comp		10061	Stool O & P	87177	
Cocci Skin Test	86490		I & D Pilonidal Cyst Simple		10080	Strep Screen	87880	
DPT	90701		Pilonidal Cyst Complex		10081	Theophylline	80198	
Hemophilus	90646		IV Therapy—To One Hour		90760	Thyroid Uptake	84479	
Influenza	90658		Each Additional Hour		90761	TSH	84443	
MMR	90707		Laceration Repair			Urinalysis	81000	
OPV	90712		Location Size Simp/Comp			Urine Culture	87088	
Pneumovax	90732		Laryngoscopy		31505	Drawing Fee	36415	X
TB Skin Test	86580		Oximetry		94760	Specimen Collection	99000	
TD	90718		Punch Biopsy			**Other:**		
Unlisted Immun	90749		Rhythm Strip		93040			
Tetanus Toxoid	90703		Treadmill		93015			
Vaccine/Toxoid Admin <8 Yr Old w/ Counseling	90465		Trigger Point or Tendon Sheath Inj.		20550			
Vaccine/Toxoid Administration for Adult	90471		Tympanometry		92567			

Diagnosis/ICD-9: **401.9, 346.10, 250.01**

I acknowledge receipt of medical services and authorize the release of any medical information necessary to process this claim for healthcare payment only. I do authorize payment to the provider.

Total Estimated Charges: _____

Payment Amount: _____

Patient Signature Murphy Bromley

Next Appointment: _____

CASE A-17

Capital City Medical—123 Unknown Boulevard, Capital City, NY 12345-2222 (555)555-1234 Phil Wells, MD, Mannie Mends, MD, Bette R. Soone, MD	Patient Information Form Tax ID: 75-0246810 Group NPI: 1513171216

Patient Information:

Name: (Last, First) Powers, Gus   ☒ Male   ☐ Female   Birth Date: 12/25/1940

Address: 3982 Cedar St, Township, NY 12345   Phone: (555) 555-1112

Social Security Number: 243-52-0069   Full-Time Student: ☐ Yes   ☒ No

Marital Status: ☐ Single   ☐ Married   ☒ Divorced   ☐ Other

Employment:

Employer: Retired   Phone: ( ) _____

Address: _____

Condition Related to: ☐ Auto Accident   ☐ Employment   ☒ Other Accident

Date of Accident: _____   State _____

Emergency Contact: _____   Phone: ( ) _____

Primary Insurance: Medicare   Phone: ( ) _____

Address: P.O Box 9834, Capital City, NY 12345

Insurance Policyholder's Name: Same   ☐ M ☐ F DOB: _____

Address: _____

Phone: _____   Relationship to Insured: ☒ Self ☐ Spouse ☐ Child ☐ Other

Employer: _____   Phone: ( ) _____

Employer's Address: _____

Policy/ID No: 366736530A   Group No: ____   Percent Covered: 80 %, Copay Amt: $____

Secondary Insurance: Aetna   Phone: ( ) _____

Address: 1625 Healthcare Bldg, Capital City, NY 12345

Insurance Policyholder's Name: Same   ☐ M ☐ F DOB: _____

Address: _____

Phone: _____   Relationship to Insured: ☒ Self ☐ Spouse ☐ Child ☐ Other

Employer: Retired   Phone: ( ) _____

Employer's Address: _____

Policy/ID No: 0059843   Group No: 312007 Percent Covered: ___%, Copay Amt: $ 15.00

Reason for Visit: I was working around the house and a nail shot into my leg

Known Allergies: _____

Were you referred here? If so, by whom?: _____

09/07/20XX
Assignment of Benefits: Y
Signature on File: Y
Referring Physician: N

S: New patient, Gus Powers, is seen today for a wound in his left thigh due to a nail gun that occurred today.

O: The wound penetrates only the epidermis layers without dermal involvement. This area was cleansed with hydrogen peroxide. There is no need for sutures, but tetanus needs updated.

A: 1. Wound; thigh—890.0, due to nail gun accident—E920.1
2. Tetanus vaccination—V03.7

P: 1. Pt. to keep wound clean and bandage.
2. To return to office if redness, swelling, pus, discoloration, or fever occur.

_____

Mannie Mends, MD
General Surgeon
NPI: 1234567890
UPIN: 012345
PIN: 654321

CASE A-17 ENCOUNTER FORM

Patient Name <u>Gus Powers</u>

Capital City Medical
123 Unknown Boulevard, Capital City, NY 12345-2222

Date of Service
09-07-20XX

New Patient			Other Invasive/Noninvasive			Laboratory	
Problem Focused	99201		Arthrocentesis/Aspiration/Injection			Amylase	82150
Expanded Problem, Focused	99202		Small Joint		20600	B12	82607
Detailed	99203	X	Interm Joint		20605	CBC & Diff	85025
Comprehensive	99204		Major Joint		20610	Comp Metabolic Panel	80053
Comprehensive/High Complex	99205		**Other Invasive/Noninvasive**			Chlamydia Screen	87110
Well Exam Infant (up to 12 mos.)	99381		Audiometry		92552	Cholesterol	82465
Well Exam 1–4 yrs.	99382		Cast Application			Digoxin	80162
Well Exam 5–11 yrs.	99383		Location Long Short			Electrolytes	80051
Well Exam 12–17 yrs.	99384		Catheterization		51701	Ferritin	82728
Well Exam 18–39 yrs.	99385		Circumcision		54150	Folate	82746
Well Exam 40–64 yrs.	99386		Colposcopy		57452	GC Screen	87070
			Colposcopy w/Biopsy		57454	Glucose	82947
			Cryosurgery Premalignant Lesion			Glucose 1 HR	82950
			Location (s):			Glycosylated HGB A1C	83036
Established Patient			Cryosurgery Warts			HCT	85014
Post-Op Follow Up Visit	99024		Location (s):			HDL	83718
Minimum	99211		Curettement Lesion			Hep BSAG	87340
Problem Focused	99212		Single		11055	Hepatitis panel, acute	80074
Expanded Problem Focused	99213		2–4		11056	HGB	85018
Detailed	99214		>4		11057	HIV	86703
Comprehensive/High Complex	99215		Diaphragm Fitting		57170	Iron & TIBC	83550
Well Exam Infant (up to 12 mos.)	99391		Ear Irrigation		69210	Kidney Profile	80069
Well exam 1–4 yrs.	99392		ECG		93000	Lead	83655
Well Exam 5–11 yrs.	99393		Endometrial Biopsy		58100	Liver Profile	80076
Well Exam 12–17 yrs.	99394		Exc. Lesion Malignant			Mono Test	86308
Well Exam 18–39 yrs.	99395		Benign			Pap Smear	88155
Well Exam 40–64 yrs.	99396		Location			Pregnancy Test	84703
Obstetrics			Exc. Skin Tags (1–15)		11200	Obstetric Panel	80055
Total OB Care	59400		Each Additional 10		11201	Pro Time	85610
Injections			Fracture Treatment			PSA	84153
Administration Sub. / IM	90772		Loc			RPR	86592
Drug			w/Reduc		w/o Reduc	Sed. Rate	85651
Dosage			I & D Abscess Single/Simple		10060	Stool Culture	87045
Allergy	95115		Multiple or Comp		10061	Stool O & P	87177
Cocci Skin Test	86490		I & D Pilonidal Cyst Simple		10080	Strep Screen	87880
DPT	90701		Pilonidal Cyst Complex		10081	Theophylline	80198
Hemophilus	90646		IV Therapy—To One Hour		90760	Thyroid Uptake	84479
Influenza	90658		Each Additional Hour		90761	TSH	84443
MMR	90707		Laceration Repair			Urinalysis	81000
OPV	90712		Location Size Simp/Comp			Urine Culture	87088
Pneumovax	90732		Laryngoscopy		31505	Drawing Fee	36415
TB Skin Test	86580		Oximetry		94760	Specimen Collection	99000
TD	90718		Punch Biopsy			**Other:**	
Unlisted Immun	90749		Rhythm Strip		93040		
Tetanus Toxoid	90703	X	Treadmill		93015		
Vaccine/Toxoid Admin <8 Yr Old w/ Counseling	90465		Trigger Point or Tendon Sheath Inj.		20550		
Vaccine/Toxoid Administration for Adult	90471		Tympanometry		92567		

Diagnosis/ICD-9: **890.0, E920.1, V03.7**

I acknowledge receipt of medical services and authorize the release of any medical information necessary to process this claim for healthcare payment only. I do authorize payment to the provider.

Patient Signature <u>Gus Powers</u>

Total Estimated Charges: _____

Payment Amount: _____

Next Appointment: _____

Capital City Medical—123 Unknown Boulevard, Capital City, NY 12345-2222 (555)555-1234

Phil Wells, MD, Mannie Mends, MD, Bette R. Soone, MD

Patient Information Form

Tax ID: 75-0246810

Group NPI: 1513171216

Patient Information:

Name: (Last, First) Acosta, Kimber   ❑ Male ☒ Female   Birth Date: 08/01/1946

Address: 821 Spruce St, Township, NY 12345   Phone: (555) 555-5678

Social Security Number: 101-19-6205   Full-Time Student: ❑ Yes ☒ No

Marital Status: ❑ Single ❑ Married ☒ Divorced ❑ Other

Employment:

Employer: Braddock Care Home   Phone: (555) 555-2060

Address: 294 Elmhurst Way, Township, NY 12345

Condition Related to: ❑ Auto Accident ❑ Employment ❑ Other Accident

Date of Accident: _____ State _____

Emergency Contact: _____ Phone: ( ) _____

Primary Insurance: Aetna   Phone: ( ) _____

Address: 1625 Healthcare Bldg, Capital City, NY 12345

Insurance Policyholder's Name: Same   ❑ M ❑ F DOB: _____

Address: _____

Phone: _____ Relationship to Insured: ☒ Self ❑ Spouse ❑ Child ❑ Other

Employer: Braddock Care Home   Phone: ( ) _____

Employer's Address: Same

Policy/ID No: 2054654   Group No: 201410   Percent Covered: ____%, Copay Amt: $ 10.00

Secondary Insurance: Medicare   Phone: ( ) _____

Address: P.O. Box 9834, Capital City, NY 12345

Insurance Policyholder's Name: Same   ❑ M ❑ F DOB: _____

Address: _____

Phone: _____ Relationship to Insured: ☒ Self ❑ Spouse ❑ Child ❑ Other

Employer: _____   Phone: ( ) _____

Employer's Address: _____

Policy/ID No: 856426598A   Group No: _____ Percent Covered: 80 %, Copay Amt: $____

Reason for Visit: I need a physical and a check on my diabetes

Known Allergies: _____

Were you referred here? If so, by whom?: _____

CASE A-18
SOAP

03/11/20XX
Assignment of Benefits: Y
Signature on File: Y
Referring Physician: N

S: Kimber Acosta is being seen for her annual physical.
O: ROS shows negative findings consistent with any disease process. Pt. does have DM II. Glucose, and U/A shows stable blood sugar levels.
A: 1. Annual PE—V70.0
  2. DM II—250.00
P: 1. Healthy female.
  2. Flu vaccine today—V04.81.

Phil Wells, MD
Family Practice
NPI: 1234567890
UPIN: 123456
PIN: 654321

Patient Name <u>Kimber Acosta</u>

Capital City Medical
123 Unknown Boulevard, Capital City, NY 12345-2222

Date of Service
03-11-20XX

CASE A-18 ENCOUNTER FORM

New Patient		Other Invasive/Noninvasive			Laboratory		
Problem Focused	99201	Arthrocentesis/Aspiration/Injection			Amylase	82150	
Expanded Problem, Focused	99202	Small Joint		20600	B12	82607	
Detailed	99203	Interm Joint		20605	CBC & Diff	85025	
Comprehensive	99204	Major Joint		20610	Comp Metabolic Panel	80053	
Comprehensive/High Complex	99205	**Other Invasive/Noninvasive**			Chlamydia Screen	87110	
Well Exam Infant (up to 12 mos.)	99381	Audiometry		92552	Cholesterol	82465	
Well Exam 1–4 yrs.	99382	Cast Application			Digoxin	80162	
Well Exam 5–11 yrs.	99383	Location Long Short			Electrolytes	80051	
Well Exam 12–17 yrs.	99384	Catheterization		51701	Ferritin	82728	
Well Exam 18–39 yrs.	99385	Circumcision		54150	Folate	82746	
Well Exam 40–64 yrs.	99386	Colposcopy		57452	GC Screen	87070	
		Colposcopy w/Biopsy		57454	Glucose	82947	X
		Cryosurgery Premalignant Lesion			Glucose 1 HR	82950	
		Location (s):			Glycosylated HGB A1C	83036	
Established Patient		Cryosurgery Warts			HCT	85014	
Post-Op Follow Up Visit	99024	Location (s):			HDL	83718	
Minimum	99211	Curettement Lesion			Hep BSAG	87340	
Problem Focused	99212	Single		11055	Hepatitis panel, acute	80074	
Expanded Problem Focused	99213	2–4		11056	HGB	85018	
Detailed	99214	>4		11057	HIV	86703	
Comprehensive/High Complex	99215	Diaphragm Fitting		57170	Iron & TIBC	83550	
Well Exam Infant (up to 12 mos.)	99391	Ear Irrigation		69210	Kidney Profile	80069	
Well exam 1–4 yrs.	99392	ECG		93000	Lead	83655	
Well Exam 5–11 yrs.	99393	Endometrial Biopsy		58100	Liver Profile	80076	
Well Exam 12–17 yrs.	99394	Exc. Lesion Malignant			Mono Test	86308	
Well Exam 18–39 yrs.	99395	Benign			Pap Smear	88155	
Well Exam 40–64 yrs.	99396 X	Location			Pregnancy Test	84703	
Obstetrics		Exc. Skin Tags (1–15)		11200	Obstetric Panel	80055	
Total OB Care	59400	Each Additional 10		11201	Pro Time	85610	
Injections		Fracture Treatment			PSA	84153	
Administration Sub. / IM	90772 X	Loc			RPR	86592	
Drug		w/Reduc		w/o Reduc	Sed. Rate	85651	
Dosage		I & D Abscess Single/Simple		10060	Stool Culture	87045	
Allergy	95115	Multiple or Comp		10061	Stool O & P	87177	
Cocci Skin Test	86490	I & D Pilonidal Cyst Simple		10080	Strep Screen	87880	
DPT	90701	Pilonidal Cyst Complex		10081	Theophylline	80198	
Hemophilus	90646	IV Therapy—To One Hour		90760	Thyroid Uptake	84479	
Influenza	90658	Each Additional Hour		90761	TSH	84443	
MMR	90707	Laceration Repair			Urinalysis	81000	X
OPV	90712	Location Size		Simp/Comp	Urine Culture	87088	
Pneumovax	90732	Laryngoscopy		31505	Drawing Fee	36415	X
TB Skin Test	86580	Oximetry		94760	Specimen Collection	99000	
TD	90718	Punch Biopsy			**Other:**		
Unlisted Immun	90749	Rhythm Strip		93040			
Tetanus Toxoid	90703	Treadmill		93015			
Vaccine/Toxoid Admin <8 Yr Old w/ Counseling	90465	Trigger Point or Tendon Sheath Inj.		20550			
Vaccine/Toxoid Administration for Adult	90471 X	Tympanometry		92567			

Diagnosis/ICD-9: **V70.0, V04.81, 250.00**

I acknowledge receipt of medical services and authorize the release of any medical information necessary to process this claim for healthcare payment only. I do authorize payment to the provider.

Total Estimated Charges: _____

Payment Amount: _____

Patient Signature <u>Kimber Acosta</u>

Next Appointment: _____

CASE A-19

Capital City Medical—123 Unknown Boulevard, Capital City, NY 12345-2222 (555)555-1234

Phil Wells, MD, Mannie Mends, MD, Bette R. Soone, MD

Patient Information Form

Tax ID: 75-0246810

Group NPI: 1513171216

Patient Information:

Name: (Last, First) Fields, Chester   ☒ Male   ☐ Female   Birth Date: 08/31/1943

Address: 1902 Birch Ave, Capital City, NY 12345   Phone: (555) 555-1112

Social Security Number: 652-91-3046   Full-Time Student: ☐ Yes   ☒ No

Marital Status: ☐ Single   ☒ Married   ☐ Divorced   ☐ Other

Employment:

Employer: Retired   Phone: ( ) _____

Address: _____

Condition Related to: ☐ Auto Accident   ☐ Employment   ☐ Other Accident

Date of Accident: _____ State _____

Emergency Contact: _____   Phone: ( ) _____

Primary Insurance: Medicare   Phone: ( ) _____

Address: P.O. Box 9834, Capital City, NY 12345

Insurance Policyholder's Name: Same   ☐ M ☐ F DOB: _____

Address: _____

Phone: _____ Relationship to Insured: ☒ Self ☐ Spouse ☐ Child ☐ Other

Employer: _____   Phone: ( ) _____

Employer's Address: _____

Policy/ID No: 359560568A   Group No: _____ Percent Covered: 80 %, Copay Amt: $_____

Secondary Insurance: Blue Cross Blue Shield Medigap   Phone: ( ) _____

Address: 379 Blue Plaza, Capital City, NY 12345

Insurance Policyholder's Name: Same   ☐ M ☐ F DOB: _____

Address: _____

Phone: _____ Relationship to Insured: ☒ Self ☐ Spouse ☐ Child ☐ Other

Employer: _____   Phone: ( ) _____

Employer's Address: _____

Policy/ID No: YYZ65281623   Group No: _____ Percent Covered: ___%, Copay Amt: $_____

Reason for Visit: Having chest pain

Known Allergies: _____

Were you referred here? If so, by whom?: _____

04/24/20XX
Assignment of Benefits: Y
Signature on File: Y
Referring Physician: N

S: Chester Fields presents with complaints of CP.

O: BP stable at 118/80, P: 94. EKG reveals normal sinus rhythm with no ST-T changes. Holter ordered. Pt. does admit to palpitations x2 days.

A: 1. Angina pectoris—413.9
2. Palpitations—785.1
3. HTN; benign—402.10

P: 1. Refill BP med Norvasc.
2. Return tomorrow for Holter monitor disconnection.
3. Refer to Dr. Iva Hart, cardiology, for possible stress test.

Phil Wells, MD
Family Practice
NPI: 1234567890
UPIN: 12345
PIN: 657891

CASE A-19 ENCOUNTER FORM

Patient Name _Chester Fields_

Capital City Medical
123 Unknown Boulevard, Capital City, NY 12345-2222

Date of Service
04-24-20XX

New Patient			Laboratory		
Problem Focused	99201	Arthrocentesis/Aspiration/Injection	Amylase	82150	
Expanded Problem, Focused	99202	Small Joint 20600	B12	82607	
Detailed	99203	Interm Joint 20605	CBC & Diff	85025	X
Comprehensive	99204	Major Joint 20610	Comp Metabolic Panel	80053	
Comprehensive/High Complex	99205	**Other Invasive/Noninvasive**	Chlamydia Screen	87110	
Well Exam Infant (up to 12 mos.)	99381	Audiometry 92552	Cholesterol	82465	
Well Exam 1–4 yrs.	99382	Cast Application	Digoxin	80162	
Well Exam 5–11 yrs.	99383	Location Long Short	Electrolytes	80051	
Well Exam 12–17 yrs.	99384	Catheterization 51701	Ferritin	82728	
Well Exam 18–39 yrs.	99385	Circumcision 54150	Folate	82746	
Well Exam 40–64 yrs.	99386	Colposcopy 57452	GC Screen	87070	
		Colposcopy w/Biopsy 57454	Glucose	82947	
		Cryosurgery Premalignant Lesion	Glucose 1 HR	82950	
		Location (s):	Glycosylated HGB A1C	83036	
Established Patient		Cryosurgery Warts	HCT	85014	
Post-Op Follow Up Visit	99024	Location (s):	HDL	83718	
Minimum	99211	Curettement Lesion	Hep BSAG	87340	
Problem Focused	99212	Single 11055	Hepatitis panel, acute	80074	
Expanded Problem Focused	99213 X	2–4 11056	HGB	85018	
Detailed	99214	>4 11057	HIV	86703	
Comprehensive/High Complex	99215	Diaphragm Fitting 57170	Iron & TIBC	83550	
Well Exam Infant (up to 12 mos.)	99391	Ear Irrigation 69210	Kidney Profile	80069	
Well exam 1–4 yrs.	99392	ECG 93000 X	Lead	83655	
Well Exam 5–11 yrs.	99393	Endometrial Biopsy 58100	Liver Profile	80076	
Well Exam 12–17 yrs.	99394	Exc. Lesion Malignant	Mono Test	86308	
Well Exam 18–39 yrs.	99395	Benign	Pap Smear	88155	
Well Exam 40–64 yrs.	99396	Location	Pregnancy Test	84703	
Obstetrics		Exc. Skin Tags (1–15) 11200	Obstetric Panel	80055	
Total OB Care	59400	Each Additional 10 11201	Pro Time	85610	
Injections		Fracture Treatment	PSA	84153	
Administration Sub. / IM	90772	Loc	RPR	86592	
Drug		w/Reduc w/o Reduc	Sed. Rate	85651	
Dosage		I & D Abscess Single/Simple 10060	Stool Culture	87045	
Allergy	95115	Multiple or Comp 10061	Stool O & P	87177	
Cocci Skin Test	86490	I & D Pilonidal Cyst Simple 10080	Strep Screen	87880	
DPT	90701	Pilonidal Cyst Complex 10081	Theophylline	80198	
Hemophilus	90646	IV Therapy—To One Hour 90760	Thyroid Uptake	84479	
Influenza	90658	Each Additional Hour 90761	TSH	84443	
MMR	90707	Laceration Repair	Urinalysis	81000	
OPV	90712	Location Size Simp/Comp	Urine Culture	87088	
Pneumovax	90732	Laryngoscopy 31505	Drawing Fee	36415	X
TB Skin Test	86580	Oximetry 94760 X	Specimen Collection	99000	
TD	90718	Punch Biopsy	**Other:**		
Unlisted Immun	90749	Rhythm Strip 93040			
Tetanus Toxoid	90703	Treadmill 93015			
Vaccine/Toxoid Admin <8 Yr Old w/ Counseling	90465	Trigger Point or Tendon Sheath Inj. 20550			
Vaccine/Toxoid Administration for Adult	90471	Tympanometry 92567			

Diagnosis/ICD-9: **413.9, 785.1, 402.10**

| | EKG | 9300 | |
| Holter Monitor | 93225 | X |

I acknowledge receipt of medical services and authorize the release of any medical information necessary to process this claim for healthcare payment only. I do authorize payment to the provider.

Patient Signature _Chester Fields_

Total Estimated Charges: _____

Payment Amount: _____

Next Appointment: _____

Capital City Medical—123 Unknown Boulevard, Capital City,
NY 12345-2222 (555)555-1234

Phil Wells, MD, Mannie Mends, MD, Bette R. Soone, MD

Patient Information Form

Tax ID: 75-0246810

Group NPI: 1513171216

Patient Information:

Name: (Last, First) Huckle, Gertrude   ☐ Male   ☒ Female   Birth Date: 04/08/1939

Address: 901 Poplar Rd, Capital City, NY 12345   Phone: (555) 555-1213

Social Security Number: 309-18-0684   Full-Time Student: ☐ Yes   ☒ No

Marital Status: ☐ Single   ☒ Married   ☐ Divorced   ☐ Other

Employment:

Employer: Retired   Phone: ( )

Address:

Condition Related to: ☐ Auto Accident   ☐ Employment   ☐ Other Accident

Date of Accident: State

Emergency Contact: Phone: ( )

Primary Insurance: Medicare   Phone: ( )

Address: P.O. Box 9834, Capital City, NY 12345

Insurance Policyholder's Name: Same   ☐ M ☐ F DOB:

Address:

Phone: Relationship to Insured: ☒ Self ☐ Spouse ☐ Child ☐ Other

Employer: Phone: ( )

Employer's Address:

Policy/ID No: 238123565A   Group No: Percent Covered: 80 %, Copay Amt: $

Secondary Insurance: Health America   Phone: ( )

Address: 2031 Healthica Center, Capital City, NY 12345

Insurance Policyholder's Name: Same   ☐ M ☐ F DOB:

Address:

Phone: Relationship to Insured: ☒ Self ☐ Spouse ☐ Child ☐ Other

Employer: Retired   Phone: ( )

Employer's Address:

Policy/ID No: 0004594   Group No: 9048000 Percent Covered: 80 %, Copay Amt: $

Reason for Visit: Check up on pilonidal cyst and possible removal of it

Known Allergies:

Were you referred here? If so, by whom?:

CASE A-20
SOAP

11/09/20XX
Assignment of Benefits: Y
Signature on File: Y
Referring Physician: N

S: Gertrude Huckle is here for a follow-up on her pilonidal cyst. She has had it ×3 weeks.

O: Pt. still complains of pain associated with sitting. She says that it is so bad, she can't even sit for 10 minutes. Upon exam, there is no change in the size of the cyst. Simple I&D will be necessary.

A: 1. Pilonidal cyst—685.1

P: 1. Keep bandaged for one week.
    2. Do not take baths, only showers.
    3. Return in 7 days for suture removal.

Mannie Mends, MD
General Surgeon
NPI: 012345689
UPIN: 012345
PIN: 446213

Patient Name _Gertrude Huckle_

Capital City Medical
123 Unknown Boulevard, Capital City, NY 12345-2222

Date of Service
11-09-20XX

**CASE A-20
ENCOUNTER
FORM**

New Patient			Arthrocentesis/Aspiration/Injection		**Laboratory**	
Problem Focused	99201		Arthrocentesis/Aspiration/Injection		Amylase	82150
Expanded Problem, Focused	99202		Small Joint	20600	B12	82607
Detailed	99203		Interm Joint	20605	CBC & Diff	85025
Comprehensive	99204		Major Joint	20610	Comp Metabolic Panel	80053
Comprehensive/High Complex	99205		**Other Invasive/Noninvasive**		Chlamydia Screen	87110
Well Exam Infant (up to 12 mos.)	99381		Audiometry	92552	Cholesterol	82465
Well Exam 1–4 yrs.	99382		Cast Application		Digoxin	80162
Well Exam 5–11 yrs.	99383		Location Long Short		Electrolytes	80051
Well Exam 12–17 yrs.	99384		Catheterization	51701	Ferritin	82728
Well Exam 18–39 yrs.	99385		Circumcision	54150	Folate	82746
Well Exam 40–64 yrs.	99386		Colposcopy	57452	GC Screen	87070
			Colposcopy w/Biopsy	57454	Glucose	82947
			Cryosurgery Premalignant Lesion		Glucose 1 HR	82950
			Location (s):		Glycosylated HGB A1C	83036
Established Patient			Cryosurgery Warts		HCT	85014
Post-Op Follow Up Visit	99024		Location (s):		HDL	83718
Minimum	99211		Curettement Lesion		Hep BSAG	87340
Problem Focused	99212		Single	11055	Hepatitis panel, acute	80074
Expanded Problem Focused	99213		2–4	11056	HGB	85018
Detailed	99214		>4	11057	HIV	86703
Comprehensive/High Complex	99215		Diaphragm Fitting	57170	Iron & TIBC	83550
Well Exam Infant (up to 12 mos.)	99391		Ear Irrigation	69210	Kidney Profile	80069
Well exam 1–4 yrs.	99392		ECG	93000	Lead	83655
Well Exam 5–11 yrs.	99393		Endometrial Biopsy	58100	Liver Profile	80076
Well Exam 12–17 yrs.	99394		Exc. Lesion Malignant		Mono Test	86308
Well Exam 18–39 yrs.	99395		Benign		Pap Smear	88155
Well Exam 40–64 yrs.	99396		Location		Pregnancy Test	84703
Obstetrics			Exc. Skin Tags (1–15)	11200	Obstetric Panel	80055
Total OB Care	59400		Each Additional 10	11201	Pro Time	85610
Injections			Fracture Treatment		PSA	84153
Administration Sub. / IM	90772		Loc		RPR	86592
Drug			w/Reduc w/o Reduc		Sed. Rate	85651
Dosage			I & D Abscess Single/Simple	10060	Stool Culture	87045
Allergy	95115		Multiple or Comp	10061	Stool O & P	87177
Cocci Skin Test	86490		I & D Pilonidal Cyst Simple	10080 X	Strep Screen	87880
DPT	90701		Pilonidal Cyst Complex	10081	Theophylline	80198
Hemophilus	90646		IV Therapy—To One Hour	90760	Thyroid Uptake	84479
Influenza	90658		Each Additional Hour	90761	TSH	84443
MMR	90707		Laceration Repair		Urinalysis	81000
OPV	90712		Location Size Simp/Comp		Urine Culture	87088
Pneumovax	90732		Laryngoscopy	31505	Drawing Fee	36415
TB Skin Test	86580		Oximetry	94760	Specimen Collection	99000
TD	90718		Punch Biopsy		**Other:**	
Unlisted Immun	90749		Rhythm Strip	93040		
Tetanus Toxoid	90703		Treadmill	93015		
Vaccine/Toxoid Admin <8 Yr Old w/ Counseling	90465		Trigger Point or Tendon Sheath Inj.	20550		
Vaccine/Toxoid Administration for Adult	90471		Tympanometry	92567		

Diagnosis/ICD-9: **685.1**

I acknowledge receipt of medical services and authorize the release of any medical information necessary to process this claim for healthcare payment only. I do authorize payment to the provider.

Patient Signature _Gertrude Huckle_

Total Estimated Charges: _____

Payment Amount: _____

Next Appointment: _____

Capital City Medical
Fee Schedule

New Patient OV			Punch Biopsy various codes	$80
Problem Focused 99201	$45		Nebulizer various codes	$45
Expanded Problem Focused 99202	$65		Cast Application various codes	$85
Detailed 99203	$85		Laryngoscopy 31505	$255
Comprehensive 99204	$105		Audiometry 92552	$85
Comprehensive/High Complex 99205	$115		Tympanometry 92567	$85
Well Exam infant (less than 1 year) 99381	$45		Ear Irrigation 69210	$25
Well Exam 1–4 yrs. 99382	$50		Diaphragm Fitting 57170	$30
Well Exam 5–11 yrs. 99383	$55		IV Therapy (up to one hour) 90760	$65
Well Exam 12–17 yrs. 99384	$65		Each additional hour 90761	$50
Well Exam 18–39 yrs. 99385	$85		Oximetry 94760	$10
Well Exam 40–64 yrs. 99386	$105		ECG 93000	$75
Established Patient OV			Holter Monitor various codes	$170
Post Op Follow Up Visit 99024	$0		Rhythm Strip 93040	$60
Minimum 99211	$35		Treadmill 93015	$375
Problem Focused 99212	$45		Cocci Skin Test 86490	$20
Expanded Problem Focused 99213	$55		X-ray, spine, chest, bone—any area various codes	$275
Detailed 99214	$65		Avulsion Nail 11730	$200
Comprehensive/High Complex 99215	$75		**Laboratory**	
Well exam infant (less than 1 year) 99391	$35		Amylase 82150	$40
Well Exam 1–4 yrs. 99392	$40		B12 82607	$30
Well Exam 5–11 yrs. 99393	$45		CBC & Diff 85025	$95
Well Exam 12–17 yrs. 99394	$55		Comp Metabolic Panel 80053	$75
Well Exam 18–39 yrs. 99395	$65		Chlamydia Screen 87110	$70
Well Exam 40–64 yrs. 99396	$75		Cholestrerol 82465	$75
Obstetrics			Digoxin 80162	$40
Total OB Care 59400	$1700		Electrolytes 80051	$70
Injections			Estrogen, Total 82672	$50
Administration 90772	$10		Ferritin 82728	$40
Allergy 95115	$35		Folate 82746	$30
DPT 90701	$50		GC Screen 87070	$60
Drug various codes	$35		Glucose 82947	$35
Influenza 90658	$25		Glycosylated HGB A1C 83036	$45
MMR 90707	$50		HCT 85014	$30
OPV 90712	$40		HDL 83718	$35
Pneumovax 90732	$35		HGB 85018	$30
TB Skin Test 86580	$15		Hep BSAG 83740	$40
TD 90718	$40		Hepatitis panel, acute 80074	$95
Tetanus Toxoid 90703	$40		HIV 86703	$100
Vaccine/Toxoid Administration for Younger Than 8 Years Old w/ counseling 90465	$10		Iron & TIBC 83550	$45
			Kidney Profile 80069	$95
Vaccine/Toxoid Administration for Adult 90471	$10		Lead 83665	$55
Arthrocentesis/Aspiration/Injection			Lipase 83690	$40
Small Joint 20600	$50		Lipid Panel 80061	$95
Interm Joint 20605	$60		Liver Profile 80076	$95
Major Joint 20610	$70		Mono Test 86308	$30
Trigger Point/Tendon Sheath Inj. 20550	$90		Pap Smear 88155	$90
Other Invasive/Noninvasive Procedures			Pap Collection/Supervision 88142	$95
Catheterization 51701	$55		Pregnancy Test 84703	$90
Circumcision 54150	$150		Obstetric Panel 80055	$85
Colposcopy 57452	$225		Pro Time 85610	$50
Colposcopy w/Biopsy 57454	$250		PSA 84153	$50
Cryosurgery Premalignant Lesion various codes	$160		RPR 86592	$55
Endometrial Biopsy 58100	$190		Sed. Rate 85651	$50
Excision Lesion Malignant various codes	$145		Stool Culture 87045	$80
Excision Lesion Benign various codes	$125		Stool O & P 87177	$105
Curettement Lesion			Strep Screen 87880	$35
Single 11055	$70		Theophylline 80198	$40
2–4 11056	$80		Thyroid Uptake 84479	$75
>4 11057	$90		TSH 84443	$50
Excision Skin Tags (1–15) 11200	$55		Urinalysis 81000	$35
Each Additional 10 11201	$30		Urine Culture 87088	$80
I & D Abscess Single/Simple 10060	$75		Drawing Fee 36415	$15
Multiple/Complex 10061	$95		Specimen Collection 99000	$10
I & D Pilonidal Cyst Simple 10080	$105			
I & D Pilonidal Cyst Complex 10081	$130			
Laceration Repair various codes	$60			

Completing the CMS-1500 Form for Physician Outpatient Billing Plus Determining the Correct Diagnostic and Procedure Codes

The case studies in this appendix are provided for additional practice in coding and in completing the CMS-1500 claim form for physician outpatient billing. By applying what you have learned in this text, your objective is to accurately code and complete each case study. In addition to completing the CMS-1500 form, you will be required to insert the correct diagnostic and procedure codes on the SOAP forms for each patient, for which you will need both the ICD and CPT® manuals. Patient demographics and a brief case history are provided. Complete the cases based on the following criteria. All patients have release of information and assignment of benefit signatures on file. All providers are participating and accept assignment. The group practice is the billing entity. The national transition to NPI numbers is complete and legacy PINs of individual payers are no longer used. 2007 ICD-9-CM and CPT codes are used. When entering procedures, enter E/M code first, followed by all other codes in descending cost order. Use these history & exam levels to determine E/M codes:

- Min = Minimal
- PF = Problem Focused
- EPF = Extended Problem Focused
- D = Detailed
- C = Comprehensive
- HC = Comprehensive with High Complexity decision making.

Use 8 digit dates for birthdates. Use 6 digit dates for all other dates. All street names should be entered using standard postal abbreviations, even if they are spelled out on the source documents. To complete each case study, copy the CMS-1500 form provided in Appendix D or download it from the CD-ROM that accompanies this text. Refer to the Capital City Medical Fee Schedule on page 638 to determine the correct fees. For a list of abbreviations used in these case studies and their meanings, please refer to the CD-ROM that accompanies this text.

CASE STUDIES

Primary

Case	Patient	Primary Payer
Case B-1	Roberto Munoz	Medicaid
Case B-2	Aaron Abner	Blue Cross Blue Shield
Case B-3	Abbie Spencer	Blue Cross Blue Shield
Case B-4	Justin Leasure	Blue Cross Blue Shield
Case B-5	Shayla Robinson	Medicaid
Case B-6	Mia Lui	Health America
Case B-7	April O'Leary	Aetna
Case B-8	Abdul Qabiz	Aetna
Case B-9	Clyde Hedberg	TRICARE
Case B-10	Kelly Campbell	Accidents Happen (auto insurance)

Primary/Secondary

Case	Patient	Primary Payer/Secondary Payer
Case B-11	Doree Marowski	Medicare/Medicaid
Case B-12	Joseph Hodreal	Medicare/Medicaid
Case B-13	Victoria Kozak	Medicare/Medicaid
Case B-14	Natasha Gubin	Medicare/Medicaid
Case B-15	Norma Casella	Medicare/Blue Cross Blue Shield (Medigap)
Case B-16	Earl Abbott	Blue Cross Blue Shield/Medicare (MSP)
Case B-17	Clifford McDavidson	Medicare/Aetna (Medigap)
Case B-18	Stewart Jenkins	Medicare/Medicaid
Case B-19	Adelphie Popazekus	Medicare/Aetna (Retiree)
Case B-20	Marsha Gambaro	Medicare/Health America (Retiree)

Capital City Medical—123 Unknown BLVD, Capital City,
NY 12345-2222 (555)555-1234
Phil Wells, MD, Mannie Mends, MD, Bette R. Soone, MD

Patient Information Form
Tax ID: 75-0246810
Group NPI: 1513171216

Patient Information:

Name: (Last, First) Munoz, Roberto   ☒ Male ☐ Female   Birth Date: 11/27/1978
Address: 1210 Sunny AVE, Township, NY 12345   Phone: (555) 555-1541
Social Security Number: 794-58-3422   Full-Time Student: ☐ Yes ☒ No
Marital Status: ☐ Single ☒ Married ☐ Divorced ☐ Other

Employment:

Employer: 24-7 Mini Mart   Phone: (555) 555-8241
Address: 7472 W. Washington St, Capital City, NY 12345
Condition Related to: ☐ Auto Accident ☐ Employment ☐ Other Accident
Date of Accident: _____ State _____
Emergency Contact: _____ Phone: ( ) _____

Primary Insurance: Medicaid   Phone: ( ) _____
Address: 4875 Capital Blvd, Capital City, NY 12345
Insurance Policyholder's Name: _____ ☐ M ☐ F DOB: _____
Address: _____
Phone: _____ Relationship to Insured: ☒ Self ☐ Spouse ☐ Child ☐ Other
Employer: _____ Phone: _____
Employer's Address: _____
Policy/ID No: 000174563256   Group No: ____ Percent Covered: ___%, Copay Amt: $5.00

Secondary Insurance: _____   Phone: ( ) _____
Address: _____
Insurance Policyholder's Name: _____ ☐ M ☐ F DOB: _____
Address: _____
Phone: _____ Relationship to Insured: ☐ Self ☐ Spouse ☐ Child ☐ Other
Employer: _____ Phone: ( ) _____
Employer's Address: _____
Policy/ID No: _____ Group No: ____ Percent Covered: ___%, Copay Amt: $____

Reason for Visit: Surgery follow-up for a keloid scar removal

Known Allergies: _____

Were you referred here? If so, by whom?: Dr. Eva N. Good, Internal Medicine, NPI: 8976453201

CASE B-1
SOAP

06/27/20XX
Assignment of Benefits: Y
Signature on File: Y
Referring Physician: N

S: Roberto Munoz presents for a follow-up on his keloid scar surgery.
O: Pt. had keloid scar on the abdomen removed seven days ago. It has healed well. Skin intact. No swelling, redness, drainage, or rash at site. Sutures to be removed today. The procedure has 10 global days for post-op follow up. The payer requires reporting of the post-up visit (no charge).
A: 1. Surgical follow-up—
      2. Post-op follow-up—
P: 1. Call office if any problems occur.

—————————————

Mannie Mends, MD
General Surgeon
NPI: 0123456789
Referral # 35877562

Capital City Medical—123 Unknown BLVD, Capital City, NY 12345-2222 (555)555-1234

Phil Wells, MD, Mannie Mends, MD, Bette R. Soone, MD

Patient Information Form

Tax ID: 75-0246810

Group NPI: 1513171216

Patient Information:

Name: (Last, First) Abner, Aaron   ☒ Male ☐ Female   Birth Date: 01/28/1976

Address: 98 N. Rosewood Dr, Township, NY 12345   Phone: (555) 555-8852

Social Security Number: 367-77-1104   Full-Time Student: ☐ Yes ☒ No

Marital Status: ☐ Single ☒ Married ☐ Divorced ☐ Other

Employment:

Employer: M Mart   Phone: (555) 555-3200

Address: 1019 County Rd, Township, NY 12345

Condition Related to: ☐ Auto Accident ☐ Employment ☐ Other Accident

Date of Accident: _____ State _____

Emergency Contact: _____ Phone: ( ) _____

Primary Insurance: Blue Cross Blue Shield   Phone: ( ) _____

Address: 379 Blue PLZ, Capital City, NY 12345

Insurance Policyholder's Name: Melissa Abner   ☐ M ☒ F DOB: 08/04/1974

Address: Same

Phone: _____ Relationship to Insured: ☐ Self ☒ Spouse ☐ Child ☐ Other

Employer: Pasta USA   Phone: (555) 555-6213

Employer's Address: 421 Eight AVE, Township, NY 12345

Policy/ID No: YYJ744258013   Group No: 015386 Percent Covered: ____%, Copay Amt: $ 10.00

Secondary Insurance: _____   Phone: ( ) _____

Address: _____

Insurance Policyholder's Name: _____   ☐ M ☐ F DOB: _____

Address: _____

Phone: _____ Relationship to Insured: ☐ Self ☐ Spouse ☐ Child ☐ Other

Employer: _____   Phone: ( ) _____

Employer's Address: _____

Policy/ID No: _____ Group No: _____ Percent Covered: ____%, Copay Amt: $_____

Reason for Visit: I am having feelings of anxiousness

Known Allergies: _____

Were you referred here? If so, by whom?: _____

CASE B-2
SOAP

12/01/20XX
Assignment of Benefits: Y
Signature on File: Y
Referring Physician: N

S: New patient, Aaron Abner, is seen in the office for anxiousness, and a feeling of "dying."

O: ROS reveals no disease process. He has family history of CAD; father. Mother has asthma. He has no siblings. He says he gets these episodes more frequently since they started about a month ago. Pt. also complains of bloating, dizziness, palpitations, and a feeling of fainting during these episodes. He is a smoker; one pack a day, and he denies any alcohol use. EKG displays normal sinus rhythm. CBC and lytes are normal values. He has been experiencing a lot of stress lately at work and with his marriage. Medical decision making (MDM) is low complexity (LC).

A: 1. Panic disorder—
2. Smoker—
3. Family history of CAD—
4. Family history of asthma—
5. E/M (D)—
6. Venipuncture—
7. CBC with diff—
8. Comprehensive Metabolic Panel (CMP)—
9. EKG—

P: 1. Start pt. on Paxil.
2. Refer pt. to psychiatrist.
3. Return after seeing the psychiatrist.
4. Xanax one p.o. t.i.d. # 10.

_____
Phil Wells, MD
Family Practice
NPI: 1234567890

Capital City Medical—123 Unknown BLVD, Capital City, NY 12345-2222 (555)555-1234

Phil Wells, MD, Mannie Mends, MD, Bette R. Soone, MD

Patient Information Form

Tax ID: 75-0246810

Group NPI: 1513171216

CASE B-3

Patient Information:

Name: (Last, First) Spencer, Abbie   ☐ Male ☒ Female   Birth Date: 03/21/1999

Address: 831 Crystal Dr, Capital City, NY 12345   Phone: (555) 555-7163

Social Security Number: 201-48-7302   Full-Time Student: ☐ Yes   ☒ No

Marital Status: ☒ Single   ☐ Married   ☐ Divorced   ☐ Other

Employment:

Employer: _____ Phone ( ) _____

Address: _____

Condition Related to: ☐ Auto Accident   ☐ Employment   ☐ Other Accident

Date of Accident: _____ State _____

Emergency Contact: _____ **Phone: ( )** _____

Primary Insurance: Blue Cross Blue Shield   Phone: ( ) _____

Address: 379 Blue PLZ, Capital City, NY 12345

Insurance Policyholder's Name: Mila Spencer   ☐ M ☒ F DOB: 09/25/1987

Address: Same

Phone: _____ Relationship to Insured: ☐ Self ☐ Spouse ☒ Child ☐ Other

Employer: Travel Plus   Phone: (555) 555-0471

Employer's Address: 1632 Getaway Ln, Capital City, NY 12345

Policy/ID No: YYZ210529333   Group No: 521036 Percent Covered: ____%, Copay Amt: $25.00

Secondary Insurance: _____ Phone: ( ) _____

Address: _____

Insurance Policyholder's Name: _____ ☐ M ☐ F DOB: _____

Address: _____

Phone: _____ Relationship to Insured: ☐ Self ☐ Spouse ☐ Child ☐ Other

Employer: _____ Phone: ( ) _____

Employer's Address: _____

Policy/ID No: _____ Group No: _____ Percent Covered: ____%, Copay Amt: $_____

Reason for Visit: Throat hurts really bad

Known Allergies: _____

Were you referred here? If so, by whom?: _____

CASE B-3
SOAP

07/19/20XX
Assignment of Benefits: Y
Signature on File: Y
Referring Physician: N

S: Abbie Spencer, an established patient, presents in the office today with complaints of a painful sore throat since this morning.

O: On exam, parotid glands swollen and the throat shows rubor. Eyes, ears, and nose clear. Chest clear. Strep screen is positive.

A: 1. Strep throat—
2. E/M (PF)—
3. Strep screen—

P: 1. Amox q.i.d.
2. Return as needed.

Phil Wells, MD
Family Practice
NPI: 1234567890

Capital City Medical—123 Unknown BLVD, Capital City,
NY 12345-2222 (555)555-1234

Phil Wells, MD, Mannie Mends, MD, Bette R. Soone, MD

Patient Information Form
Tax ID: 75-0246810
Group NPI: 1513171216

Patient Information:

Name: (Last, First) Leasure, Justin   ☒ Male   ☐ Female   Birth Date: 12/07/1973

Address: 1820 Grandview AVE, Capital City, NY 12345   Phone: (555) 555-6043

Social Security Number: 329-81-7402   Full-Time Student: ☐ Yes   ☒ No

Marital Status: ☐ Single   ☒ Married   ☐ Divorced   ☐ Other

Employment:

Employer: _____ Phone ( ) _____

Address: _____

Condition Related to: ☐ Auto Accident   ☐ Employment   ☐ Other Accident

Date of Accident: _____ State _____

Emergency Contact: _____ **Phone: ( )** _____

Primary Insurance: Blue Cross Blue Shield   Phone: ( ) _____

Address: 379 Blue PLZ, Capital City, NY 12345

Insurance Policyholder's Name: Tiffany Leasure   ☐ M ☒ F DOB: 11/13/1977

Address: Same

Phone: _____ Relationship to Insured: ☐ Self ☒ Spouse ☐ Child ☐ Other

Employer: Capital Junior/Senior High School   Phone: (555) 555-6986

Employer's Address: 1400 School House Rd, Capital City, NY 12345

Policy/ID No: YYJ426812684   Group No: 158386 Percent Covered: ___%, Copay Amt: $10.00

Secondary Insurance: _____ Phone: ( ) _____

Address: _____

Insurance Policyholder's Name: _____ ☐ M ☐ F DOB: _____

Address: _____

Phone: _____ Relationship to Insured: ☐ Self ☐ Spouse ☐ Child ☐ Other

Employer: _____ Phone: ( ) _____

Employer's Address: _____

Policy/ID No: _____ Group No: _____ Percent Covered: ___%, Copay Amt: $_____

Reason for Visit: My blood pressure has been running higher than normal

Known Allergies: _____

Were you referred here? If so, by whom?: _____

CASE B-4
SOAP

07/16/20XX
Assignment of Benefits: Y
Signature on File: Y
Referring Physician: N

S: Justin Leasure, an established patient, presents today complaining that his BP has been running above normal x one week.

O: On exam, pt. denies any stress. Pt. does have family history of HTN. BP today 162/94. ROS unremarkable, except for his BP reading.

A: 1. Elevated BP—
2. Family history of HTN—
3. E/M (EPF)—
4. CBC with diff—
5. Comprehensive Metabolic Panel (CMP)—

P: 1. CBC and CMP today.
2. Return to the office for the next 3 days for BP check.
3. If consistently above normal, start pt. on hypertensive medicine.
4. Appointment on Monday.

_____

Phil Wells, MD
Family Practice
NPI: 1234567890

Capital City Medical—123 Unknown BLVD, Capital City,
NY 12345-2222 (555)555-1234
Phil Wells, MD, Mannie Mends, MD, Bette R. Soone, MD

Patient Information Form
Tax ID: 75-0246810
Group NPI: 1513171216

Patient Information:

Name: (Last, First) Robinson, Shayla   ❑ Male ☒ Female   Birth Date: 11/20/2006

Address: 621 Bluff St, Capital City, NY 12345   Phone: (555) 555-2080

Social Security Number: 553-680-0125   Full-Time Student: ❑ Yes ☒ No

Marital Status: ☒ Single ❑ Married ❑ Divorced ❑ Other

Employment:

Employer: _____ Phone ( ) _____

Address: _____

Condition Related to: ❑ Auto Accident ❑ Employment ❑ Other Accident

Date of Accident: _____ State _____

Emergency Contact: _____ **Phone: ( )** _____

Primary Insurance: Medicaid   Phone: ( ) _____

Address: 4875 Capital Blvd, Capital City, NY 12345

Insurance Policyholder's Name: Same   ❑ M ❑ F DOB: _____

Address: Same

Phone: _____ Relationship to Insured: ☒ Self ❑ Spouse ❑ Child ❑ Other

Employer: _____ Phone: _____

Employer's Address: _____

Policy/ID No: 643566862   Group No: _____ Percent Covered: ___%, Copay Amt: $ 5.00

Secondary Insurance: _____ Phone: ( ) _____

Address: _____

Insurance Policyholder's Name: _____ ❑ M ❑ F DOB: _____

Address: _____

Phone: _____ Relationship to Insured: ❑ Self ❑ Spouse ❑ Child ❑ Other

Employer: _____ Phone: ( ) _____

Employer's Address: _____

Policy/ID No: _____ Group No: _____ Percent Covered: ___%, Copay Amt: $_____

Reason for Visit: Here for first year check _____

Known Allergies: _____

Were you referred here? If so, by whom?: _____

CASE B-5
SOAP

01/23/20XX
Assignment of Benefits: Y
Signature on File: Y
Referring Physician: N

S: Shayla Robinson returns for her one-year-old well-child exam. Her mother has no complaints.

O: ROS: unremarkable. Ht. and Wt. appropriate for age and gender. There is no evidence of illness.

A: 1. Healthy child exam—
2. MMR vaccine—
3. Administration of vaccination (with counseling)—
4. Vaccine—

P: 1. Return p.r.n.
2. Make appointment for next well checkup.

_____

Phil Wells, MD
Family Practice
NPI: 1234567890

CASE B-6

Capital City Medical—123 Unknown BLVD, Capital City,
NY 12345-2222 (555)555-1234
Phil Wells, MD, Mannie Mends, MD, Bette R. Soone, MD

Patient Information Form
Tax ID: 75-0246810
Group NPI: 1513171216

Patient Information:

Name: (Last, First) Lui, Mia ___ ❑ Male ☒ Female Birth Date: 05/25/1957

Address: 51 Orchard Ln, Township, NY 12345 ___ Phone: (555) 555-4798

Social Security Number: 660-89-5353 ___ Full-Time Student: ❑ Yes ☒ No

Marital Status: ❑ Single ☒ Married ❑ Divorced ❑ Other

Employment:

Employer: Township County Court ___ Phone: (555) 555-7000

Address: One Court St, Suite 201, Township, NY 12345

Condition Related to: ❑ Auto Accident ❑ Employment ❑ Other Accident

Date of Accident: ___ State ___

Emergency Contact: ___ **Phone: ( )** ___

Primary Insurance: Health America ___ Phone: ( ) ___

Address: 2031 Healthica CTR, Capital City, NY 12345

Insurance Policyholder's Name: Same ___ ❑ M ❑ F DOB: ___

Address: ___

Phone: ___ Relationship to Insured: ☒ Self ❑ Spouse ❑ Child ❑ Other

Employer: ___ Phone: ___

Employer's Address: ___

Policy/ID No: YYJ062054621 ___ Group No: 319521 Percent Covered: ___%, Copay Amt: $ 20.00

Secondary Insurance: ___ Phone: ( ) ___

Address: ___

Insurance Policyholder's Name: ___ ❑ M ❑ F DOB: ___

Address: ___

Phone: ___ Relationship to Insured: ❑ Self ❑ Spouse ❑ Child ❑ Other

Employer: ___ Phone: ( ) ___

Employer's Address: ___

Policy/ID No: ___ Group No: ___ Percent Covered: ___%, Copay Amt: $___

Reason for Visit: I haven't been having a period ___

Known Allergies: ___

Were you referred here? If so, by whom?: ___

CASE B-6
SOAP

07/16/20XX
Assignment of Benefits: Y
Signature on File: Y
Referring Physician: N

S: Mia Lui is here for a follow-up on menopausal screen.
O: Pt. still experiencing absence of menstruation. Estrogen and progesterone levels have decreased since last visit. Pt. was informed of hormone replacement therapy, its risks, and benefits. Pt. has agreed to proceed.
A: 1. Menopausal—
   2. E/M (PF)—
   3. Total estrogen—
   4. Venipuncture—
P: 1. Premarin one p.o. daily
   2. Follow up in six months.

_____

Bette R. Soone, MD
Obstetrics/Gynecology
NPI: 0987654321

CASE B-7

Capital City Medical—123 Unknown BLVD, Capital City,
NY 12345-2222 (555)555-1234
Phil Wells, MD, Mannie Mends, MD, Bette R. Soone, MD

Patient Information Form
Tax ID: 75-0246810
Group NPI: 1513171216

Patient Information:

Name: (Last, First) O'Leary, April   ☐ Male   ☒ Female   Birth Date: 04/03/1970

Address: 872 Hickory Pl, Capital City, NY 12345   Phone: (555) 555-4289

Social Security Number: 102-84-2471   Full-Time Student: ☐ Yes   ☒ No

Marital Status: ☒ Single   ☐ Married   ☐ Divorced   ☐ Other

Employment:

Employer: _____ Phone ( ) _____

Address: _____

Condition Related to: ☐ Auto Accident   ☐ Employment   ☐ Other Accident

Date of Accident: _____ State _____

Emergency Contact: _____ **Phone: ( )** _____

Primary Insurance: Medicaid   Phone: ( ) _____

Address: 4875 Capital Blvd, Capital City, NY 12345

Insurance Policyholder's Name: Same   ☐ M ☐ F DOB: _____

Address: _____

Phone: _____ Relationship to Insured: ☒ Self ☐ Spouse ☐ Child ☐ Other

Employer: _____ Phone: _____

Employer's Address: _____

Policy/ID No: 9839505   Group No: _____ Percent Covered: ____%, Copay Amt: $35.00

Secondary Insurance: _____ Phone: ( ) _____

Address: _____

Insurance Policyholder's Name: _____ ☐ M ☐ F DOB: _____

Address: _____

Phone: _____ Relationship to Insured: ☐ Self ☐ Spouse ☐ Child ☐ Other

Employer: _____ Phone: ( ) _____

Employer's Address: _____

Policy/ID No: _____ Group No: _____ Percent Covered: ____%, Copay Amt: $_____

Reason for Visit: Here for check up on pregnancy _____

Known Allergies: _____

Were you referred here? If so, by whom?: _____

CASE B-7
SOAP

10/07/20XX
Assignment of Benefits: Y
Signature on File: Y
Referring Physician: N

S: April O'Leary presents for her 8-week prenatal exam. (LMP 7/29/XX)
O: Pt. hasn't had any problems so far. Obstetric panel is normal. She is still considered high risk. (Medicaid pays separately for prenatal visits until patient has selected a participating OB)
A: 1. High-risk pregnancy—
2. E/M (PF)—
3. Venipuncture—
4. Obstetric panel—
P: 1. Register with an OB on your Medicaid managed care plan so you can get on a regular program.

_____

Phil Wells, MD
Family Practice
NPI: 1234567890

CASE B-8

Capital City Medical—123 Unknown BLVD, Capital City,
NY 12345-2222 (555)555-1234
Phil Wells, MD, Mannie Mends, MD, Bette R. Soone, MD

Patient Information Form
Tax ID: 75-0246810
Group NPI: 1513171216

Patient Information:

Name: (Last, First) Qabiz, Abdul   ☒ Male   ☐ Female   Birth Date: 02/17/1976

Address: 278 Covert Rd, Township, NY 12345   Phone: (555) 555-8725

Social Security Number: 655-34-4385   Full-Time Student: ☐ Yes   ☒ No

Marital Status: ☐ Single   ☒ Married   ☐ Divorced   ☐ Other

Employment:

Employer: Goodhealth Unlimited, Inc.   Phone ( ) _____

Address: 13 Mile Blvd, Capital City, NY 12345

Condition Related to: ☐ Auto Accident   ☐ Employment   ☐ Other Accident

Date of Accident: _____ State _____

Emergency Contact: _____ **Phone: ( )** _____

Primary Insurance: Aetna   Phone: ( ) _____

Address: 1625 Healthcare Bldg, Capital City, NY 12345

Insurance Policyholder's Name: Same   ☐ M ☐ F DOB: _____

Address: _____

Phone: _____ Relationship to Insured: ☒ Self ☐ Spouse ☐ Child ☐ Other

Employer: _____ Phone: _____

Employer's Address: _____

Policy/ID No: 6523483   Group No: 85624 Percent Covered: 90 %, Copay Amt: $_____

Secondary Insurance: _____ Phone: ( ) _____

Address: _____

Insurance Policyholder's Name: _____   ☐ M ☐ F DOB: _____

Address: _____

Phone: _____ Relationship to Insured: ☐ Self ☐ Spouse ☐ Child ☐ Other

Employer: _____ Phone: ( ) _____

Employer's Address: _____

Policy/ID No: _____ Group No: _____ Percent Covered: ___%, Copay Amt: $_____

Reason for Visit: Need a physical _____

Known Allergies: _____

Were you referred here? If so, by whom?: _____

CASE B-8
SOAP

10/26/20XX
Assignment of Benefits: Y
Signature on File: Y
Referring Physician: N

S: New patient, Abdul Qabiz, is being seen today for an annual check up. He is 32 years old and has no complaints at this time.

O: ROS: Unremarkable. Vitals: T: 98.6°F, P: 74, R: 18, BP: 114/70. Pt. has no complaints. U/A shows no evidence of WBCs, glucose, or any other abnormality. CBC, CMP, and lipid panels present unremarkable. MDM is SF.

A: 1. General health check up—
   2. E/M—
   3. Venipuncture—
   4. CBC with diff—
   5. Comprehensive Metabolic Panel (CMP)—
   6. Lipid panel—
   7. U/A dipstick—

P: 1. Return p.r.n.

_____

Phil Wells, MD
Family Practice
NPI: 1234567890

Capital City Medical—123 Unknown BLVD, Capital City,
NY 12345-2222 (555)555-1234
Phil Wells, MD, Mannie Mends, MD, Bette R. Soone, MD

Patient Information Form
Tax ID: 75-0246810
Group NPI: 1513171216

Patient Information:

Name: (Last, First) Hedberg, Clyde   ☒ Male   ☐ Female   Birth Date: 05/02/1969

Address: 939 Freedom Rd, Township, NY 12345   Phone: (555) 555-4546

Social Security Number: 897-51-7831   Full-Time Student: ☐ Yes   ☒ No

Marital Status: ☐ Single   ☒ Married   ☐ Divorced   ☐ Other

Employment:

Employer: _____ Phone ( ) _____

Address: _____

Condition Related to: ☐ Auto Accident   ☐ Employment   ☐ Other Accident

Date of Accident: _____ State _____

Emergency Contact: _____ **Phone: ( )** _____

Primary Insurance: Tricare   Phone: ( ) _____

Address: 7594 Forces-Run Rd, Militaryville, NY 12345

Insurance Policyholder's Name: Same   ☐ M ☐ F DOB: _____

Address: _____

Phone: _____ Relationship to Insured: ☒ Self ☐ Spouse ☐ Child ☐ Other

Employer: United States Army Reserves   Phone: _____

Employer's Address: 43 S. Army Blvd, Militaryville, NY 12345

Policy/ID No: 897517831   Group No: _____ Percent Covered: _80_%, Copay Amt: $_____

Secondary Insurance: _____ Phone: ( ) _____

Address: _____

Insurance Policyholder's Name: _____ ☐ M ☐ F DOB: _____

Address: _____

Phone: _____ Relationship to Insured: ☐ Self ☐ Spouse ☐ Child ☐ Other

Employer: _____ Phone: ( ) _____

Employer's Address: _____

Policy/ID No: _____ Group No: _____ Percent Covered: ___%, Copay Amt: $_____

Reason for Visit: I have been having a burning sensation in my throat

Known Allergies: _____

Were you referred here? If so, by whom?: _____

CASE B-9
SOAP

12/30/20XX
Assignment of Benefits: Y
Signature on File: Y
Referring Physician: N

S: New patient, Clyde Hedberg, presents with complaints of a burning sensation in his esophagus.

O: ROS shows no visceromegaly; sounds are normal. Vitals normal. Pt. says that for about 2 months he has been experiencing a burning sensation in his throat, as if his esophagus was eroding. He says that it is worse after meals, especially fried foods.

A: 1. GERD—
2. E/M (EPF)—

P: 1. Nexium daily.
2. Schedule an upper GI and esophageal x-ray.
3. Return in one week.
4. Avoid fatty and fried foods.
5. Avoid caffeine.
6. Give pamphlet on GERD.

Phil Wells, MD
Family Practice
NPI: 1234567890

CASE B-10

Capital City Medical—123 Unknown BLVD, Capital City,
NY 12345-2222 (555)555-1234

Phil Wells, MD, Mannie Mends, MD, Bette R. Soone, MD

Patient Information Form

Tax ID: 75-0246810

Group NPI: 1513171216

Patient Information:

Name: (Last, First) Campbell, Kelly   ❑ Male   ☒ Female   Birth Date: 09/12/1985

Address: 565 Cottage Ln, Capital City, NY 12345   Phone: (555) 555-2631

Social Security Number: 598-77-5432   Full-Time Student: ❑ Yes   ☒ No

Marital Status: ☒ Single   ❑ Married   ❑ Divorced   ❑ Other

Employment:

Employer: Quick Fill Pharmacy   Phone: (555) 555-2683

Address: Brier Rd, Township, NY 12345

Condition Related to: ❑ Auto Accident   ❑ Employment   ❑ Other Accident

Date of Accident: 12/17/20XX   State NY

Emergency Contact: _____   **Phone: ( )** _____

Primary Insurance: Accidents Happen Insurance Co.   Phone: ( ) _____

Address: 8100 Crash Blvd, Capital City, NY 12345

Insurance Policyholder's Name: Same   ❑ M ❑ F DOB: _____

Address: _____

Phone: _____   Relationship to Insured: ☒ Self ❑ Spouse ❑ Child ❑ Other

Employer: _____   Phone: _____

Employer's Address: _____

Policy/ID No: 658235476   Group No: ____ Percent Covered: ___%, Copay Amt: $____

Secondary Insurance: Health America (if denied by Auto)   Phone: ( ) _____

Address: 2031 Healthica Ctr, Capital City, NY 12345

Insurance Policyholder's Name: Same   ❑ M ❑ F DOB: _____

Address: _____

Phone: _____   Relationship to Insured: ☒ Self ❑ Spouse ❑ Child ❑ Other

Employer: _____   Phone: ( ) _____

Employer's Address: _____

Policy/ID No: 658235476   Group No: QFP624 Percent Covered: ___%, Copay Amt: $ 35.00

Reason for Visit: Here to get checked out for a car accident that happened yesterday

Known Allergies: _____

Were you referred here? If so, by whom?: _____

CASE B-10
SOAP

12/18/20XX
Assignment of Benefits: Y
Signature on File: Y
Referring Physician: N

S: Kelly Campbell, an established patient, presents in office today after a motor vehicle collision yesterday around 2 p.m. She was driving and slid on ice through a stop sign, hitting a tree on the opposite side of the road. She was at the ER yesterday afternoon following the accident.

O: Pt. complains of cervical vertebrae pain. She is not wearing the neck support because she says that it hurts more with it on. X-rays from the ER show cervical sprain at C-3 and C-4.

A: 1. Cervical sprain—
2. MVA—
3. E/M (EPF)—

P: 1. Continue Ibuprofen as ordered by the hospital.
2. Vicodin one q 6 h p.r.n. # 20.
3. Refer to physical therapy 3 x week x 4 weeks.
4. Return after therapy is completed.
5. Off work until further notice:
Claim # CK856312007

_____
Phil Wells, MD
Family Practice
NPI: 1234567890

Capital City Medical—123 Unknown BLVD, Capital City, NY 12345-2222 (555)555-1234

Phil Wells, MD, Mannie Mends, MD, Bette R. Soone, MD

Patient Information Form

Tax ID: 75-0246810

Group NPI: 1513171216

Patient Information:

Name: (Last, First) Marowski, Doree   ☐ Male   ☒ Female   Birth Date: 11/02/1944

Address: 3940 Holiday Way, Capital City, NY 12345   Phone: (555) 555-2007

Social Security Number: 494-61-7105   Full-Time Student: ☐ Yes   ☒ No

Marital Status: ☐ Single   ☐ Married   ☒ Divorced   ☐ Other

Employment:

Employer: Retired   Phone ( )

Address:

Condition Related to: ☐ Auto Accident   ☐ Employment   ☐ Other Accident

Date of Accident: _____ State _____

Emergency Contact: _____ **Phone: ( )** _____

Primary Insurance: Medicare   Phone: ( ) _____

Address: P.O. Box 9834, Capital City, NY 12345

Insurance Policyholder's Name: Same   ☐ M ☐ F DOB: _____

Address:

Phone: _____ Relationship to Insured: ☐ Self ☐ Spouse ☐ Child ☐ Other

Employer: _____ Phone: _____

Employer's Address: _____

Policy/ID No: 953255475A   Group No: _____ Percent Covered: 80 %, Copay Amt: $_____

Secondary Insurance: Medicaid   Phone: ( ) _____

Address: 4875 Capital Blvd, Capital City, NY 12345

Insurance Policyholder's Name: Same   ☐ M ☐ F DOB: _____

Address:

Phone: _____ Relationship to Insured: ☒ Self ☐ Spouse ☐ Child ☐ Other

Employer: _____ Phone: ( ) _____

Employer's Address: _____

Policy/ID No: 00008776732   Group No: _____ Percent Covered: ___%, Copay Amt: $5.00

Reason for Visit: Here to find out what my EMG results are for pain in both arms

Known Allergies: _____

Were you referred here? If so, by whom?: _____

CASE B-11
SOAP

03/24/20XX
Assignment of Benefits: Y
Signature on File: Y
Referring Physician: N

S: Doree Marowski is being seen for a follow-up on an EMG of B/L arms.
O: On exam, edema is still present bilaterally. She still complains of pain, tingling, and weakness. EMG is consistent with CTS.
A: 1. Carpal tunnel syndrome; bilateral—
   2. E/M (EPF)—
P: 1. Continue ibuprofen.
   2. Set up surgery with Dr. Mends.

_____

Phil Wells, MD
Family Practice
NPI: 1234567890

Capital City Medical—123 Unknown BLVD, Capital City, NY 12345-2222 (555)555-1234
Phil Wells, MD, Mannie Mends, MD, Bette R. Soone, MD

Patient Information Form
Tax ID: 75-0246810
Group NPI: 1513171216

CASE B-12

Patient Information:

Name: (Last, First) Hodreal, Joseph   ☒ Male   ☐ Female   Birth Date: 09/06/1938

Address: 11 Round St, Capital City, NY 12345   Phone: (555) 555-9798

Social Security Number: 153-96-2004   Full-Time Student: ☐ Yes   ☒ No

Marital Status: ☐ Single   ☒ Married   ☐ Divorced   ☐ Other

Employment:

Employer: Retired   Phone ( )

Address:

Condition Related to: ☐ Auto Accident   ☐ Employment   ☐ Other Accident

Date of Accident: _____ State _____

Emergency Contact: _____ **Phone: ( )** _____

Primary Insurance: Medicare   Phone: ( ) _____

Address: P.O. Box 9834, Capital City, NY 12345

Insurance Policyholder's Name: Same   ☐ M ☐ F DOB: _____

Address:

Phone: _____ Relationship to Insured: ☒ Self ☐ Spouse ☐ Child ☐ Other

Employer: _____ Phone: _____

Employer's Address: _____

Policy/ID No: 153521115A   Group No: _____ Percent Covered: 80 %, Copay Amt: $_____

Secondary Insurance: Medicaid   Phone: ( ) _____

Address: 4875 Capital Blvd, Capital City, NY 12345

Insurance Policyholder's Name: Same   ☐ M ☐ F DOB: _____

Address:

Phone: _____ Relationship to Insured: ☒ Self ☐ Spouse ☐ Child ☐ Other

Employer: _____ Phone: ( ) _____

Employer's Address: _____

Policy/ID No: 00235883216   Group No: _____ Percent Covered: ____%, Copay Amt: $ 5.00

Reason for Visit: To see how my prostate and blood pressure are doing

Known Allergies:

Were you referred here? If so, by whom?:

CASE B-12
SOAP

05/05/20XX
Assignment of Benefits: Y
Signature on File: Y
Referring Physician: N

S: Joseph Hodreal, an established patient, is in the office for a checkup on his prostate and HTN.

O: ROS shows no bladder or colon incontinence at this time. BP: 122/86. PSA has increased by 0.2.

A: 1. Benign prostatic hypertrophy—
     2. HTN—
     3. E/M (EPF)—
     4. Venipuncture—
     5. PSA—

P: 1. Repeat PSA in 2 months.
     2. Return in 2 months.

_____

Phil Wells, MD
Family Practice
NPI: 1234567890

Capital City Medical—123 Unknown BLVD, Capital City,
NY 12345-2222 (555)555-1234
Phil Wells, MD, Mannie Mends, MD, Bette R. Soone, MD

Patient Information Form
Tax ID: 75-0246810
Group NPI: 1513171216

Patient Information:

Name: (Last, First) Kozak, Victoria ☐ Male ☒ Female   Birth Date: 09/03/1937

Address: 501 Locust St, Capital City, NY 12345   Phone: (555) 555-3374

Social Security Number: 156-73-0953   Full-Time Student: ☐ Yes ☒ No

Marital Status: ☐ Single ☐ Married ☒ Divorced ☐ Other

Employment:

Employer: Retired   Phone ( )

Address:

Condition Related to: ☐ Auto Accident ☐ Employment ☐ Other Accident

Date of Accident: State

Emergency Contact: **Phone: ( )**

Primary Insurance: Medicare   Phone: ( )

Address: P.O. Box 9834, Capital City, NY 12345

Insurance Policyholder's Name: Same   ☐ M ☐ F DOB:

Address:

Phone: Relationship to Insured: ☒ Self ☐ Spouse ☐ Child ☐ Other

Employer: Phone:

Employer's Address:

Policy/ID No: 698334572A   Group No: Percent Covered: 80 %, Copay Amt: $

Secondary Insurance: Medicaid   Phone: ( )

Address: 4875 Capital Blvd, Capital City, NY 12345

Insurance Policyholder's Name: Same   ☐ M ☐ F DOB:

Address:

Phone: Relationship to Insured: ☒ Self ☐ Spouse ☐ Child ☐ Other

Employer: Phone: ( )

Employer's Address:

Policy/ID No: 00060268359   Group No: Percent Covered: %, Copay Amt: $ 5.00

Reason for Visit: Follow-up on cancer of the pancreas

Known Allergies:

Were you referred here? If so, by whom?:

CASE B-13
SOAP

08/11/20XX
Assignment of Benefits: Y
Signature on File: Y
Referring Physician: N

S: Victoria Kozak presents for a checkup on chronic pancreatitis and cancer of the pancreas that I have been following.

O: Pt. starts chemotherapy and radiation next week. Amylase and lipase unchanged. Abdomen reveals enlargement of the pancreas due to the cancer. Pt. still drinks excessively every day. Everything is clear to proceed with the chemo and radiation.

A: 1. Pancreatic cancer of islet cells (neoplasm)—
   2. Chronic pancreatitis—
   3. Continuing alchol abuse—
   4. E/M (EPF)—
   5. Venipuncture—
   6. Amylase—
   7. Lipase—

P: 1. Clearance o.k. for chemo and radiation therapy.
   2. Return in one week.
   3. Stop drinking.

_____

Phil Wells, MD
Family Practice
NPI: 1234567890

Capital City Medical—123 Unknown BLVD, Capital City,
NY 12345-2222 (555)555-1234

Phil Wells, MD, Mannie Mends, MD, Bette R. Soone, MD

Patient Information Form

Tax ID: 75-0246810

Group NPI: 1513171216

CASE B-14

Patient Information:

Name: (Last, First) Gubin, Natasha   ❑ Male   ☒ Female   Birth Date: 04/18/1946

Address: 1589 Ridge AVE, Capital City, NY 12345   Phone: (555) 555-4142

Social Security Number: 253-00-6295   Full-Time Student: ❑ Yes   ☒ No

Marital Status: ❑ Single   ☒ Married   ❑ Divorced   ❑ Other

Employment:

Employer: Retired   Phone ( )

Address:

Condition Related to: ❑ Auto Accident   ❑ Employment   ❑ Other Accident

Date of Accident: _____ State _____

Emergency Contact: _____ **Phone: ( )** _____

Primary Insurance: Medicare   Phone: ( )

Address: P.O. Box 9834, Capital City, NY 12345

Insurance Policyholder's Name: Same   ❑ M ❑ F DOB:

Address:

Phone: _____ Relationship to Insured: ☒ Self ❑ Spouse ❑ Child ❑ Other

Employer: _____ Phone:

Employer's Address:

Policy/ID No: 53168465A   Group No: ____ Percent Covered: 80 %, Copay Amt: $____

Secondary Insurance: Medicaid   Phone: ( )

Address: 4875 Capital Blvd, Capital City, NY 12345

Insurance Policyholder's Name: Same   ❑ M ❑ F DOB:

Address:

Phone: _____ Relationship to Insured: ☒ Self ❑ Spouse ❑ Child ❑ Other

Employer: _____ Phone: ( )

Employer's Address:

Policy/ID No: 001544358706   Group No: ____ Percent Covered: ___%, Copay Amt: $ 5.00

Reason for Visit: I think I have a sinus infection causing me shortness of breath

Known Allergies: _____

Were you referred here? If so, by whom?: _____

CASE B-14
SOAP

09/09/20XX
Assignment of Benefits: Y
Signature on File: Y
Referring Physician: N

S: Natasha Gubin comes in today complaining of a sinus infection and SOB.

O: On exam, pt. has fever; T: 99.9°F. Nares are patent, but there is mucosal drainage. Chest reveals wheezes. Pt. does have asthma. Pt. was here a month ago with same complaints. Inhaled treatment with albuterol given. CXR negative.

A: 1. Asthma, exacerbated—
   2. Chronic sinusitis—
   3. E/M (EPF)—
   4. CXR—
   5. Nebulizer—

P: 1. Levaquin one daily for seven days.
   2. Prednisone 2 sprays q 6 h.
   3. Return p.r.n.

_____

Phil Wells, MD
Family Practice
NPI: 1234567890

Appendix B   Completing the CMS-1500 Form for Physician Outpatient Billing   669

CASE B-15

Capital City Medical—123 Unknown BLVD, Capital City,
NY 12345-2222 (555)555-1234
Phil Wells, MD, Mannie Mends, MD, Bette R. Soone, MD

Patient Information Form
Tax ID: 75-0246810
Group NPI: 1513171216

Patient Information:

Name: (Last, First) Casella, Norma   ❑ Male ☒ Female   Birth Date: 03/19/1945

Address: 200 Liberty AVE, Capital City, NY 12345   Phone: (555) 555-7183

Social Security Number: 8622-29-3546   Full-Time Student: ❑ Yes ☒ No

Marital Status: ☒ Single ❑ Married ❑ Divorced ❑ Other

Employment:

Employer: Retired   Phone ( )

Address:

Condition Related to: ❑ Auto Accident   ❑ Employment   ❑ Other Accident

Date of Accident: _____ State _____

Emergency Contact: _____ **Phone: ( )** _____

Primary Insurance: Medicare   Phone: ( )

Address: P.O. Box 9834, Capital City, NY 12345

Insurance Policyholder's Name: Same   ❑ M ❑ F DOB:

Address:

Phone: _____ Relationship to Insured: ☒ Self ❑ Spouse ❑ Child ❑ Other

Employer: _____ Phone:

Employer's Address:

Policy/ID No: 216933650A   Group No: _____ Percent Covered: 80 %, Copay Amt: $_____

Secondary Insurance: Blue Cross Blue Shield Medigap   Phone: ( )

Address: 379 Blue PLZ, Capital City, NY 12345

Insurance Policyholder's Name: Same   ❑ M ❑ F DOB:

Address:

Phone: _____ Relationship to Insured: ☒ Self ❑ Spouse ❑ Child ❑ Other

Employer: _____ Phone: ( )

Employer's Address:

Policy/ID No: YYZ007893521   Group No: _____ Percent Covered: ___%, Copay Amt: $_____

Reason for Visit: My left heel is hurting all the time

Known Allergies:

Were you referred here? If so, by whom?:

CASE B-15
SOAP

04/24/20XX
Assignment of Benefits: Y
Signature on File: Y
Referring Physician: N

S: Norma Casella, an established patient, presents today for complaints of pain in her left heel.

O: Exam shows that pt. has pain when walking or standing. She says it is worse when she has been sitting, and then gets up. The first couple of steps feels like she's walking on a broken heel. X-ray reveals a spur on the heel bone. I would like to see if steroids will help before operating.

A: 1. Heel spur—
2. E/M (PF)—
3. X-ray; heel—
4. Administration of injection—

P: 1. Cortisone injection at site.
2. Return in 2 weeks to evaluate status.

_____

Mannie Mends, MD
General Surgeon
NPI: 0123456789

CASE B-16

Capital City Medical—123 Unknown BLVD, Capital City,
NY 12345-2222 (555)555-1234
Phil Wells, MD, Mannie Mends, MD, Bette R. Soone, MD

Patient Information Form
Tax ID: 75-0246810
Group NPI: 1513171216

Patient Information:

Name: (Last, First) Abbott, Earl ☒ Male ☐ Female Birth Date: 08/30/1932

Address: 34 Diamond Ln, Capital City, NY 12345 Phone: (555) 555-4608

Social Security Number: 410-11-6293 Full-Time Student: ☐ Yes ☒ No

Marital Status: ☐ Single ☒ Married ☐ Divorced ☐ Other

Employment:

Employer: Retired Phone ( )

Address:

Condition Related to: ☐ Auto Accident ☐ Employment ☐ Other Accident

Date of Accident: State

Emergency Contact: **Phone: ( )**

Primary Insurance: Blue Cross Blue Shield Phone: ( )

Address: 379 Blue PLZ, Capital City, NY 12345

Insurance Policyholder's Name: Sheila Abbott ☐ M ☒ F DOB: 09/05/1944

Address: Same

Phone: Relationship to Insured: ☐ Self ☒ Spouse ☐ Child ☐ Other

Employer: Spotless Cleaning Co. Phone:

Employer's Address: 624 Dust Rd, Capital City, NY 12345

Policy/ID No: XYZ4427895235 Group No: 490003 Percent Covered: ____%, Copay Amt: $ 25.00

Secondary Insurance: Medicare Phone: ( )

Address: P.O. Box 9834, Capital City, NY 12345

Insurance Policyholder's Name: Same ☐ M ☐ F DOB:

Address:

Phone: Relationship to Insured: ☒ Self ☐ Spouse ☐ Child ☐ Other

Employer: Phone: ( )

Employer's Address:

Policy/ID No: 800563798A Group No: Percent Covered: 80 %, Copay Amt: $

Reason for Visit: Heart check up

Known Allergies:

Were you referred here? If so, by whom?:

CASE B-16
SOAP

03/11/20XX
Assignment of Benefits: Y
Signature on File: Y
Referring Physician: N

S: Earl Abbott is in for a checkup on his heart. He is an established patient.
O: Pt. has old MI, s/p CABG for CAD, and HTN. BP: 136/78. Pt. denies angina, SOB, or any other symptoms. EKG shows old MI, otherwise normal. No carotid bruits. Lipid panel shows mild elevation.
A: 1. CAD—
2. HTN—
3. Old MI—
4. Status post CABG—
5. E/M (EPF)—
6. EKG—
7. Venipuncture—
8. Lipid panel—
P: 1. Refill medications.
2. Return in 2 months.

_____

Phil Wells, MD
Family Practice
NPI: 1234567890

CASE B-17

Capital City Medical—123 Unknown BLVD, Capital City,
NY 12345-2222 (555)555-1234
Phil Wells, MD, Mannie Mends, MD, Bette R. Soone, MD

Patient Information Form
Tax ID: 75-0246810
Group NPI: 1513171216

Patient Information:

Name: (Last, First) McDavidson, Clifford   ☒ Male   ☐ Female   Birth Date: 05/23/1947

Address: 717 Hillcrest Dr, Capital City, NY 12345   Phone: (555) 555-7585

Social Security Number: 673-51-1149   Full-Time Student: ☐ Yes   ☒ No

Marital Status: ☒ Single   ☐ Married   ☐ Divorced   ☐ Other

Employment:

Employer: Retired   Phone ( ) _____

Address: _____

Condition Related to: ☐ Auto Accident   ☐ Employment   ☐ Other Accident

Date of Accident: _____   State _____

Emergency Contact: _____   **Phone: ( )** _____

Primary Insurance: Medicare   Phone: ( ) _____

Address: P.O. Box 9834, Capital City, NY 12345

Insurance Policyholder's Name: Same   ☐ M   ☐ F   DOB: _____

Address: _____

Phone: _____   Relationship to Insured: ☒ Self   ☐ Spouse   ☐ Child   ☐ Other

Employer: _____   Phone: _____

Employer's Address: _____

Policy/ID No: 468752139A____   Group No: _____   Percent Covered: 80__%, Copay Amt: $_____

Secondary Insurance: Aetna Medigap   Phone: ( ) _____

Address: 1625 Healthcare Bldg, Capital City, NY 12345

Insurance Policyholder's Name: Same   ☐ M   ☐ F   DOB: _____

Address: _____

Phone: _____   Relationship to Insured: ☒ Self   ☐ Spouse   ☐ Child   ☐ Other

Employer: _____   Phone: ( ) _____

Employer's Address: _____

Policy/ID No: 0321227____   Group No: _____   Percent Covered: ___%, Copay Amt: $_____

Reason for Visit: I have a cough and I'm really congested

Known Allergies: _____

Were you referred here? If so, by whom?: _____

CASE B-17
SOAP

09/07/20XX
Assignment of Benefits: Y
Signature on File: Y
Referring Physician: N

S: Clifford McDavidson is being seen today for cough and congestion.

O: Chest sounds are that of his COPD, but with congestion. CXR shows this disorder. He is on oxygen therapy, 2 L/min.

A: 1. Chronic bronchitis with acute exacerbation of COPD—
   2. E/M (EPF)—
   3. CXR—

P: 1. Augmentin one b.i.d. for 10 days.
   2. Plenty of rest and fluids.
   3. Return for normal appointment scheduled in October.

_____

Phil Wells, MD
Family Practice
NPI: 1234567890

CASE B-18

Capital City Medical—123 Unknown BLVD, Capital City,
NY 12345-2222 (555)555-1234

Phil Wells, MD, Mannie Mends, MD, Bette R. Soone, MD

Patient Information Form

Tax ID: 75-0246810

Group NPI: 1513171216

Patient Information:

Name: (Last, First) Jenkins, Stewart   ☒ Male   ☐ Female   Birth Date: 07/29/1947

Address: 27 Highland AVE, Capital City, NY 12345   Phone: (555) 555-9475

Social Security Number: 429-66-0631   Full-Time Student: ☐ Yes   ☒ No

Marital Status: ☐ Single   ☒ Married   ☐ Divorced   ☐ Other

Employment:

Employer: Retired   Phone ( )

Address:

Condition Related to: ☐ Auto Accident   ☐ Employment   ☐ Other Accident

Date of Accident: State

Emergency Contact: **Phone: ( )**

Primary Insurance: Medicare   Phone: ( )

Address: P.O. Box 9834, Capital City, NY 12345

Insurance Policyholder's Name: Same   ☐ M ☐ F DOB:

Address:

Phone: Relationship to Insured: ☒ Self   ☐ Spouse   ☐ Child   ☐ Other

Employer: Phone:

Employer's Address:

Policy/ID No: 238823364A   Group No: Percent Covered: 80 %, Copay Amt: $

Secondary Insurance: Medicaid   Phone: ( )

Address: 4875 Capital Blvd, Capital City, NY 12345

Insurance Policyholder's Name: Same   ☐ M ☐ F DOB:

Address:

Phone: Relationship to Insured: ☒ Self   ☐ Spouse   ☐ Child   ☐ Other

Employer: Phone: ( )

Employer's Address:

Policy/ID No: 00005733268   Group No: Percent Covered: %, Copay Amt: $ 5.00

Reason for Visit: I have a wart on my right index finger

Known Allergies:

Were you referred here? If so, by whom?:

CASE B-18
SOAP

11/09/20XX
Assignment of Benefits: Y
Signature on File: Y
Referring Physician: N

S: Stewart Jenkins, an established patient, presents today with complaints of a wart on his right index finger.

O: Pt. says that he tried to "cut it out," but it only made it 2 times bigger. He would like it removed.

A: 1. Wart; right index finger—
2. Cryosurgery; wart—

P: 1. Ibuprofen b.i.d.

_____

Mannie Mends, MD
General Surgeon
NPI: 0123456789

Capital City Medical—123 Unknown BLVD, Capital City,
NY 12345-2222 (555)555-1234
Phil Wells, MD, Mannie Mends, MD, Bette R. Soone, MD

Patient Information Form
Tax ID: 75-0246810
Group NPI: 1513171216

CASE B-19

Patient Information:

Name: (Last, First) Popazekus, Adelphie   ❑ Male   ☒ Female   Birth Date: 09/08/1942

Address: 333 Violet CIR, Capital City, NY 12345   Phone: (555) 555-0853

Social Security Number: 729-04-6278   Full-Time Student: ❑ Yes   ☒ No

Marital Status: ❑ Single   ☒ Married   ❑ Divorced   ❑ Other

Employment:

Employer: Retired   Phone ( ) _____

Address: _____

Condition Related to: ❑ Auto Accident   ❑ Employment   ❑ Other Accident

Date of Accident: _____   State _____

Emergency Contact: _____   **Phone: ( )** _____

Primary Insurance: Medicare   Phone: ( ) _____

Address: P.O. Box 9834, Capital City, NY 12345

Insurance Policyholder's Name: Same   ❑ M   ❑ F   DOB: _____

Address: _____

Phone: _____   Relationship to Insured: ☒ Self   ❑ Spouse   ❑ Child   ❑ Other

Employer: _____   Phone: _____

Employer's Address: _____

Policy/ID No: 653284563A   Group No: ____ Percent Covered: 80 %, Copay Amt: $____

Secondary Insurance: Aetna   Phone: ( ) _____

Address: 1625 Healthcare Bldg, Capital City, NY 12345

Insurance Policyholder's Name: Samuel Popazekus   ☒ M   ❑ F   DOB: 10/14/1941

Address: Same

Phone: _____   Relationship to Insured: ❑ Self   ☒ Spouse   ❑ Child   ❑ Other

Employer: Retired   Phone: ( ) _____

Employer's Address: _____

Policy/ID No: 210805   Group No: 496000 Percent Covered: ____%, Copay Amt: $ 30.00

Reason for Visit: Checkup on diabetes

Known Allergies: _____

Were you referred here? If so, by whom?: _____

CASE B-19
SOAP

03/17/20XX
Assignment of Benefits: Y
Signature on File: Y
Referring Physician: N

S: Adelphie Popazekus is being seen for evaluation of her DM II.

O: Pt. only complains of symptoms related to her diabetic neuropathy. Her pedal pulses are 2+. There is no evidence of wounds. Glucose 174. She says that she ate within the past hour. She has gained 7 lbs. since her last visit. Pt. instructed to lose weight.

A: 1. DM II—
2. Diabetic polyneuropathy—
3. Obesity—
4. E/M (EPF)—
5. Venipuncture—
6. Glucose—

P: 1. Continue medications.
2. Recheck in one month.
3. Refer to hospital dietary services for weight loss.

_____

Phil Wells, MD
Family Practice
NPI: 1234567890

Capital City Medical—123 Unknown BLVD, Capital City,
NY 12345-2222 (555)555-1234
Phil Wells, MD, Mannie Mends, MD, Bette R. Soone, MD

Patient Information Form
Tax ID: 75-0246810
Group NPI: 1513171216

CASE B-20

Patient Information:

Name: (Last, First) Gambaro, Marsha   ☐ Male ☒ Female   Birth Date: 04/15/1932

Address: 19 Crestview PL, Capital City, NY 12345   Phone: (555) 555-4737

Social Security Number: 873-12-9784   Full-Time Student: ☐ Yes ☒ No

Marital Status: ☐ Single ☒ Married ☐ Divorced ☐ Other

Employment:

Employer: Retired   Phone ( )

Address:

Condition Related to: ☐ Auto Accident ☐ Employment ☐ Other Accident

Date of Accident: _____ State _____

Emergency Contact: _____ **Phone: ( )** _____

Primary Insurance: Medicare   Phone: ( )

Address: P.O. Box 9834, Capital City, NY 12345

Insurance Policyholder's Name: Same   ☐ M ☐ F DOB: _____

Address:

Phone: _____ Relationship to Insured: ☒ Self ☐ Spouse ☐ Child ☐ Other

Employer: _____ Phone:

Employer's Address:

Policy/ID No: 231481483A   Group No: ____ Percent Covered: 80 %, Copay Amt: $____

Secondary Insurance: Health America   Phone: ( )

Address: 2031 Healthica CTR, Capital City, NY 12345

Insurance Policyholder's Name: Same   ☐ M ☐ F DOB: _____

Address:

Phone: _____ Relationship to Insured: ☒ Self ☐ Spouse ☐ Child ☐ Other

Employer: Retired   Phone: ( )

Employer's Address:

Policy/ID No: 0548726   Group No: 6843 Percent Covered: ____%, Copay Amt: $ 15.00

Reason for Visit: Checkup on Alzheimer's and thyroid

Known Allergies:

Were you referred here? If so, by whom?:

CASE B-20
SOAP

11/09/20XX
Assignment of Benefits: Y
Signature on File: Y
Referring Physician: N

S: Marsha Gambaro presents in the office for a regular checkup on Alzheimer's and hypothyroidism.

O: Pt. is brought in by daughter Ann, whom says that her mother has been doing well. Pt. is in no acute distress. TSH shows stable functioning.

A: 1. Alzheimer's disease—
    2. Hypothyroidism—
    3. E/M (PF)—
    4. TSH—
    5. Venipuncture—

P: 1. Refill Synthroid and Aricept.
    2. Return in 3 months.

Phil Wells, MD
Family Practice
NPI: 1234567890

Completing the UB-04 Form for Hospital Billing

The case studies in this appendix are provided for additional practice in completing the UB-04 claim form for hospital billing. By applying what you have learned in this text, your objective is to accurately complete each case study. All of the information you need is provided, including patient demographics, diagnostic and procedure codes, and a brief case history of each patient's health problem. Complete the cases based on the following criteria. All patients have release of information and assignment of benefit signatures on file. All physicians and hospitals participate in all of the health care plans listed, and all physicians and hospitals accept assignment for these plans. The hospital is the billing entity. The national transition to NPI numbers is complete and legacy PINs of individual payers are no longer used. 2007 ICD-9-CM, ICD-9-PCS and CPT codes are used. Use 6 digit dates for ALL dates. All street names should be entered using standard postal abbreviations, even if they are spelled out on the source documents. Room charges reflect the daily rate and should be multiplied times the number of days to get the total room charge for the stay. All other services reflect the total charges for all units provided. To complete each case study, copy the UB-04 form provided in Appendix D or download it from the CD-ROM that accompanies this text. For a list of abbreviations used in these case studies and their meanings, please refer to the CD-ROM that accompanies this text.

CASE STUDIES

Inpatient Hospital

Case	Patient	Primary Payer
C-1	Nestor Willis	Medicaid
C-2	Melvin Lyles	Blue Cross Blue Shield
C-3	Emilio Mendez	Blue Cross Blue Shield
C-4	Harold Janovich	Aetna
C-5	Ramesh Kedar	Health America
C-6	Arthur Zbegan	Medicare
C-7	Rita Mangino	Aetna
C-8	Dorothy Greer	Medicare
C-9	Virginia Moore	Medicaid
C-10	Albert Kim	Medicare

Outpatient Hospital

Case	Patient	Primary Payer
C-11	Olivia Marselle	Medicaid
C-12	Antonio Rodriquez	Blue Cross Blue Shield
C-13	Randall Paul	Aetna
C-14	Megan Bishop	Blue Cross Blue Shield
C-15	Patricia Vlah	Aetna
C-16	Bryson Chung	Health America
C-17	Keith Lombardo	Medicare
C-18	Tyrone Clark	Medicaid
C-19	Dawn Hunt	Medicare
C-20	Jenna Masters	Medicare

Optional Additional Case Study Exercises

Using the information from the above case studies, prepare a CMS-1500 claim form for professional physician billing. Copy the CMS-1500 form from Appendix D or download it from the CD-ROM that accompanies this text.

CASE C-1

Township Memorial Hospital
700 Shady Street
Township, NY 12345
(555)555-0700

Patient Information:	Nestor Willis 63 Park Avenue, Capital City, NY 12345 (555)555-2901
DOB:	09-29-1952
Sex:	Female
SSN:	873-02-6447
Status:	Married **Student:** No
Employer:	Retired
Responsible Party:	Nestor Willis Address—same as above

Insurance Information:	Medicaid 4875 Capital Boulevard, Capital City, NY 12345
ID #:	322654921345 **Group #:**
Insured's Name:	Same **Relationship to Patient:** Self
Insured's Address:	

Insured's Employer:

Authorization:	3.2191321 **Approved # of Days:** 4
Attending Physician:	Phil Wells, MD
Federal Tax ID #:	75-1234567
NPI:	1234567890
Group NPI:	1513171216

Reason for visit: I'm having chest pain and I am short of breath.

CASE C-1

HPI: This is an African American female admitted on July 28, 20XX, at 1:17 am with CP and SOB. Pt. has emphysema, has smoked 2 packs a day for 34 years and still smokes. Pt. denies N&V. Mouth breathing noted. CXR reveals pneumonia in the RLL of lung. Sputum cultures ordered. Pt. was discharged on August 1, 20XX, at 3:20 pm.

Patient Control #:	56139844	**Type of Admission:**	1
MR #:	659431896	**Source of Admission:**	1
Hospital NPI:	3434343434	**Discharge Status:**	01
Hospital Tax ID:	75-0750750	**Type of Bill Code:**	111

Fees:

Revenue Codes	Units	Total Charges	Date of Service
120 Room/Board/Semi	4	$ 450.00/day	07/28/20XX–08/01/20XX
260 IV Therapy	4	$1000.00	07/28/20XX–07/31/20XX
300 Lab	1	$ 235.00	07/28/20XX
320 Radiology	1	$ 250.00	07/28/20XX
900 Respiratory Services	4	$ 400.00	07/28/20XX–07/31/20XX
001 TOTAL		$3685.00	

Principal DX:	486, 492.8, 305.11
Admitting DX:	786.59
Principal Procedure Code:	87.44

CASE C-2

Capital City General Hospital
1000 Cherry Street
Capital City, NY 12345
(555)555-1000

Patient Information:	Melvin Lyles
	2001 Meadow Road, Capital City, NY 12345
	(555)555-1342
DOB:	05-14-1972
Sex:	Male
SSN:	178-37-2456
Status:	Married **Student:** No
Employer:	None
Responsible Party:	Melvin Lyles
	Address—same as above

Insurance Information:	Blue Cross Blue Shield
	379 Blue Plaza Capital City, NY 12345
ID #:	YYJ561319821 **Group #:** 025648
Insured's Name:	Shelby Lyles **Relationship to Patient:** Spouse
Insured DOB:	05/03/1971 **Insured Party's Sex:** Female
Insured's Address:	Same

Insured's Employer:	Green Landscaping Co.
	1315 Green Avenue, Capital City, NY 12345
	(555)555-8503
Authorization:	846465315 **Approved # of Days:** 3
Attending Physician:	Elby Alright, MD
Federal Tax ID #:	75-7654321
NPI:	9876543210

Reason for visit: My sugar has been running high.

CASE C-2

HPI: This is a Caucasian male admitted on October 10, 20XX, at 8:44 pm for uncontrolled DM II. Pt. has had a recent change in medicines and these may be the contributor to his condition. Pt. does admit to noncompliance with diet. Pt. was discharged on October 13, 20XX, at 7:45 am.

Patient Control #:	6132198	**Type of Admission:**	1
MR #:	ML18913	**Source of Admission:**	1
Hospital NPI:	1212121212	**Discharge Status:**	01
Hospital Tax ID:	75-7575757	**Type of Bill Code:**	111

Fees:

Revenue Codes	Units	Total Charges	Date of Service
120 Room/Board/Semi	3	$ 400.00/day	10/10/20XX–10/13/20XX
250 Pharmacy	8	$ 375.00	10/10/20XX–10/13/20XX
260 IV Therapy	2	$ 850.00	10/10/20XX–10/12/20XX
300 Lab	5	$ 450.00	10/10/20XX–10/12/20XX
320 Radiology	1	$ 900.00	10/11/20XX
001 TOTAL		$3775.00	

Principal DX:	250.42; 583.81, 278.00, V65.3, V85.32
Admitting DX:	250.02
Principal Procedure Code:	88.48, 88.66

CASE C-3

Capital City General Hospital
1000 Cherry Street
Capital City, NY 12345
(555)555-1000

Patient Information: Emilio Mendez
                              3009 River Road, Capital City, NY 12345
                              (555)555-3839

DOB: 09-30-1984
Sex: Male
SSN: 548-37-0081
Status: Married   **Student:** Yes
Employer: Tough Guy's Gym
                              79 W. Boron Avenue, Township, NY 12345
                              (555)555-4816

Responsible Party: Emilio Mendez
                              Address—same as above

Insurance Information: Blue Cross Blue Shield
                              379 Blue Plaza, Capital City, NY 12345
ID #:   YYZ156349873   **Group #:** 252354
Insured's Name: Same   **Relationship to Patient:** Self
Insured's Address:

Insured's Employer:

Authorization: 5168431313   **Approved # of Days:** 4
Attending Physician: Elby Alright, MD
Federal Tax ID #:   75-7654321
NPI: 9876543210

Reason for visit: I think that I have an infection from my wisdom tooth surgery.

HPI: This is a Latin American male admitted on June 7, 20XX, at 5:42 pm for an infected wisdom tooth. Pt. recently underwent wisdom tooth extraction and now has septicemia. He says that he stopped taking his antibiotic because he felt better. Pt. was discharged on June 10, 20XX, at 11:00 am.

CASE C-3

Patient Control #:	646413	Type of Admission:	1
MR #:	84616489	Source of Admission:	7
Hospital NPI:	1212121212	Discharge Status:	01
Hospital Tax ID:	75-7575757	Type of Bill Code:	111

Fees:

Revenue Codes	Units	Total Charges	Date of Service
120 Room/Board/Semi	3	$ 400.00/day	06/07/20XX–06/10/20XX
250 Pharmacy	7	$ 400.00	06/07/20XX–06/09/20XX
260 IV Therapy	3	$ 900.00	06/07/20XX–06/09/20XX
300 Lab	6	$ 700.00	06/07/20XX–06/09/20XX
001 TOTAL		$3600.00	

Principal DX:	038.10, 526.5
Admitting DX:	526.5
Principal Procedure Code:	90.52

CASE C-4

County Community Hospital
1600 Clover Street
Capital City, NY 12345
(555)555-1600

Patient Information: Harold Janovich
532 Creek Street, Township, NY 12345
(555)555-8824

DOB: 12-12-1971

Sex: Male

SSN: 401-64-7228

Status: Single   **Student:** No

Employer: Buy 'N Save Grocer's, Ltd.
927 Interstate Plaza, Township, NY 12345
(555)555-8193

Responsible Party: Harold Janovich
Address—same as above

Insurance Information: Aetna
1625 Heath Care Building
Capital City, NY 12345

ID #:   65321313   **Group #:** 97390

Insured's Name: Same   **Relationship to Patient:** Self

Insured's Address:

Insured's Employer:

Authorization: 10564598   **Approved # of Days:** 2

Attending Physician: Mannie Mends, MD

Federal Tax ID #:   75-1234567

NPI: 0123456789

Group NPI: 1513171216

Reason for visit: My stomach hurts, I've been vomiting, and I have the chills.

HPI: Pt. presents in the ER on November 22, 20XX, at 6:19 pm. He is complaining of N&V, chills, and RLQ pain. Pt. tolerated appendectomy well and was discharged on November 24, 20XX, at 5:15 pm.

CASE C-4

Patient Control #:	564321	Type of Admission:	1
MR #:	005332496	Source of Admission:	7
Hospital NPI:	6767676767	Discharge Status:	01
Hospital Tax ID:	70-707070	Type of Bill Code:	111
Fees:	$950.00		

Revenue Codes	Units	Total Charges	Date of Service
120 Room/Board/Semi	2	$ 400.00/day	11/22/20XX–11/24/20XX
250 Pharmacy	5	$ 400.00	11/22/20XX–11/23/20XX
260 IV Therapy	2	$ 950.00	11/22/20XX–11/23/20XX
270 Med/Surg Supplies	1	$ 500.00	11/22/20XX
300 Lab	2	$ 300.00	11/22/20XX–11/23/20XX
320 Radiology	1	$ 650.00	11/22/20XX
360 OR Services	1	$1200.00	11/22/20XX
370 Anesthesia	1	$ 600.00	11/22/20XX
001 TOTAL		$5400.00	

Principal DX:	540.9
Admitting DX:	789.03
Principal Procedure Code:	47.09, 88.76

CASE C-5

Township Memorial Hospital
700 Shady Street
Township, NY 12345
(555)555-0700

Patient Information: Ramesh Kedar
14 Berry Lane, Township, NY 12345
(555)555-2624

DOB: 03-07-1967

Sex: Male

SSN: 534-69-7184

Status: Divorced   **Student:** No

Employer: Wholsale Electronics, Inc.
5634 Electric Boulevard, Capital City, NY 12345
(555)555-1476

Responsible Party: Ramesh Kedar
Address—same as above

Insurance Information: Health America
2031 Healthica Center, Capital City, NY 12345

ID #:   65432678   **Group #:** 6649

Insured's Name: Same   **Relationship to Patient:** Self

Insured's Address:

Insured's Employer:

Authorization: 545777888   **Approved # of Days:** 2

Attending Physician: Iva Hart, MD

Federal Tax ID #:   75-0246802

NPI: 0246802468

Reason for visit: I feel anxious and my chest hurts.

CASE C-5

HPI: This is an Asian male admitted on December 12, 20XX, at 12:25 pm for CP and anxiousness. Pt. is hypertensive. CXR showed no abnormalities. Labs positive for clotting issues. VQ scan of lung reveals pulmonary embolism. Pt. was discharged on December 14, 20XX, at 10:30 am.

Patient Control #:	594313	Type of Admission:	1
MR #:	RK654142	Source of Admission:	1
Hospital NPI:	3434343434	Discharge Status:	01
Hospital Tax ID:	75-0750750	Type of Bill Code:	111

Fees:

Revenue Codes	Units	Total Charges	Date of Service
120 Room/Board/Semi	2	$ 400.00/day	12/12/20XX–12/14/20XX
250 Pharmacy	3	$ 375.00	12/12/20XX–12/14/20XX
260 IV Therapy	3	$1200.00	12/12/20XX–12/14/20XX
300 Lab	6	$ 450.00	12/12/20XX–12/14/20XX
320 Radiology	1	$1000.00	12/12/20XX
730 EKG	1	$ 150.00	12/12/20XX
001 TOTAL		$3975.00	

Principal DX:	415.19, 300.00, 401.9
Admitting DX:	786.05
Principal Procedure Code:	92.15, 89.52

CASE C-6

Capital City General Hospital
1000 Cherry Street
Capital City, NY 12345-2222
(555)555-1000

Patient Information:	Arthur Zbegan
	9832 Grass Road, Capital City, NY 12345
	(555)555-6549
DOB:	04-11-1939
Sex:	Male
SSN:	457-67-2470
Status:	Married **Student:** No
Employer:	Retired
Responsible Party:	Arthur Zbegan
	Address—same as above

Insurance Information:	Medicare
	P.O. Box 9834, Capital City, NY 12345
ID #:	629417113A **Group #:**
Insured's Name:	Same **Relationship to Patient:** Self
Insured's Address:	

Insured's Employer:

Authorization:	5463664535 **Approved # of Days:** 4
Attending Physician:	Iva Hart, MD
Federal Tax ID #:	75-0246802
NPI:	0246802468

Reason for visit: I can't breathe. I feel winded very easily.

CASE C-6

HPI: This is a Caucasian male admitted on September 1, 20XX, at 2:39 am for coronary artery disease, HTN, and angina. Pt. had s/p CABG 12 years ago. Coronary artery blockage requires CABG. Pt. was discharged on September 5, 20XX, at 11:00 am.

Patient Control #:	4616549		**Type of Admission:**	1
MR #:	ZA16836401		**Source of Admission:**	7
Hospital NPI:	1212121212		**Discharge Status:**	01
Hospital Tax ID:	75-7575757		**Type of Bill Code:**	0111

Fees:

Revenue Codes	Units	Total Charges	Date of Service
0210 Coronary Care	4	$ 650.00/day	09/01/20XX–09/05/20XX
0250 Pharmacy	5	$ 425.00	09/01/20XX–09/05/20XX
0260 IV Therapy	4	$ 1200.00	09/01/20XX–09/04/20XX
0270 Med/Surg Supplies	1	$ 800.00	09/02/20XX
0300 Lab	5	$ 450.00	09/01/20XX–09/05/20XX
0360 OR Services	1	$2300.00	09/02/20XX
0370 Anesthesia	1	$ 675.00	09/02/20XX
0730 EKG	1	$ 175.00	09/01/20XX
0001 TOTAL		$8625.00	

Principal DX:	411.81, 414.00, 402.00, V45.81
Admitting DX:	413.9
Principal Procedure Code:	36.12, 89.52

CASE C-7

Capital City General Hospital
1000 Cherry Street
Capital City, NY 12345
(555)555-1000

Patient Information:	Rita Mangino
	4 S. Orange Way, Township, NY 12345
	(555)555-5776
DOB:	02-08-1957
Sex:	Female
SSN:	243-51-6328
Status:	Married **Student:** No
Employer:	Retired
Responsible Party:	Rita Mangino
	Address—same as above

Insurance Information:	Aetna
	1625 Healthcare Building, Capital City, NY 12345
ID #:	4783900 **Group #:** 493
Insured's Name:	Bruce Mangino **Relationship to Patient:** Husband
DOB:	11/06/1957 **Sex:** Male
Insured's Address:	Same

Insured's Employer:	Critter's Campus
	6291 Grove Boulevard, Township, NY 12345
	(555)555-3374
Authorization:	5331648 **Approved # of Days:** 2
Attending Physician:	Phil Wells, MD
Federal Tax ID #:	75-1234567
NPI:	1234567890

Reason for visit: I'm having an asthma attack.

HPI: Caucasian female admitted on January 14, 20XX, at 6:05 am for exacerbation of asthma. Chest auscultation and percussion show severe wheezes, and SpO_2 is 86%. CXR revealed atelectasis, and a thoracentesis was performed to expand the right lung. Thoracentesis was performed without complications. Pt. was discharged on January 16, 20XX, at 1:30 pm.

CASE C-7

Patient Control #:	0063259	**Type of Admission:** 1
MR #:	000233168	**Source of Admission:** 1
Hospital NPI:	1212121212	**Discharge Status:** 01
Hospital Tax ID:	75-7575757	**Type of Bill Code:** 111

Fees:

Revenue Codes	Units	Total Charges	Date of Service
120 Room/Board/Semi	2	$ 450.00/day	01/14/20XX–01/16/20XX
250 Pharmacy	3	$ 375.00	01/14/20XX–01/16/20XX
260 IV Therapy	2	$ 820.00	01/14/20XX–01/15/20XX
270 Med/Surg Supplies	1	$ 400.00	01/14/20XX
300 Lab	1	$ 105.00	01/14/20XX
320 Radiology	2	$ 500.00	01/14/20XX–01/15/20XX
900 Respiratory Services	3	$ 600.00	01/14/20XX–01/16/20XX
001 TOTAL		$3700.00	

Principal DX:	493.92
Admitting DX:	493.92
Principal Procedure Code:	34.91, 87.44

CASE C-8

Capital City General Hospital
1000 Cherry Street
Capital City, NY 12345-2222
(555)555-1000

Patient Information: Dorothy Greer
                                  777 Sycamore Circle, Capital City, NY 12345
                                  (555)555-5682

DOB: 10-02-1949

Sex: Female

SSN: 738-53-2081

Status: Married   **Student:** No

Employer: Retired

Responsible Party: Dorothy Greer
                                  Address—same as above

Insurance Information: Medicare
                                  P.O. Box 9834, Capital City, NY 12345

ID #:   629417113A   **Group #:**

Insured's Name: Same   **Relationship to Patient:** Self

Insured's Address:

Insured's Employer:

Authorization: 198131332   **Approved # of Days:** 5

Attending Physician: Iva Hart, MD

Federal Tax ID #:   75-0246802

NPI: 0246802468

Reason for visit: I fainted this morning.

CASE C-8

HPI: This is an African American female admitted on August 14, 20XX, at 9:15 am for syncope. Pt. has history of SSS and has a pacemaker. Pacemaker has failed, and a new one needs to be implanted. Pt. was discharged on August 18, 20XX, at 2:00 pm.

Patient Control #:	198761	**Type of Admission:**	1
MR #:	00025643189	**Source of Admission:**	7
Hospital NPI:	1212121212	**Discharge Status:**	01
Hospital Tax ID:	75-7575757	**Type of Bill Code:**	0111

Fees:

Revenue Codes	Units	Total Charges	Date of Service
0210 Coronary Care	4	$ 600.00/day	08/14/20XX–08/18/20XX
0250 Pharmacy	5	$ 350.00	08/14/20XX–08/18/20XX
0260 IV Therapy	4	$1000.00	08/14/20XX–08/17/20XX
0270 Med/Surg Supplies	1	$ 900.00	08/14/20XX
0300 Lab	4	$ 600.00	08/14/20XX–08/17/20XX
0360 OR Services	1	$1950.00	08/14/20XX
0370 Anesthesia	1	$ 700.00	08/14/20XX
0730 EKG	1	$ 150.00	08/14/20XX
0001 TOTAL		$8050.00	

Principal DX:	996.01, 780.2
Admitting DX:	780.2
Principal Procedure Code:	00.50, 89.44, 88.72, 89.52

CASE C-9

Capital City General Hospital
1000 Cherry Street
Capital City, NY 12345
(555)555-1000

Patient Information:	Virginia Moore
	934 Smithfield Street, Capital City, NY 12345
DOB:	01-27-1944
Sex:	Female
SSN:	237-02-3331
Status:	Divorced **Student:** No
Employer:	Retired
Responsible Party:	Virginia Moore
	Address—same as above

Insurance Information:	Medicaid
	4875 Capital Boulevard, Capital City, NY 12345
ID #:	629417113972 **Group #:**
Insured's Name:	Same **Relationship to Insured:** Self
Insured's Address:	

Insured's Employer:

Authorization:	519843131 **Approved # of Days:** 5
Attending Physician:	Arthur I. Tiss, MD
Federal Tax ID #:	75-1135791
NPI:	1357613579

Reason for visit: I am having hip surgery.

CASE C-9

HPI: This white female admitted on March 11, 20XX, at 5:30 pm for left hip replacement; total. Pt. has history of HTN, osteoporosis, and osteoarthritis. She tolerated the procedure well. Pt. was discharged on March 15, 20XX, at 2:00 pm.

Patient Control #:	578877	Type of Admission:	2
MR #:	654943233	Source of Admission:	1
Hospital NPI:	1212121212	Discharge Status:	62
Hospital Tax ID:	75-7575757	Type of Bill Code:	111

Fees:

Revenue Codes	Units	Total Charges	Date of Service
120 Room/Board/Semi	4	$ 650.00/day	03/11/20XX–03/15/20XX
250 Pharmacy	5	$ 400.00	03/11/20XX–03/15/20XX
260 IV Therapy	4	$1200.00	03/11/20XX–03/14/20XX
270 Med/Surg Supplies	1	$1200.00	03/12/20XX
300 Lab	2	$ 400.00	03/11/20XX–03/12/20XX
320 Radiology	1	$ 250.00	03/11/20XX
360 OR Services	1	$2600.00	03/12/20XX
370 Anesthesia	1	$ 800.00	03/12/20XX
730 EKG	1	$ 175.00	03/11/20XX
001 TOTAL		$9775.00	

Principal DX:	820.20, 733.10, 715.09, 401.9
Admitting DX:	820.20
Principal Procedure Code:	81.51, 88.26, 89.52

CASE C-10

Capital City General Hospital
1000 Cherry Street
Capital City, NY 12345-2222
(555)555-1000

Patient Information: Albert Kim
601 Sunflower Drive, Capital City, NY 12345
(555)555-6843

DOB: 06-02-1930

Sex: Male

SSN: 563-56-7031

Status: Married   **Student:** No

Employer: Retired

Responsible Party: Albert Kim
Address—same as above

Insurance Information: Medicare
P.O. Box 9834, Capital City, NY 12345

ID #: 629417113A   **Group #:**

Insured's Name: Same   **Relationship to Patient:** Self

Insured's Address:

Insured's Employer:

Authorization: 646819900   **Approved # of Days:** 5

Attending Physician: Iva Hart, MD

Federal Tax ID #: 75-0246802

NPI: 0246802468

Reason for visit: I'm having trouble breathing and I'm very tired

HPI: This Asian male presents in the ER on April 3, 20XX, at 4:43 pm. He is complaining of SOB and excessive tiredness. Exam revealed increased BP, respiration, and pulse rate. Pt. denies any CP. Says it just feels uncomfortably full. B/L pitting ankle edema 2+. Pt. does have a history of malignant HTN. Pt. was admitted for further workup. Over the course of the stay, CXR revealed pleural effusion. Thoracentesis was performed without complications. Pt. was discharged on April 7, 20XX, at 12:30 pm.

CASE C-10

Patient Control #:	015356		**Type of Admission:**	1
MR #:	AK45329		**Source of Admission:**	7
Hospital NPI:	1212121212		**Discharge Status:**	03
Hospital Tax ID:	75-5757575		**Type of Bill Code:**	0111

Fees:

Revenue Codes	Units	Total Charges	Date of Service
0210 Coronary Care	4	$ 650.00/day	04/03/20XX–04/07/20XX
0250 Pharmacy	5	$ 375.00	04/03/20XX–04/07/20XX
0260 IV Therapy	4	$1000.00	04/03/20XX–04/06/20XX
0270 Med/Surg Supplies	1	$ 400.00	04/05/20XX
0300 Lab	2	$ 220.00	04/03/20XX; 04/06/20XX
0320 Radiology	2	$ 550.00	04/03/20XX; 04/05/20XX
0730 EKG	1	$ 150.00	04/03/20XX
0900 Respiratory Services	1	$ 400.00	04/05/20XX
0001 TOTAL		$5695.00	

Principal DX:	402.01, 428.0
Admitting DX:	786.05
Principal Procedure Code:	34.91, 87.44

CASE C-11

Capital City General Hospital Outpatient Services
1000 Cherry Street
Capital City, NY 12345
(555)555-1000

Patient Name: Olivia Marselle
                           4142 Valley Road, Capital City, NY 12345
                           (555)555-1037

DOB: 10-29-1975
Sex: Female
SSN: 993-92-7046
Status: Married   **Student:** No
Employer: Sandwiches Plus
                           26 Seneca Boulevard, Capital City, NY 12345
                           (555)555-3300

Responsible Party: Olivia Marselle
                           Address—same as above

Insurance Information: Medicaid
                            4875 Capital Boulevard, Capital City, NY 12345

ID #:   0564616665659   **Group #:**
Insured's Name: Same   **Relationship to Patient:** Self
Insured's Address:

Insured's Employer:

Authorization:
Emergency Physician: Karen A. Lotts, MD
Federal Tax ID #:   75-1471471
NPI: 1471471471

Reason for visit: Nausea & Vomiting

Capital City General Hospital Emergency Services

CASE C-11

Patient's Name: Olivia Marselle

Date of Procedure: 08/23/20XX

Emergency Physician: Karen A. Lotts, MD

DOB: 10/29/1975

PCP: Phil Wells, MD

MR#: OM 24965

This is a white female who presents to the ER on August 23, 20XX, at 6:32 pm with complaints of N&V. She is asthmatic and has recently started prednisone and tetracycline for exacerbation and bronchitis. She says that she has taken prednisone before without any problems. Patient denies any possibility of being pregnant. Lab values are negative. She is advised to stop the tetracycline. Augmentin given, and clear liquid diet x2 days. Follow up with PCP.

Reason for Visit: 787.01

DX Code: 960.4, E930.4, 493.22

CPT Procedure Code: 85025, 80053, 36415

Source of Admission: 7

Discharge Status: 01

Hospital NPI:	1212121212	**Type of Bill Code:** 131
Hospital Tax ID:	75-7575757	**Patient Control #:** 313652

Fees:

Revenue Codes	Units	Total Charges	Date of Service
300 Lab 36415	1	$ 20.00	08/23/20XX
301 Lab 80053	2	$230.00	08/23/20XX
305 Lab 85025	1	$ 25.00	08/23/20XX
450 ER	1	$350.00	08/23/20XX
001 TOTAL		$625.00	

CASE C-12

Capital City General Hospital Outpatient Services
1000 Cherry Street
Capital City, NY 12345
(555)555-1000

Patient Name:	Antonio Rodriguez
	32 Plank Circle, Township, NY 12345
	(555)555-2015
DOB:	04-28-1954
Sex:	Male
SSN:	259-70-0732
Status:	Married **Student:** No
Employer:	The Builder's Outlet
	6391 Graceland Highway, Capital City, NY 12345
	(555)555-7439
Responsible Party:	Antonio Rodriguez
	Address—same as above

Insurance Information:	Blue Cross Blue Shield
	379 Blue Plaza, Capital City, NY 12345
ID #:	YYZ94004954 **Group #:** 727524
Insured's Name:	Cassandra Rodriguez **Relationship to Patient:** Spouse
DOB:	07/30/1959 **Sex:** Female
Insured's Address:	Same

Insured's Employer:	Richie Rich Bank of USA
	7384 Dollar Avenue, Capital City, NY 12345
	(555)555-0195
Operating Physician:	Mannie Mends, MD
Federal Tax ID #:	75-0123456
NPI:	0123456789
Group NPI:	1513171216

Reason for visit: I am scheduled for a colonoscopy.

Capital City General Hospital Outpatient Surgery

CASE C-12

Patient Name: Antonio Rodriguez

DOB: 04/28/1954

Date of Procedure: 05/18/20XX

Surgeon: Mannie Mends, MD

PCP: Elby Alright, MD

Anesthesia: Twilight

MR#: AR 3461

Preoperative Diagnosis: Melena

Postoperative Diagnosis: Carcinoma of the Colon; In Situ

PROCEDURE: COLONOSCOPY

Patient is prepped and draped in the usual sterile fashion. The scope is entered up and through the rectum for visualization. There are 3 polyps noted. Both were excised by and sent to pathology for further evaluation. Patient tolerated the procedure well with minimal blood loss.

Exam is consistent with carcinoma.

Source of Admission: 1

Discharge Status: 01

DX Code: 230.3

Type of Bill Code: 131

CPT Procedure Code: 45384

Patient Control #: 869244

Hospital NPI:	1212121212
Hospital Tax ID:	75-7575757

Fees:

Revenue Codes	Units	Total Charges	Date of Service
260 IV Therapy	1	$ 400.00	05/18/20XX
270 Med/Surg Supplies	1	$ 500.00	05/18/20XX
500 Ambul Surg	1	$2200.00	05/18/20XX
001 TOTAL		$3100.00	

CASE C-13

County Community Hospital Outpatient Services
1600 Clover Street
Capital City, NY 12345
(555)555-1600

Patient Name: Randall Paul
                      231 Boston Avenue, Apt. 5, Capital City, NY 12345
                      (555)555-3644

DOB: 12-09-1959

Sex: Male

SSN: 468-37-9631

Status: Divorced   **Student:** No

Employer: Randy's Gaming Stop
                      118 Swellsville Square, Capital City, NY 12345
                      (555)555-1941

Responsible Party: Randall Paul
                      Address—same as above

Insurance Information: Aetna
                      1625 Healthcare Building, Capital City, NY 12345

ID #:   YYZ204753589   **Group #:** 200754

Insured's Name: Same   **Relationship to Patient:** Self

Insured's Address:

Insured's Employer:

Authorization:

Ordering Physician: Elby Alright, MD

Federal Tax ID #:   75-7654321

NPI: 9876543210

Reason for visit:

County Community Hospital Outpatient Radiology

Patient's Name: Randall Paul

Date of Procedure: 11/25/20XX

Ordering Physician: Elby Alright, MD

Report #: RP-0251

Diagnosis: Mass, kidney

Procedure: CT OF THE ABDOMEN

DOB: 12/09/1959

PCP: Elby Alright, MD

MR #: MR 1297

Exam is performed with the administration of oral and IV contrast. Noncontrast studies are performed of the kidneys and liver before the contrast introduction.

Liver presents normal in size and mass. There is, however, a 5- x 5.2-cm mass noted in the caudad lobe of the left kidney. The gallbladder presents as normal. Kidneys, spleen, and abdominal aorta are negative of any findings.

Source of Admission:	1
Discharge Status:	01
DX Code: 789.30 / **Type of Bill Code:**	131
CPT Procedure Code: 74170 / **Patient Control #:**	04698

Hospital NPI:	6767676767
Hospital Tax ID:	70-7070707

Fees:

Revenue Codes	Units	Total Charges	Date of Service
250 Pharmacy	1	$ 90.00	11/25/20XX
260 IV Therapy	1	$ 575.00	11/25/20XX
320 Radiology	1	$ 850.00	11/25/20XX
001 TOTAL		$1515.00	

CASE C-14

Capital City General Hospital Outpatient Services
1000 Cherry Street
Capital City, NY 12345
(555)555-1000

Patient Name: Megan Bishop
                         5834 Cliff Street, Capital City, NY 12345
                         (555)555-1107

DOB: 10-31-1962

Sex: Female

SSN: 501-18-6349

Status: Single   **Student:** No

Employer: Videos Plus
                         800 Mead Boulevard, Capital City, NY 12345
                         (555)555-3275

Responsible Party: Megan Bishop
                         Address—same as above

Insurance Information: Blue Cross Blue Shield
                             379 Blue Plaza, Capital City, NY 12345

ID #:   YYJ846168930   **Group #:** 688112

Insured's Name: Same   **Relationship to Patient:** Self

Insured's Address:

Insured's Employer:

Authorization:

Ordering Physician: Bette R. Soone, MD

Federal Tax ID #:   75-7654321

NPI: 0987654321

Reason for visit:

Capital City General Hospital Outpatient Radiology

CASE C-14

Patient's Name: Megan Bishop

Date of Procedure: 09/16/20XX

Ordering Physician: Bette R. Soone, MD

Report #: MG-82206

Diagnosis: Routine yearly exam

Procedure: BILATERAL MAMMOGRAM

DOB: 10/31/1962

PCP: Elby Alright, MD

MR #: MB 8020

Comparison is made using patient's mammogram films from last year's exam. The mammary are primarily fatty. Margins are well defined, and there is no evidence of any suspicious masses.

Both breasts present unremarkable.

Source of Admission:	1
Discharge Status:	01
Type of Bill Code:	131
Patient Control #:	462013

DX Code: V76.12

CPT Procedure Code: 77057

Hospital NPI: 1212121212

Hospital Tax ID: 75-7575757

Fees:

Revenue Codes	Units	Total Charges	Date of Service
320 Radiology	1	$775.00	09/16/20XX
972 Radiologist	1	$100.00	09/16/20XX
001 TOTAL		$875.00	

CASE C-15

County Community Hospital Outpatient Surgery
1600 Clover Street
Capital City, NY 12345
(555)555-1600

Patient Name:	Patricia Vlah
	988 Mill Run Road, Township, NY 12345
	(555)555-2015
DOB:	02-11-2000
Sex:	Female
SSN:	747-03-6473
Status:	Single **Student:** Yes
Employer:	None
Responsible Party:	Patricia Vlah
	Address—same as above

Insurance Information:	Aetna
	1625 Health Care Building, Capital City, NY 12345
ID #:	6561946
Group #:	649104
Insured's Name:	Suzanne Vlah **Relationship to Patient:** Mother
DOB:	10/18/1982 **Sex:** Female
Insured's Address:	Same

Insured's Employer:	Cut 'N Curls Salon
	53 Second Avenue, Township, NY 12345
Authorization:	
Operating Physician:	Mannie Mends, MD
Federal Tax ID #:	75-0123456
NPI:	0123456789
Group NPI:	1513171216

Reason for visit:

County Community Hospital Outpatient Surgery

CASE C-15

Patient Name: Patricia Vlah   **DOB:** 02/11/2000

Date of Procedure: 06/19/20XX

Surgeon: Mannie Mends, MD   **PCP:** Elby Alright, MD

Anesthesia: General   **MR #:** PV 7539

Preoperative Diagnosis: Adenotonsillitis; chronic

Postoperative Diagnosis: Adenotonsillitis; chronic

PROCEDURE: TONSILLECTOMY WITH ADENOIDECTOMY

Patient is prepped and draped in the usual sterile fashion. There is severe swelling of the tonsils and adenoidal tissue. This area is grasped and excised. Patient tolerated the procedure well.

Source of Admission:	1
Discharge Status:	01
DX Code: 474.02	**Type of Bill Code:** 131
CPT Procedure Code: 42820	**Patient Control #:** 665090

Hospital NPI:	6767676767
Hospital Tax ID:	70-7070707

Fees:

Revenue Codes	Units	Total Charges	Date of Service
250 Pharmacy	1	$ 150.00	06/19/20XX
260 IV Therapy	1	$ 750.00	06/19/20XX
270 Med/Surg Supplies	1	$ 400.00	06/19/20XX
370 Anesthesia	1	$ 700.00	06/19/20XX
500 Ambul Surg	1	$1500.00	06/19/20XX
001 TOTAL		$3500.00	

CASE C-16

Capital City General Hospital Outpatient Services
1000 Cherry Street
Capital City, NY 12345
(555)555-1000

Patient Name: Bryson Chung
                       205 Glass Road, Capital City, NY 12345
                       (555)555-3749

DOB: 01-21-1997
Sex: Male
SSN: 115-84-5974
Status: Single   **Student:** Yes
Employer: None
Responsible Party: Melissa Chung
                       Address—same as above

Insurance Information: Health America
                            2031 Healthica Center, Capital City, NY 12345

ID #:   4684646   **Group #:** 5215
Insured's Name: Michael Chung   **Relationship to Patient:** Father,
                                         not financially responsible

DOB: 04/28/1978   **Sex:** Male
Insured's Address: Same

Insured's Employer: Best Furniture
                        8999 Wood Road, Capital City, NY 12345
                        (555)555-0012

Authorization:
Emergency Physician: Karen A. Lotts, MD
Federal Tax ID #:   75-1471471
NPI: 1471471471

Reason for visit: Having diarrhea all morning.

Capital City General Hospital Emergency Services

Patient's Name: Bryson Chung

Date of Procedure: 11/01/20XX

Emergency Physician: Karen A. Lotts, MD

DOB: 01/21/1997

PCP: Phil Wells, MD

MR #: BC 69281

This is an Asian American male presenting to the ER on November 1, 20XX, at 10:18 am with complaints of diarrhea all morning. He has a fever of 101°F. Lab values are negative for dehydration or any other processes. Patient is to rest, drink clear liquids, take children's Tylenol, and follow up with his pediatrician for abdominal flu.

Source of Admission:	7
Discharge Status:	01
DX Code: 487.8	**Type of Bill Code:** 131
CPT Procedure Code: 36415, 85025, 80053	**Patient Control #:** 925259

Hospital NPI:	1212121212
Hospital Tax ID:	75-7575757

Fees:

Revenue Codes	Units	Total Charges	Date of Service
250 Pharmacy	1	$ 75.00	11/01/20XX
300 Lab 36415	1	$ 20.00	11/01/20XX
301 Lab 80053	1	$250.00	11/01/20XX
305 Lab 85025	1	$ 30.00	11/01/20XX
450 ER	1	$350.00	11/01/20XX
001 TOTAL		$725.00	

CASE C-17

Township Memorial Hospital Outpatient Services
700 Shady Street
Township, NY 12345-2222
(555)555-0700

Patient Name: Keith Lombardo
174 Jefferson Street, Township, NY 12345
(555)555-8413

DOB: 05-13-1933

Sex: Male

SSN: 165-40-3199

Status: Married   **Student:** No

Employer: Retired

Responsible Party: Keith Lombardo
Address—same as above

Insurance Information: Medicare
P.O. Box 9834, Capital City, NY 12345

ID #: 649331304A   **Group #:**

Insured's Name: Same   **Relationship to Patient:** Self

Insured's Address:

Insured's Employer:

Authorization:

Ordering Physician: Phil Wells, MD

Federal Tax ID #: 75-1234567

NPI: 1234567890

Group NPI: 1513171216

Reason for visit:

Township Memorial Hospital Outpatient Radiology

CASE C-17

Patient's Name: Keith Lombardo

Date of Procedure: 01/06/20XX

Ordering Physician: Phil Wells, MD

Report #: KL-56460

Diagnosis: Renal calculi

Procedure: RENAL ULTRASOUND

DOB: 05/13/1933

PCP: Phil Wells, MD

MR #: KL 693321

Ultrasound reveals a small area of echogenicity with some shadowing in the midportion of the right kidney that is consistent with renal calculus diagnosis. Otherwise, both kidneys are unremarkable.

There is no visualization of the urinary bladder.

Source of Admission:	1
Discharge Status:	01
Type of Bill Code:	0131
Patient Control #:	728438

DX Code: 592.0

CPT Procedure Code: 76770

Hospital NPI:	3434343434
Hospital Tax ID:	75-0750750

Fees:

Revenue Codes	Units	Total Charges	Date of Service
0320 Radiology	1	$300.00	01/06/20XX
0972 Radiologist	1	$125.00	01/06/20XX
0001 TOTAL		$425.00	

Information on File

CASE C-18

Township Memorial Hospital Outpatient Services
700 Shady Street
Township, NY 12345
(555)555-0700

Patient Name:	Tyrone Clark
	55 Lockwood Drive, Township, NY 12345
	(555)555-7578
DOB:	06-15-1980
Sex:	Male
SSN:	817-39-6220
Status:	Single **Student:** No
Employer:	Suzie's Styles
	42 West Deer Road, Capital City, NY 12345
	(555)555-6776
Responsible Party:	Tyrone Clark
	Address—same as above

Insurance Information:	Medicaid
	4875 Capital Boulevard, Capital City, NY 12345
ID #:	498481614 **Group #:**
Insured's Name:	Same **Relationship to Patient:** Self
Insured's Address:	

Insured's Employer:

Authorization:
Emergency Physician: Karen A. Lotts, MD
Federal Tax ID #:   75-1471471
NPI: 1471471471

Reason for visit: I have poison ivy really bad near my eye.

Township Memorial Hospital Emergency Services

CASE C-18

Patient's Name: Tyrone Clark

Date of Procedure: 08/21/20XX

Emergency Physician: Karen A. Lotts, MD

DOB: 06/15/1980

PCP: Phil Wells, MD

MR #: TC 11720

This is an African American male presenting to the ER on August 21, 20XX, at 7:55 pm for poison ivy. He thinks that he had gotten it when he took his grandson for a walk in the woods 2 days ago. Since then, it has "gotten out of hand." He says that he used OTC medicine on it without any relief. It has now spread to the outer aspects of his right eyelid. Depo-Medrol injection given for systemic reaction.

Source of Admission:	1
Discharge Status:	01
Type of Bill Code:	131
Patient Control #:	210158

DX Code: 692.6

CPT Procedure Code: None

Hospital NPI:	3434343434
Hospital Tax ID:	75-0750750

Fees:

Revenue Codes	Units	Total Charges	Date of Service
250 Pharmacy	1	$ 50.00	08/21/20XX
450 ER	1	$275.00	08/21/20XX
001 TOTAL		$325.00	

CASE C-19

Capital City General Hospital Outpatient Services
1000 Cherry Street
Capital City, NY 12345-2222
(555)555-1000

Patient Name:	Dawn Hunt
	46 Harley Drive, Capital City, NY 12345
	(555)555-8852
DOB:	09-21-1943
Sex:	Female
SSN:	341-67-5051
Status:	Married **Student:** No
Employer:	Retired
Responsible Party:	Dawn Hunt
	Address—same as above

Insurance Information:	Medicare
	P.O. Box 9834, Capital City, NY 12345
ID #:	532865149A **Group #:**
Insured's Name:	Same **Relationship to Patient:** Self
Insured's Address:	

Insured's Employer:

Authorization:	
Emergency Physician:	Karen A. Lotts, MD
Federal Tax ID #:	75-1471471
NPI:	1471471471

Reason for visit: Fell down my stairs and hurt my left arm.

Capital City General Hospital Emergency Services

CASE C-19

Patient's Name: Dawn Hunt

Date of Procedure: 11/25/20XX

Emergency Physician: Karen A. Lotts, MD

DOB: 09/21/1943

PCP: Phil Wells, MD

MR #: DH 40195

This is a white female presenting to the ER on November 25, 20XX, at 3:30 pm with complaints of falling down her basement stairs about an hour ago. She has since experienced pain and swelling in her left arm and wrist. On exam she has limited ROM. X-ray of the left arm and wrist are consistent with fracture with ulnar and radial involvement toward the distal aspect of the arm. Casting was applied. Ibuprofen and Tylenol #3 given. Follow up with orthopedist ASAP.

DX Code: 813.44, E880.9

CPT Procedure Code: 73090, 73100, 29075

Source of Admission: 7

Discharge Status: 01

Type of Bill Code: 0131

Patient Control #: 319654

Hospital NPI:	1212121212
Hospital Tax ID:	75-7575757

Fees:

Revenue Codes	Units	Total Charges	Date of Service
0320 Radiology 73090	1	$200.00	11/25/20XX
0320 Radiology 73100	1	$200.00	11/25/20XX
0450 ER	1	$300.00	11/25/20XX
0700 Casting 29075	1	$ 95.00	11/25/20XX
0001 TOTAL		$795.00	

CASE C-20

Township Memorial Hospital Outpatient Services
700 Shady Street
Township, NY 12345-2222
(555)555-0700

Patient Name: Jenna Masters
                            388 Atlantic Avenue, Township, NY 12345
                            (555)555-9751

DOB: 03-12-1950

Sex: Female

SSN: 485-72-3982

Status: Divorced   **Student:** No

Employer: Retired

Responsible Party: Jenna Masters
                            Address—same as above

Insurance Information: Medicare
                            P.O. Box 9834, Capital City, NY 12345

ID #:   853614253A   **Group #:**

Insured's Name: Same   **Relationship to Patient:** Self

Insured's Address:

Insured's Employer:

Authorization:

Operating Physician: Mannie Mends, MD

Federal Tax ID #:   75-0123456

NPI: 0123456789

Group NPI: 1513171216

Reason for visit:

Township Memorial Hospital Outpatient Surgery

CASE C-20

Patient Name: Jenna Masters   **DOB:** 03/12/1950

Date of Procedure: 07/20/20XX

Surgeon: Mannie Mends, MD   **PCP:** Phil Wells, MD

Anesthesia: General   **MR #:** JM 820135

Preoperative Diagnosis: Lymph node enlargement; cervical

Postoperative Diagnosis: Left cervical lymphadenopathy

PROCEDURE: CERVICAL LYMPH NODE EXCISION FOR BIOPSY

Patient is prepped and draped in the usual sterile fashion. Incision is made into the left region of the left cervical nodes. The node is grasped and excised and sent to pathology for examination.

Source of Admission:	1
Discharge Status:	01
DX Code: 785.6 **Type of Bill Code:**	131
CPT Procedure Code: 38510 **Patient Control #:**	751259

Hospital NPI:	3434343434
Hospital Tax ID:	75-0750750

Fees:

Revenue Codes	Units	Total Charges	Date of Service
0250 Pharmacy	1	$ 175.00	07/20/20XX
0260 IV Therapy	1	$ 825.00	07/20/20XX
0270 Med/Surg Supplies	1	$ 450.00	07/20/20XX
0300 Lab	1	$ 375.00	07/20/20XX
0310 Lab/Path	1	$ 300.00	07/20/20XX
0370 Anesthesia	1	$ 750.00	07/20/20XX
0500 Ambul Surg	1	$1700.00	07/20/20XX
0001 TOTAL		$4575.00	

Medical Forms

The forms included in this appendix are documents that medical office specialists use. The format may vary from one facility to another; however, the information is universal. Exercises in the textbook will require students to utilize these forms.

Patient's Name: _____   Medicare # (HICN): _____

ADVANCE BENEFICIARY NOTICE (ABN)

NOTE: You need to make a choice about receiving these healthcare items or services.

We expect that Medicare will not pay for the item(s) or service(s) that are described below. Medicare does not pay for all of your healthcare costs. Medicare only pays for covered items and services when Medicare rules are met. The fact that Medicare may not pay for a particular item or service does not mean that you should not receive it. There may be a good reason your doctor recommended it. Right now, in your case, **Medicare probably will not pay for—**

Items or Services:
Because:

The purpose of this form is to help you make an informed choice about whether or not you want to receive these items or services, knowing that you might have to pay for them yourself. Before you make a decision about your options, you should **read this entire notice carefully.**

- Ask us to explain, if you don't understand why Medicare probably won't pay.
- Ask us how much these items or services will cost you (**Estimated Cost: $_____**), in case you have to pay for them yourself or through other insurance.

PLEASE CHOOSE ONE OPTION. CHECK ONE BOX. SIGN and DATE YOUR CHOICE.

☐ **Option 1. YES.   I want to receive these items or services.**
I understand that Medicare will not decide whether to pay unless I receive these items or services. Please submit my claim to Medicare. I understand that you may bill me for items or services and that I may have to pay the bill while Medicare is making its decision. If Medicare does pay, you will refund to me any payments I made to you that are due to me. If Medicare denies payment, I agree to be personally and fully responsible for payment. That is, I will pay personally, either out of pocket or through any other insurance that I have. I understand I can appeal Medicare's decision.

☐ **Option 2.   NO.   I have decided not to receive these items or services.**
I will not receive these items or services. I understand that you will not be able to submit a claim to Medicare and that I will not be able to appeal your opinion that Medicare won't pay.

_____   _____
        Date   **Signature of patient or person acting on patient's behalf**

NOTE: Your health information will be kept confidential. Any information that we collect about you on this form will be kept confidential in our offices. If a claim is submitted to Medicare, your health information on this form may be shared with Medicare. Your health information, which Medicare sees, will be kept confidential by Medicare.

OMB Approval No. 0938-0566   Form No. CMS-R-131-G   (June 2002)

ASSIGNMENT OF BENEFITS (SAMPLE)

I authorize payment of medical benefits to Allied Medical Center or the specified physician below.

Elizabeth S. Braceland, M.D.   Samson Westheimer, M.D.

_____   _____

Patient/Guarantor's Signature   **Date**

LIFETIME ASSIGNMENT OF BENEFITS (SAMPLE)

Financial Responsibility

All professional services rendered are charged to the patient and are due at the time of service, unless other arrangements have been made in advance with our business office. Necessary forms will be completed to file for insurance carrier payments.

Assignment of Benefits

I hereby assign all medical and surgical benefits, to include major medical benefits to which I am entitled. I hereby authorize and direct my insurance carrier(s), including Medicare, private insurance, and any other health/medical plan, to issue payment check(s) directly to Dr. Sean Robin Kirk for medical services rendered to myself and/or my dependents regardless of my insurance benefits, if any. I understand that I am responsible for any amount not covered by insurance.

Authorization to Release Information

I hereby authorize Dr. Sean Robin Kirk to: (1) release any information necessary to insurance carriers regarding my illness and treatments; (2) process insurance claims generated in the course of examination or treatment; and (3) allow a photocopy of my signature to be used to process insurance claims for the period of lifetime. This order will remain in effect until revoked by me in writing.

I have requested medical services from Dr. Sean Robin Kirk on behalf of myself and/or my dependents, and understand that by making this request, I become fully financially responsible for any and all charges incurred in the course of the treatment authorized.

I further understand that fees are due and payable on the date that services are rendered and agree to pay all such charges incurred in full immediately upon presentation of the appropriate statement. A photocopy of this assignment is to be considered as valid as the original.

_____   _____
Patient/Responsible Party Signature   Date

_____   _____
Witness   Date

CMS-1500 CLAIM FORM

(1500)

HEALTH INSURANCE CLAIM FORM
APPROVED BY NATIONAL UNIFORM CLAIM COMMITTEE 08/05

☐☐ PICA   PICA ☐☐

1. MEDICARE MEDICAID TRICARE CHAMPVA GROUP FECA OTHER	1a. INSURED'S I.D. NUMBER (For Program in Item 1)

☐ (Medicare #) ☐ (Medicaid #) ☐ (Sponsor's SSN) ☐ (Member ID#) ☐ (SSN or ID) ☐ (SSN) ☐ (ID)

2. PATIENT'S NAME (Last Name, First Name, Middle Initial)
3. PATIENT'S BIRTH DATE MM DD YY SEX M☐ F☐
4. INSURED'S NAME (Last Name, First Name, Middle Initial)

5. PATIENT'S ADDRESS (No, Street)
6. PATIENT RELATIONSHIP TO INSURED Self☐ Spouse☐ Child☐ Other☐
7. INSURED'S ADDRESS (No, Street)

CITY   STATE
8. PATIENT STATUS Single☐ Married☐ Other☐
CITY   STATE

ZIP CODE   TELEPHONE (Include Area Code) ( )
Employed☐ Full-Time Student☐ Part-Time Student☐
ZIP CODE   TELEPHONE (Include Area Code) ( )

9. OTHER INSURED'S NAME (Last Name, First Name, Middle Initial)
10. IS PATIENT'S CONDITION RELATED TO:
11. INSURED'S POLICY GROUP OR FECA NUMBER

a. OTHER INSURED'S POLICY OR GROUP NUMBER
a. EMPLOYMENT? (Current or Previous) ☐YES ☐NO
a. INSURED'S DATE OF BIRTH MM DD YY SEX M☐ F☐

b. OTHER INSURED'S DATE OF BIRTH MM DD YY SEX M☐ F☐
b. AUTO ACCIDENT? PLACE (State) ☐YES ☐NO
b. EMPLOYER'S NAME OR SCHOOL NAME

c. EMPLOYER'S NAME OR SCHOOL NAME
c. OTHER ACCIDENT? ☐YES ☐NO
c. INSURANCE PLAN NAME OR PROGRAM NAME

d. INSURANCE PLAN NAME OR PROGRAM NAME
10d. RESERVED FOR LOCAL USE
d. IS THERE ANOTHER HEALTH BENEFIT PLAN? ☐YES ☐NO If yes, return to and complete item 9 a-d

READ BACK OF FORM BEFORE COMPLETING & SIGNING THIS FORM.
12. PATIENT'S OR AUTHORIZED PERSON'S SIGNATURE I authorize the release of any medical or other information necessary to process this claim. I also request payment of government benefits either to myself or to the party who accepts assignment below.
SIGNED _____ DATE _____
13. INSURED'S OR AUTHORIZED PERSON'S SIGNATURE I authorize payment of medical benefits to the undersigned physician or supplier for services described below.
SIGNED _____

14. DATE OF CURRENT ILLNESS (First symptom) OR INJURY (Accident) OR PREGNANCY (LMP) MM DD YY
15. IF PATIENT HAS HAD SAME OR SIMILAR ILLNESS. GIVE FIRST DATE MM DD YY
16. DATES PATIENT UNABLE TO WORK IN CURRENT OCCUPATION FROM MM DD YY TO MM DD YY

17. NAME OF REFERRING PHYSICIAN OR OTHER SOURCE
17a.
17b. NPI
18. HOSPITALIZATION DATES RELATED TO CURRENT SERVICES FROM MM DD YY TO MM DD YY

19. RESERVED FOR LOCAL USE
20. OUTSIDE LAB? ☐YES ☐NO $ CHARGES

21. DIAGNOSIS OR NATURE OF ILLNESS OR INJURY (Relate Items 1,2,3 or 4 to Item 24E by Line)
1. ___ 3. ___
2. ___ 4. ___
22. MEDICAID RESUBMISSION CODE   ORIGINAL REF. NO.
23. PRIOR AUTHORIZATION NUMBER

24. A. DATE(S) OF SERVICE From MM DD YY To MM DD YY	B. PLACE OF SERVICE	C. EMG	D. PROCEDURES, SERVICES, OR SUPPLIES (Explain Unusual Circumstances) CPT/HCPCS MODIFIER	E. DIAGNOSIS POINTER	F. $ CHARGES	G. DAYS OR UNITS	H. EPSDT Family Plan	I. ID. QUAL.	J. RENDERING PROVIDER ID. #
1								NPI	
2								NPI	
3								NPI	
4								NPI	
5								NPI	
6								NPI	

25. FEDERAL TAX ID NUMBER SSN EIN ☐☐
26. PATIENT'S ACCOUNT NO.
27. ACCEPT ASSIGNMENT? (For govt. claims, see back) ☐YES ☐NO
28. TOTAL CHARGE $
29. AMOUNT PAID $
30. BALANCE DUE $

31. SIGNATURE OF PHYSICIAN OR SUPPLIER INCLUDING DEGREES OR CREDENTIALS (I certify that the statements on the reverse apply to this bill and are made a part thereof)
SIGNED _____ DATE _____
32. SERVICE FACILITY LOCATION INFORMATION
a.   b.
33. BILLING PROVIDER INFO & PH. # ( )
a.   b.

NUCC Instruction Manual available at: www.nucc.org
WCMS-1500CS
APPROVED OMB 0938-0999 FORM CMS-1500 (08/05)

E/M Audit Tool
Patient Information

Patient: Visit Date: History Level
Examined By: Exam Level
Patient Status: DOB: Decision Making
Service Type: Sex: Insurance Carrier

CPT® Code(s) Billed   DOCUMENTED   DIAGNOSIS CODE(S) BILLED   DOCUMENTED

History

History of Present Illness
- ❑ location
- ❑ quality
- ❑ severity
- ❑ duration
- ❑ timing
- ❑ context
- ❑ modifying factors
- ❑ associated signs and symptoms
- ❑ No. of chronic diseases

History _____

Review of Systems
- ❑ Constitutional symptoms
- ❑ Eyes
- ❑ Ears, nose, mouth, throat
- ❑ Cardiovascular
- ❑ Respiratory
- ❑ Gastrointestinal
- ❑ Genitourinary
- ❑ Integumentary
- ❑ Musculoskeletal

- ❑ Neurologic
- ❑ Psychiatric
- ❑ Endocrine

- ❑ Hematologic/lymphatic
- ❑ Allergic/immunologic

Past, Family & Social History

PAST
- ❑ current medication
- ❑ prior illnesses and injuries
- ❑ operations and hospitalizations
- ❑ age-appropriate immunizations
- ❑ allergies   ❑ dietary status

FAMILY
- ❑ health status or cause of death of parents, siblings, and children
- ❑ hereditary or high-risk diseases
- ❑ diseases related to CC, HPI, ROS

SOCIAL
- ❑ living arrangements
- ❑ marital status   ❑ sexual history
- ❑ occupational history
- ❑ use of drugs, alcohol, or tobacco
- ❑ extent of education
- ❑ current employment   ❑ other

❑ PFSH Form reviewed, no change   ❑ PFSH form reviewed, updated   ❑ PFSH form new

General Multi-System Examination

Constitutional
- ❑ 3 of 7 (2 BP, pulse, respir, tmp, hgt, wgt)
- ❑ General Appearance

Eyes
- ❑ Conjunctivac, Lids
- ❑ Eyes: Pupils, Irises
- ❑ Opthal exam—Optic discs, Pos Seg

ENT
- ❑ Ears, Nose
- ❑ Oto exam—Aud canals, Tymp membr
- ❑ Hearing
- ❑ Nasal mucosa, Septum, Turbinates
- ❑ ENTM: Lips, Teeth, Gums
- ❑ Oropharynx—oral mucosa, palates

Neck
- ❑ Neck
- ❑ Thyroid

Respiratory
- ❑ Respiratory effort
- ❑ Percussion of chest
- ❑ Palpation of chest
- ❑ Auscultation of lungs

Cardiovascular
- ❑ Palpation of heart
- ❑ Auscultation of heart (& sounds)
- ❑ Carotid arteries, Abdominal aorta
- ❑ Femoral arteries
- ❑ Pedal pulses
- ❑ Extrem for periph edema/varicosities

Chest
- ❑ Inspect Breasts
- ❑ Palpation of Breasts & Axillae

Gastrointestinal
- ❑ Abd (+/− masses or tenderness)
- ❑ Liver, Spleen
- ❑ Hernia (+/−)
- ❑ Anus, Perineum, Rectum
- ❑ Stool for occult blood

GU/Female
- ❑ Female: Genitalia, Vagina
- ❑ Female Urethra
- ❑ Bladder
- ❑ Cervix
- ❑ Uterus
- ❑ Adnexa/parametria

GU/Male
- ❑ Scrotal Contents
- ❑ Penis
- ❑ Digital Rectal of Prostate

Lymphatic
- ❑ Lymph: Neck
- ❑ Lymph: Axillae
- ❑ Lymph: Groin
- ❑ Lymph: Other

Musculoskeletal
- ❑ Gait (. . . ability to exercise)
- ❑ Palpation Digits, Nails
- ❑ Head/Neck: Inspect, Percuss, Palp
- ❑ Head/Neck: Motion (+/− pain, crepit)
- ❑ Head/Neck: Stability (+/− lux, sublux)
- ❑ Head/Neck: Muscle strength & tone
- ❑ Spine/Rib/Pelv: Inspect, Percuss, Palp
- ❑ Spine/Rib/Pelv: Motion
- ❑ Spine/Rib/Pelv: Stability
- ❑ Spine/Rib/Pelv: Strength and tone

- ❑ R. Up Extrem: Inspect, Percuss, Palp
- ❑ R. Up Extrem: Motion (+/− pain, crepit)
- ❑ R. Up Extrem: Stability (+/− lux, sublux)
- ❑ R. Up Extrem: Muscle strength & tone
- ❑ L. Up Extrem: Inspect, Percuss, Palp
- ❑ L. Up Extrem: Motion (+/− pain, crepit)
- ❑ L. Up Extrem: Muscle strength & tone
- ❑ R. Low Extrem: Inspect, Percuss, Palp
- ❑ R. Low Extrem: Motion (+/− pain, crepit)
- ❑ R. Low Extrem: Stability (+/− lux, laxity)
- ❑ R. Low Extrem: Muscle strength & tone
- ❑ L. Low Extrem: Inspect, Percuss, Palp
- ❑ L. Low Extrem: Motion (+/− pain, crepit)
- ❑ L. Low Extrem: Sability (+/− lux, sublux)
- ❑ L. Low Extrem: Muscle strength & tone

Skin
- ❑ Skin: Inspect Skin & Subcut tissues
- ❑ Skin: Palpation Skin & Subcut tissues

Neuro
- ❑ Neuro: Cranial nerves (+/− deficits)
- ❑ Neuro: DTRs (+/− pathological reflexes)
- ❑ Neuro: Sensations

Psychiatry
- ❑ Psych: Judgment, Insight
- ❑ Psych: Mood, Affect (depression, anxiety)

Exam Documented _____

(continued)

Number of Diagnoses/ Management Options	Points
Self-limited or minor (Stable, improved, or worsened)—Maximum 2 points in this category.	1
Established problem (to examining MD); stable or improved	1
Established problem (to examining MD); worsening	2
New problem (to examining MD); no additional workup planned—Maximum 1 point in this category.	3
New problem (to examining MD); additional workup (eg., admit/transfer)	4
Total	

Table of Risk

Level of Risk	Presenting Problem(s)	Diagnostic Procedure(s) Ordered	Management Options Selected
Minimal	• One self-limited or minor problem, e.g., cold, insect bite, tinea corporis	• Laboratory tests requiring venipuncture • Chest x-rays • EKG/EEG • Urinalysis • Ultrasound, eg, echocardiography • KOH prep	• Rest • Gargles • Elastic bandages • Superficial dressings
Low	• Two or more self-limited or minor problem • One stable chronic illness, e.g., well-controlled hypertension, non-insulin-dependent diabetes, cataract, BPH • Acute uncomplicated illness or injury, e.g., cystitis allergic rhinitis, simple sprain	• Physiologic tests not under stress, e.g., pulmonary functions tests • Noncardiovascular imaging studies with contrast, e.g., barium enema • Superficial needle biopsies • Clinical laboratory tests requiring arterial puncture • Skin biopsies	• Over-the-counter drugs • Minor surgery with no identified risk factors • Physical therapy • Occupational therapy • IV fluids without additives
Moderate	• One or more chronic illnesses with mild exacerbation, progression, or side effects of treatment • Two or more stable chronic illness • Undiagnosed new problem with uncertain prognosis, e.g., lump in breast • Acute illness with systemic symptoms, e.g., pyelonephritis, pneumonitis, colitis • Acute complicated injury, e.g., head injury with brief loss of consciousness	• Physiologic tests under stress, e.g., cardiac stress tests, fetal contraction stress test • Diagnostic endoscopies with no identified risk factors • Deep needle or incisional biopsy • Cardiovascular imaging studies with contrast and no identified risk factors, eg, arteriogram, cardiac catheterization • Obtain fluid from body cavity, e.g., lumbar puncture, thoracentesis, culdocentesis	• Minor surgery with identified risk factors • Elective major surgery (open, percutaneous, or endoscopic) with no identified risk factors • Prescription drug management • Therapeutic nuclear medicine • IV fluids with additives • Closed treatment of fracture or dislocation without manipulation
High	• One or more chronic illnesses with severe exacerbation, progression, or side effects of treatment • Acute or chronic illnesses or injuries that pose a threat to life or bodily function, eg, multiple trauma, acute MI, pulmonary embolus, severe respiratory distress, progressive severe rheumatoid arthritis, psychiatric illness with potential threat to self or others, peritonitis, acute renal failure • An abrupt change in neurologic status, e.g., seizure, TIA, weakness, sensory loss	• Cardiovascular imaging studies with contrast with identified risk factors • Cardiac electrophysiological tests • Diagnostic endoscopies with identified risk factors • Discography	• Elective major surgery (open, percutaneous, or endoscopic) with identified risk factors • Emergency major surgery (open, percutaneous, or endoscopic) • Parenteral controlled substances • Drug therapy requiring intensive monitoring for toxicity • Decision not to resuscitate or to deescalate care because of poor prognosis

Amount and/or Complexity of Data Reviewed	Points
Lab ordered and/or reviewed (regardless of # ordered)	1
X-ray ordered and/or reviewed (regardless of # ordered)	1
Medicine section (90701–99199) ordered and/or reviewed	1
Discussion of test results with performing physician	1
Decision to obtain old record and/or obtain hx from someone other than patient	1
Review and summary of old records and/or obtaining hx from someone other than patient and/or discussion with other health provider	2
Independent visualization of image, tracing, or specimen (not simply review of report)	2
Total	

Medical Decision Making	SF	LOW	MOD	HIGH
Number of Diagnoses or Treatment Options	1	2	3	4
Amount and/or Complexity of Data to be Reviewed	1	2	3	4
Risk of Complications, Morbidity, Mortality	Minimal	Low	Moderate	High
E/M Level=2 out of 3				

MDM_____

Chart Note
❑ Dictated   ❑ Handwritten
❑ Form   ❑ Illegible
❑ Note signed
❑ Signature missing

Other Services or Modalities:

Auditor:

EXPLANATION OF BENEFITS (SAMPLE)

For Students Use Only.

Payer's Name and Address

Today's Date:

Provider's Name and Address

This statement covers payments for the following patient(s):

Claim Detail Section (if there are number in the "SEE REMARKS" column, see the Remarks Section for explanation)

Patient Name	Patient Account Number:
Patient ID Number:	Insured's Name:
Group Number:	
Provider Name:	Inventory Number: Claim Control Number:

Service Date(s)	Procedure	Charges	Adjustment	Allowed	Copay	Deduct/Not Covered	Coins	Paid Amt.	Provider Paid/Remarks
TOTALS									

BALANCE DUE FROM PATIENT: PT'S DED/NOT COV $_____

PT'S COINSURANCE $_____

PAYMENT SUMMARY SECTION (TOTALS)

Charges	Adjustment	Allowed	Copay	Deduct/Not Covered	Coins	Total Paid

Financial Agreement (Sample)
Allied Medical Center
1933 E. Frankford Road
Suite 110
Carrollton, TX 12345
Phone: 910-555-1717
FAX: 910-555-1716

Please read the following carefully and sign below that you understand and accept Allied Medical Center's basic operating policies and agree to the financial terms:

Payment is expected at time of service:

Unless insurance is verified by the office or a treatment payment plan is arranged, clients are responsible for making full payment at the time of service.

Schedule of Fees:

Clients will be provided a schedule of fees regarding their treatment and payment options.

Health Insurance:

Allied Medical Center participates (in-network) with several major insurers, and the practice will make every reasonable effort to work with your insurance plan to file for all covered services.

Until the office can verify your coverage, full payment at time of service is required. In-network coverage can usually be verified in less than one week. After the office receives an Explanation of Benefits from your insurer, any surplus payment for services will be credited to your account or refunded promptly.

Once insurance coverage is verified, clients are responsible for payment of all copays, coinsurance, deductibles, and uncovered balances at time of service.

If insurance is used, please understand that it is the client's (or client's legal guardian's) responsibility to notify Allied Medical Center of any changes in insurance coverage. You are responsible for prompt and full payment of services not covered by insurance. When insurance is used to pay for services, the client agrees to assign any insurance benefit payments to Allied Medical Center for services rendered.

Limitations of Insurance:

Not all insurance plans cover all services, and Allied Medical Center does not participate in all plans. Some plans require preauthorization, referrals, or justification of medical necessity which limit or deny reimbursement. Also, some insurance companies regard therapy, including biofeedback, for medical conditions to be reimbursed under mental health coverage which frequently has less coverage than medical benefits. Please check with your carrier to determine specifics of your policy and your mental health coverage for this type of treatment.

If you participate in an insurance plan in which Allied Medical Center is not in-network, it is strongly recommended that you provide a physician referral letter so the practice can better assist you to advocate for payment by your insurance company. Allied Medical Center will provide you with a statement that can be submitted to the insurance carrier for consideration of out-of-network reimbursement, but full payment is your responsibility.

(continued)

Prompt Payment:

The practice provides the most cost-effective, high-quality care possible. To do this, costs related to billing overhead are kept to a minimum. Therefore clients are obliged to make prompt payment for all fees due. Charges for late payment, collections, or missed appointments will be assessed as needed to recover these costs.

Late Charges:

All outstanding balances are due within 30 days of services rendered or by the date due for prearranged payment plans. A 5% per month fee is assessed for overdue balances. Balances that exceed 90 days are considered delinquent and will be assigned to collections. Clients are responsible for payment of all fees related to collecting the unpaid balance.

Returned Checks:

There is a $50.00 fee for returned checks.

Missed Appointments:

Scheduled appointments are time that is blocked out for you, and the practice does not overbook appointments that might limit or delay your appointment. Therefore, clients are responsible for payment for their reserved time.

Late Cancellations:

Appointments must be cancelled or rescheduled by 5 pm of the prior day, or the client will be charged the full appointment charge (even if the client does not show for the appointment). Allied Medical Center will make every reasonable effort to forgive unforeseen emergency missed appointments, but all missed or late cancelled appointments need to be discussed and approved. After two missed appointments without adequate notification or explanation, Allied Medical Center reserves the right to terminate treatment.

Appointment Notification:

Allied Medical Center will remind you of your scheduled appointment by telephone or e-mail. (Please state your preference of e-mail or telephone or neither). However, it is your responsibility to keep your appointment as scheduled or notify the practice as outlined above if you need to cancel or reschedule.

Telephone Consults:

The services that Allied Medical Center offers are elective in nature. Allied Medical Center does not offer emergency medical or psychiatric care. Therefore, emergency telephone calls are generally not accepted. Clients should contact their medical providers for any medically oriented emergencies. Telephone calls outside of prearranged consultations or as a medical consultation scheduled by the client will be billed at the hourly rate in 15-minute increments. Telephone consults are typically not reimbursable by insurance.

Ancillary Services:

Legal and disability support is offered through the practice, with advance arrangement and approval only. Court appearances, correspondence, report writing, and other efforts

Financial Agreement (Sample) (continued)

for legal action or disability work are not reimbursable by health insurance and will be billed on a time and materials basis.

Questions about Payment or Insurance:

For payment or insurance questions or concerns, contact the practice administrator via e-mail at (billing@alliedmedcenter.com) or phone (910-555-1717).

I received a copy of the current Allied Medical Center fee schedule.
I have read, understand, and agree to the policies outlined in this agreement.

_____
Patient's Name

_____   _____
Patient/Guardian Signature   Date

INSURANCE VERIFICATION WORKSHEET (SAMPLE)

Patient's Name: _____ Chart Number: _____ Appt. Date: _____

D.O.B. _____ Policy ID Number _____ Group Number _____

Policyholder: _____ DOB: _____

Insurance Co. Name: _____ Referral Number Required: ❑ No ❑ Yes

Telephone Number _____ Referral Number: _____

Mailing Address: _____

Employer's Name: _____

Employer's Phone Number: _____

Effective Date: _____ Lifetime maximum: _____

Pre-Cert Required: ❑ Yes   ❑ No

Deductible Met:

Copay _____ Deductible _____ ❑ No ❑ Yes

Pays @ _____%

Exclusion/Preexisting: _____

Chief Complaint/Diagnosis: _____

Insurance Rep's Name: _____ Ext Number _____

Voice Tracking Number: _____ Date: _____ Time: _____

Verified by_____ Date: _____

MEDICAL RECORD RELEASE FORM (SAMPLE)

I, _____ ACTING ON
BEHALF OF: (Print Name of Patient or Legally Authorized Representative)

_____ HEREBY AUTHORIZE THE RELEASE
(Print Name of Patient)
OF INFORMATION AS INDICATED:

My Healthcare Information

_____ I authorize disclosure of healthcare information (related to my medical history, diagnosis, treatment, or prognosis) to all inquiries or only to the following people or entities (for example, family friends, employer, insurance companies, clergy):

<u>List Names</u>:

_____

_____

Limited Healthcare Information

_____ I wish to limit disclosure of only certain kinds of healthcare information (related to my medical history, diagnosis, treatment, or prognosis) to the following people or entities:

<u>List Names</u>   <u>List information that may be released</u>

_____   _____

_____   _____

No Information

_____ I do not authorize release of any information regarding my admission or treatment. I wish to be a "no information" patient, and I realize that flowers, telephone calls, and visitors will be refused on my behalf.

_____   _____

(Signature of Patient or Legally Authorized Representative)   (Date)

MEDICARE LIMITING CHARGE FORM

Limiting Charge
Overview

Note: This form will only be sent if the beneficiary requests it.

We were advised by TrailBlazer Health Enterprises, LLC on (<u>insert date</u>) that the services described below were billed with charges that exceeded the amounts permitted under Medicare rules. In accordance with their instructions, we are refunding the excess amount or posting a credit to your account.

TODAY'S DATE: _____

BENEFICIARY (PATIENT) NAME: _____

BENEFICIARY HICN: _____

DATE(S) OF SERVICE: _____

PROCEDURE CODE(S): _____

DESCRIPTION OF THE PROCEDURE(S): _____

_____

AMOUNT OF REFUND: _____

NAME AND ADDRESS OF PHYSICIAN OR NON-PHYSICIAN PRACTITIONER:

_____

_____

_____

_____

Medicare Questionnaire Form

1. Are you receiving Black Lung (BL) Benefits?
   - ◆ The Black Lung Benefits Act of 1981 provides benefits to miners totally disabled due to pneumoconiosis arising out of coal mine employment. Black Lung IS PRIMARY ONLY FOR CLAIMS RELATED TO Black Lung diagnosis.

      _____ If no, write "N" and go to the next question.
      _____ If yes, write "Y" and document the date benefits began: CCYY/MM/DD. Black Lung is primary, only for claims related to Black Lung.

2. Will this be paid by a government program (i.e., research grant)?
   - ◆ If the services provided are part of any government **program,** they may be paid by a source other than Medicare. Your patient will know whether it is a research grant or another program is paying for their services.

      _____ If no, write "N" and go to the next question.
      _____ If yes, write "Y" and determine who the primary payer is. Government programs will be primary for these services.

3. Has Veterans Affairs (DVA) authorized and agreed to pay?
   - ◆ If the Department of Veterans Affairs (DVA) has authorized and agreed to pay, ask the patient for the authorization.

      _____ If no, write "N" and go to the next question.
      _____ If yes, write "Y" and enter as the primary insurance. DVA is primary for these services.

4. Was the illness/injury due to a work-related accident/condition?
   - ◆ If the illness/injury is due to a work-related accident MEDICARE IS NOT PRIMARY, WORKERS' COMPENSATION IS THE PRIMARY PAYER ONLY FOR CLAIMS RELATED TO WORK-RELATED INJURIES OR ILLNESS. GO TO PART III.

      _____ If no, this is not a work-related illness/accident. GO TO PART II.
      _____ If yes, write "Y" and enter the date of injury/illness: CCYY/MM/DD. Workers' Compensation is primary payer only for claims related to work-related injury or illness. STOP

   Date of injury/illness. _____
   _____
   _____
   _____
   Record the policy or identification number _____
   Document the name and address of the patient's employer _____
   _____
   _____
   _____
   _____

Part II

1. Was the illness/injury due to a non-work-related accident?
   - ◆ (i.e., automobile, fall in the home, fall in business)
      _____ If no, GO TO PART III.
      _____ If yes, record the date of accident: CCYY/MM/DD.
2. Was the accident automobile related?
      _____ If no, GO TO PART III.
      _____ If yes, record the name and address of no-fault or liability insurer.
   _____
   _____
   Insurance Claim Number _____

(continued)

3. Was another party responsible for this accident?

_____ If no, GO TO PART III.

_____ If yes, record the name and address of the liability insurer.

LIABILITY INSURER IS PRIMARY ONLY FOR THOSE RELATED TO THE ACCIDENT. GO TO PART III.

Name and address of any liability insurer

_____

_____

_____

_____

Insurance claim number_____

Part III

1. Are you entitled to Medicare based on:
   - ◆ Age (people 65 years of age and older). GO TO PART IV.
   - ◆ Disability (some people with disabilities under 65 years of age). GO TO PART V.
   - ◆ ESRD (end-stage renal disease—(permanent kidney failure treated with dialysis or a transplant). GO TO PART VI.

Part IV

If you are entitled to Medicare based on age

1. Are you currently employed?

   _____If no, record the date of retirement: CCYY/MM/DD.

   _____If yes, record the name and address of your employer.

   _____

   _____

   _____

2. Is your spouse currently employed?

   _____If no, record the date of their retirement: CCYY/MM/DD.

   _____If yes, record the name and address of your spouse's employer:

   _____

   _____

   _____

   _____

   IF THE PATIENT ANSWERED NO TO BOTH QUESTIONS 1 AND 2, MEDICARE IS PRIMARY. DO NOT PROCEED ANY FURTHER. IF YES TO QUESTIONS 1 AND 2, GO TO QUESTIONS 3 AND 4.

3. If either you or your spouse is employed, do you have Group Health Plan (GHP) coverage?

   _____ If no, STOP. MEDICARE IS PRIMARY.

   _____ If yes, does the employer that sponsors your GHP employ 20 or more employees?

   _____ If no, STOP. MEDICARE IS PRIMARY.

   _____ If yes, the GROUP HEALTH PLAN IS PRIMARY. RECORD THE FOLLOWING INFORMATION.

   Name and address of GHP:

   _____

   _____

   _____

   _____

   Policy ID Number: _____

   Group ID Number: _____

   Name of Policy Holder: _____

   Relationship to Patient: _____

Part V

If you are entitled to Medicare based on a disability

1. Are you currently employed?

   _____ If no, record the date of retirement: CCYY/MM/DD.

   _____ If yes, record the name and address of your employer:

   _____

   _____

   _____

Medicare Questionnaire Form (continued)

2. Is a family member currently employed?

_____ IF THE PATIENT ANSWERS NO TO BOTH QUESTIONS 1 AND 2, MEDICARE IS PRIMARY, DO NOT PROCEED ANY FURTHER.

_____ If yes, record the name and address of employer:

_____

_____

_____

_____

3. Do you have group health plan (GHP) coverage based on your own or a family member's current employment?

_____ If no, STOP. MEDICARE IS PRIMARY.

_____ If yes, does the employer that sponsors your GHP employ 100 or more employees?

_____ If no, STOP. MEDICARE IS PRIMARY.

_____ If yes, the Group Health Plan is PRIMARY. OBTAIN THE FOLLOWING INFORMATION:

Name and address of GHP:

_____

_____

_____

_____

Policy ID Number: _____

Group ID Number: _____

Name of Policy Holder: _____

Relationship to Patient: _____

Part VI

Are you entitled to Medicare based on ESRD?

1. Do you have group health plan (GHP) coverage?

_____ If no, STOP. MEDICARE IS PRIMARY.

_____ If yes, record the name and address of GHP:

_____

_____

_____

_____

Policy ID Number: _____

Group ID Number: _____

Name of Policy Holder: _____

Relationship to Patient: _____

Name and address of employer, if any, from which you receive GHP

coverage: _____

2. Have you received a kidney transplant?

_____ If no,

_____ If yes, record the date of transplant: CCYY/MM/DD. GO TO QUESTION 3.

3. Have you received maintenance dialysis treatments? These are dialysis treatments relating to transplant and should be billed as part of the transplant cost.

_____ If no,

_____ If yes, record the date dialysis began: CCYY/MM/DD. GO TO QUESTION 4.

If you participated in a self-dialysis program, provide date training started: CCYY/MM/DD.

4. Are you within the 30-month coordination period?

When a patient is diagnosed with ESRD their GHP must pay claims for the first 30 months after diagnosis.

_____ If no, STOP. MEDICARE IS PRIMARY.

_____ If yes, GO TO QUESTION 5.

5. Are you entitled to Medicare on the basis of either ESRD and age or ESRD and disability?

_____ If no, STOP. GHP IS PRIMARY DURING THE 30-MONTH COORDINATION PERIOD.

_____ If yes, GO TO QUESTION 6.

(continued)

6. Was your initial entitlement to Medicare (including simultaneous entitlement) based on ESRD?
   _____ If no, INITIAL ENTITLEMENT BASED ON AGE OR DIABILITY.
   _____ If yes, STOP. GHP CONTINUES TO PAY PRIMARY DURING THE
   30-MONTH COORDINATION PERIOD.

7. Does the working aged or disability MSP provision apply (i.e., is the GHP primary based on age or disability entitlement)?
   _____ If no, MEDICARE CONTINUES TO PAY PRIMARY.
   _____ If yes, GHP CONTINUES TO PAY PRIMARY DURING THE 30-MONTH
   COORDINATION PERIOD.

A. If beneficiary provides information which is different from that found on the Common Working File (CWF).
   If, as a result of asking the preceding questions, the beneficiary provides information to you that is different from that found in CWF, it is important to provide that information on the bill with the proper uniform billing codes. This information will then be used to update CWF through the billing process.

   FAILURE TO OBTAIN THE INFORMATION LISTED IN THESE SECTIONS IS A VIOLATION OF YOUR PROVIDER AGREEMENT WITH MEDICARE. (SEE§142.3F.) THE INFORMATION YOU MUST OBTAIN IS ESSENTIAL TO FILING A PROPER CLAIM WITH MEDICARE OR A PRIMARY PAYER. FAILURE TO FILE A PROPER CLAIM CAN RESULT IN THE UNNECESSARY DENIAL OR DEVELOPMENT OF CLAIMS.

B. If there is no MSP data on available on CWF for beneficiary.
   If no MSP data are found in CWF for the beneficiary, you must still ask the questions found in §301.2A and provide any MSP information on the bill using the proper uniform billing codes. This information will then be used to update CWF through the billing process.

Medicare Questionnaire Form (continued)

DEPARTMENT OF HEALTH AND HUMAN SERVICES
CENTERS FOR MEDICARE & MEDICAID SERVICES

MEDICARE REDETERMINATION REQUEST FORM

1. Beneficiary's Name: _____

2. Medicare Number: _____

3. Description of Item or Service in Question: _____

4. Date the Service or Item Was Received: _____

5. I do not agree with the determination of my claim. MY REASONS ARE:

_____

_____

_____

6. Date of the Initial Determination Notice: _____
   (If you received your initial determination notice more than 120 days ago, include your reason for not making this request earlier.)

_____

_____

7. Additional Information Medicare Should Consider: _____

_____

_____

_____

8. Requester's Name: _____

9. Requester's Relationship to the Beneficiary: _____

10. Requester's Address: _____

_____

11. Requester's Telephone Number: _____

12. Requester's Signature: _____

13. Date Signed: _____

14. ❑ I have evidence to submit. (Attach such evidence to this form.)
   ❑ I do not have evidence to submit.

NOTICE: Anyone who misrepresents or falsifies essential information requested by this form may upon conviction be subject to fine or imprisonment under Federal Law.

Form CMS-20027 (05/05) EF 05/2005

PATIENT INFORMATION/REGISTRATION FORM (SAMPLE)

Allied Medical Center
REGISTRATION FORM

(Please Print)

Today's date: _____   PCP: _____

PATIENT INFORMATION

Patient's last name:	First:	Middle:	❏ Mr. ❏ Mrs.	❏ Miss ❏ Ms.	Marital status (circle one) Single / Mar / Div / Sep / Wid

Is this your legal name? ❏ Yes ❏ No	If not, what is your legal name?	(Former name):	Birth date:	Age:	Sex: ❏ M ❏ F

Street address:	Social Security no.:	Home phone no.:

P.O. box:	City:	State:	ZIP Code:

Occupation:	Employer:	Employer phone no.: ( )

Chose clinic because/Referred to clinic by (please choose one):	❏ Dr.	❏ Insurance Plan	❏ Hospital
❏ Family ❏ Friend ❏ Close to home/work	❏ Yellow Pages	❏ Other	

Other family members seen here:	**REASON FOR THIS VISIT:**

INSURANCE INFORMATION

(Please give your insurance card to the receptionist.)

Person responsible for bill:	Birth date: / /	Address (if different):	Home phone no.: ( )

Is this person a patient here? ❏ Yes ❏ No

Occupation:	Employer:	Employer address:	Employer phone no.: ( )

Is this patient covered by insurance? ❏ Yes ❏ No

Please indicate primary insurance		Claims Mailing Address:			
			PHONE:		

Subscriber's name:	Subscriber's S.S. no.:	Birth date:	❏ M ❏ F	Group no.:	Policy no.:	Co-payment:

Patient's relationship to subscriber: ❏ Self ❏ Spouse ❏ Child ❏ Other

Name of secondary insurance (if applicable):	Subscriber's name and DOB:	❏ M ❏ F	Group no.:	Policy no.:

Patient's relationship to subscriber: ❏ Self ❏ Spouse ❏ Child ❏ Other   Claims Address:

IN CASE OF EMERGENCY

Name of local friend or relative (not living at same address):	Relationship to patient:	Home phone no.:	Work phone no.:

The above information is true to the best of my knowledge. I authorize my insurance benefits be paid directly to the physician. I understand that I am financially responsible for any balance. I also authorize ALLIED MEDICAL CENTER or insurance company to release any information required to process my claims.

Patient/Guardian signature _____   _Date_ _____

PATIENT INFORMATION/REGISTRATION FORM (SAMPLE)

Capital City Medical—123 Unknown BLVD, Capital City, NY 12345-2222 (555)555-1234 Phil Wells, MD, Mannie Mends, MD, Bette R. Soone, MD	Patient Information Form Tax ID: 75-0246810 Group NPI: 1513171216

Patient Information:

Name: (Last, First) _____ ❑ Male ❑ Female Birth Date: _____

Address: _____ Phone: ( ) _____

Social Security Number: _____ Full-Time Student: ❑ Yes ❑ No

Marital Status: ❑ Single ❑ Married ❑ Divorced ❑ Other

Employment:

Employer: _____ Phone: ( ) _____

Address: _____

Condition Related to: ❑ Auto Accident ❑ Employment ❑ Other Accident

Date of Accident: _____ State _____

Emergency Contact: _____ **Phone: ( )** _____

Primary Insurance: _____ Phone: ( ) _____

Address: _____

Insurance Policyholder's Name: _____ ❑ M ❑ F DOB: _____

Address: _____

Phone: _____ Relationship to Insured: ❑ Self ❑ Spouse ❑ Child ❑ Other

Employer: _____ Phone: ( ) _____

Employer's Address: _____

Policy/ID No: _____ Group No: _____ Percent Covered: ___%, Copay Amt: $_____

Secondary Insurance: _____ Phone: ( ) _____

Address: _____

Insurance Policyholder's Name: _____ ❑ M ❑ F DOB: _____

Address: _____

Phone: _____ Relationship to Insured: ❑ Self ❑ Spouse ❑ Child ❑ Other

Employer: _____ Phone: ( ) _____

Employer's Address: _____

Policy/ID No: _____ Group No: _____ Percent Covered: ___%, Copay Amt: $_____

Reason for Visit: _____

Known Allergies: _____

Were you referred here? If so, by whom?: _____

Pre-Certification Form (Sample)

Name: _____   DOB: _____

Chart: _____   DOS: _____

Policy Holder: _____   Policy ID: _____

Group Number: _____

PTS DX: _____   Procedure to be done: _____

Insurance Co: _____   Phone: _____

Pre-Cert Rep's Name: _____   Phone: _____

Authorization Number: _____   Time: _____

OPS or IP _____

Global Period (how many days): _____

Other Comments: _____

Voice Tracking Number: _____

Verified by: _____   Date: _____

Requested verification in writing to fax number or e-mail: _____

Preoperative Verification Form (Hospital Outpatient Benefits Form) (Sample)

PATIENT NAME _____   ACCT NUMBER _____

POLICY ID NUMBER _____   GROUP NUMBER _____

POLICY HOLDER _____   RELATION _____

SERVICE DATE _____   PROCEDURE _____

CONTRACTED WITH _____ PLAN

PLAN TYPE: HMO _____ PPO _____ POS _____ EPO _____ MC _____ INDEM _____
WORKERS' COMP _____ SUBSCRIBER/NON-SUBSCRIBER _____

COVERAGE EFFECTIVE DATE _____   LIFETIME MAXIMUM _____

COPAY _____ DOES PREEXISTING APPLY? ❑ YES ❑ NO   What _____

DEDUCTIBLE: _____ MET ❑ YES ❑ NO   HOW MUCH? _____

INS PAYS _____%   PATIENT PAYS _____%

OOP _____ MET: ❑ YES ❑ NO   HOW MUCH? _____ THEN PAYS _____

BENEFITS REP. NAME _____   TELEPHONE # _____

DATE YOU SPOKE TO REP: _____   TIME: _____

Submit claims to: _____

VOICE TRACKING NUMBER _____

REFERAL NEEDED? ❑ YES ❑ NO   REFFERAL NUMBER: _____

PCP NAME _____   PHONE NUMBER _____

ADDITIONAL
COMMENTS _____

PRE CERT REP NAME _____   PHONE NUMBER _____

AUTHORIZATION NUMBER _____ IS THIS OPS (outpatient surgery) or CLI (clinical admission inpatient)?

If this is for a surgery, is 23-hour observation included? ❑ YES ❑ NO

Exclusions: ❑ Y ❑ N   What _____

Verified by: _____ Date: _____

Privacy Policy/HIPAA Form (Sample)

ALLIED MEDICAL CENTER
Notice of Privacy Policies and Practices

This Notice of Privacy and Practices (the "Notice") tells you about the ways we may use and disclose medical information about you and your rights and our obligations regarding the use and disclosure of your medical information. This Notice applies to Allied Medical Center and its employees and it is effective beginning April 14, 2003.

I. <u>OUR OBLIGATIONS</u>.

We are required by law to:

- Make sure that the medical information we have about you is kept private, to the extent required by state and federal law;

- Give you this Notice explaining our legal duties and privacy practices with respect to medical information about you; and

- Follow the terms of the version of the Notice that is currently in effect at the time we acquire medical information about you.

II. <u>HOW WE MAY USE AND DISCLOSE MEDICAL INFORMATION ABOUT YOU</u>.

The following categories describe the different reasons that we typically use and disclose medical information. These categories are intended to be generic descriptions only, and not a list of every instance in which we may use or disclose medical information. Please understand that for these categories, the law generally does not require us to get your consent in order for us to release your medical information.

A. **<u>For Treatment</u>**. We may use medical information about you to provide you with medical treatment and services, and we may disclose medical information about you to doctors, nurses, technicians, medical students, or hospital personnel who are providing or involved in providing medical care to you. For example, we will provide information about the results of your test to your physicians and his or her office staff.

B. **<u>For Payment</u>**. We may use and disclose medical information about you so that we may bill and collect from you, an insurance company, or a third party for the services we provided. This may also include the disclosure of medical information to obtain prior authorization for treatment and procedures from your insurance plan. For example, we may send a claim for payment to your insurance company, and that claim may have a code on it that describes your diagnosis.

C. **<u>For Healthcare Operations</u>.** We may use and disclose medical information about you for our healthcare operations. These uses and disclosures are necessary to operate our practice appropriately and make sure all of our patients receive quality care. For example, we may need to use or disclose your medical information in order to conduct certain cost-management practices, or to provide information to our insurance carriers.

(continued)

D. **Quality Assurance.** We may need to use or disclose your medical information for our internal processes to determine that we are providing appropriate care to our patients.

E. **Utilization Review.** We may need to use or disclose your medical information about you in order for us to review the credentials and actions of physicians to ensure they meet our qualifications and standards.

F. **Peer Review.** We may need to use or disclose your medical information about you in order for us to review the credentials and actions of physicians to ensure they meet our qualifications and standards.

G. **Treatment Alternatives.** We may use and disclose medical information to tell you about or recommend possible treatment options or alternatives that we believe may be of interest to you.

H. **Health-Related Benefits and Services.** We may use and disclose medical information to tell you about health-related benefits or services that we believe may be of interest to you.

I. **Individuals Involved in Your Care or Payment for Your Care.** We may release medical information about you to a friend or family member who is involved in your medical care, as well as to someone who helps pay for your care, but we will do so only as allowed by state or federal law, or in accordance with your prior authorization.

J. **As Required by Law.** We will disclose medical information about you when required to do so by federal, state, or local law.

K. **To Avert a Serious Threat to Health or Safety.** We may use and disclose medical information about you when necessary to prevent or decrease a serious and imminent threat to your health or safety or the health and safety of the public or another person. Such disclosure would only be to someone able to help prevent the threat, or to appropriate law enforcement officials.

L. **Organ and Tissue Donation.** If you are an organ donor, we may release medical information to organizations that handle organ procurement or organ, eye, or tissue transplantation or to an organ donation bank as necessary to facilitate organ or tissue donation and transplantation.

M. **Research.** We may use or disclose your medical information to an Institutional Review Board or other authorized research body if it has obtained your consent as required by law, or if the information we provide them is "de-identified."

N. **Military and Veterans.** If you are or were a member of the armed forces, we may release medical information about you as required by the appropriate military authorities.

O. **Workers' Compensation.** We may release medical information about you for your employer's workers' compensation or similar program. These programs provide benefits for work-related injuries. For example, if your injuries result from your employment, workers' compensation insurance or a state workers' compensation program may be responsible for payment for your care, in which case we might be required to provide information to the insurer or program.

(continued)

P. Public Health Risks. We may disclose medical information about you to public health authorities for public health activities. As a general rule, we are required by law to disclose the following types of information to public health authorities, such as the Texas Department of Health. These types of information generally include the following:

- To prevent or control disease, injury, or disability (including the reporting of a particular disease or injury).

- To report births and deaths.

- To report suspected child abuse or neglect.

- To report reactions to medications or problems with medical devices and supplies.

- To notify people of recalls or products they may be using.

- To notify a person who may have been exposed to a disease or may be at risk for contracting or spreading a disease or condition.

- To notify the appropriate government authority if we believe a patient has been the victim of abuse, neglect, or domestic violence. We will only make this disclosure if you agree or when required or authorized by law.

- To provide information on certain medical devices.

- To assist in public health investigations, surveillance, or interventions.

Q. Health Oversight Activities. We may disclose medical information to a health oversight agency for activities authorized by law. These oversight activities include audits, civil, administrative, or criminal investigations and proceedings, inspections, licensure and disciplinary actions, and other activities necessary for the government to monitor the healthcare system, certain governmental benefit programs, certain entities subject to government regulation which relates to health information, and compliance with civil rights laws.

R. Lawsuits and Legal Proceedings. If you are involved in a lawsuit or a legal dispute, we may disclose medical information about you in response to a court or administrative order, subpoena, discovery request, or other lawful process. In addition to lawsuits, there may be other legal proceedings for which we may be required or authorized to use or disclose your medical information, such as investigations of healthcare providers, competency hearings on individuals, or claims over the payment of fees for medical services.

S. Law Enforcement. We may disclose your medical information if we are asked to do so by law enforcement officials, or if we are required by law to do so. Examples of these situations are:

- In response to a court order, subpoena, warrant, summons, or similar process.

- To identify or locate a suspect, fugitive, material witness, or missing person.

- About the victim of a crime.

- About a death we believe may be the result of criminal conduct.

- About criminal conduct in our office.

Privacy Policy/HIPAA Form (Sample) (continued)

- In emergency circumstances to report a crime, the location of the crime of victims, or the identity, description, or location of the person who committed the crime.

- To report certain types of wounds or physical injuries (for example, gunshot wounds).

T. <u>Coroners, Medical Examiners, and Funeral Home Directors</u>. We may disclose your medical information to a coroner or medical examiner. This may be necessary, for example, to identify a deceased person or determine the cause of death. We may also release medical information about our patients to funeral home directors as necessary to carry out their duties.

U. <u>National Security and Intelligence Activities</u>. We may disclose medical information about you to authorized federal officials for intelligence, counterintelligence, and other national security activities authorized by law.

V. <u>Inmates</u>. If you are an inmate of a correctional institution or under custody of a law enforcement official, we may disclose medical information about you to the correctional institution or the law enforcement official. This would be necessary for the institution to provide you with health care, to protect your health and safety and the health and safety of others, or for the safety and security of the correctional institution or law enforcement official.

III. <u>OTHER USES OF MEDICAL INFORMATION</u>.

There are times we may need or want to use or disclose your medical information other than for the reasons listed above, but to do so we will need your prior permission. If you provide us permission to use or disclose medical information about you for such other purposes, you may revoke that permission in writing at any time. If you revoke your permission, we will no longer use or disclose medical information about you for the reasons covered by your written authorization. You understand that we are unable to take back any disclosures we have already made with your permission, and that we are required to retain our records of the care that we provided to you.

IV. <u>YOUR RIGHTS REGARDING MEDICAL INFORMATION ABOUT YOU</u>.

Federal and state laws provide you with certain rights regarding the medical information we have about you. The following are a summary of those rights.

A. <u>Right to Inspect and Copy</u>. Under most circumstances, you have the right to inspect and/or copy your medical information that we have in our possession, which generally includes your medical and billing records. To inspect or copy your medical information, you must submit your request to do so in writing to the Allied Medical Center's HIPAA Officer at the address listed in Section VI below.

If you request a copy of your information, we may charge a fee for the costs of copying, mailing, or other supplies associated with your request. The fee we may charge will be the amount allowed by state law.

In certain very limited circumstances allowed by law, we may deny your request to review or copy your medical information. Under federal law, you may not inspect or copy psychotherapy notes. We will give you any such denial in writing. If you are denied access to medical information, you may request that the denial be reviewed.

(continued)

Another licensed healthcare professional chosen by the Allied Medical Center will review your request and the denial. The person conducting the review will not be the person who denied your request. We will abide by the outcome of the review.

B. **Right to Amend.** If you feel the medical information we have about you is incorrect or incomplete, you may ask us to amend the information. You have the right to request an amendment for as long as the information is kept by Allied Medical Center. To request an amendment, your request must be in writing and submitted to the HIPAA Officer at the address listed in Section VI below. In your request, you must provide a reason as to why you want this amendment. If we accept your request, we will notify you of that in writing.

We may deny your request for an amendment if it is not in writing or does not include a reason to support the request. In addition, we may deny your request if you ask us to amend information that (i) was not created by us, (ii) is not part of the information kept by Allied Medical Center, (iii) is not part of the information which you would be permitted to inspect and copy, or (iv) is accurate and complete. If we deny your request, we will notify you of that denial in writing.

C. **Right to an Accounting of Disclosures.** You have the right to request an "accounting of disclosures" of your medical information. This is a list of the disclosures we have made for up to six years prior to the date of your request of your medical information, but does not include disclosures for treatment, payment, or healthcare operations (as described in Sections II A, B, and C of this Notice), or certain other disclosures. To request this list of accounting, you must submit your request in writing to the Allied Medical Center's HIPAA Officer at the address set forth in Section VI below. Your request must state a time period, which may not be longer than six years and may not include dates before April 14, 2003. Your request should indicate in what form you want the list (for example, on paper or electronically). The first list you request within a twelve-month period will be free. For additional lists, we may charge you a reasonable fee for the costs of providing the list. We will notify you of the cost involved and you may choose to withdraw or modify your request at that time before any costs are incurred.

D. **Right to Request Restrictions.** You have the right to request a restriction or limitation on the medical information we use or disclose about you in various situations. You also have the right to request a limit on the medical information we disclose about you to someone who is involved in your care or the payment for your care, like a family member or friend. We are not required to agree to your request. If we do agree, we will comply with your request unless the information is needed to provide you with emergency treatment. In addition, there are certain situations where we won't be able to agree to your request, such as when we are required by law to use or disclose your medical information. To request restrictions, you must make your request in writing to Allied Medical Center's HIPAA Officer at the address listed in Section VI below. In your request, you must specifically tell us what information you want to limit, whether you want us to limit our use, disclosure, or both, and to whom you want the limits to apply.

E. **Right to Request Confidential Communications.** You have the right to request that we communicate with you about medical matters in a certain way or at a certain location. For example, you can ask that we only contact you at home, not at work or conversely, only at work and not at home. To request such confidential communications, you must make your request in writing to Allied Medical Center's HIPAA Officer at the address listed in Section VI below.

Privacy Policy/HIPAA Form (Sample) (continued)

We will not ask the reason for your request, and we will use our best efforts to accommodate all reasonable requests, but there are some requests with which we will not be able to comply. Your request must specify how and where you wish to be contacted.

F. **Business Associates.** These are some services provided in our organization through contracts with business associates. When these services are contracted, we may disclose your medical information to our business associates so that they can perform the job we have asked them to do. To protect your medical information, however, we require the business associate to appropriately safeguard your information.

G. **Right to a Paper Copy of This Notice.** You have the right to a paper copy of this Notice. You may ask us to give you a copy of this Notice at any time. To obtain a copy of this Notice, you must make your request in writing to Allied Medical Center's HIPAA Officer at the address set forth in Section VI below.

V. CHANGES TO THIS NOTICE.

We reserve the right to change this Notice at any time, along with our privacy policies and practices. We reserve the right to make the revised or changed Notice effective for medical information we already have about you as well as any information we receive in the future. We will post a copy of the current notice, along with an announcement that changes have been made, as applicable, in our offices. When changes have been made to the Notice, you may obtain a revised copy by sending a letter to Allied Medical Center's HIPAA Officer at the address listed in Section VI below or by asking the office receptionist for a current copy of the Notice.

VI. COMPLAINTS.

If you believe that your privacy rights as described in this notice have been violated, you may file a complaint with Allied Medical Center at the following address or phone number:

Allied Medical Center
Attn: HIPAA Officer
1933 E. Frankford Road, Suite 110
Carrollton, TX 12345
(972) 555-5482

To file a complaint, you may either call or send a written letter. Allied Medical Center will not retaliate against any individual who files a complaint. If you do not want to file a complaint with Allied Medical Center, you may file one with the Secretary of the Department of Health and Human Services.

In addition, if you have any questions about this Notice, please contact Allied Medical Center's HIPAA Officer at the address or phone number listed above.

I hereby certify and state that I have read, and that I fully and completely understand the HIPAA policy above.

_____

Signature   (Patient)   Date

_____

Signature (Patient Representative)   (Relationship to Patient)   Witness

SUPERBILL/ENCOUNTER FORM (SAMPLE)

Patient Information		Payment Method		Visit Information	
Patient ID number		**Primary**		Visit date	
Patient name		Primary ID number		Visit number	
Address		Primary group number		Rendering physician	
City/State		**Secondary**		Referring physician	
Phone number		Secondary ID number		Reason for visit	
Date of birth		Secondary group no.			
Age		Cash/credit card			
		Other billing			

E/M Modifiers	Procedure Modifiers	DIAGNOSIS:
21 — Prolonged E & M Service	22 — Unusual, excessive procedure	
24 — Unrelated E/M service during postop.	50 — Bilateral procedure	
25 — Significant, separately identifiable E/M	51 — Multiple surgical procedures in same day	
32 — Mandated Service	52 — Reduced/incomplete procedure	
57 — Decision for surgery	55 — Postop, management only	
	59 — Distinct multiple procedures	

CATEGORY	CODE	MOD	FEE	CATEGORY	CODE	MOD	FEE
Office Visit — New Patient				**Wound Care**			
Minimal office visit	99201			Debride partial thick burn	11040		
20 minutes	99202			Debride full thickness burn	11041		
30 minutes	99203			Debride wound, not a burn	11000		
45 minutes	99204			Unna boot application	29580		
60 minutes	99205			Unna boot removal	29700		
Other				Other			
Office Visit — Established				**Supplies**			
Minimal office visit	99211			Ace bandage, 2"	A6448		
10 minutes	99212			Ace bandage, 3"-4"	A6449		
15 minutes	99213			Ace bandage, 6"	A6450		
25 minutes	99214			Cast, fiberglass	A4590		
40 minutes	99215			Coban wrap	A6454		
Other				Foley catheter	A4338		
General Procedures				Immobilizer	L3670		
Anoscopy	46600			Kerlix roll	A6220		
Audiometry	92551			Oxygen mask/cannula	A4620		
Breast aspiration	19000			Sleeve, elbow	E0191		
Cerumen removal	69210			Sling	A4565		
Circumcision	54150			Splint, ready-made	A4570		
DDST	96110			Splint, wrist	S8451		
Flex sigmoidoscopy	45330			Sterile packing	A6407		
Flex sig. w/ biopsy	45331			Surgical tray	A4550		
Foreign body removal—foot	28190			Other			
Nail removal	11730			**OB Care**			
Nail removal/phenol	11750			Routine OB care	59400		
Trigger point injection	20552			Ante partum 4–6 visits	59425		
Tympanometry	92567			Ante partum 7 or more visits	59426		
Visual acuity	99173			Postpartum care only (separate procedure)	59430		
Other				Other			
Other				Other			

Other Visit Information:
Lab Work to Order: _____
Referral to: _____
Provider Signature: _____
Next Appointment: _____

Fees:
Total Charges: $
Copay Received: $
Other Payment: $
Total Due: $

Allied Medical Center 1933 E. Frankford Rd. Carrollton, TX 12345 **972-555-5482**

SUPERBILL/ENCOUNTER FORM (SAMPLE)

Patient Name _____

Capital City Medical
123 Unknown Boulevard, Capital City, NY 12345-2222

Date of Service _____

New Patient			Arthrocentesis/Aspiration/Injection		Laboratory	
Problem Focused	99201		Small Joint	20600	Amylase	82150
Expanded Problem, Focused	99202		Interm Joint	20605	B12	82607
Detailed	99203		Major Joint	20610	CBC & Diff	85025
Comprehensive	99204		**Other Invasive/Noninvasive**		Comp Metabolic Panel	80053
Comprehensive/High Complex	99205		Audiometry	92552	Chlamydia Screen	87110
Well Exam Infant (up to 12 mos.)	99381		Cast Application		Cholesterol	82465
Well Exam 1–4 yrs.	99382		Location Long Short		Digoxin	80162
Well Exam 5–11 yrs.	99383		Catheterization	51701	Electrolytes	80051
Well Exam 12–17 yrs.	99384		Circumcision	54150	Ferritin	82728
Well Exam 18–39 yrs.	99385		Colposcopy	57452	Folate	82746
Well Exam 40–64 yrs.	99386		Colposcopy w/Biopsy	57454	GC Screen	87070
			Cryosurgery Premalignant Lesion		Glucose	82947
			Location (s):		Glucose 1 HR	82950
			Cryosurgery Warts		Glycosylated HGB A1C	83036
Established Patient			Location (s):		HCT	85014
Post-Op Follow Up Visit	99024		Curettement Lesion		HDL	83718
Minimum	99211		Single	11055	Hep BSAG	87340
Problem Focused	99212		2–4	11056	Hepatitis panel, acute	80074
Expanded Problem Focused	99213		>4	11057	HGB	85018
Detailed	99214		Diaphragm Fitting	57170	HIV	86703
Comprehensive/High Complex	99215		Ear Irrigation	69210	Iron & TIBC	83550
Well Exam Infant (up to 12 mos.)	99391		ECG	93000	Kidney Profile	80069
Well exam 1–4 yrs.	99392		Endometrial Biopsy	58100	Lead	83655
Well Exam 5–11 yrs.	99393		Exc. Lesion Malignant		Liver Profile	80076
Well Exam 12–17 yrs.	99394		Benign		Mono Test	86308
Well Exam 18–39 yrs.	99395		Location		Pap Smear	88155
Well Exam 40–64 yrs.	99396		Exc. Skin Tags (1–15)	11200	Pregnancy Test	84703
Obstetrics			Each Additional 10	11201	Obstetric Panel	80055
Total OB Care	59400		Fracture Treatment		Pro Time	85610
Injections			Loc		PSA	84153
Administration Sub. / IM	90772		w/Reduc w/o Reduc		RPR	86592
Drug			I & D Abscess Single/Simple	10060	Sed. Rate	85651
Dosage			Multiple or Comp	10061	Stool Culture	87045
Allergy	95115		I & D Pilonidal Cyst Simple	10080	Stool O & P	87177
Cocci Skin Test	86490		Pilonidal Cyst Complex	10081	Strep Screen	87880
DPT	90701		IV Therapy—To One Hour	90760	Theophylline	80198
Hemophilus	90646		Each Additional Hour	90761	Thyroid Uptake	84479
Influenza	90658		Laceration Repair		TSH	84443
MMR	90707		Location Size Simp/Comp		Urinalysis	81000
OPV	90712		Laryngoscopy	31505	Urine Culture	87088
Pneumovax	90732		Oximetry	94760	Drawing Fee	36415
TB Skin Test	86580		Punch Biopsy		Specimen Collection	99000
TD	90718		Rhythm Strip	93040	**Other:**	
Unlisted Immun	90749		Treadmill	93015		
Tetanus Toxoid	90703		Trigger Point or Tendon Sheath Inj.	20550		
Vaccine/Toxoid Admin <8 Yr Old w/ Counseling	90465		Tympanometry	92567		
Vaccine/Toxoid Administration for Adult	90471					

Diagnosis/ICD-9:

I acknowledge receipt of medical services and authorize the release of any medical information necessary to process this claim for healthcare payment only. I do authorize payment to the provider.

Patient Signature _____

Total Estimated Charges: _____

Payment Amount: _____

Next Appointment: _____

Tool to Determine Correct CPT® Code

1 HISTORY

		Status of 1-2 chronic conditions ☐	Status of 1-2 chronic conditions ☐	Status of 3 chronic conditions ☐	Status of 3 chronic conditions ☐
HPI (History of Present Illness): Characterize HPI by considering either the status of chronic conditions or the number of elements recorded. ☐ 1 condition ☐ 2 conditions ☐ 3 conditions **OR** ☐ Location ☐ Severity ☐ Timing ☐ Modifying factors ☐ Quality ☐ Duration ☐ Context ☐ Associated signs and symptoms		☐ Brief (1-3)	☐ Brief (1-3)	☐ Extended (4 or more)	☐ Extended (4 or more)
ROS (Review of Systems): ☐ Constitutional (wt loss, etc.) ☐ Ears, nose, mouth, throat ☐ GI ☐ Integumentary (skin, breast) ☐ Endo ☐ Eyes ☐ Card/vasc ☐ GU ☐ Hem/lymph ☐ Musculo ☐ Neuro ☐ All/immuno ☐ Resp ☐ Psych		N/A	☐ Pertinent to problem (1 system)	☐ Extended (Pert and others) (2-9 systems)	☐ Complete (Pert and all others) (10 systems)
PFSH (Past Medical, Family, Social History) areas: ☐ Past history (the patient's past experiences with illnesses, operation, injuries and treatments) ☐ Family history (a review of medical events in the patient's family, including diseases that may be hereditary or place the patient at risk) ☐ Social history (an age-appropriate review of past and current activities)		N/A	N/A	☐ Pertinent (1 history area)	☐ *Complete (2 or 3 history areas)
*Complete PFSH: 2 history areas: a) established patients - office (outpatient) care, domiciliary care, home care; b) emergency department; c) subsequent nursing facility care; d) subsequent hospital care; and, e) follow-up consultations. 3 history areas: a) new patients - office (outpatient) care, domiciliary care, home care; b) initial consultations; c) initial hospital care; d) hospital observation; and, e) comprehensive nursing facility assessments.		**PROBLEM-FOCUSED**	**EXP. PROBLEM-FOCUSED**	**DETAILED**	**COMPREHENSIVE**
				Final History requires all 3 components above met or exceeded	

2 EXAMINATION

CPT Exam Description	95 Guideline Requirements	97 Guideline Requirements	CPT Type of Exam
Limited to affected body area or organ system	One body area or organ system	1-5 bulleted elements	**PROBLEM-FOCUSED EXAM**
Affected body area or organ system and other symptomatic or related organ systems	2-7 body areas and/or organ systems	6-11 bulleted elements	**EXPANDED PROBLEM-FOCUSED EXAM**
Extended exam of affected body area or organ system and other symptomatic or related organ systems	2-7 body areas and/or organ systems	12-17 bulleted elements for 2 or more systems	**DETAILED EXAM**
General multi-system	8 or more body areas and/or organ systems	18 or more bulleted elements for 9 or more systems	**COMPREHENSIVE EXAM**
Complete single organ system exam	Not defined	See requirements for individual single system exams	

3 MEDICAL DECISION-MAKING

Final Result of Complexity for Medical Decision-Making Level				
A. Number of diagnoses and/or management options	≤ 2 Minimal	3-4 Limited	5-6 Multiple	≥ 7 Extensive
B. Amount and complexity of data reviewed/ordered	≤ 1 None/Minimal	2 Limited	3 Multiple	≥ 4 Extensive
C. Risk	Minimal	Low	Moderate	High
Type of medical decision-making	Straightforward	Low Complexity	Moderate Complexity	High Complexity
Final Medical Decision-Making requires 2 of 3 components above met or exceeded				

A. Number of Diagnoses and/or Management Options (see Table A.1)	#DX	#TX	#DX + #TX
New or est problem(s), no evaluation/management mentioned and problem **is not** clearly co-morbid condition.	0	0	0
New or est problem(s), no evaluation/management mentioned and problem **is** a co-morbid condition.		0	
New or established problem(s), evaluation/management mentioned.			
		TOTAL	

(continued)

3 MEDICAL DECISION-MAKING (continued)

A.1 Treatments and Therapeutic Options

DO NOT COUNT AS TREATMENT OPTIONS NOTATIONS SUCH AS Continue "same" therapy or "no change" in therapy (including drug management) without further description (record does not document what the current therapy plan is nor that the physician reviewed it)	0
Continue "same" therapy or "no change" in therapy without further description (record clearly documents what the current therapy plan is and that the physician reviewed it); or scheduled monitoring without specific therapy	1
Drug management, new prescriptions, or changes in dosing for current medications	1
Complex drug management (more than 3 medications/prescriptions and/or over-the-counter) new prescriptions or changes in dosing for current medications	2
Open or percutaneous therapeutic cardiac, surgical, or radiological procedure – minor or major	1
Physical, occupational, or speech therapy or other manipulation	1
Closed treatment for fracture or dislocation	1
IV fluids	1
Complex insulin prescription (SC or combo of SC/IV), hyperalimentation, insulin drip, or other complex IV admix prescription	2
Conservative measures such as rest, ice, bandages, dietary	1
Radiation therapy	1
IM injection/aspiration or other pain management procedure	1
Patient educated on self or home care topics/techniques	1
Hospital admit	1
Hospital admit – other physician(s) contacted	2
Referral to another physician, consultation	1
Other – specify	
TOTAL	

B. Amount and/or Complexity of Data Reviewed or Ordered

Order and/or review results of clinical lab tests	1
Order and/or review results of tests in Radiology section of CPT	1
Order and/or review results of tests in Medical section of CPT	1
Discuss case with consultant or order consultation or discuss case with other physician also managing the patient	1
Discuss test results with performing physician	1
Order (identify specific source of records ordered) and/or summarize old or other health care records (simple statements to the effect that other or old outside records were reviewed is insufficient to count)	1
Physiologic monitoring	1
Independently visualize and report findings from images, tracings, pathological specimens themselves (not the reports) for procedures and tests for which interpretation not separately billed by the provider	1
TOTAL	

C. Risk of Complication and/or Mortality (see Table C.1)

Nature of the presenting illness	Minimal	Low	Moderate	High
Risk conferred by diagnostic options	Minimal	Low	Moderate	High
Risk conferred by therapeutic options	Minimal	Low	Moderate	High

Final Risk determined by highest of 3 components above

C.1 Risk of Complications and/or Morbity or Mortality

LEVEL OF RISK	PRESENTING PROBLEM(S)	DIAGNOSTIC PROCEDURE(S) ORDERED	MANAGEMENT OPTIONS SELECTED
Minimal	• One self-limited or minor problem, e.g., cold, insect bite, tinea corporis	• Laboratory tests requiring venipuncture • Chest x-rays • EKG/EEG • Urinalysis • Ultrasound, e.g., echo • KOH prep	• Rest • Gargles • Elastic bandages • Superficial dressings
Low	• Two or more self-limited or minor problems • One stable chronic illness, e.g., well-controlled hypertension or non-insulin dependent diabetes, cataract, BPH • Acute uncomplicated illness or injury, e.g., cystitis, allergic rhinitis, simple sprain	• Physiologic tests not under stress, e.g., pulmonary function tests • Non-cardiovascular imaging studies with contrast, e.g., barium enema • Superficial needle biopsies • Clinical laboratory tests requiring arterial puncture • Skin biopsies	• Over-the-counter drugs • Minor surgery with no identified risk factors • Physical therapy • Occupational therapy • IV fluids without additives

C.1 Risk of Complications and/or Morbidity or Mortality

LEVEL OF RISK	PRESENTING PROBLEM(S)	DIAGNOSTIC PROCEDURE(S) ORDERED	MANAGEMENT OPTIONS SELECTED
Moderate	• One or more chronic illnesses with mild exacerbation, progression or side effects of treatment • Two or more stable chronic illnesses • Undiagnosed new problem with uncertain prognosis, e.g., lump in breast • Acute illness with systemic symptoms, e.g., pyelonephritis, pneumonitis, colitis • Acute complicated injury, e.g., head injury with brief loss of consciousness	• Physiologic tests under stress, e.g., cardiac stress test, fetal contraction stress test • Diagnostic endoscopies with no identified risk factors • Deep needle or incisional biopsy • Cardiovascular imaging studies with contrast and no identified risk factors, e.g., arteriogram cardiac cath • Obtain fluid from body cavity, e.g., lumbar procedure, thoracentesis, culdocentesis	• Minor surgery with identified risk factors • Elective major surgery (open, percutaneous or endoscopic) with no identified risk factors • Prescription drug management • Therapeutic nuclear medicine • IV fluids with additives • Closed treatment of fracture or dislocation without manipulation
High	• One or more chronic illnesses with severe exacerbation, progression, or side effects of treatment • Acute or chronic illnesses or injuries that may pose a threat to life or bodily function, e.g., multiple trauma, acute MI, pulmonary embolus, severe respiratory distress, progressive severe rheumatoid arthritis, psychiatric illness with potential threat to self or others, peritonitis, acute renal failure • An abrupt change in neurologic status, e.g., seizure, TIA, weakness or sensory loss	• Cardiovascular imaging studies with contrast with identified risk factors • Cardiac electrophysiological tests • Diagnostic endoscopies with identified risk factors • Discography	• Elective major surgery (open, percutaneous or endoscopic with identified risk factors) • Emergency major surgery (open, percutaneous or endoscopic) • Parenteral controlled substances • Drug therapy requiring intensive monitoring for toxicity • Decision not to resuscitate or to de-escalate care because of poor prognosis

(continued)

4   LEVEL OF SERVICE

OUTPATIENT, CONSULTS (OUTPATIENT AND INPATIENT) AND ER

	New Office/Consults/ER — Requires 3 components within shaded area						Established Office — Requires 2 components within shaded area			
History	PF / ER: PF	EPF / ER: EPF	D / ER: EPF	C / ER: D	C / ER: C	Minimal problem that may not require presence of physician	PF	EPF	D	C
Examination	PF / ER: PF	EPF / ER: EPF	D / ER: EPF	C / ER: D	C / ER: C		PF	EPF	D	C
Complexity of Medical Decision	SF / ER: SF	SF / ER: L	L / ER: M	M / ER: M	H / ER: H		SF	L	M	H
Average Time (minutes) (ER have no average time)	10 New (99201) 15 Outpt cons (99241) 20 Inpat cons (99251) ER (99281)	20 New (99202) 30 Outpt cons (99242) 40 Inpat cons (99252) ER (99282)	30 New (99203) 40 Outpt cons (99243) 55 Inpat cons (99253) ER (99283)	45 New (99204) 60 Outpt cons (99244) 80 Inpat cons (99254) ER (99284)	60 New (99205) 80 Outpt cons (99245) 100 Inpat cons (99255) ER (99285)	5 (99211)	10 (99212)	15 (99213)	25 (99214)	40 (99215)
Level	I	II	III	IV	V	I	II	III	IV	V

INPATIENT

	Initial Hospital/Observation — Requires 3 components within shaded area			Subsequent Inpatient/Follow-up — Requires 2 components within shaded area		
History	D or C	C	C	PF interval	EPF interval	D interval
Examination	D or C	C	C	PF	EPF	D
Complexity of Medical Decision	SF/L	M	H	SF/L	M	H
Average Time (minutes) (Observation care has no average time)	30 Init hosp (99221) Observ care (99218)	50 Init hosp (99222) Observ care (99219)	70 Init hosp (99223) Observ care (99220)	15 Subsequent (99231)	25 Subsequent (99232)	35 Subsequent (99233)
Level	I	II	III	I	II	III

NURSING FACILITY

	Annual Assessment/Admission — Requires 3 components within shaded area			Subsequent Nursing Facility — Requires 2 components within shaded area			
	Old Plan Review	New Plan	Admission				
History	D/C	C	C	PF interval	EPF interval	D interval	C interval
Examination	D/C	C	C	PF	EPF	D	C
Complexity of Medical Decision	SF	M	M	SF	L	M	H
No Average Time Established (Confirmatory consults and ER have no average time)	(99304)	(99305)	(99306)	(99307)	(99308)	(99309)	(99310)
Level	I	II	III	I	II	III	IV

DOMICILIARY (REST HOME, CUSTODIAL CARE) AND HOME CARE

	New — Requires 3 components within shaded area					Established — Requires 2 components within shaded area			
History	PF	EPF	D	C	C	PF interval	EPF interval	D interval	C
Examination	PF	EPF	D	C	C	PF	EPF	D	C
Complexity of Medical Decision	SF	L	M	M	H	SF	L	M	H
Average Time (minutes)	20 Domiciliary (99324) 20 Home care (99341)	30 Domiciliary (99325) 30 Home care (99342)	45 Domiciliary (99326) 45 Home care (99343)	60 Domiciliary (99327) 60 Home care (99344)	75 Domiciliary (99328) 75 Home care (99345)	15 Domiciliary (99334) 15 Home care (99347)	25 Domiciliary (99335) 25 Home care (99348)	40 Domiciliary (99336) 40 Home care (99349)	60 Domiciliary (99337) 60 Home care (99350)
Level	I	II	III	IV	V	I	II	III	IV

PF = Problem focused   EPF = Expanded problem focused   D = Detailed   C = Comprehensive   SF = Straightforward   L = Low   M = Moderate   H = High

Tool to Determine Correct CPT® Code (continued)

UB-04 (CMS-1450) FORM

1	2	3a PAT CNTL #	4 TYPE OF BILL
		b MED REC #	
		5 FED. TAX. NO.	6 STATEMENT COVERS PERIOD FROM THROUGH	7

| 8 PATIENT NAME | a | 9 PATIENT ADDRESS | a |
| b | | b | c | d | e |

| 10 BIRTHDATE | 11 SEX | 12 DATE | ADMISSION 13 HR 14 TYPE 15 SRC | 16 DHR | 17 STAT | 18 | 19 | 20 | 21 | CONDITION CODES 22 23 24 25 26 27 28 | 29 ACDT STATE | 30 |

| 31 OCCURRENCE CODE   DATE | 32 OCCURRENCE CODE   DATE | 33 OCCURRENCE CODE   DATE | 34 OCCURRENCE CODE   DATE | 35 CODE | OCCURRENCE SPAN FROM   THROUGH | 36 CODE | OCCURRENCE SPAN FROM   THROUGH | 37 |
| a |
| b |

38		39 CODE VALUE CODES AMOUNT	40 CODE VALUE CODES AMOUNT	41 CODE VALUE CODES AMOUNT
		a		
		b		
		c		
		d		

42 REV.CD.	43 DESCRIPTION	44 HCPCS/RATE/HPPS CODE	45 SERV. DATE	46 SERV. UNIT	47 TOTAL CHARGES	48 NON-COVERED CHARGES	49
1							
2							
3							
4							
5							
6							
7							
8							
9							
10							
11							
12							
13							
14							
15							
16							
17							
18							
19							
20							
21							
22							
23	PAGE ____ OF ____	CREATION DATE	TOTALS				

50 PAYER NAME	51 HEALTH PLAN ID	52 REL INFO	53 ASG BEN	54 PRIOR PAYMENTS	55 EST. AMOUNT DUE	56 NPI	
A						57 OTHER PRV. ID	
B							
C							

58 INSURED'S NAME	59	60 INSURED'S UNIQUE ID	61 GROUP NAME	62 INSURANCE GROUP NO.
A				
B				
C				

63 TREATMENT AUTHORIZATION CODES	64 DOCUMENT CONTROL NUMBER	65 EMPLOYER NAME
A		
B		
C		

| 66 | 67 | A | B | C | D | E | F | G | H | 68 |
| | I | J | K | L | M | N | O | P | Q | |

| 69 ADMIT DX | 70 PATIENT REASON DX a b c | 71 PPS CODE | 72 ECI a b c | 73 |

74 PRINCIPAL PROCEDURE CODE DATE	a OTHER PROCEDURE CODE DATE	b OTHER PROCEDURE CODE DATE	75	76 ATTENDING	NPI	QUAL
				LAST		FIRST
c OTHER PROCEDURE CODE DATE	d OTHER PROCEDURE CODE DATE	e OTHER PROCEDURE CODE DATE		77 OPERATING	NPI	QUAL
				LAST		FIRST

80 REMARKS	81CC a		78 OTHER	NPI	QUAL
	b		LAST		FIRST
	c		79 OTHER	NPI	QUAL
	d		LAST		FIRST

Appendix E

Acronyms and Abbreviations

ABN	advanced beneficiary notice
AFDC	Aid to Families with Dependent Children
AHA	American Hospital Association
AMA	American Medical Association; against medical advice
ANSI	American National Standards Institute
APC	Ambulatory Payment Classification
ASC	ambulatory surgical center
ASU	ambulatory surgical unit
BCBSA	Blue Cross Blue Shield Association
CC	chief complaint; comorbidities and complications
CDM	charge description master
CHAMPUS	Civilian Health and Medical Program of the Uniformed Services
CHAMPVA	Civilian Health and Medical Program of the Department of Veterans Affairs
CLIA	Clinical Laboratory Improvement Amendments
CMN	certificate of medical necessity
CMP	competitive medical plan
CMS	Centers for Medicare and Medicaid Services
COB	coordination of benefits
COBRA	Consolidated Omnibus Budget Reconciliation Act of 1985
CPU	central processing unit
CSRS	Civil Service Retirement System
DEERS	Defense Enrollment Eligibility Reporting System
DHHS	Department of Health and Human Services
DME	durable medical equipment
DMERC	durable medical equipment resource center
DOB	date of birth
DOJ	Department of Justice
DRG	diagnosis-related group
ER	emergency department
EDI	electronic data interchange
EIN	employer identification number
EOB	Explanation of Benefits
EPO	exclusive provider organization
EPSDT	early and periodic screening, diagnosis, and treatment
ESRD	end-stage renal disease
FDA	Food and Drug Administration
FECA	Federal Employees' Compensation Act
FFS	fee for service
FICA	Federal Insurance Contribution Act
FPN	facility provider number
GHP	group health plan
g, gm	gram
GTIN	global trade item number
HCFA	Health Care Financing Administration
HCPCS	Healthcare Care Procedure Coding System

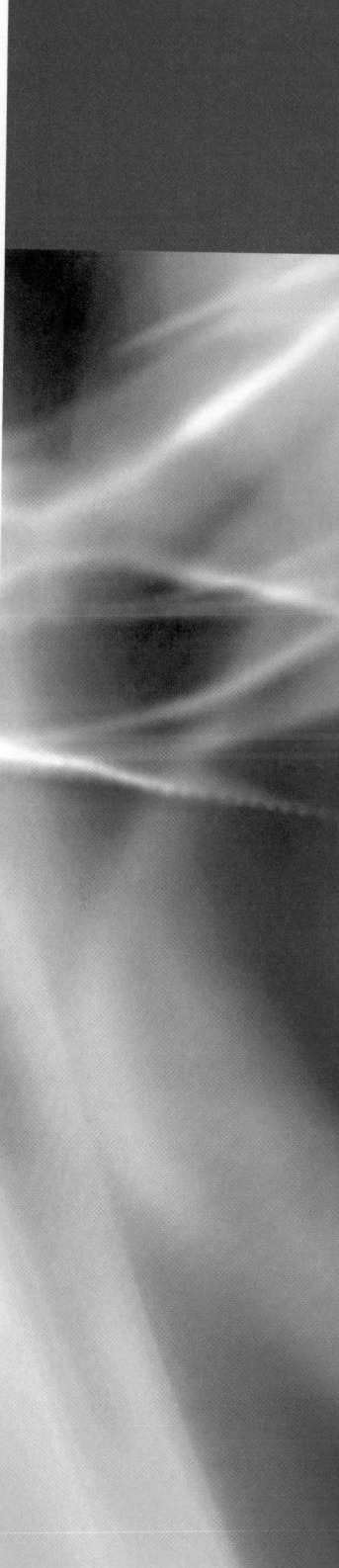

HIAA	Health Insurance Association of America
HIBCC	Health Industry Business Communications Council
HIC	health insurance claim
HIM	health information management
HIPAA	Health Insurance Portability and Accountability Act of 1996
HMO	health maintenance organization
HPI	history of present illness
ICD-9	International Classification of Diseases, Ninth Revision
ICD-9-CM	International Classification of Diseases, Ninth Revision, Clinical Modification
IDDM	insulin-dependent diabetes mellitus
LCD	Local Coverage Determination
LMRP	local Medicare review policy
LTR	lifetime reserve days
MCO	managed care organization
MDC	Major Diagnostic Categories
MFS	Medicare Fee Schedule
mL	milliliter
MOS	medical office specialist
MPM	medical practice management (software)
MQGE	Medicare qualified government employment
MRN	Medicare Remittance Notice
MSA	medical savings account
MSN	Medicare Summary Notice
MSP	Medicare secondary payer
NCCI	National Correct Coding Initiative
NDC	national drug codes
NIDDM	non-insulin-dependent diabetes mellitus
NOC	not otherwise classified
NPI	National Provider Identifier
NUCC	National Uniform Claim Committee
OCR	optical character recognition
OIG	Office of Inspector General
OPPS	outpatient prospective payment system
OTAF	obligated to accept as payment in full
PAR	participating provider
PAS	patient account services
PCN	patient control number
PCP	primary care physician
PFSH	past family social history
PIN	provider identification number
PMPM	per member per month
POS	point of service, place of service
PPIN	preferred provider identification number
PPO	preferred provider organization
PQRI	Physicians Quality Reporting Initiative
PSO	provider sponsored organization
QIC	qualified independent contractor
RBRVS	resource-based relative value scale
ROS	review of systems
RVU	relative value unit

SMI	supplemental medical insurance
SNF	skilled nursing facility
SOF	signature on file
SSA	Social Security Administration
SSDI	Social Security Disability Insurance
SSI	Supplemental Security Income
SSN	Social Security number
TANF	Temporary Assistance for Needy Families
TEFRA	Tax Equity Fiscal Responsibility Act
TRHCA	Tax Relief and Healthcare Act of 2006
UPC	Universal Product Code
UPIN	Unique Provider Identification Number
VOB	verification of benefits

Medical Terminology Word Parts

Medical terms are like individual jigsaw puzzles. Once you divide the terms into their component parts and learn the meaning of the individual parts, you can use that knowledge to understand many other new terms. Four basic component parts are used to create medical terms:

Root	The basic, or core, part that makes up the essential meaning of the term. The root usually, but not always, denotes a body part. Root words usually come from the Greek or Latin languages. For example, *bronch* is a root word that means "the air passages in the lungs" or "bronchial tubes." *Cephal* means "head." An extensive list of root words is given on page 770.
Prefix	One or more letters placed before the root to change its meaning. Prefixes usually, but not always, indicate location, time, number, or status. For example, the prefix *bi-* means "two" or "twice." When *bi* is placed before the root *lateral* ("side"), to form *bilateral*, the meaning is "having two sides." An extensive list of prefixes is given on page 770.
Suffix	One or more letters placed after the root to change its meaning. Suffixes usually, but not always, indicate the procedure, condition, disorder, or disease. For example, the suffix *-itis* means "inflammation," that is, damaged tissue that is red and painful. The medical term *bronchitis* means "inflammation of the bronchial tubes." Another example is the suffix *-ectomy*, which means "removal." Hence, *appendectomy* means "removal of the appendix." An extensive list of suffixes is given on page 773.
Combining vowel	A letter used to combine roots with other word parts. The vowel is usually an *o*, but sometimes it is an *a* or *i*. When a combining vowel is added to a root, the result is called a combining form. For example, in the word encephalogram, the root is *cephal* ("head"), the prefix is *en-* ("inside"), and the suffix is *-gram* ("something recorded"). These word parts are joined by the combining vowel *o* to make a word more easy to pronounce. *Cephal/o* is the combining form. An *encephalogram* is an x-ray of the inside of the head.

Analyzing a Medical Term

You can often decipher the meaning of a medical term by breaking it down into its separate parts. Consider the following examples:

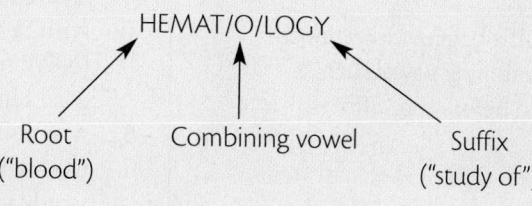

HEMAT/O/LOGY

Root
("blood")   Combining vowel   Suffix
("study of")

The term *hematology* is divided into three parts. When you analyze a medical term, begin at the end of the word. The ending is called the suffix. Almost all medical terms contain suffixes. The suffix in *hematology* is *-logy*, which means "study of." Now look at the beginning of the word. *Hemat* is the root word, which means "blood." The root word gives the essential meaning of the term.

The third part of this term, which is the letter *o*, has no meaning of its own, but is an important connector between the root (*hemat*) and the suffix (*logy*). It is the combining vowel. The letter *o* is the combining vowel usually found in medical terms.

Putting together the meanings of the suffix and the root, the term *hematology* means "the study of blood."

The combining vowel plus the root is called the combining form. A medical term can have more than one root word; therefore, there can be two combining forms. For example:

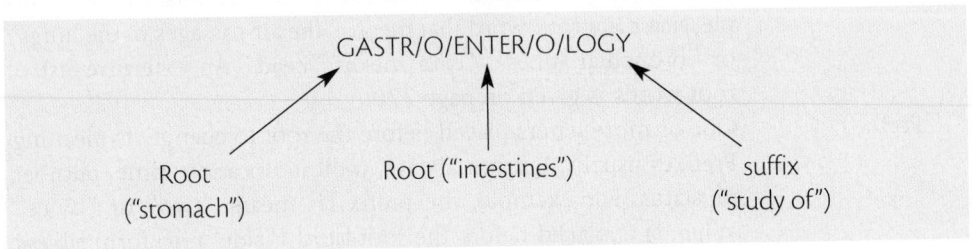

GASTR/O/ENTER/O/LOGY

Root   Root ("intestines")   suffix
("stomach")   ("study of")

The two combining forms are *gastr/o* and *enter/o*. The entire term (reading from the suffix, back to the beginning of the term, and across) means "the study of the stomach and the intestines."

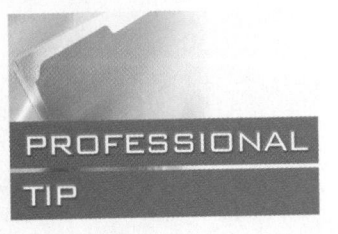

PROFESSIONAL TIP

A prefix does not require a combining vowel. Do not place a combining vowel between a prefix and a root word.

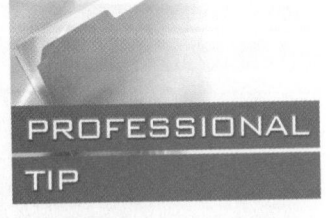

PROFESSIONAL TIP

Word Part Guidelines

1. A single root word with a combining form cannot stand alone. A suffix must be added to complete the term.
2. The rules for the use of combining vowels apply when adding a suffix.
3. When a suffix begins with a consonant, a combining vowel such as O, is placed before the suffix.

Rules for Using Combining Vowels

1. A combining vowel is not used when the suffix begins with a vowel (a-e-i-o-u). For example, when *neur/o* (nerve) is joined with the suffix *-itis* (inflammation), the combining vowel is not used because *-itis* begins with a vowel. *Neuritis* (new-RYE-tis) is an inflammation of a nerve or nerves.

2. A combining vowel is used when the suffix begins with a consonant. For example, when *neur/o* (nerve) is joined with the suffix *-plasty* (surgical repair), the combining vowel *o* is used because *-plasty* begins with a consonant. *Neuroplasty* (NEW-roh-plas-tee) is the surgical repair of a nerve.

3. A combining vowel is always used when two or more root words are joined. As an example,

when *gastr/o* (stomach) is joined with *enter/o* (small intestine), the combining vowel is used with *gastr/o*. *Gastroenteritis* (gas-troh-en-ter-EYE-tis) is an inflammation of the stomach and small intestine.

Suffixes and Medical Terms Related to Pathology

Pathology is the study of disease and the following suffixes describe specific disease conditions. (A more complete list of suffixes appears on page 773.)

Suffix	Meaning
-algia	pain and suffering
-dynia	pain
-ectomy	surgical removal
-graphy	process of recording a picture or record
-gram	record or picture
-necr/osis	death (tissue death)
-scler/osis	abnormal hardening
-sten/osis	abnormal narrowing
-centesis	surgical puncture to remove fluid for diagnostic purposes or to remove excess fluid
-plasty	surgical repair
-scopy	visual examination with an instrument

The Double RRs Suffixes

The following suffixes are often referred to as the "double RRs,"

* -rrhage and -rrhagia	Bursting form; an abnormal excessive discharge or bleeding. *Note: -rrhage* and *-rhagia* refer to the flow of blood.
* -rrhaphy	To suture or stitch.
* -rrhea	Abnormal flow or discharge; refers to the abnormal flow of most bodily fluids. *Note:* Although -rrhea and -rrhage both refer to abnormal flow, they are not used interchangeably.
* -rrhexis	Rupture.

Contrasting and Confusing Prefixes

The following contrasting prefixes can be confusing. Study this list to make sure you know the differences between the contrasting terms. (A more complete list of prefixes begins on page 770.)

Ab- Means "away from." *Abnormal* means not normal or away from normal.
Ad- Means "toward" or "in the direction." *Addiction* means drawn toward or a strong dependence on a drug or substance.

Dys- Means "bad," "difficult," "painful." *Dysfunctional* means an organ or body that is not working properly.
Eu- Means "good," normal, well, or easy. Euthyroid (you-THIGH-roid) means a normally functioning thyroid gland.

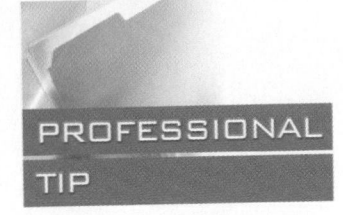

Learning to use a medical dictionary is an important part of mastering the correct use of medical terms. Some dictionaries use categories such as "Diseases and Syndromes" to group disorders with these terms in the titles. For example:

- Venereal disease would be found under "disease, venereal."
- Fetal alcohol syndrome would be found under "syndrome, fetal alcohol."

When you come across a term and cannot find it listed by the first word, the next step is to look under the appropriate category.

Hyper- Means "excessive" or "increased." *Hypertension* (high-per-TEN-shun) is higher than normal blood pressure.

Hypo- Means "deficient" or "decreased." *Hypotension* (high-poh-TEN-shun) is lower than normal blood pressure.

Inter- Means "between" or "among." *Interstitial* (in-ter-STISH-al) means between, but not within, the parts of a tissue.

Intra- Means "within" "into." *Intramuscular* (in-trah-MUS-kyou-lar) means within the muscle.

Sub- Means "under," "less," or "below." *Subcostal* (sub-KOS-tal) means below a rib or ribs.

Supra- Means "above." *Supracostal* (sue-prah-KOS-tal) means above or outside the ribs.

Singular and Plural Endings

Many medical terms have Greek or Latin origins. As a result of these different origins, the rules for changing a singular word into a plural form are unusual. Additionally, English endings have been adopted for some commonly used terms.

Guidelines to Unusual Plural Forms

Guideline	Singular	Plural
1. If the term ends in an *a*, the plural is usually formed by adding an *e*.	bursa vertebra	bursae vertebrae
2. If the term ends in *ex* or *ix*, the plural is usually formed by changing the *ex* or *ix* to *ices*.	appendix index	appendices indices
3. If the term ends in *is*, the plural is usually formed by changing the *is* to *es*.	diagnosis metastasis	diagnoses metastases
4. If the term ends in *itis*, the plural is usually formed by changing the *is* to *ides*.	arthritis meningitis	arthritides meningitides
5. If the term ends in *nx*, the plural is usually formed by changes the *x* to *ges*.	phalanx meninx	phalanges meninges
6. If the term ends in *on*, the plural is usually formed by changing the *on* to *a*.	criterion ganglion	criteria ganglia

7. If the term ends in *um*, the plural is usually formed by changing the *um* to *a*.

diverticulum   diverticula
ovum   ova

8. If the term ends in *us*, the plural is usually formed by changing the *us* to *i*.

alveolus   alveoli
malleolus   malleoli

Basic Medical Terms

The following subsections discuss basic medical terms that are used to describe diseases and disease conditions, major body systems, and body direction.

Terms Used to Describe Diseases and Disease Conditions

The basic medical terms used to describe diseases and disease conditions are listed here:

- A *sign* is evidence of disease, such as fever, that can be observed by the patient and others. A sign is objective because it can be evaluated or measured by others.
- A *symptom*, such as pain or a headache, can only be experienced or defined by the patient. A symptom is subjective because it can be evaluated or measured only by the patient.
- A *syndrome* is a set of signs and symptoms that occur together as part of a specific disease process.
- *Diagnosis* is the identification of disease. To diagnose is the process of reaching a diagnosis.
- A *differential diagnosis* attempts to determine which of several diseases may be producing the symptoms.
- A *prognosis* is a forecast or prediction of the probable course and outcome of a disorder.
- An *acute* disease or symptom has a rapid onset, a severe course, and relatively short duration.
- A *chronic* symptom or disease has a long duration. Although chronic symptoms or diseases may be controlled, they are rarely cured.
- A *remission* is the partial or complete disappearance of the symptoms of a disease without having achieved a cure. A remission is usually temporary.
- Some diseases are named for the condition described. For example, *chronic fatigue syndrome* (CFS) is a persistent overwhelming fatigue that does not resolve with bed rest.
- An *eponym* is a disease, structure, operation, or procedure that is named for the person who discovered or described it first.

> Accuracy in spelling medical terms is extremely important! Changing just one or two letters can completely change the meaning of the word—and this difference could literally be a matter of life or death for the patient.

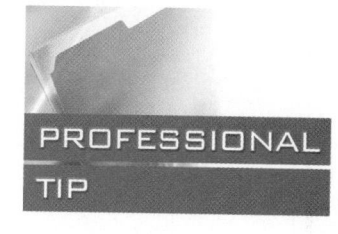

For example, Alzheimer's disease is named for Alois Alzheimer, a German neurologist who lived from 1864 to 1915.

- An *acronym* is a word formed from the initial letter or letters of the major parts of a compound term. For example, the acronym AMA stands for American Medical Association.

Terms Used to Describe Major Body Systems

The following is a list of the major body systems and some common related combining forms used with each.

Major Structures and Body System	Related Roots with Combining Forms

Skeletal system	bones (oste/o)
	  joints (arthr/o)
	  cartilage (chondr/o)

Muscular system	muscles (my/o)
	  ligaments (syndesm/o)
	  tendons (ten/o, tend/o, tendin/o)

Cardiovascular system	heart (card/o, cardi/o)
	  arteries (arteri/o)
	  veins (phleb/o, ven/o)
	  blood (hem/o, hemat/o)

Lymphatic and immune systems	lymph, lymph vessels, and lymph
	  nodes (lymph/o), (lymphangi/o)
	  tonsils (tonsill/o)
	  spleen (splen/o)
	  thymus (thym/o)

Respiratory system	nose (nas/o, rhin/o)
	  pharynx (pharyng/o)
	  trachea (trache/o)
	  larynx (laryng/o)
	  lungs (pneum/o, pneumon/o)

Digestive system	mouth (or/o)
	  esophagus (esophag/o)
	  stomach (gastr/o)
	  small intestines (enter/o)
	  large intestines (col/o)
	  liver (hepat/o)
	  pancreas (pancreat/o)

Urinary system	kidneys (nephr/o, ren/o)
	  ureters (ureter/o)
	  urinary bladder (cyst/o, visic/o)
	  urethra (urethr/o)

Integumentary system	glands (aden/o)
	  skin (cutane/o, dermat/o, derm/o)
	  sebaceous glands (seb/o)
	  sweat glands (hidraden/o)

Nervous system	nerves (neur/o)
	  brain (encephal/o)
	  spinal cord (myel/o)
	  eyes (ocul/o, ophthalm/o)
	  ears (acoust/o, ot/o)

Endocrine system	adrenals (adren/o)
	  pancreas (pancreat/o)
	  pituitary (pituit/o)
	  thyroid (thyr/o, thyroid/o)

parathyroids (parathyroid/o)
thymus (thym/o)

Reproductive system

Male:

testicles (orch/o, orchid/o)

Female:

ovaries (oophor/o, ovari/o)
uterus (hyster/o, metr/o, metri/o, uter/o)

Terms Used to Describe Body Direction

Certain terms are used to describe the location of body parts relative to the trunk or other parts of the anatomy.

Ventral (VEN-tral) refers to the front or belly side of the body or organ (*ventr* means "belly side" of the body and *al* means "pertaining to").

Dorsal (DOR-sal) refers to the back of the body or organ (*dors* means "back of body" and *al* means "pertaining to").

Anterior (an-TEER-ee-or) means situated in the front. It also means on the forward part of an organ (*anter* means "front" or "before" and *ior* means "pertaining to"). For example, the stomach is located anterior to (in front of) the pancreas. Anterior is also used in reference to the ventral surface of the body.

Posterior (pos-TEER-ee-or) means situated in the back. It also means on the back portion of an organ (*poster* means "back" or "after" and *ior* means "pertaining to"). For example, the pancreas is located posterior to (behind) the stomach. Posterior is also used in reference to the dorsal surface of the body.

Superior means uppermost, above, or toward the head. For example, the lungs are superior to (above) the diaphragm.

Inferior means lowermost, below, or toward the feet. For example, the stomach is located inferior to (below) the diaphragm.

Cephalic (seh-FAL-ick) means toward the head (*cephal* means "head" and *ic* means "pertaining to").

Caudal (KAW-dal) means toward the lower part of the body (*caud* means "tail" or "lower part" of the body and *al* means "pertaining to").

Proximal (PROCK-sih-mal) means situated nearest the midline or beginning of a body structure. For example, the proximal end of the humerus (the bone of the upper arm) forms part of the shoulder. Or, it may be easier for you to think of it as "closer to the origin of the body part or the point of attachment of a limb to the body trunk."

Distal (DIS-tal) means situated farthest from the midline or beginning of a body structure. For example, the distal end of the humerus forms part of the elbow.

Medial means the direction toward or nearer the midline. For example, the medial ligament of the knee is near the inner surface of the leg.

Lateral means the direction toward or nearer the side and away from the midline. For example, the lateral ligament of the knee is near the side of the leg.

Bilateral means relating to, or having, two sides.

Prefixes, Root Words, and Suffixes

The most common medical prefixes, root words, and suffixes are listed here. Knowing these common prefixes, roots, and suffixes will help you decipher medical terms.

Prefixes

a	without or absence of		inter	between
ab	from; away from		intra	within
ad	to; toward		mal	bad
an	without or absence of		meso	middle
ante	before		meta	after; beyond; change
anti	against		micro	small
bi	two		multi	many
bin	two		neo	new
brady	slow		nulli	none
con	together		pan	all; total
contra	against		para	outside; beyond; around
de	from; down from; lack of		per	through
dia	through; complete; between; apart		peri	surrounding (outer)
			poly	many; much
dis	to undo; free from		post	after
dys	difficult; labored; painful; abnormal		pre	before; in front of
			pro	before
ec	out		quadri	four
ecto	outside		re	back
endo	within		retro	back; behind
epi	on; upon; over		semi	half
eso	inward		sub	under; below
eu	normal; good		super	over; above
ex	outside; outward		supra	above; beyond; on top
exo	outside; outward		sym	together; joined
extra	outside of; beyond		syn	together; joined
hemi	half		tachy	fast; rapid
hyper	above; excessive		tetra	four
hypo	below; incomplete; deficient		trans	through; across; beyond
			tri	three
in	in; into; not		ultra	beyond; excess
infra	under; below		uni	one

Root Words

abdomin	abdomen		aur	ear
aden	gland		aut	self
adren	adrenal gland		bil	bile
adrenal	adrenal gland		bio	life
aer	air; oxygen; gas		blephar	eyelid
alveol	alveolus		bronch	airway; bronchus
angi	(blood) vessel; (lymph) vessel		bronchiol	bronchiole
			burs	bursa
ankyl	crooked; stiff; bent		carcin	cancer
appendic	appendix		cardi	heart
arteri, arter	artery		caud	tail; toward lower part of the body
arteriol	arteriole (small artery)			
arthr	joint		cephal	head
ather	yellowish; fatty plaque		cerebell	cerebellum
			cerebr	cerebrum; brain

cervic	neck; cervix	gingiv	gums
cheil	lip	glauc	gray
chiro	hand	gloss	tongue
cholangi	bile duct	gluc	sweetness; sugar
chole	gall; bile	glyc	sugar; glucose
chondr	cartilage	glycos	sugar; glucose
coccyg	coccyx; tailbone	gnos	knowledge; a knowing
col	colon; large intestine	gonad	gonad; sex glands
conjunctiv	conjunctiva	gyn	woman
corne	cornea	gynec	woman
coron	heart; crown of the head	gyr	turning; folding
		hem	blood
cost	rib	hemat	blood
crani	cranium; skull	hepat	liver
cutane	skin	hidr	sweat
cyan	blue	hist	tissue
cyst	bladder; sac	hom	same
cyt, cyte	cell	home	sameness; unchanging
dacry	tears; tear duct	hydr	water
dactyl	fingers or toes	hyster	uterus
dent	tooth	ile	ileum
derm	skin	ili	ilium
dermat	skin	immun	immune
dipl	two; double	irid	iris
diverticul	diverticulum	kerat	horny tissue; hard
dors	back (of the body)	kin	movement
duoden	duodenum	kinesi	movement; motion
ectop	located away from usual place	labi	lips
		lacrim	tear duct; tear
edema	swelling	lact	milk
electr	electricity; electrical activity	lapar	abdomen
		laryng	larynx
encephal	brain	later	side
endocrin	endocrine	lei	smooth
enter	intestines (usually small intestine)	leuk	white
		lingu	tongue
epiglott	epiglottis	lip	fat
epitheli	epithelium	lith	stone; calculus
erythr	red	lob	lobe
esophag	esophagus	lymph	lymph
esthesi	sensation; feeling; sensitivity	macr	abnormal largeness
		mamm	breast
eti	cause (of disease)	mast	breast
exocrin	secrete out of	meat	opening or passageway
faci	face	melan	black
fasci	fascia; fibrous band	men	menstruation
fract	break; broken	mening	meninges
galact	milk	ment	mind
gastr	stomach	mes, meso	middle
ger	old age; aged	metr	uterus
geront	old age; aged	mon	one

morbid	disease; sickness	pneum	lung; air
muc	mucus	pneumat	lung; air
my, myos	muscle	pneumon	lung; air
myc	fungus	pod	foot
myel	bone marrow; spinal cord	poli	gray matter
		polyp	polyp; small growth
myelon	bone marrow	poster	back (of body)
myring	eardrum	prim	first
narc	stupor; numbness	proct	rectum
nas	nose	pseud	fake; false
nat	birth	psych	mind
necr	death (cells; body)	pulmon	lung
nephr	kidney	py	pus
neur	nerve	pyel	renal pelvis
noct	night	pylor	pylorus
nyct	night	pyr	fever; heat
nyctal	night	quadr	four
ocul	eye	rect	rectum
onc	tumor	ren	kidney
onych	nail	retin	retina
oophor	ovary	rhin	nose
ophthalm	eye	sacr	sacrum fallopian (uterine)
or	mouth		
orth	straight	salping	tube
oste	bone	sanit	soundness; health
ot	ear	sarc	flesh; connective tissue
ox	oxygen	scler	sclera; white of eye; hard
palpat	touch; feel; stroke		
pancreat	pancreas	scoli	crooked; curved
par, part	bear; give birth to; labor	seb	sebum; oil
		seps	infection
parathyroid	parathyroid	sept	infection; partition; septum
path	disease; suffering		
pector	chest; muscle	sial	saliva
ped	child; foot	sinus	inus
pelv	pelvis; pelvic bone	somat	body
pen	penis	somn	sleep
perine	perineum	son	sound
peritone	peritoneum	sopor	sleep
petr	stone; portion of temporal bone	sperm	sperm, spermatazoa; seed
phac, phak	lens of the eye	spermat	sperm, spermatazoa; seed
phag	eat; swallow		
phalang	finger or toe bone	spher	round; sphere; ball
pharyng	pharynx, throat	sphygm	pulse
phas	speech	spin	spine; backbone to
phleb	vein	spir	breathe
phot	light	splen	spleen
phren	mind	spondyl	vertebra; spinal or vertebral column
physi	nature		
pleur	pleura	staphyl	grapelike clusters

stern	(breastbone)	urin	urine or urinary organs
steth	chest (muscles)	uter	uterus
stoma	mouth; opening	uvul	vula; little grape
stomat	mouth; opening	vagin	vagina
strab	squint; squint-eyed	valv	valve
synovi	synovia; synovial membrane	valvul	valve
		vas	vessel; duct
system	system	vascul	blood vessel; little vessel
ten, tend	tendon	ven	vein
tendin	tendon	versicul	seminal vesicles; blister
test	testis; testicle	vertebr	vertebra; backbone
therm	heat	vesic	urinary bladder
thorac	thorax; chest	vir	poison; virus
thromb	clot	viril	masculine; manly
thym	thymus gland; soul	vis	seeing; sight
thyr	thyroid gland	visc	sticky
thyroid	thyroid gland	viscer	viscera; internal organs sternum
tom	cut; section		
ton	tension; pressure	viscos	sticky
tone	to stretch	vit	life
tonsill	tonsils	xanth	yellow
top	place; position; location	xen	strange; foreign
		xer	dry
tox, toxic	poison; poisonous	zygot	joined together
trach, trache	trachea; windpipe		
trachel	neck; necklike		
trich	hair		
tubercul	little knot; swelling		
tympan	eardrum; middle ear		
ulcer	sore; ulcer		
ungu	nail		
ur	urine; urinary tract		
ureter	ureter		
urethr	urethra		
uria	urination; urine		

Additional Rootwords

caus	burning sensation; capable of burning
cusp	point; cusp
flexion	bending
genital	pertaining to birth
lumb	lumbar; loin region
mediastin	mediastinum
tens, tensi	pressure, force, stretching

Suffixes

Suffixes Meaning "Pertaining to"

ac		eal	ous
al	ine	ial	
ar	ior	ic	
ary	ory	ical	tic

Suffixes Meaning "Abnormal Conditions"

ago	abnormal condition, disease
esis	abnormal condition, disease
ia	abnormal condition, disease
iasis	abnormal condition, disease
ion	condition

ism	condition, state of abnormal condition		
osis	disease		

Common Suffixes Used in Medical Terminology

algia	pain, suffering	meter	instrument used to measure
asthenia	weakness		
cele	hernia, protrusion	metry	measurement
centesis	surgical puncture to remove fluid	morph	form; shape
		oid, ode	resembling
cidal	killing	oma	tumor; mass
clasia	break	opia	vision (condition)
clasis	break	opsy	to view
clast	break	oxia	oxygen
clysis	irrigating; washing	paresis	slight paralysis
coccus	berry shaped (a form of bacterium)	pathy	disease
		penia	abnormal reduction in number; lack of
crine	separate; secrete		
crit	to separate		
cyte	cell	peps, pepsia	digestion
desis	fusion; to bind; tie together	pexy	surgical fixation; suspension
drome	run; running	phagia	eating; swallowing
ductor	to lead or pull	philia	love
dynia	pain	phily	love
ectasis	stretching out; dilation; expansion	phobia	abnormal fear of or adversion to specific objects or things
ectomy	excision or surgical removal		
ectopia	displacement	phonia	sound or voice
emesis	vomiting	phoria	feeling
emia	blood; blood condition	physis	growth
gen	producing, forming	plasia	formation; development; a growth
genesis	producing; forming		
genic	producing, forming	plasm	growth; formation; substance
gnosis	a knowing		
gram	record; x-ray	plasty	plastic or surgical repair
graph	instrument used to record		
graphy	process of recording; x-ray filming	plegia	paralysis; stroke
		pnea	breathing
ictal	seizure; attack	porosis	lessening in density; porous condition
ism	state of		
itis	inflammation		
lepsy	seizure	praxia	in front of; before
logist	specialist	ptosis	drooping; sagging; prolapse
logy	study of		
lysis	destruction; reduce; separation	ptysis	spitting
		rrhage	bursting forth, an abnormal excessive discharge or bleeding
malacia	softening		
mania	madness; insane desire		
megaly	enlargement		

rrhagia	bursting forth, an abnormal excessive discharge or bleeding	stalsis	contraction; con-striction
rrhaphy	to suture or stitch	stasis	control; stop; standing still
rrhea	abnormal flow or dis-charge	stat	to stop
rrhexis	rupture	stenosis	narrowing; con-striction
schisis	split; fissure	stomy	new artificial opening
sclerosis	hardening		
scope	instrument used for visual exam	therapy	treatment
		tome	instrument used to cut
scopic	visual exam		
scopy	visual exam with an instrument	tomy	cutting into; sur-gical incision
sepsis	infection	tripsy	crushing
sis	state of	trophy	nourishment
spasm	sudden involuntary muscle contraction	ule	little
		uria	urine; urination

Helpful Websites

Chapter 1: Introduction to Professional Billing and Coding Careers

Alliance of Claims Assistance Professionals	*www.claims.org*
American Academy of Professional Coders	*www.aapc.com*
American Association for Medical Transcription	*www.aamt.org*
American Health Information Management Association	*www.ahima.org*
American Medical Billing Association	*www.ambanet.net*
Health Professions Institute	*www.hpisum.com*
Healthcare Information and Management Systems Society	*www.himss.org*
Medical Association of Billers	*www.physicianswebsites.com*
Medical Coding and Billing	*www.medicalcodingandbilling.com*
Medical Group Management Association	*www.mgma.com*
Medical Records Institute	*www.medrecinst.com*
MT Jobs	*www.mtjobs.com*
MT Monthly	*www.mtmonthly.com*
National Center for Competency Testing	*www.NCCTinc.com*
National Health Career Association	*www.nha2000.com*
Professional Association of Health Care Office Managers	*www.pahcom.com*

Chapter 2: Managed Care Terminology

Blue Cross Blue Shield Association: "Blues History"	*www.bcbs.com*
California Health Care Foundation: "Making Sense of Managed Care Regulations in California"	*www.chcf.org*
Centers for Medicare and Medicaid Services: "Key Milestones in CMS Programs"	*www.cms.gov*
Damir Wallener, WiseGeek	*www.wisegeek.com/what-are-the-different-type-of-health-insurance.htm*

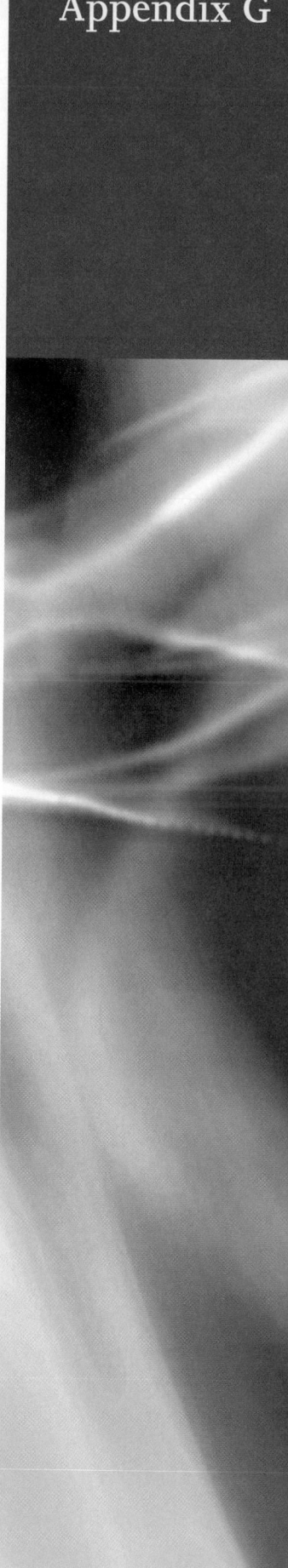

Kaiser Permanente: "History of Kaiser Permanente"	*www.kp.org*
Managed Care Museum	*www.managedcaremuseum.com*
MCOL Managed Care Fact Sheets	*www.mcol.com*
NCQA Timelines	*www.ncqa.org/about/timeline.htm*
Public's Library and Digital Archive	*www.ibiblio.org*
Tufts Managed Care Institute: "A Brief History of Managed Care"	*www.thci.org*

Chapter 3: Understanding Managed Care: Medical Contracts and Ethics

American Cancer Society	*www.cancer.org*
Federal Government: Resources for Consumers	*www.consumer.gov*
Healthcare Fraud	*http://atlanta.fbi.gov/dojpressrel/ pressrel06/healthcarefraud060206 .htm*
Office of Inspector General	*www.oig.hhs.gov*

Chapter 4: ICD-9 Medical Coding

Assistance with Coding and Medical Terminology	*www.icd9.chrisendres.com*
Bills of Mortality	*www.davidorme.demon.co.uk/ plague10.htm*
ICD-9-CM and ICD-10-CM Development	*www.cdc.gov/nchs/icd9.htm*
ICD-9-CM Encoder	*www.icd9coding.com*

Chapter 5: Introduction to CPT and Place of Service Coding

American Medical Association-current procedural terminology	*www.ama-assn.org/go/CPT*
American Medical Association-CPT network	*www.cptnetwork.com*

Chapter 6: Coding Procedures and Services

American Association of Anesthesiologists	*www.asahq.org*

Chapter 7: HCPCS and Coding Compliance

Compliance Training Manual	*www.usc.edu/health/uscp/ compliance/tm1.html#1*

Chapter 8: Auditing

American Academy of Neurology   www.aan.com/professionals/
                                             coding/Internal_Auditing.pdf

Chapter 9: Physician Medical Billing

Healthcare Financial Management Association   www.hfma.org/library/revenue/
                                               PatientFriendlyBilling/

Chapter 10: Hospital Medical Billing

Healthcare Financial Management Association   www.hfma.org/library/revenue/
                                               PatientFriendlyBilling/

Chapter 11: Medicare Medical Billing

TrailBlazer Health Enterprises, L.L.C.   www.trailblazerhealth.com

Chapter 12: Medicaid Medical Billing

Medicaid Billing/Claim Handbook   www.oms.nysed.gov/medicaid/
                                               guidebook/guideboo.htm

Chapter 13: TRICARE Medical Billing

TRICARE—Military Health System   www.tricare.mil/provider.aspx

TRICARE—Military Explanation of Benefits   www.tricare.mil/eob/

Chapter 14: Explanation of Benefits and Payment Adjudication

How to read and explain your   www.beneplan.com
   Explanation of Benefits

Chapter 15: Refunds and Appeals

Aetna   www.aetna.com

Claims Resolution for Healthcare Providers   www.appealsolutions.com

Chapter 16: Workers' Compensation

U.S. Department of Labor: Federal Workers'   www.dol.gov/dol/topic/
   Compensation   workcomp

U.S. Department of Labor: OSHA   www.osha.gov

U.S. Department of Labor: State   www.dol.gov/esa/regs/compliance
   Workers' Compensation

Chapter 17: Electronic Medical Claims Processing

Retrieving and Processing medical provider payments	*http://www.freepatentsonline.com/ 20030120632.html*

Government Websites

Agency for Healthcare Policy and Research	*www.ahcpr.gov*
Centers for Medicare and Medicaid (CMS)	*www.hcfa.gov*
Coverage Issues Manual for Medical Procedures	*www.hcfa.gov/pubforms*
Department of Health and Human Services	*www.dhhs.gov*
Health Insurance Portability and Accountability Act	*http://aspe.os.dhhs.gov; http://www.cms.hhs.gov/hipaa*
Healthfinder	*www.healthfinder.gov*
Joint Commission on Accreditation of Healthcare Organizations	*www.jcaho.org*
Social Security Online	*www.ssa.gov*
U.S. Department of Health and Human Services' Office of the Inspector General	*www.dhhs.gov/progorg/oig*

Medicolegal

American Health Lawyer Association	*www.healthlawyers.org*
Health Insurance Portability and Accountability Act	*http://aspe.os.dhhs.gov*
MediRegs a Government search engine	*www.mediregs.com/index.html*
MedNets Government Searchable Databases	*www.internets.com/mednets/ smedgovt.htm*
National Healthcare Antifraud Association	*www.nhcaa.org*

Coding Resources

American Academy of Professional Coders	*www.aapcnatl.org*
American College of Healthcare Executives	*www.ache.org*
American College of Legal Medicine	*www.aclm.org*
Appeal Letter (published quarterly by Appeal Solutions to assist medical providers in appealing denied insurance claims)	*www.integsoft.com/appeals/ tal/index.htm*
Health Care Compliance Association	*www.hcca-info.org*
Just Coding.com	*www.justcoding.com*

Medical Professionals, Inc.	*www.medprofs.com*
Medline (U.S. National Library of Medicine)	*www.nlm.nih.gov/databases/ freemedl.html*
Medsite's clinical information search tool	*http://206.132.0.133/medline/ basic.cfm*
Online Medicare Coding & Billing Training from First Coast Service Options	*www.medicaretraining.com/ cbt.htm*

HIPAA Regulations

The Health Insurance Portability and Accountability Act (Public Law 104–191), or HIPAA, was passed in 1996. There is much involved in HIPAA, but the part that is the most important to the medical office specialist (MOS) is the Administrative Simplification subsection, or Title II. The Administrative Simplification subsection (Title II, Subtitle F) (hereafter referred to simply as HIPAA) has four distinct components:

1. Transactions and code sets
2. Uniform identifiers
3. Privacy
4. Security

HIPAA regulates health plans, clearinghouses, and healthcare providers as "covered entities" with regard to these four areas.

Transactions and Code Sets

HIPAA standardized the formats for electronic data interchange (EDI) by requiring specific transaction standards. These standards are currently used for eight types of electronic health transactions between covered entities: (1) health plan eligibility, (2) enrollment and disenrollment in a health plan, (3) health claims, (4) payments for care and health plan premiums, (5) claim status, (6) First Report of Injury reports, (7) coordination of benefits, and (8) related transactions.

Historically, medical providers and insurance plans used many different electronic formats to exchange, or transact, medical claims and related business. Implementing a national standard will result in the use of one format, thereby simplifying, improving, and making transactions more efficient nationwide. This standardization of formats was the first part of the Administrative Simplification subsection to be implemented. This section also requires standardized code sets such as the HCPCS, CPT-4®, ICD-9-CM, and other codes to be used.

Uniform Identifiers

HIPAA also established uniform identifier standards, which will be used on all claims and other data transmissions. These standard identifiers include the following:

- The *National Provider Identifier* (NPI) is assigned to doctors, nurses, and other healthcare providers. The use of the NPI has been in effect since May 2007 for Medicare providers.
- The *Federal Employer Identification Number* is used to identify employer-sponsored health insurance. The EIN, or tax identification number, is used.
- The *National Health Plan Identifier* is a unique identification number that will be assigned to each insurance plan, and to the organizations that administer insurance plans, such as payers and third-party administrators.

CPT is a registered trademark of the American Medical Association.

Privacy Standards

The HIPAA privacy standards are designed to protect a patient's identifiable health information from unauthorized disclosure or use in any form, while permitting the practice to deliver the best health care possible. To comply with the law that became effective April 14, 2003, privacy activities in the average medical office might include these:

- Providing a copy of the office privacy policy informing patients about their privacy rights and how their information can be used.
- Asking the patient to acknowledge receiving a copy of the policy or signing a consent form.
- Obtaining signed authorization forms and in some cases tracking the disclosures of patient health information when it is to be given to a person or organization outside the practice for purposes other than treatment, billing, or payment.
- Adopting clear privacy procedures for its practice.
- Training employees so that they understand the privacy procedures.
- Designating an individual to be responsible for seeing that the privacy procedures are adopted and followed.
- Securing patient records containing individually identifiable health information so that they are not readily available to those who do not need them.

The privacy and security rules use two acronyms that the MOS should learn: PHI, which stands for protected health information, and EPHI, which stands for protected health information in an electronic format.

One example of implementation. Before HIPAA's privacy rule went into effect, medical practices routinely kept a sign-in sheet or registration sheet at the receptionist's desk. Multiple lines on this sheet allowed each patient arriving for an appointment to sign his or her name. This not only let patients see how many others had arrived before them that day but also gave them the name of each patient who had arrived before them. To protect the privacy of all patients, covered entities now use a single-page sign-in sheet or registration sheet. One patient writes his or her name on the sheet and it is then torn off or removed from the pad. Some practices use self-stick labels to serve the same purpose and save paper.

When the privacy rule initially was issued, it required providers to obtain patient "consent" to use and disclose PHI for purposes of treatment, payment, and healthcare operations, except in emergencies. The rule was almost immediately revised to make consent optional. In general, the practice can use PHI for almost anything related to treating the patient, running the medical practice, and getting paid for services. This means doctors, nurses, and other staff can share the patient's chart within the practice.

Authorization differs from consent in that it does require the patient's permission to disclose PHI. Some examples of instances that would require an authorization would include sending the results of an employment physical to an employer or sending immunization records or the results of an athletic physical to a school.

The authorization form must include the date signed, an expiration date, to whom the information may be disclosed, what information is permitted to be disclosed, and for what purpose the information may be used. The authorization must be signed by the patient or a representative appointed by the patient. Unlike the open concept of consent, authorizations are not global. A new authorization is signed each time there is a different purpose or need for the patient's information to be disclosed.

Practices are permitted to disclose PHI without a patient's authorization or consent when it is requested by an authorized government agency. Generally such requests are for legal (law enforcement, subpoena, court orders, etc.) public health purposes or for enforcement of the privacy rule itself. Providers also are permitted to disclose PHI concerning on-the-job injuries to workers' compensation insurers, state administrators, and other entities to the extent required by state law.

Whether the practice has disclosed PHI based on a signed authorization or to comply with a government agency, the patient is entitled to know about it. The privacy rule gives individuals the right to receive a report of all disclosures made for purposes other than treatment, payment, or operations. Therefore, in most cases the medical office must track the disclosure and keep the records for at least 6 years.

Most healthcare providers and health plans use the services of a variety of other persons or businesses. HIPAA's privacy rule allows covered providers and health plans to disclose protected health information to these "business associates." The privacy rule requires a covered entity to obtain a written agreement from its business associate, which states that the business associate will appropriately safeguard the protected health information it receives or creates on behalf of the covered entity.

Congress provided civil and criminal penalties for covered entities that misuse personal health information. The privacy rule is enforced by the Department of Health and Human Services' Office for Civil Rights (OCR).

Security Standards

Whereas the privacy rule applies to all forms of patients' protected health information, whether electronic, written, or oral, the security rule covers only protected health information that is in electronic form.

Security standards were designed to provide guidelines to all types of covered entities, while affording them flexibility regarding how to implement the standards. Covered entities may use appropriate security measures that enable them to reasonably implement a standard. Security standards were designed to be "technology neutral." That is, the rule does not prescribe the use of specific technologies, so that the healthcare community will not be bound by specific systems or software that may become obsolete.

The security standards are divided into the categories of administrative, physical, and technical safeguards:

- *Administrative safeguards.* In general, these are the administrative functions that should be implemented to meet the security standards. These include assignment or delegation of security responsibility to an individual and security training requirements.
- *Physical safeguards.* In general, these are the mechanisms required to protect electronic systems—their equipment and the data they hold—from threats, environmental hazards, and unauthorized intrusion. They include restricting access to EPHI and retaining off-site computer backups.
- *Technical safeguards.* In general, these are primarily the automated processes used to protect data and control access to data. They include using authentication controls to verify that the person signing onto a computer is authorized to access that EPHI, or encrypting and decrypting data as it is being stored or transmitted.

Computer passwords and software security levels are some examples of technical safeguards. Not everyone in an organization needs access to EPHI. Software program security levels establish which user may or may not access certain information in the software program. For EPHI, the registrar may need to enter insurance and demographic information on the patient, but may not need access to actual medical record documentation areas. A locked filing cabinet or locked room containing the filing cabinets for paper medical charts is another security measure.

The original security rule also proposed a standard for electronic signatures. The final rule, however, covered only security standards. In 2000, President Clinton signed into federal law the Electronic Signatures in Global and National Commerce Act, which made digital signatures as binding as their paper-based counterparts. Although the law made digital signatures valid for commerce, HIPAA does not require the use of electronic signatures. Electronic signature standards will eventually be necessary to achieve a completely paperless health electronic record (HER). A rule for electronic signature standards may be proposed at a later date. For now, a valid electronic signature must meet three criteria:

1. *Message integrity.* The recipient must be able to confirm that the document has not been altered since it was signed.
2. *Nonrepudiation.* The signer must not be able to deny signing the document.
3. *User authentication.* The recipient must be able to confirm that the signature was in fact "signed" by the real person.

Digital signatures meet all three of these criteria. Digital signatures use a branch of mathematics called cryptography and PKI, which stands for Public Key Infrastructure. Each PKI user has two "keys," a private key for signing documents and a public key for verifying his or her signature. A computer software program performs a mathematical calculation on the entire contents of the electronic document to be signed. The result is a unique "message digest," which is then encrypted using the private key.

The digital signature is then attached to or sent with the document. When the recipient wishes to validate the signature, a similar computer program regenerates the "message digest" and decodes the digital signature with the public key. Comparing the two, the program determines if the message digest is identical to that which was originally sent. In this way digital signatures not only confirm that you are the signer but also that the document has not been altered since it was signed.

Compliance

Continued, ongoing training is required for HIPAA compliance. A one-time introduction is not sufficient. A medical office or facility will assign a designated person to fill the role as a Compliance Officer. A Compliance Officer is responsible for reviewing office policies and procedures to assure that all applicable HIPAA laws, rules and regulations are being followed. HIPAA regulations may change over time, so it is important for the compliance officer to be up to date on current regulations and conduct training seminars throughout the year. In a small and medium size facility the Office Manager is usually assigned this responsibility. A large facility or hospital may assign a staff member to act as the Compliance Officer. In a hospital setting it is common for there to be a Director of Compliance who reviews policies and procedures with a compliance committee. It is imperative that each medical office and facility commit to comply day-to-day with the ethical and legal standards established in the applicable laws and regulations.

Introduction to Medisoft Advanced (version 12) and Office Simulation

Medisoft Advanced is a medical practice management software program that offers choices of actions through a series of menus. Commands are issued by clicking an option on the menu bar or by clicking a shortcut button on the toolbar. All data, whether a patient's address or a charge for a procedure, is entered into Medisoft through menus on the menu bar or through the buttons on the toolbar. Selecting an option from the menus or toolbar brings up a dialog box. The TAB key is used to move between text boxes within a dialog box.

The menu bar lists the names of the menus in Medisoft: File, Edit, Activities, Lists, Reports, Tools, Window, Services, and Help. Beneath each menu name is a pull-down menu of one or more options.

Menu Bar Titles

The purpose of each menu is briefly described as follows:

File Menu The File menu is used to enter information about the medical office practice when first setting up Medisoft. It is also used to back up data, maintain files, and set up program options.

Edit Menu The Edit menu contains the basic commands needed to move, change, or delete information. These commands are Undo, Cut, Copy, Paste, and Delete.

Activities Menu Most medical office data collected on a day-to-day basis is entered through options on the Activities menu. This menu is used to enter information about patients' office visits, including diagnoses and procedures performed. Transactions, including charges, payments, and adjustments, are also entered via the Activities menu.

Lists Menu Information on new patients, such as name, address, and employer, is entered through the Lists menu. The Lists menu also provides access to lists of codes, insurance carriers, and providers.

Reports Menu The Reports menu is used to print reports about patients' accounts and other reports about the practice.

Tools Menu The calculator is accessed through the Tools menu. Other options on the Tools menu can be used to view the contents of a file as well as a profile of the computer system.

Window Menu Using the Window menu, it is possible to switch back and forth between several open windows.

Services Menu This menu contains links for electronic transmission of insurance claims, electronic prescriptions, and electronic eligibility verification.

Help Menu The Help menu is used to access Medisoft's Help feature.

Basic Medisoft Actions

In this section we discuss some of the basic tasks that all medical office specialists should be able to perform with the Medisoft software.

Saving Data

Information entered into Medisoft is saved by clicking the Save button that appears in most dialog boxes (those in which data is input).

Deleting Data

The majority of Medisoft dialog boxes have buttons for the purpose of deleting data.

Exiting Medisoft

Medisoft is exited by clicking Exit on the File menu or by clicking the Exit button on the toolbar.

Entering Patient Information into Medisoft

Patient information is entered in the Patient/Guarantor dialog box, accessed by clicking Patient/Guarantors and Cases on the **Lists** menu. The Patient List dialog box displays a list of established patients. Information on a new patient is entered by clicking the *New Patient* button at the bottom of the dialog box. The Patient/Guarantor dialog box contains four tabs: the **Name, Address** tab, **Other Information** tab, **Payment Plan** tab, and **Custom** tab (Figure I.1).

Name, Address Tab. This tab is completed with information provided by a new patient on the practice's patient information form. Most of the information is demo-

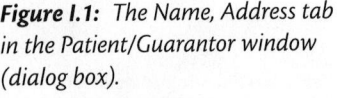

Figure I.1: *The Name, Address tab in the Patient/Guarantor window (dialog box).*

graphic: name, address, phone numbers, birth date, gender, and Social Security number. Phone numbers must be entered without parentheses or hyphens. The birth date is entered using the eight-digit MMDDCCYY format. The nine-digit Social Security number should be entered with hyphens. Some of the boxes, such as the cell phone number and fax number boxes, are optional.

Chart Number: The chart number is a unique number that identifies each patient. The most common method of assigning a number is to use the first three letters of the last name, the first two letters of the first name, and the digit 0, which represents head of household. If the last name has less than five letters, use more letters of the first name and even of the middle name if necessary. It is not necessary to enter a chart number when entering a new patient. If you choose not to enter one, Medisoft will assign one for you. It is important to note that once the Chart Number is set it cannot be changed. To correct an incorrect chart number, the patient and case information would have to be deleted then re-created with the correct Chart Number.

Other Information Tab. The Other Information tab (Figure I.2) contains facts about a patient's employment and other miscellaneous information. The major fields in the Other Information tab are:

Type: The Type drop-down list designates whether, for billing purposes, an individual is a patient or a guarantor. A guarantor is someone who is responsible for insurance and payment.

Assigned Provider: The code for the specific doctor who provides care to this patient is selected.

Signature on File: A check mark in the Signature on File check box means that the patient's signature is on file for the purpose of submitting insurance claims.

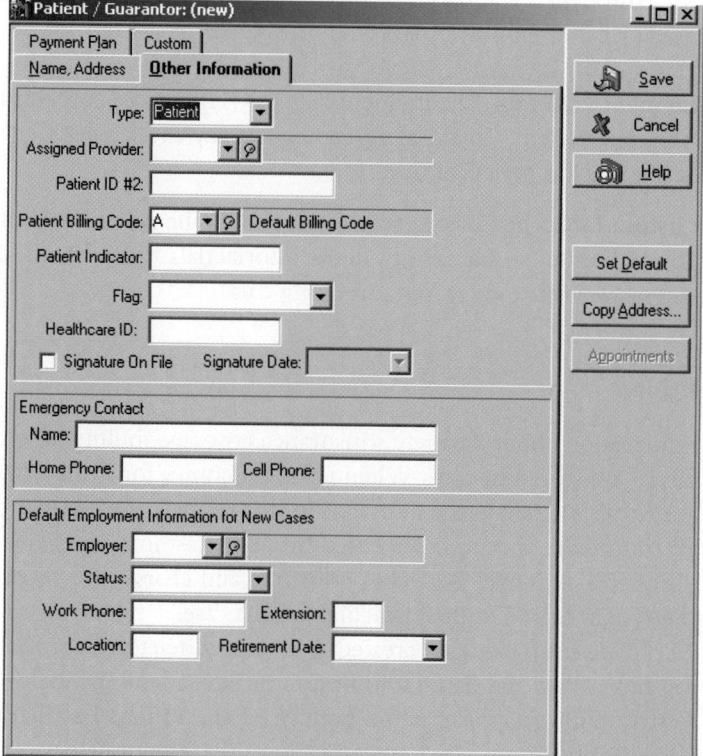

Figure I.2: *The Other Information tab in the Patient/Guarantor window.*

Figure I.3: The Payment Plan tab in the Patient/Guarantor window.

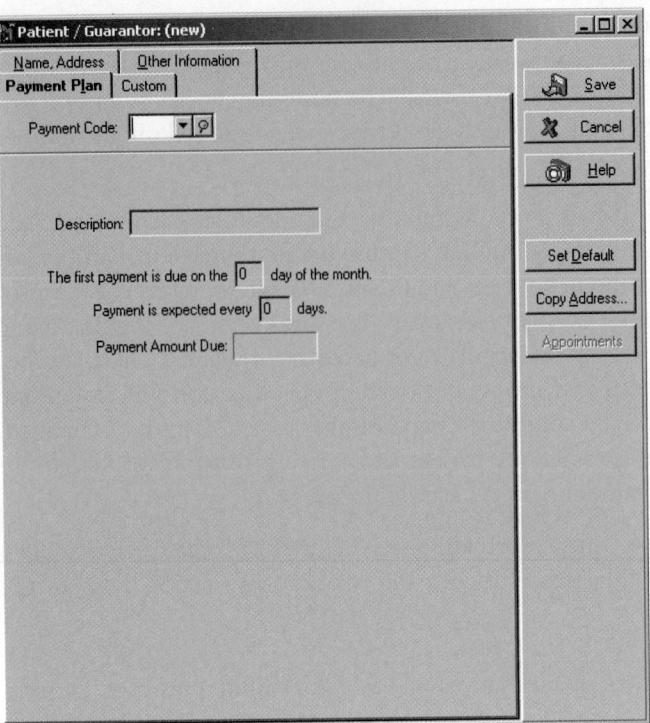

Signature Date: The date keyed in the Signature Date box is the date the patient signed the release of information form.

Emergency Contact: The name the patient/guarantor has written on the patient information form as an emergency contact is keyed in here, along with any phone numbers provided.

Employer: The name of the patient's employer is selected from the drop-down list of employers stored in the database.

Payment Plan Tab. The Payment Plan tab (Figure I.3) contains data regarding a patient who has signed a financial agreement to pay the facility the balance on the account over a specific period of time.

Custom Tab. The Custom tab is designed by the particular facility to contain information important to that facility. In the tutorial data for Medisoft, the Custom tab contains height, weight, and cigarette smoking data.

Cases

Information about a patient's insurance coverage, billing account, diagnosis, and condition are stored in cases. When a patient comes for treatment, a case is created. Cases are set up to contain the transactions that relate to a particular condition. For example, all treatments and procedures for bronchial asthma would be stored in a case called "Bronchial Asthma." Services performed and charges for those services are entered in the system linked to the bronchial asthma case.

In Medisoft cases are created, edited, and deleted from within the **Patient List** dialog box. When the Case radio button in the Patient List dialog box is clicked, the following buttons appear at the bottom of the Patient List dialog box: Edit Case, New Case, Delete Case, Copy Case, and Close. These buttons perform their respective functions on cases. For example, to create a new case, the New Case button is clicked. Data recorded in the Case dialog box is stored by clicking the Save button on the right side of the Case dialog box.

Entering Case Information

Information on a patient is entered in 11 different tabs within the Case dialog box: Personal, Account, Diagnosis, Policy 1, Policy 2, Policy 3, Condition, Miscellaneous, Medicaid and Tricare, Comment, and EDI. A 12th tab, Custom One, allows the facility to create and design its own Custom tabs as well.

Personal Tab

The Personal tab (Figure I.4) contains basic information about a patient and his or her employment. The most important boxes that must be completed in the Personal tab are as follows:

Case Number: The case number is a unique sequential number *assigned by Medisoft*.
Description: Information entered in the Description box indicates a patient's complaint, or reason for seeing the physician.
Guarantor: The Guarantor box lists the name of the person responsible for paying the bill.

Account Tab

The Account tab includes information on a patient's assigned provider, referring provider, referral source, as well as other information that may be used in some medical

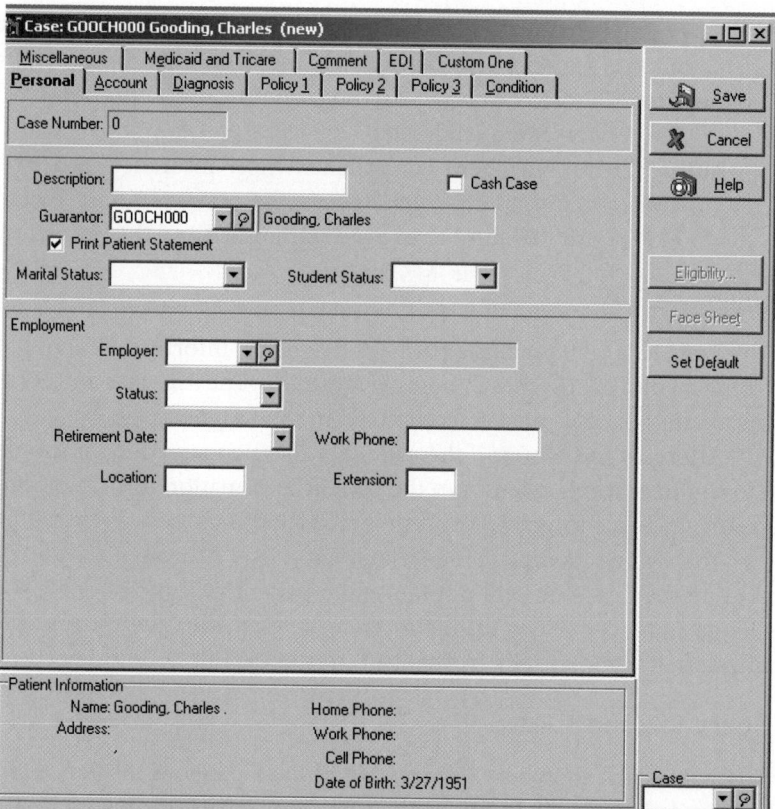

Figure I.4: *Case window, Personal tab.*

Figure I.5: *Case window, Account tab.*

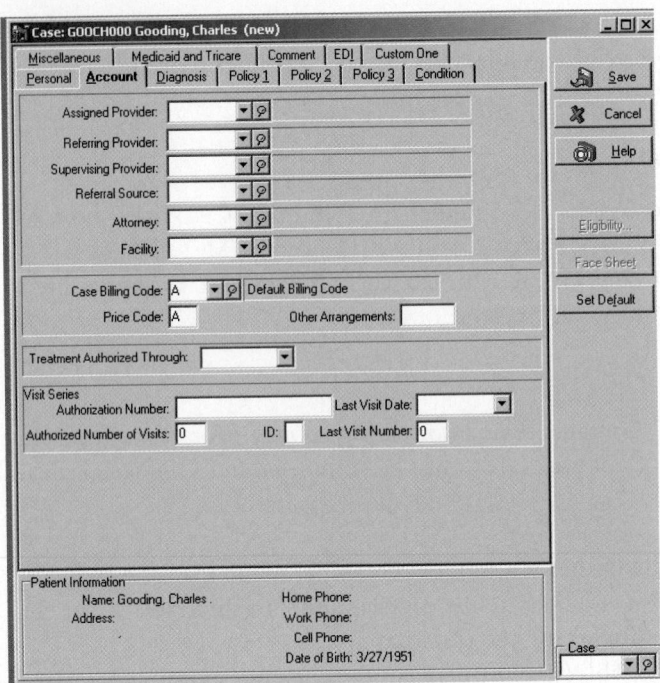

practices but not others (Figure I.5). The most important boxes that must be completed in the Account tab are as follows:

> **Assigned Provider:** The Assigned Provider box is automatically filled in with the code number and name of the assigned provider listed in the Patient/Guarantor dialog box.
>
> **Referring Provider:** If the patient was referred to the facility by another provider, choose the referring provider's name from the drop-down list.
>
> **Facility:** Choose the correct facility name from the drop-down box for the place the services were rendered.
>
> **Authorization Number:** For patients whose insurance carrier requires a referral/authorization number for services, the number issued should be entered here along with the number of visits authorized and the referral expiration date.

Diagnosis Tab

The Diagnosis tab contains a patient's diagnosis, information about allergies, and electronic medical claim (EMC) notes (Figure I.6). The Allergies and Notes box is the most important box that must be completed in the Diagnosis tab.

> **Allergies and Notes:** If the patient is allergic to anything it should be entered here. This information is taken from the patient information form. Notes regarding payment arrangements, a forgotten copayment, or anything else are entered in this area as well.

You will not complete the Default Diagnosis 1 through 4 boxes. When you are setting up the case, you will not know the patient's diagnosis. After you have posted the charge transaction, the diagnosis code entered into the charge information will be transferred automatically by Medisoft to the Default Diagnosis boxes in this tab.

Policy 1, 2, and 3 Tabs

The Policy tabs are where information about a patient's insurance carrier and coverage is recorded (Figure I.7). If a patient has more than one insurance policy, the Policy 2

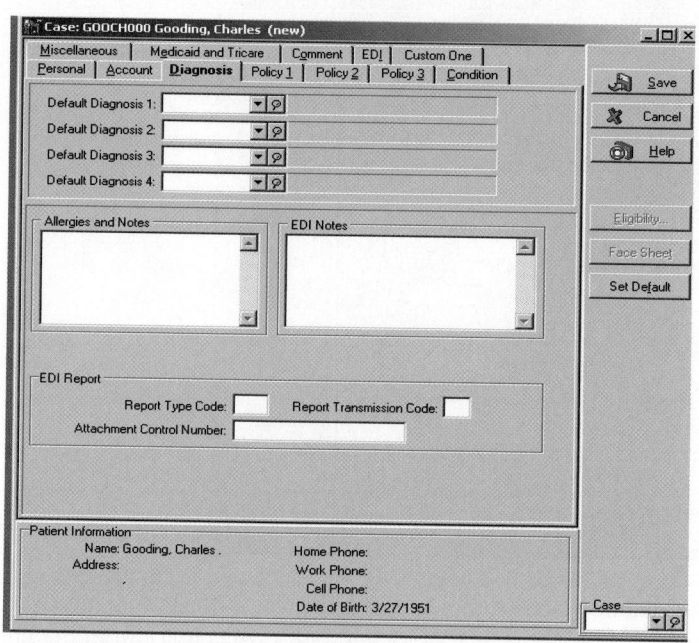
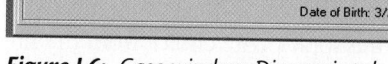

Figure I.6: *Case window, Diagnosis tab.*

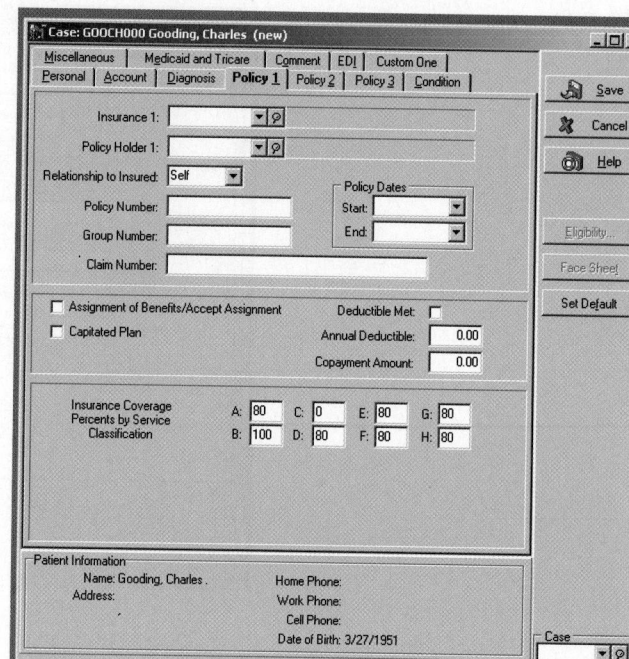

Figure I.7: *Case window, Policy 1 tab.*

and 3 tabs are used. The following boxes are the most important ones to be completed in the Policy tabs:

Insurance 1: The Insurance 1 box lists the patient's insurance carrier name, which is chosen from the drop-down list.

Policy Holder 1: This box shows the name of the insured person, which is chosen from the drop-down list. (This may or may not be the patient.) The guarantor must be entered in to the Patient List so that he or she can be chosen from the drop-down list here.

Relationship to Insured: This box indicates the patient's relationship to the individual listed in the Policy Holder 1 box.

Policy Number: The patient's insurance policy or ID number is entered in the Policy Number box.

Group Number: If there is a group number for a patient's policy, it is entered in the Group Number box.

Assignment of Benefits/Accept Assignment: Check this box if the patient has assigned insurance benefits to the provider.

Insurance Coverage Percents by Service Classification: The percentage of fees that an insurance carrier covers is entered in the Insurance Coverage Percents by Service Classification box. The default entry in this box is 80. The default can be changed by highlighting the default entry and keying the correct percentage over the default. Some insurance policies pay different percentages of charges based on the type of service rendered. For example, a carrier may pay 100% for well-man or well-woman exams and 50% for lab charges.

Condition Tab

The Condition tab stores data about a patient's illness, accident, disability, and hospitalization. This information is used by insurance carriers to process claims (Figure I.8).

Figure I.8: *Case window, Condition tab.*

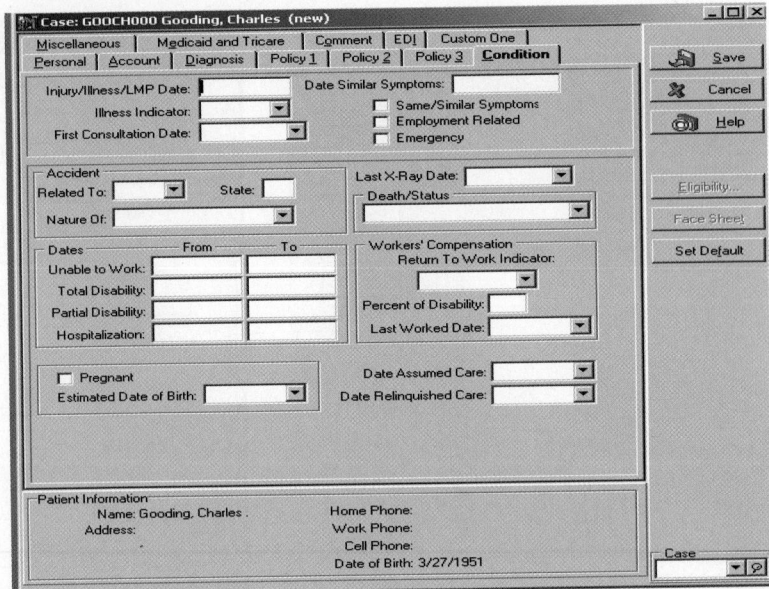

The top portion of the Condition tab is completed with the date of the illness, injury, or last menstrual period (if the patient is pregnant). Make the appropriate choice from the Illness Indicator drop-down list. If treatment rendered was for an emergency condition, check the box next to Emergency. If the case is for treatment of an accident, select the correct type from the Accident drop-down list. If the "accident" was just a fall at home, it is not considered a true accident. If the Accident box is marked, the insurance carrier may delay processing of the claim to research whether another insurance carrier should be the primary payer. If the case/treatment is workers' compensation related, the boxes for Unable to Work, Total Disability, Partial Disability, and Hospitalization may be completed. The Return To Work Indicator, Percent of Disability, and Last Worked Date all relate to workers' compensation cases.

Miscellaneous Tab

The Miscellaneous tab records a variety of miscellaneous information about the patient and his or her treatment, including outside lab work, prior authorization numbers, and other information (Figure I.9). For the authorization number to print out on the CMS-1500 form, it must be entered in the Miscellaneous tab.

Figure I.9: *Case window, Miscellaneous tab.*

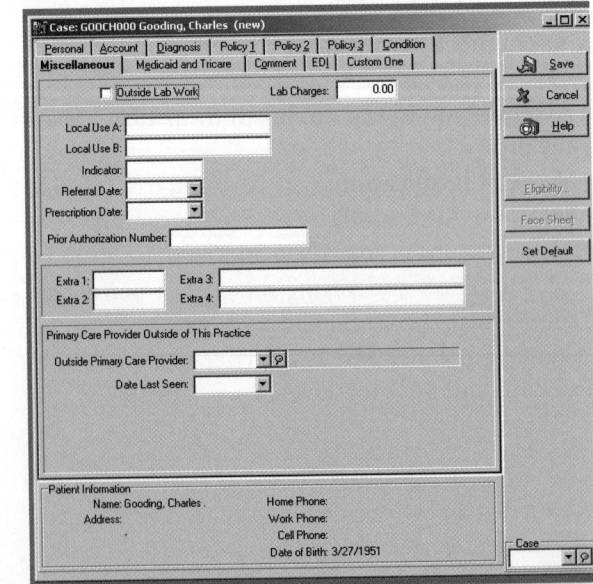

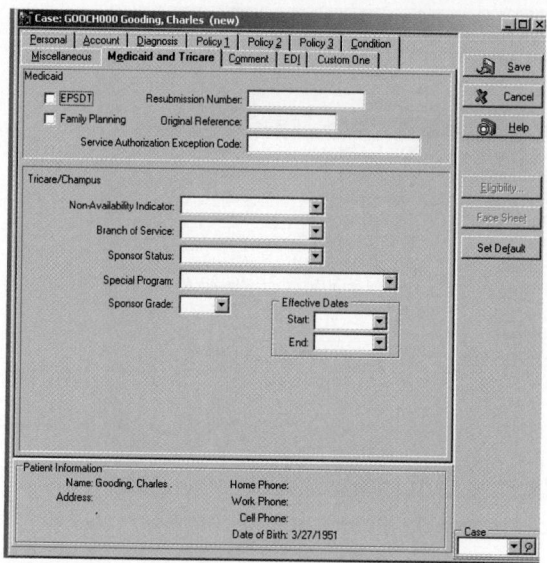

Figure I.10: *Case window, Medicaid and Tricare tab.*

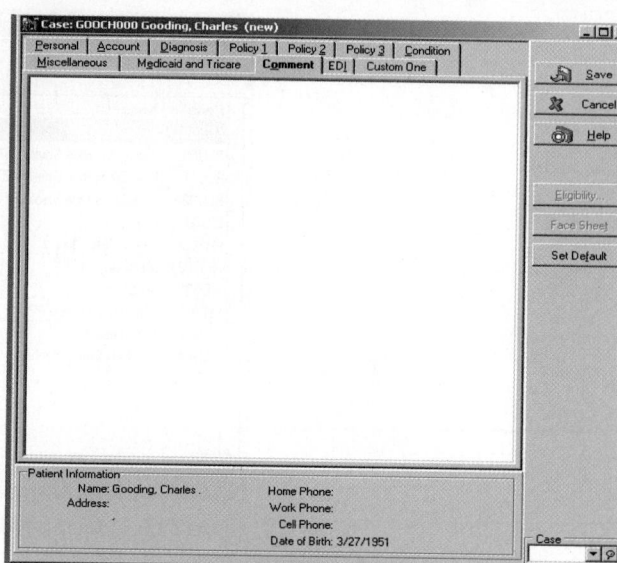

Figure I.11: *Case window, Comment tab.*

Medicaid and Tricare Tab

For patients covered by Medicaid or TRICARE, the Medicaid and Tricare tab is used to enter additional information about the government program (Figure I.10).

Comment Tab

Any comments or notes pertinent to this patient's case may be entered into the Comment tab (Figure I.11).

EDI Tab

Information necessary for the processing or transmission of electronic data interchange (EDI) data is entered in the EDI tab (Figure I.12).

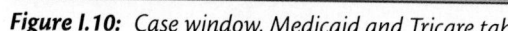

Figure I.12: *Case Window, EDI tab.*

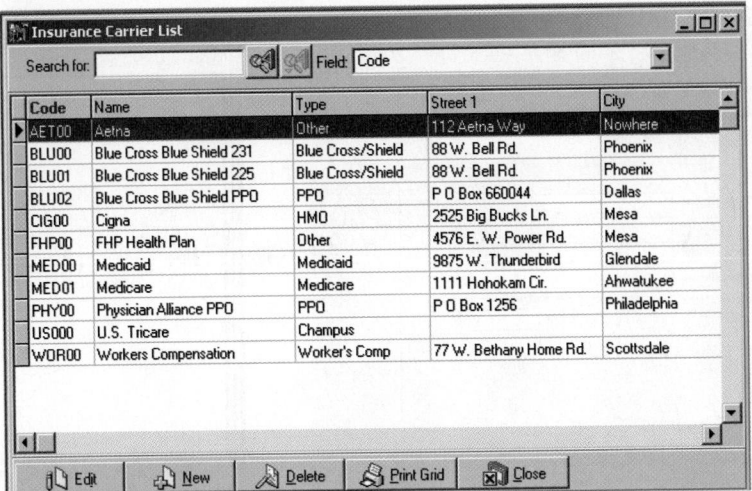

Figure I.13: *Adding an insurance carrier in the Insurance Carrier window.*

Adding the Insurance Carriers

If, when you are in the patient's Case window and entering the insurance carrier name, you notice the insurance carrier you are looking for is not in the drop-down list, you must go to the **Insurance Carrier List** to add it (Figure I.13). This can be accessed via a shortcut button or the Lists menu.

Click on the **New** button to add a new carrier name and address.

In the **Address** tab of the new Insurance Carrier window, enter the insurance carrier's name, address, telephone number, fax number, and contact name if you have one (Figure I.14).

The **Options** tab in the new Insurance Carrier window is vitally important because it is here that you choose the insurance plan type and indicate whether or not "Signature On File" (SOF) should appear on the claim form. SOF indicates that you have the patient's authorization to release this information and that the patient has assigned

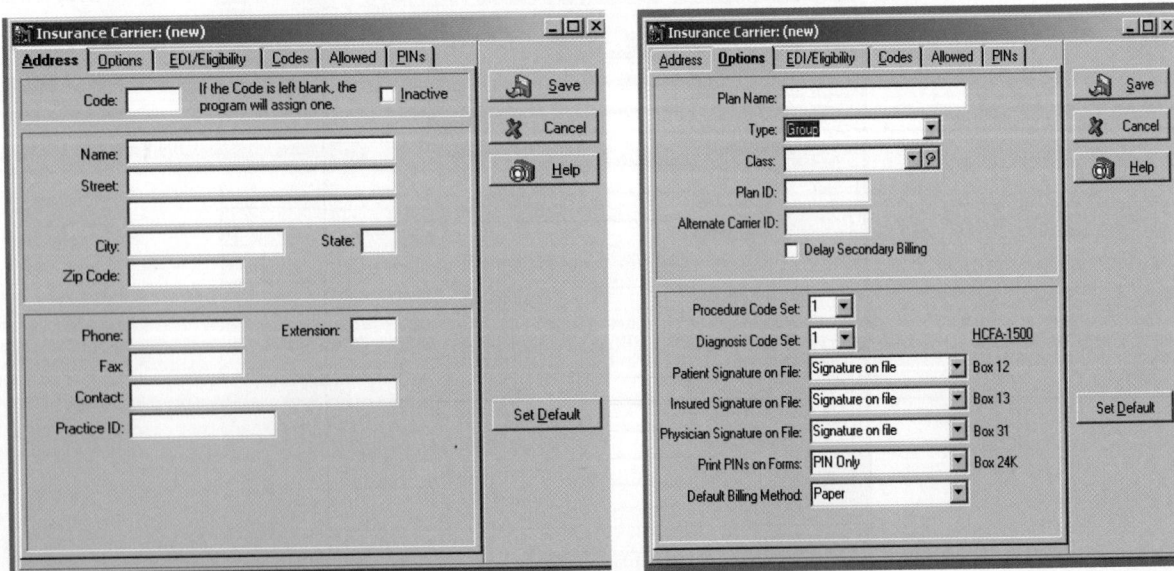

Figure I.14: *New Insurance Carrier window, Address tab (left) and Options tab (right).*

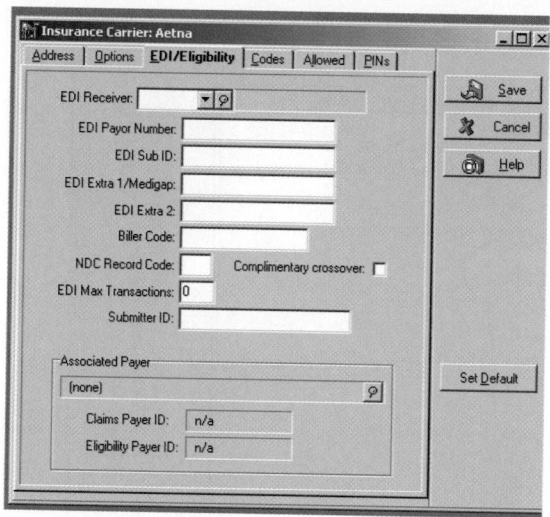

Figure I.15: *Insurance Carrier window, EDI/Eligibility tab.*

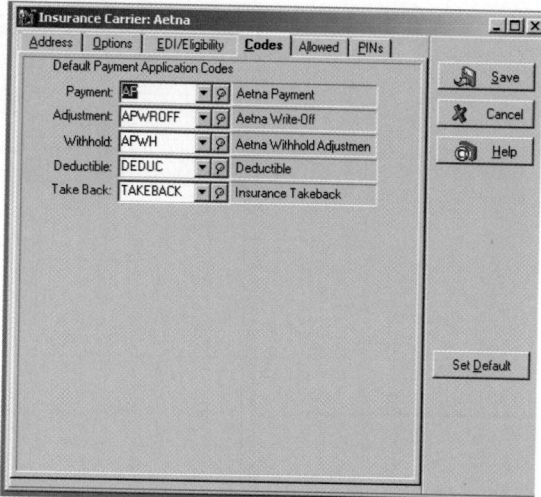

Figure I.16: *Insurance Carrier window, Codes tab.*

benefits directly to the provider (Figure I.14). (So the payment for the claim will be sent directly to your provider and not the patient.) "Signature on File" should *always* appear on the claim forms you submit.

The **EDI/Eligibility** tab is used to enter important EDI information for that insurance carrier (Figure I.15).

The Codes tab is for entering default transactions codes (Figure I.16).

The Allowed tab may be used to enter the contractual allowed amount per procedure code for that particular insurance carrier (Figure I.17).

The **PINs** tab in the Insurance Carrier List is also very important (Figure I.18). You must first Save your new carrier, then go back in and Edit it to add the provider PINs. PINs are specific to each carrier. Be sure to enter the correct insurance carrier PIN for

Code	Procedure	Allowed
17110	Wart Removal	0.00
29130	App. of Finger Splint, Static	0.00
36215	Lab Drawing Fee	0.00
43220	Esophageal Endoscopy	0.00
70250	X-Ray, Skull, 4 Views	0.00
70360	X-Ray, Neck	0.00
70373	X-Ray, Laryngography	0.00
71020	X-Ray, Chest, 2 Views	0.00
71030	X-Ray, Chest, Min 4 Views	0.00
71040	Contrast X-Ray of Bronchitis	0.00
72052	X-Ray, Spinal, Complete	0.00
73130	X-Ray, Hand, Min 3 Views	0.00
73562	X-Ray, Knee, Mn 3 Views	0.00
73610	X-Ray, Ankle, Complete	0.00
74246	MRI-Gastrointestinal Tract	0.00
74283	Barium Enema, Therapeutic	0.00
76818	U. S. Fetal Age	0.00
80050	General Health Screen Panel	0.00
81000	Urinalysis, Routine	0.00
82947	Blood Sugar Lab Test	0.00
82954	Glucose Test	0.00

Figure I.17: *Insurance Carrier window, Allowed tab.*

Figure I.18: *Insurance Carrier window, PINs tab.*

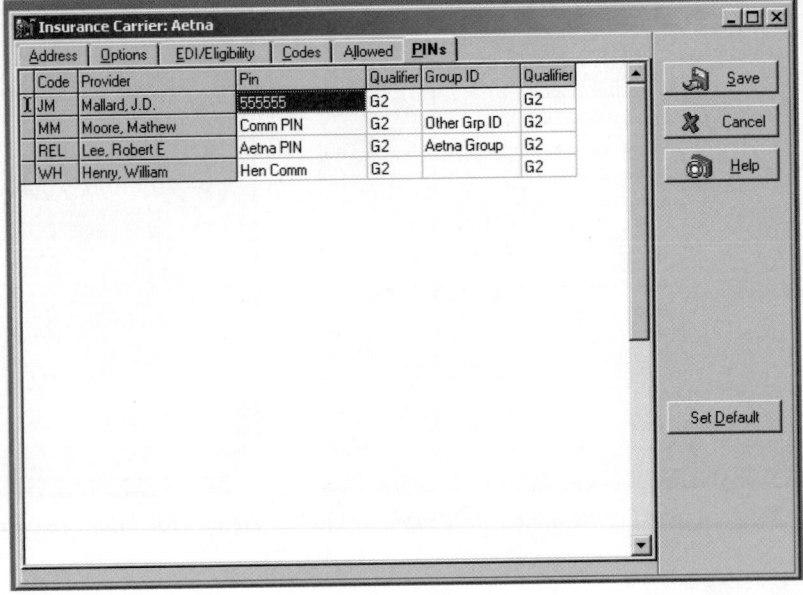

each participating provider. The appropriate qualifier should also be entered so that it prints on the CMS-1500 claim form.

Entering Employers

When entering patient and case information, it will be necessary to add the patient's or guarantor's employer name/address into Medisoft. This is accomplished in the **Address List,** which is accessed from the taskbar using the Address List shortcut button (Figure I.19).

The Address List contains not only employer addresses, but also referral sources (other than physicians), facility addresses, and attorney addresses (Figure I.20).

Click on the **New** button to begin (Figure I.21). Add the employer name, address and telephone number.

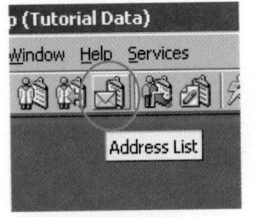

Figure I.19: *Address List shortcut button on the taskbar.*

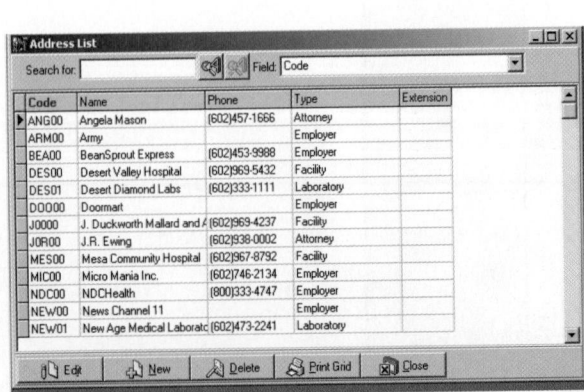

Figure I.20: *Address List window.*

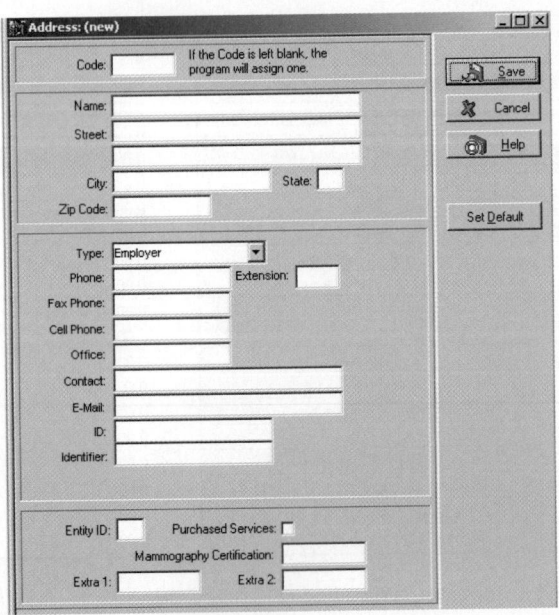

Figure I.21: *New Address window.*

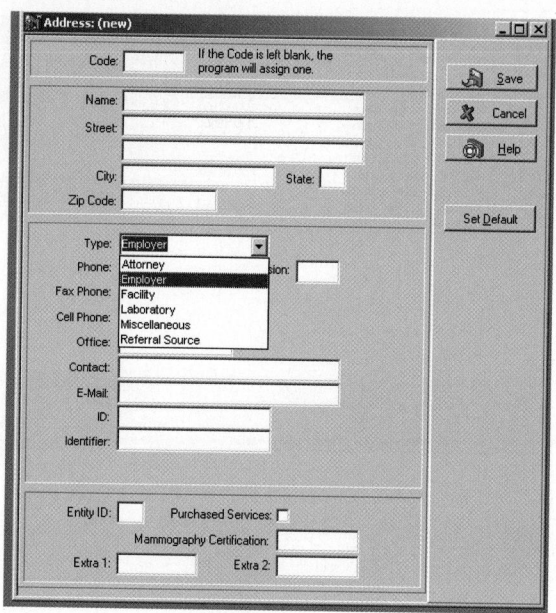

Figure I.22: *In the Type field of the new Address window, be sure to choose "Employer" when entering a new employer.*

If you are entering an employer (and not a referral source, etc.), in the Type field, be sure Employer is shown (Figure I.22). Click Save when you have finished entering the information.

You can now select the Employer name from the drop-down list in the Patient List or Case windows.

Reviewing a Completed Superbill

The completed superbill is the primary source of information a medical office specialist needs to record procedure charges. The completed superbill includes the following information: the provider's name, patient's name and chart/account number, date the services were performed, diagnosis, charge amounts, amount of payment received at the time of service, and the next appointment time needed.

After a physician completes a patient exam, he or she will place a check mark (or an X or circle) on the superbill next to the procedures performed. As you may recall, the superbill includes only the most common procedures provided by the medical office. If the physician performs a procedure not listed on the superbill, he or she writes the procedure in the "Other Procedures" area or in a blank space on the form.

Insurance carriers will not pay for treatment without a diagnosis code. The *diagnosis* is the physician's opinion of the patient's condition based on the examination. Therefore, the physician must record this information on the superbill so that it may be included as part of the procedure charge. If a procedure code or diagnosis is not marked on the superbill, you will need to ask the physician to mark it. Never demand that the physician do so and never accuse the physician of forgetting to mark the superbill. Always use respect and tact when addressing members of your medical practice.

Entering a Procedure Charge

After you review a patient's superbill, you are ready to enter the transaction into Medisoft to record the procedure charge and diagnosis code. You will process all transactions (charges, payments, and adjustments) in the **Transaction Entry** window. To access this window, you can use the **Activities** menu and click on Enter Transactions, click the **Transaction Entry** shortcut button or click the **Accounting** menu on the **Medisoft** side bar and choose Enter Transactions.

Figure I.23: *Begin working in the Transaction Entry window by choosing a patient chart number and case number.*

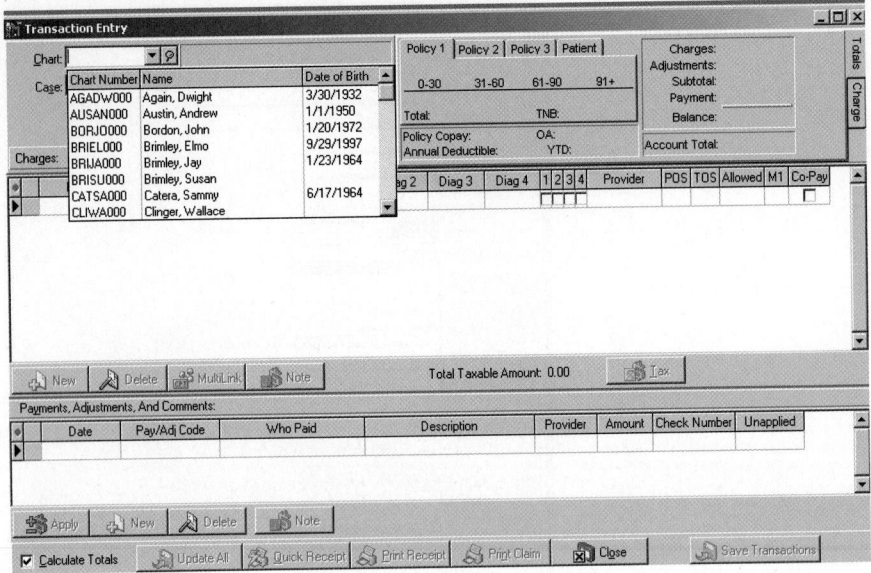

After you have opened the Transaction Entry window, the first thing you must do is choose the correct patient's chart number and case number to post a charge to.

STEP 1   Choose a patient chart number and case number (Figure I.23).

STEP 2   After the correct patient and case have been chosen, click on the **New** button in the middle of the screen (to access the top of the screen) (Figure I.24).

Medisoft will add today's date by default to the screen. If the date of service is not today's date, type the correct date in the Date field.

Click your mouse inside the **Procedure** field next to the date. A drop-down menu will be shown. You may either search for the correct procedure code marked on the superbill or type it in.

Figure I.24: *After choosing the correct patient and case, choose the New button from the middle of the screen.*

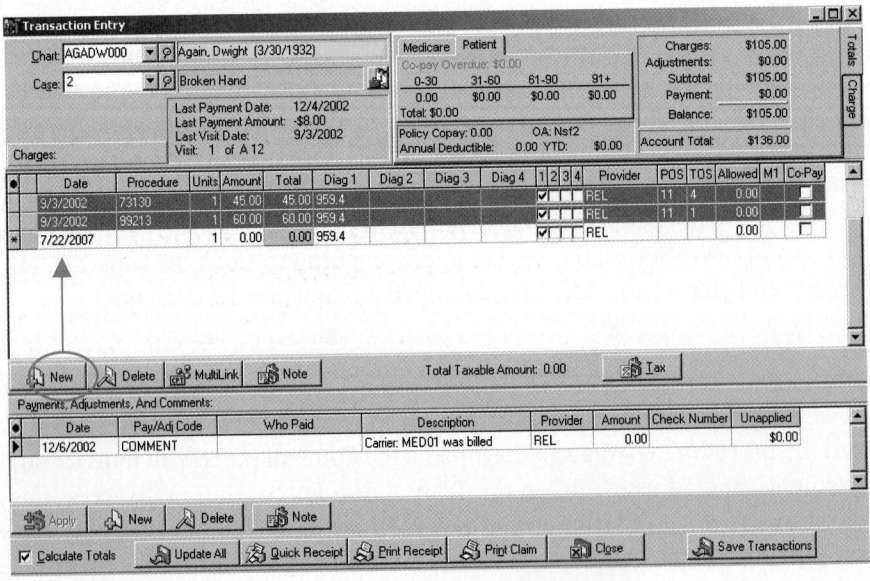

Once you have entered the CPT® code, press Enter or Tab to be taken to the Units field. Most of the time you will not need to change the default units entry.

Press Tab or Enter to move to the **Amount** field. Medisoft has already entered a dollar amount associated with that CPT code. If this amount is incorrect, key in the correct amount.

Press Tab or Enter again to be taken to the **DIAG1** field. Type in the primary diagnosis code or use the drop-down menu to search for the correct diagnosis. You may enter up to four diagnosis codes per charge transaction.

Tab over to the **Provider** field to make sure the correct provider is being credited with seeing this patient.

The **POS** (place of service) and **TOS** (type of service) fields will automatically be filled in based on the information in the CPT code database.

The **Allowed** amount field is also completed by default per information in the CPT code and insurance database.

The **M1** field is used to enter a two-character CPT modifier if one is marked on the patient superbill.

Complete all of these steps again to enter another procedure charge.

When you have finished entering charges, click on the **Save Transactions** button at the lower right of the screen or the **Update All** button near the lower left side of the window. When the Update All button is used to save transactions, the Medisoft program checks all fields for missing or invalid information and will display a message if information is needed or invalid.

Posting a Payment

When the patient (or his or her insurance carrier) makes a payment on the patient's account, you must enter this into the accounting software. Payments are posted in the **Transaction Entry** window (Figure I.25). Remember, you cannot enter a transaction

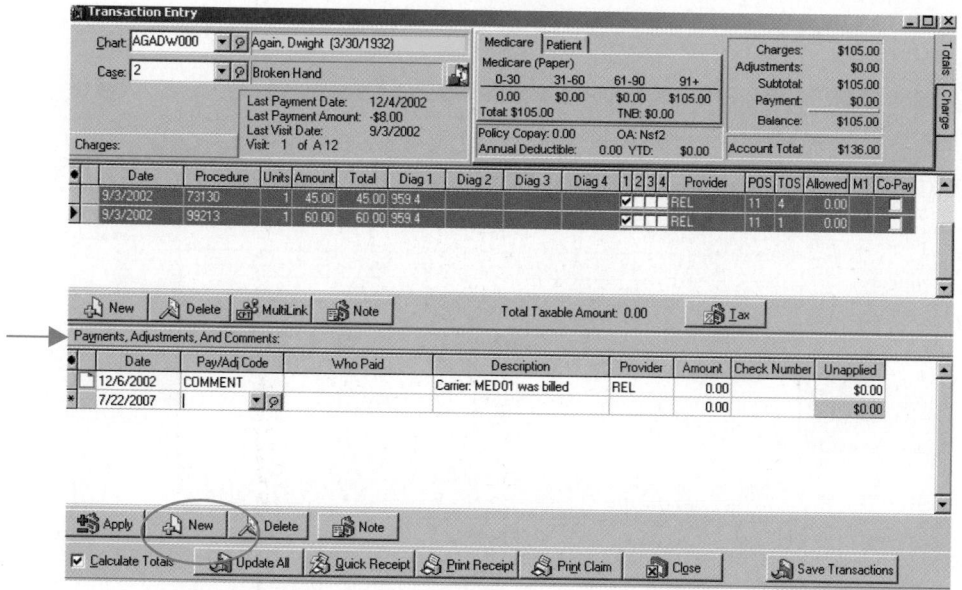

Figure I.25: *Posting payments in the Transaction Entry window.*

CPT is a registered trademark of the American Medical Association.

without first choosing a patient chart number and case number. It is important to make sure you have chosen the correct case—especially when posting payments from insurance carriers.

After opening the Transaction Entry window and choosing the appropriate chart and case number, click on the **New** button toward the *bottom* of the window within the Payments, Adjustments, And Comments section.

Medisoft will start a new entry by adding today's date.

Click in the **Pay/Adj Code** field and choose the method of payment (personal check, cash, Aetna payment, etc.).

Tab over to the **Who Paid** field and choose the party that is making the payment.

Enter a description if necessary.

Make sure the correct provider is shown in the **Provider** field.

Enter the amount of the payment in the **Amount** field. Enter a check number if appropriate in the next field.

Next, *you must apply the payment to the correct charge(s).* To do this, click on the **Apply** button at the bottom left-hand side of the window, to the left of the New button (Figure I.26).

A new window will open on top of your Transaction Entry window. This is the **Apply Payment to Charges** window. It is here that you can apply the payment to a specific charge or charges. This is called *line item posting.*

It is most important to post the payment to the correct date of service and the correct procedure code. One payment can be divided among many charges if it is "broken down" that way on the EOB/ERA or the patient has many separate charges and is paying for all of them.

When you have applied the payment to the correct charge(s), click the **Close** button at the bottom of the Apply Payment to Charges window.

Your **Unapplied** column in the Payment, Adjustment, And Comments section of the Transaction Entry window should read $0.00 if you applied the entire payment. (A patient's account may have an unapplied balance if he or she is prepaying on surgery, for example.) You must now save the payment transaction.

Click on the **Update All** or **Save Transactions** button at the bottom of the window.

Figure I.26: *Applying a payment to the correct charges.*

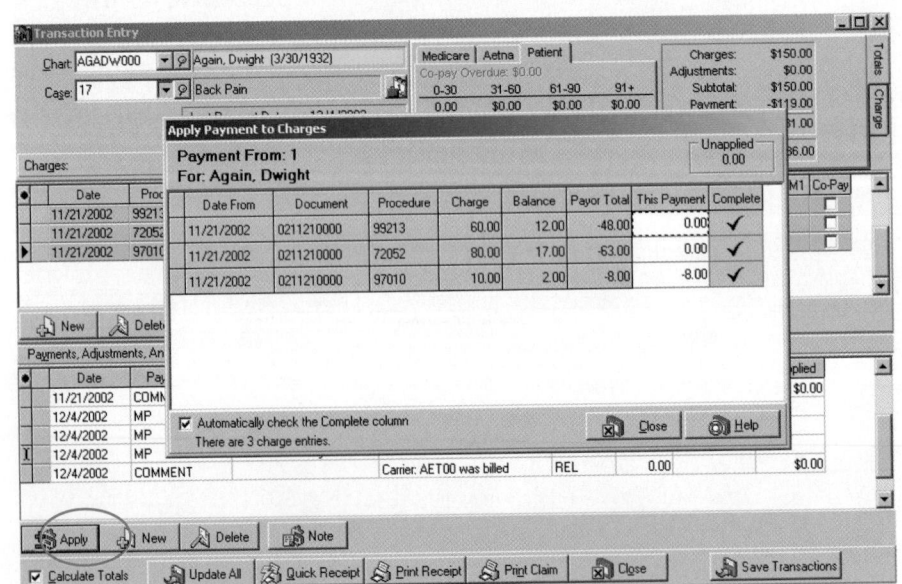

Posting an Adjustment

Entering an adjustment into a patient's account is similar to entering a payment and is also performed in the **Transaction Entry** window. To begin, you must first choose the patient chart number and case number.

Click on the **New** button towards the *bottom* of the window.

Medisoft will start a new transaction by entering today's date by default.

In the **Pay/Adj Code** field, select the correct type of adjustment (insurance write-off, charge reversal, courtesy discount, etc.).

Tab over to the **Description** entry field and type a note about why the adjustment is needed.

Tab over to the **Provider** field and choose the correct provider, then tab over to the **Amount** field.

If you are *subtracting* an amount from the patient's account, you will need to enter a minus (−) sign before typing the amount. If you are adding an amount to a patient's account, you do not need to enter a plus sign before the amount.

Note: Medisoft will assume all adjustments are positive unless you type in a minus (−) sign before the amount.

When you have entered the amount, click on the **Apply** button at the bottom left of the Transaction Entry window.

When you are applying the adjustment, make sure to choose the correct date(s) of service and CPT code(s). *You must enter a minus sign before the amount in the Apply Adjustment to Charges window.* If you do not, Medisoft will *add* the amount to the patient's account.

When you have entered all of the adjustments, click on the **Close** button to take you back to the Transaction Entry window.

To save all of your hard work, be sure to click on **Update All** or **Save Transactions.**

Using the Enter Deposits and Apply Payments Window

It is easiest to post payments that patients make at the time of service in the Transaction Entry window. However, if you receive a large insurance check that covers claims for many different patients, it is easier to post this in the **Enter Deposits and Apply Payments** window. This window can be accessed by clicking the **Enter Deposits and Apply Payments** shortcut button, opening the **Activities** menu and choosing Apply Deposits/Payments, or by clicking on the **Accounting** shortcut button on the **Medisoft** side bar and choosing Enter Deposits/Payments. A Deposit List window will open (Figure I.27) that contains the following fields:

Deposit Date: The current date is automatically entered. It can be changed by typing a different date in the field.

Show All Deposits: This check box displays all payments entered regardless of date.

Show Unapplied Only: If this box is checked, only the payments that have not been fully applied to charges are shown.

Sort By: This is a drop-down list that allows you to sort deposits by amount, patient chart number, and payer.

Locate and **Locate Next:** These shortcut buttons allow you to search for a particular deposit.

Detail: This button is used to view a specific deposit in more detail. Highlight the deposit in the window and then click the Detail button.

Figure I.27: *Deposit List window (Enter Deposits and Apply Payments).*

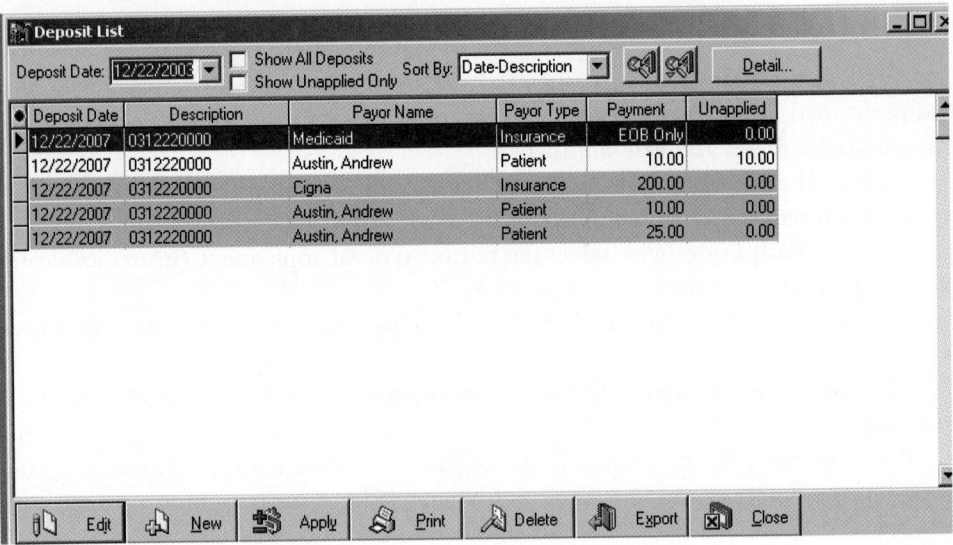

To enter a new deposit, click on the **New** button at the bottom of the Deposit List window. After the New Deposit window opens (Figure I.28), you must choose a **Payor Type** (patient, insurance carrier, capitation).

Choose the **Payment Method** (check, cash, credit card, electronic) and Enter or Tab over to the **Check Number** field to enter the check number.

The **Description/Bank No.** field is used to enter an (optional) description of the check.

Enter the dollar amount of the payment in the **Payment Amount** field.

The **Deposit Code** drop-down menu is used by some practices to sort deposits according to practice-defined categories.

Select the insurance carrier making payment from the drop-down menu in the **Insurance** field.

After you have selected the carrier, the other **Code** fields are automatically completed (Figure I.29).

When finished, click **Save.**

After entering the check information, the next step is to apply the payment.

Click the **Apply** button at the bottom of the Deposit List window.

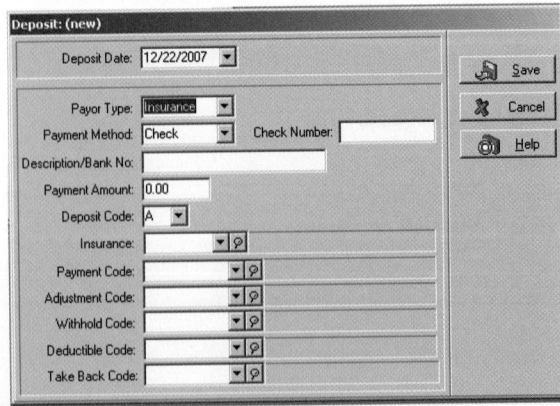

Figure I.28: *New Deposit window.*

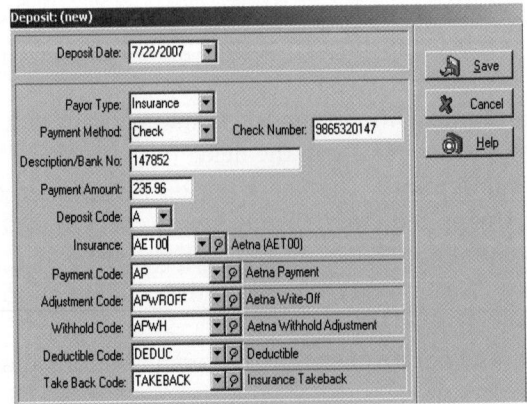

Figure I.29: *The various code fields are filled in automatically when the insurance carrier is selected from the Insurance drop-down box.*

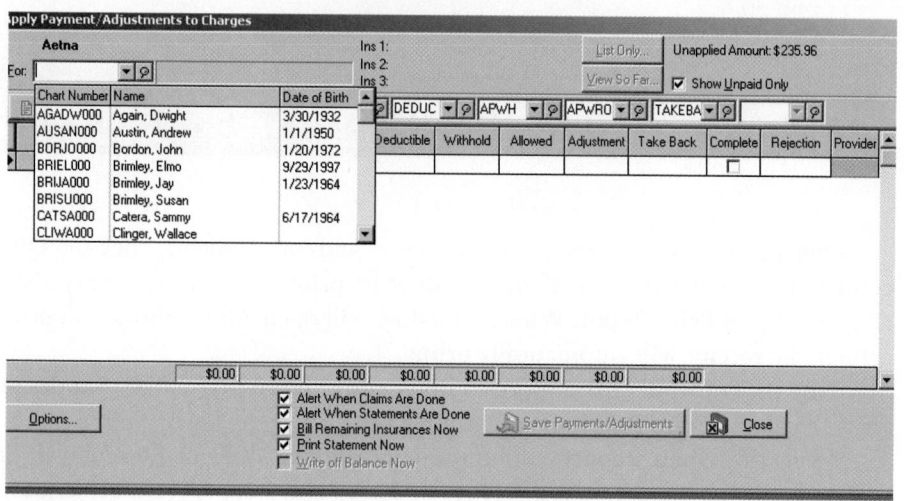

Figure I.30: *The Apply Payments/Adjustments to Charges window.*

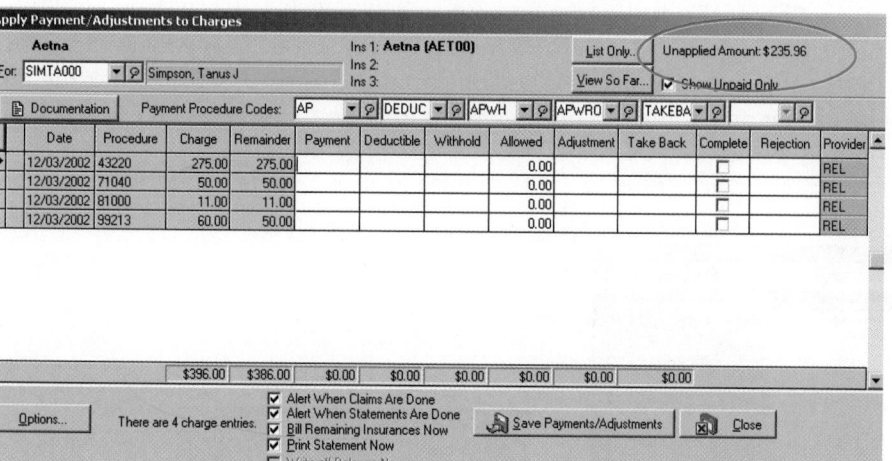

Figure I.31: *The Unapplied Amount indicator tells you how much of a deposit remains to be posted.*

The **Apply Payment/Adjustments to Charges** window (Figure I.30) is where you will apply payments and adjustments (if needed) to specific patient accounts. You are able to enter payments and adjustments as well as deductibles and withhold information at virtually the same time.

When you have finished entering payment information on one patient, click the **Save Payments/Adjustments** button at the bottom right side of the window.

If you have the **Print Statements Now** box at the bottom of the window checked, after clicking Save, Medisoft will ask what type of statement you would like to print.

If you have another patient to apply payments to, follow the same steps as before.

The **Unapplied Amount** indicator in the top right-hand corner of the window will allow you to keep track of how much you have posted and how much you still have to post (Figure I.31).

Walkout Receipts

Throughout the office simulation at the end of this appendix, you will be responsible for printing a walkout receipt for each patient who has seen the provider. This task is performed in the Transaction Entry window.

Figure I.32: *Quick Receipt button.*

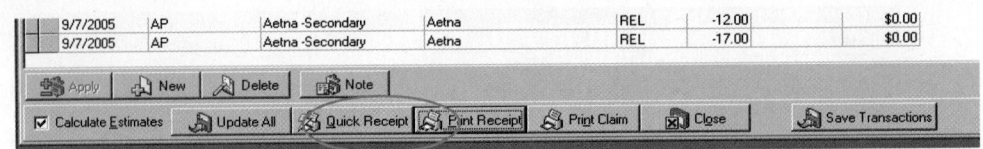

After you have posted the patient's charges and/or payments, click the **Quick Receipt** button at the bottom of the window to print a receipt for today's visit only (Figure I.32). A **Print Report Where?** window will open. After choosing to print to the printer, the receipt will automatically print.

If the patient would like a more comprehensive receipt (one that includes previous visits), click the **Print Receipt** button instead.

When the **Open Report** window opens, choose Walkout Receipt (All Transactions), then click the OK button (Figure I.33). A **Print Report Where?** window opens after you have clicked OK (Figure I.34).

After selecting where to print the report, a **Data Selection Questions** window opens. Choose the date ranges for your receipt and click the OK button.

If you choose to preview the report on the screen, you will see a screen similar to that shown in Figure I.35. To print from the preview screen, click the picture of the printer across the top of the screen. To close the preview screen, click the Close button.

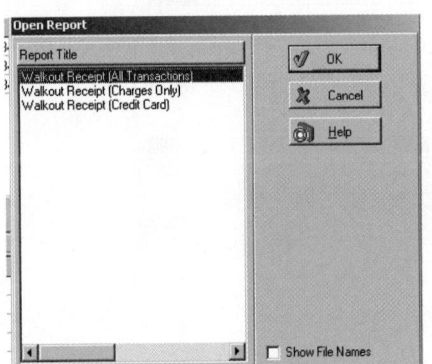

Figure I.33: *Open Report window.*

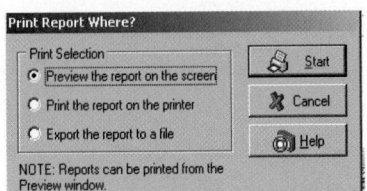

Figure I.34: *Print Report Where? window.*

Figure I.35: *Sample walkout receipt.*

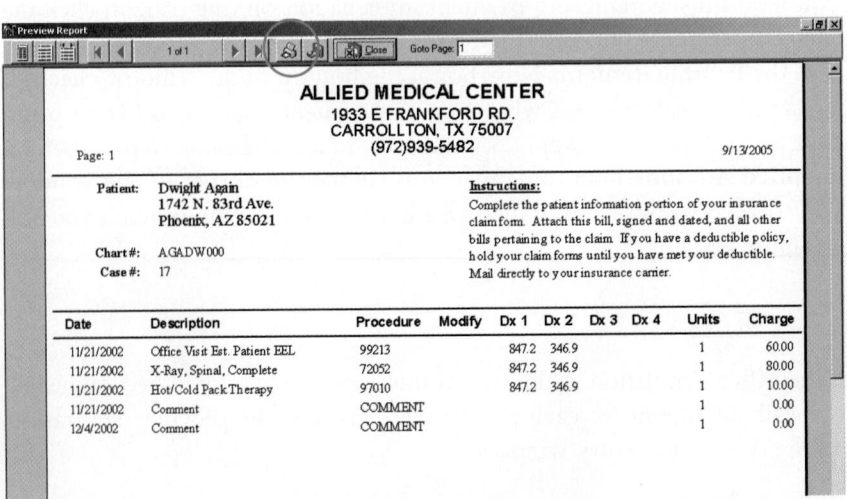

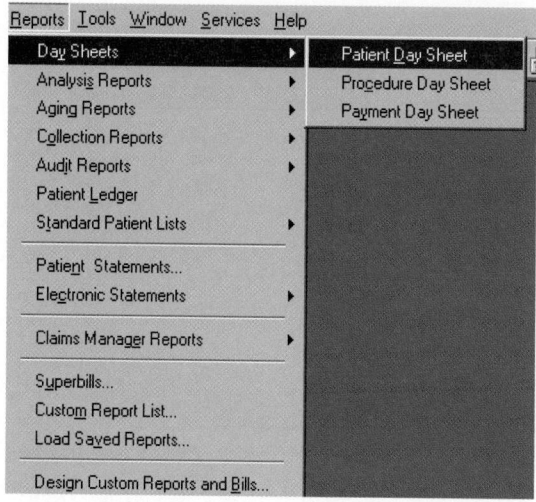

Figure I.36: *Selecting the Patient Day Sheet report from the Reports drop-down menu.*

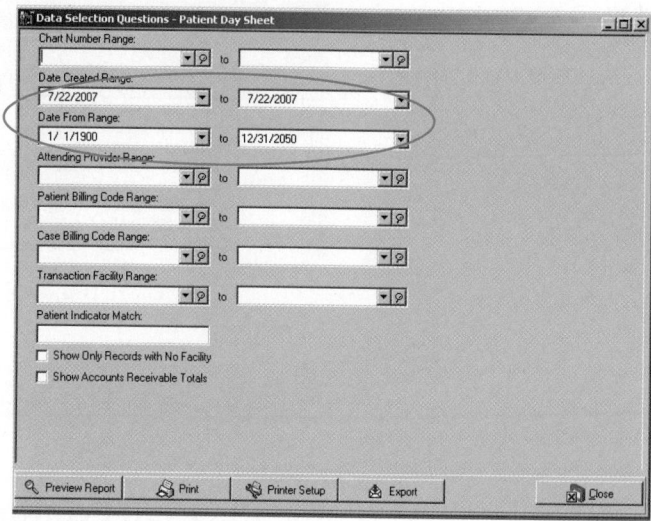

Figure I.37: *Data Selection Questions for Patient Day Sheet Reports.*

Printing Reports in Medisoft

Let's take a moment to discuss the different reports available in Medisoft version 12.

Patient Day Sheet Report

The Patient Day Sheet report can be accessed in either of two ways: by clicking on the **Reports** menu or by clicking the **Daily Reports** menu on the **Medisoft** side bar.

For the office simulation that follows, you will be instructed to stop entering transactions and "batch out." You will need to compile and run the Patient Day Sheet report. This report, as stated earlier in the text, shows all transactions posted in the database for the day. For our purposes, we will use "today's" date.

After clicking on **Patient Day Sheet** in the Reports menu (Figure I.36), a **Print Report Where?** window will open. After choosing where to print the report (our example printed it to the screen), another window/dialog box will open: **Data Selection Questions: Patient Day Sheet** (Figure I.37).

Click in the **Date Created Range** field and choose **today's date** for both the From and To boxes, then click the OK button.

Using the arrows at the top of the screen, go to the last page of the report for your totals. Your totals here should match your totals from all the superbills/EOBs you posted throughout the day (Figure I.38).

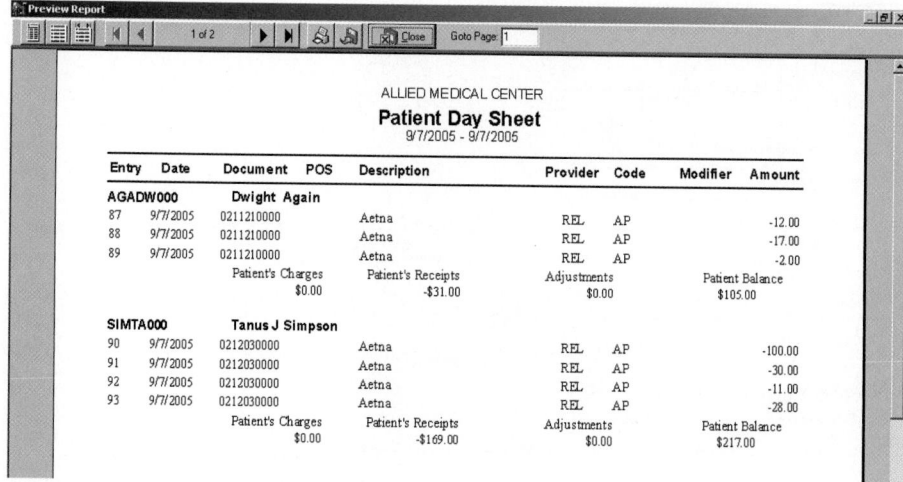

Figure I.38: *Sample Patient Day Sheet report.*

Figure I.39: To process new insurance claims, click the Create Claims button in the Claim Management window.

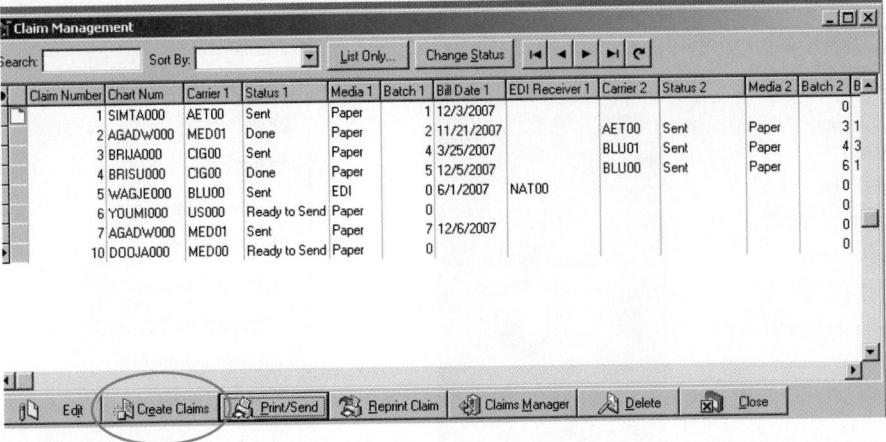

Creating and Printing Insurance Claims

During the office simulation that follows, you will be responsible for printing paper CMS-1500 claim forms at the end of each day for the patients' accounts you posted charges to. This task is accomplished in the **Claim Management** window.

The Claim Management window can be accessed by clicking the **Claim Management** shortcut button, clicking the **Accounting** button on the **Medisoft** side bar, or by opening the **Activities** menu and clicking Claim Management.

After opening the Claim Management window, the first thing to do is create the insurance claims you want to send. To do this you click the **Create Claims** button at the bottom of the window (Figure I.39).

The majority of medical practices print claims several times a week. You will notice, again, that you can sort your claim report many different ways: by transaction dates, chart numbers, primary insurance carrier—you can even create claims for one particular provider name. For the office simulation you will be using today's date in the **Transaction Dates** field (Figure I.40). After entering the dates, click the **Create** button on the right side of the window.

As you create a claim, the Claim Management window will be automatically updated. It will show the claims you've just created as "Ready to Send" in the Status 1 column of the Claim Management window.(Figure I.41).

The next step is to look over your claims *before* you print them to make sure they are "clean" claims (meaning no information is missing and all information is correct).

Figure I.40: The Transaction Dates field in the Create Claims window.

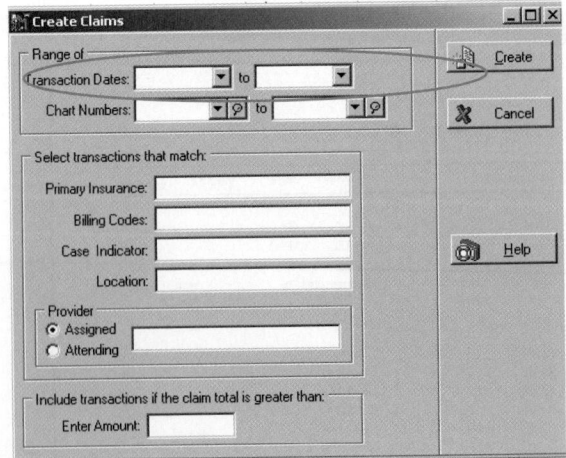

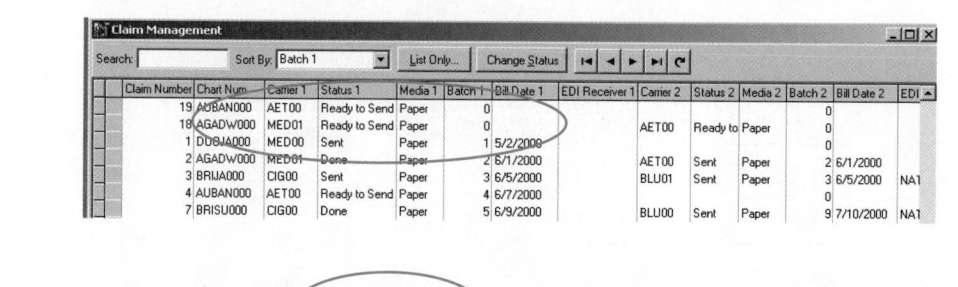

Figure I.41: *The Status 1 column indicates which newly created claims are ready to send to insurance carriers.*

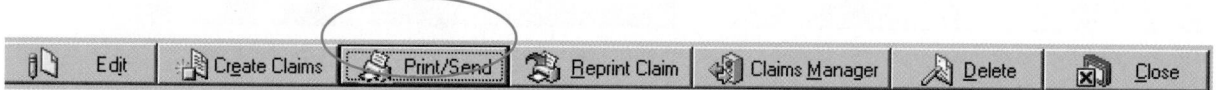

Figure I.42: *Print/Send button at the bottom of the Claim Management window.*

To do this, click on the **Print/Send** button at the bottom of the Claim Management window (Figure I.42).

A Print/Send Claims window will open asking you to choose how you wish to send the claims, either on paper or electronically. For our simulation, you will choose the Paper method for claims. Click the OK button on the right side of the window (Figure I.43).

An Open Report window will open next (Figure I.44). If you are printing Medicare claims, you will need to choose the CMS-1500 (Primary) Medicare Century report option. If you are printing claims for any other carrier, choose the CMS-1500 (Primary) report option. It is important to choose the correct report type for claims. Medicare prefers a minimum of information on claims, so be sure to choose the correct report/claim format when submitting claims to Medicare. After choosing the report style, click the OK button.

When the **Print Report Where?** window opens, choose to **Preview the report on the screen** and click Start (Figure I.45). You will look over the claims on the screen to be sure they are clean before printing.

A Data Selection Questions dialog box will open for you to choose which claims you want to preview. Use today's date in the **Date Created Range** fields. You can "filter" those claims you would like to review. Filtering is selecting certain criteria. For example, you may choose to only review claims for a particular insurance carrier (e.g. Medicaid). In order to do that, you would select the name of the insurance carrier from the drop down menu from the Insurance Carrier 1 Range boxes. This would filter out all the other insurance carrier claims and only show you the claims for the carrier you chose from the drop down menu. You can filter claims by Chart Number Range, Claim Billing

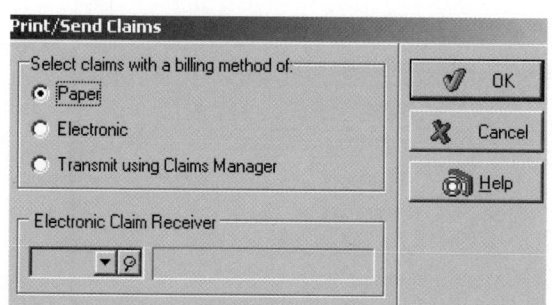

Figure I.43: *Print/Send Claims window.*

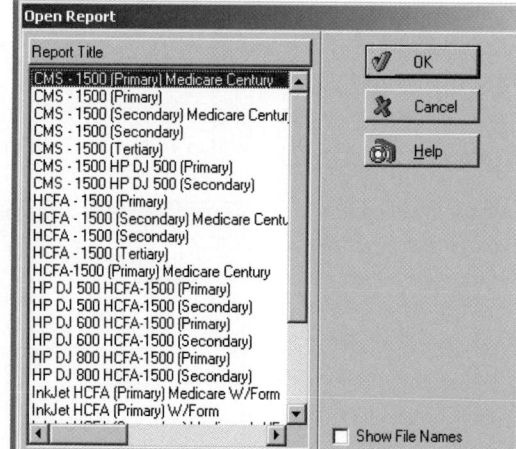

Figure I.44: *Open Report window.*

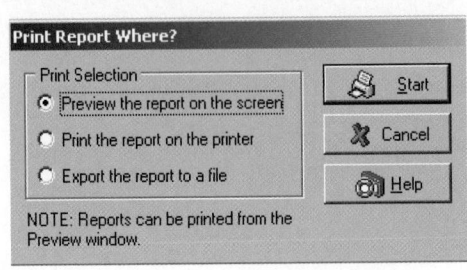

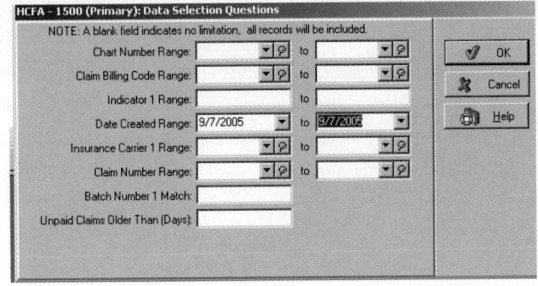

Figure I.45: *Preview the report on the screen.*

Figure I.46: *Data Selection Questions dialog box.*

Code Range or Claim Number Range. After choosing your filters, click OK (Figure I.46). If you want to see all claims created, complete only the Date Created Range boxes.

The claims will be shown on the screen in the format you chose. Note that the CMS-1500 locator boxes will not actually show on the screen because they are instead printed on the blank claim form originals that you will insert into your printer when you're ready to print claims. However, you may want to refer to a blank printed claim form while checking your claims on screen to see if any information is missing (Figure I.47).

Once you have checked all of your claims and corrected any mistakes if necessary, you are ready to print your claims on CMS-1500 forms that you have loaded into your printer's paper tray.

After you have printed your claims, Medisoft will update your Claim Management window (Status 1 column) to show that the claims have been sent (on paper or electronically) (Figure I.48).

Table I.1 shows the relationship between the form locators on the CMS-1500 claim form and the dialog boxes in Medisoft. If, when looking over the claim forms before

Figure I.47: *Sample CMS-1500 Primary claim printed to screen. Note that the locator boxes do not show on screen.*

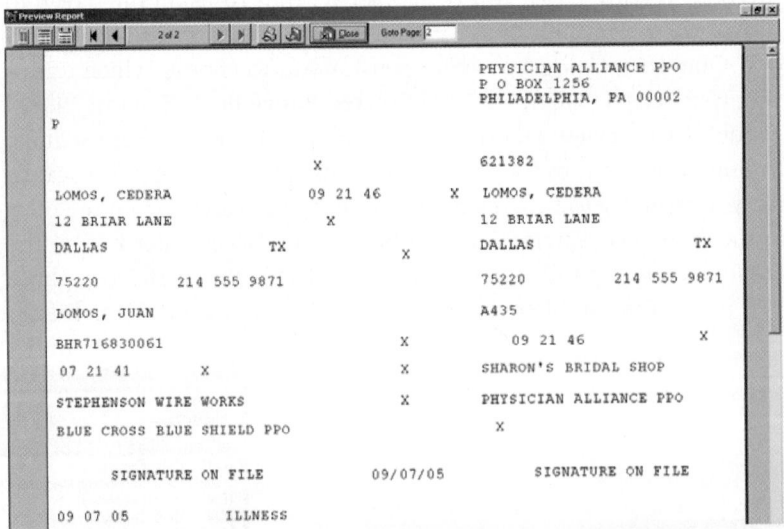

Figure I.48: *Medisoft will update your Claim Management window to indicate that the claims have been sent.*

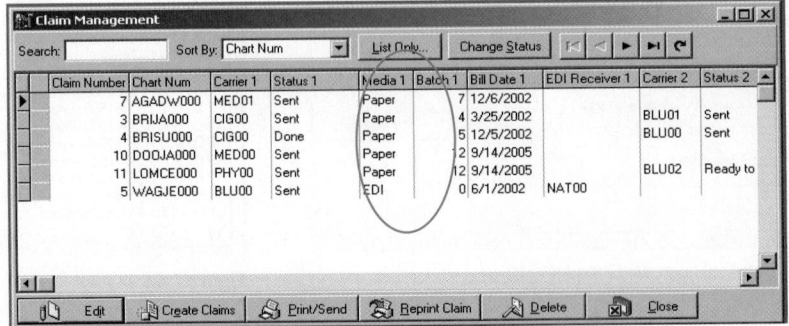

Table I.1   Patient/Guarantor and Provider Information and the CMS-1500 Form

Patient/Guarantor Information and the CMS-1500 Form

CMS Form Locator	Medisoft		
	Dialog Box	TAB (in Dialog Box)	FIELD (in Dialog Box)
1	Insurance Carrier	Options	Type
1a	Case	Policy	Policy Number
2	Patient/Guarantor	Name, Address	Last Name, First Name, Middle Initial
3	Patient/Guarantor	Name, Address	Birth Date, Sex
4	Case	Policy	Policy Holder
5	Patient/Guarantor	Name, Address	Street, City, State, Zip Code, Phones
6	Case	Policy	Relationship to Insured
7	Patient/Guarantor	Name, Address	Street, City, State, ZIP Code, Phones
8	Case	Personal	Marital Status
8	Patient/Guarantor	Other Information	Employment Status
9	Patient/Guarantor	Name, Address	Last Name, First Name, Middle Initial
9a	Case	Policy	Policy Number
9b	Patient/Guarantor	Name, Address	Birth Date, Sex
9c	Patient/Guarantor	Other Information	Employer
9d	Insurance Carrier	Options	Plan Name
10a	Case	Condition	Employment Related
10b	Case	Condition	Accident Related To
10c	Case	Condition	Accident Related To
10d	Case	Miscellaneous	Local Use A, Local Use B
11	Case	Policy	Policy Number
11a	Patient/Guarantor	Name, Address	Birth Date, Sex
11b	Patient/Guarantor	Other Information	Employer
11c	Insurance Carrier	Options	Plan Name
11d	Case	Policy 2	Insurance 2
12	Patient/Guarantor	Other Information	Signature on File
13	Patient/Guarantor	Other Information	Signature on File

(continued)

Table I.1   Patient/Guarantor and Provider Information and the CMS-1500 Form (continued)

Provider information and the CMS-1500 Form

| CMS Form Locator | Medisoft | | |
	Dialog Box	TAB (in Dialog Box)	FIELD (in Dialog Box)
14	Case	Condition	Injury/Illness/LMP Date
15	Case	Condition	Same/Similar Symptoms and First Consultation Date
16	Case	Condition	Dates Unable to Work
17	Referring Provider	Address	First Name, Middle Initial, Last Name
17a 17b	Referring Provider	NPI, Qualifiers, PINs, and IDs	Varies with carrier
18	Case	Condition	Hospitalization
19	Case	Miscellaneous	Local Use A, Local Use B
20	Case	Miscellaneous	Outside Lab Work and Lab Charges
21	Case	Diagnosis	Default Diagnosis 1–4
22	Case	Medicaid	Resubmission Number and Original Reference
23	Case	Miscellaneous	Prior Authorization Number
24a	Transaction Entry	Charge	Dates
24b	Procedure Code	General	Place of Service
24c	Emergency	Condition	Emergency check box
24d	Transaction Entry	Charge	Procedure and Modifiers
24e	Transaction Entry	Charge	Default Diagnosis 1–4
24f	Transaction Entry	Charge	Amount
24g	Transaction Entry	Charge	Units
24h 24ij	Case Provider List/ Insurance Carrier List	Medicaid PINS	EPSDT PINs/National Identifier
25	Provider	PINs and IDs	Social Security number/Federal Tax ID
26	Patient/Guarantor	Name, Address or Other Information	Chart Number or Patient ID #2
27	Case	Policy	Accept Assignment or Transaction Default
28	Transaction Entry	Charge	Amount
29	Transaction Entry	Payment	Amount
30	Transaction Entry		Case Balance
31	Provider	Address	Signature on File
32	Case	Account	Facility
33	Provider	PINs and IDs	Last Name, Middle Initial, First Name, Street, City, State, Zip Code, Phone

printing, you notice data missing on the claim, consult Table I.1 to discern where to enter it in Medisoft.

Medisoft Shortcut Buttons

The Shortcut Button toolbar is a quick way to navigate to the most commonly used windows/areas within Medisoft. As a helpful reminder, each button is labeled here with a brief description of what the window is used for.

TRANSACTION ENTRY—Use this window to post charges, payments, and adjustments in patient accounts.

CLAIM MANAGEMENT—Use this window to create, print, and send insurance claims.

STATEMENT MANAGEMENT—Use this window to print and send statements.

COLLECTION LIST—Use this window to check on open accounts that require collection follow-up and add tickler notes.

ADD COLLECTION LIST ITEMS—Use this window to add multiple collection items at once to the Collection List based on specific criteria chosen from the screen.

APPOINTMENT BOOK—Use this window to set appointments for the practice's providers.

VIEW ELIGIBILITY VERIFICATION RESULTS—This feature allows the facility to check a patient's insurance coverage online. It is a fee-based service for which the facility must enroll.

PATIENT/CASE (GUARANTOR) LIST—Use this window to add or edit patient, guarantor, or case information.

INSURANCE CARRIER LIST—Use this window to add or edit insurance carriers in the Medisoft database.

PROCEDURE CODE LIST—Use this window to edit or add procedure, payment, or adjustment codes in the Medisoft database.

DIAGNOSIS CODE LIST—Use this window to add or edit diagnostic codes in the Medisoft database.

PROVIDER LIST—Use this window to add or edit practice providers in the Medisoft database.

REFERRING PROVIDER LIST—Use this window to add or edit names of physicians that refer patients to the practice.

ADDRESS LIST—Use this window to add or edit patient/guarantor, employer, attorney, or facility names to the Medisoft database.

PATIENT RECALL LIST—Use this window to enter appointment recall information.

CUSTOM REPORT LIST—Use this window to view every report choice in Medisoft database.

QUICK LEDGER—Use this window to quickly view any patient's full financial ledger.

QUICK BALANCE—Use this window to view any patient's financial balance.

ENTER DEPOSITS AND APPLY PAYMENTS—Use this window as an alternative way to enter patient/guarantor or insurance payments to patients' accounts.

SHOW/HIDE HINTS

MEDISOFT HELP MENU

EDIT PATIENT NOTES IN FINAL DRAFT—If notes were entered anywhere in the system, they may be edited here.

LAUNCH ADVANCED REPORTING—Advanced Reporting provides users with enhanced reporting and data viewing capabilities including ad hoc reporting and a set of standard reports that may be customized by users with the report writer.

LAUNCH WORK ADMINISTRATOR—The Work Administrator program lets the staff streamline the wok process. Use this feature to organize tasks for users and user groups.

EXIT MEDISOFT PROGRAM

Medisoft Menus

Each Medisoft menu is shown here as a navigation reminder. Each menu was explained on page 787.

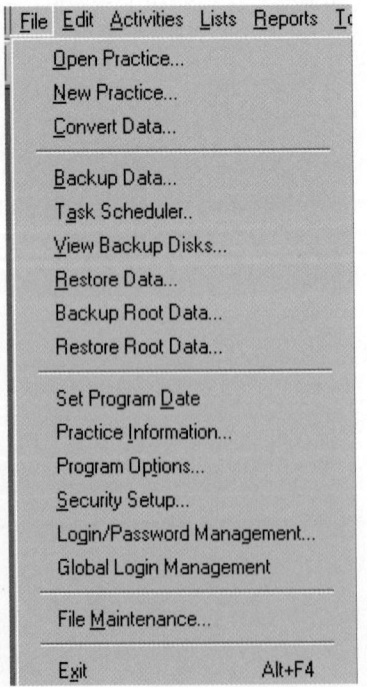

File menu.

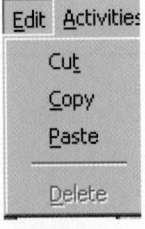

Edit menu.

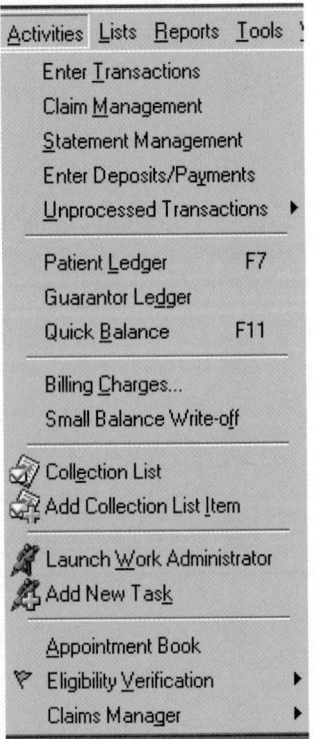

Activities menu.

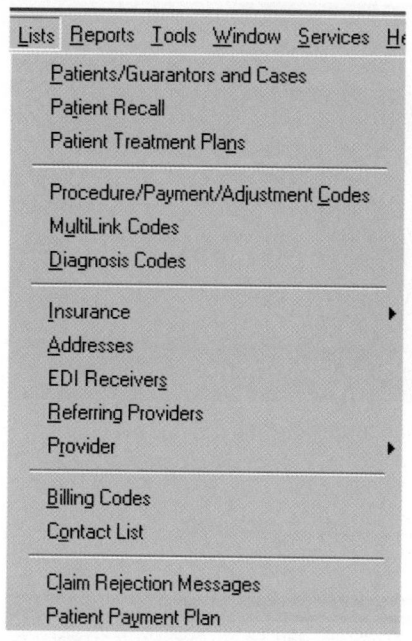

Lists menu.

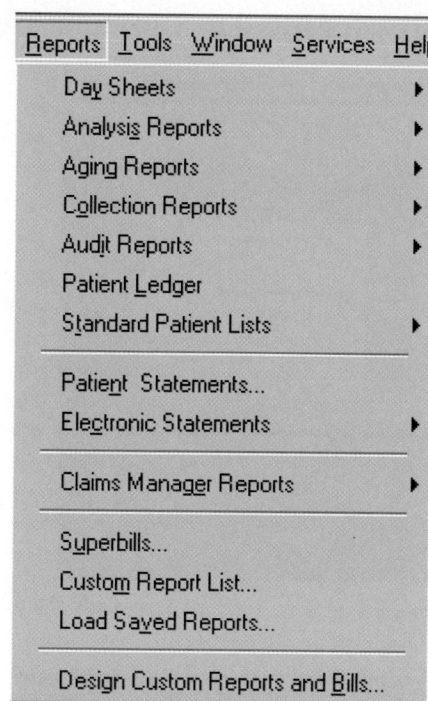

Reports menu.

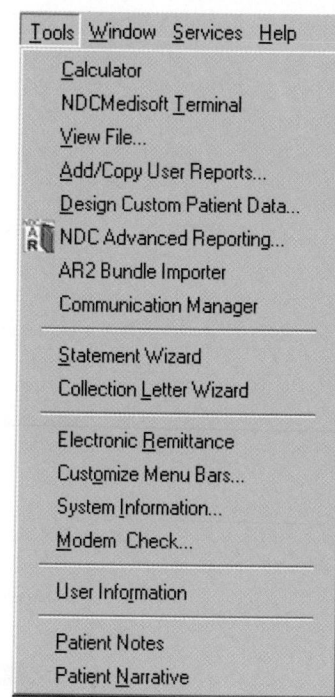

Tools menu.

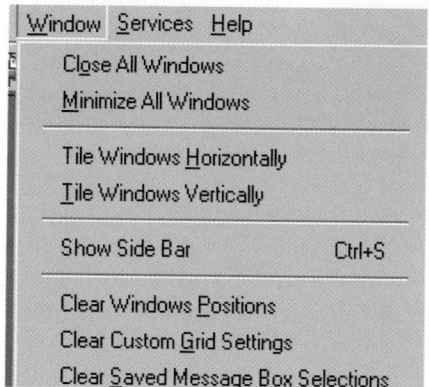

Window menu.

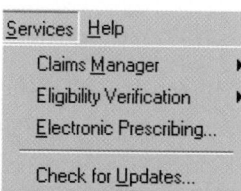

Services menu.

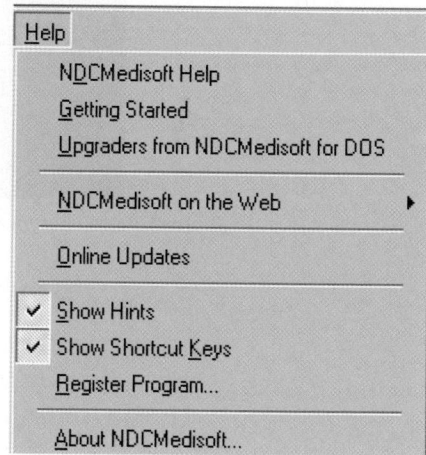

Help menu.

Medisoft Side Bar Shortcut Menus

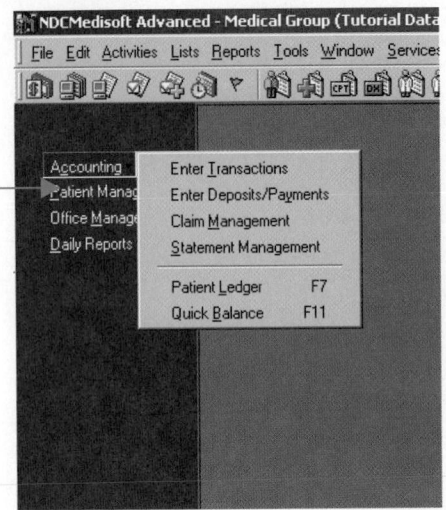

Accounting menu.

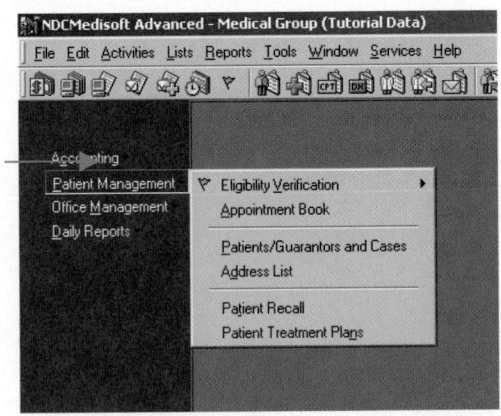

Patient Management menu.

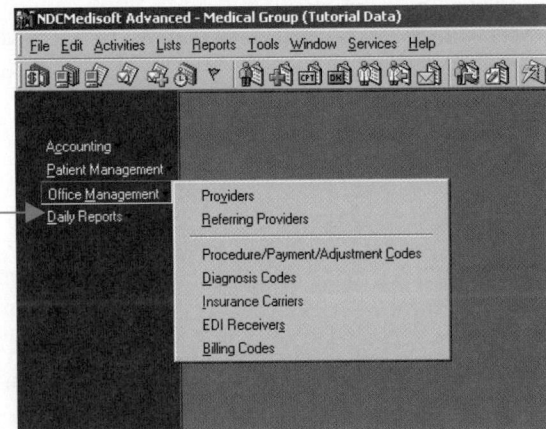

Office Management menu.

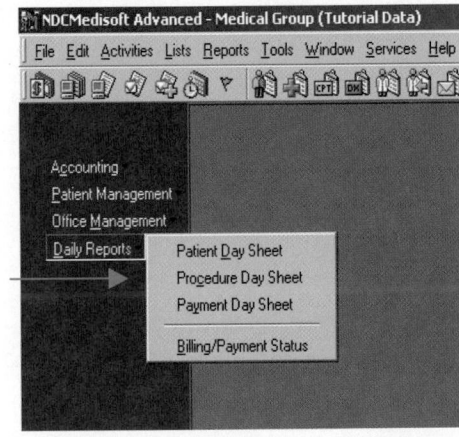

Daily Reports menu.

Simulation Instructions

Please refer to Chapter 17 and use the patient information forms, encounter forms, and Explanation of Benefits forms located at the end of the chapter to complete this simulation exercise.

For this simulation, you are the medical business office specialist for your medical practice. It is your job to enter all patient demographic information, post charges, payments, and adjustments. **It is necessary to enter the ICD-9 and CPT® codes and charges exactly as they appear on the superbills.** This may require you to enter them into the Medisoft database (as a new code) as well as the specific patient's account.

You are responsible for printing a walkout receipt for each patient's account to which you post charges. It is your responsibility to balance your batch at the end of each day and to print insurance claim forms for the patients with insurance.

Some patients may need to come back to the office for follow-up appointments. This will be noted at the bottom of the superbill. If a return appointment is needed, you will need to schedule the appointment for the patient (in Office Hours).

CPT is a registered trademark of the American Medical Association.

Before class ends each day, you may be instructed to stop posting transactions and "batch out." Access the **Reports** menu and run the **Patient Day Sheet** report for today's date. After printing your report, you will use it to make sure you "balance." To do this, you must separately add up all the charges, payments, and adjustments from all the superbills (or EOBs) you posted during the day. Your charges should add up to the amount on the **Total Charges** line on the Patient Day Sheet report. Your payments should equal the negative amount on the **Total Receipts** line of the report, and your adjustments should match the **Total Adjustments** line. If the amounts you totaled from your superbills/EOBs do not match the report totals, you will need to go over the report patient by patient as you look at each patient superbill/EOB to find the discrepancy.

After you have balanced your totals, your instructor may require you to batch your superbills/EOBs and correct Patient Day Sheet report together and turn them in before you leave each day. If this is the case, it means you will have to remove or copy the superbills/EOBs you posted from your textbook. The Patient Day Sheet report is to be placed on top of your superbills/EOBs, followed by your walkout receipts, and stapled together.

Once your batch is complete, it is time to create insurance claims for the patients for whom you entered transaction information. Medisoft allows you to view your insurance claims on screen prior to printing them or sending them electronically. You must look over the claims on the computer screen to make sure there are no errors. If you find any errors, close the claims window and go back to the specific patient's account in the computer and correct it. The claim will automatically be updated with the corrected information. Check your electronic claim batch again to make sure all claims are correct. When you are sure there are no errors, print the claims.

Paper clip your CMS-1500 forms to the bottom of your batch material and turn it in to your instructor.

Tips for Entering Information into Medisoft Advanced

1. First, look over the patient information form. Check the Address List to see if the employer name is already listed in Medisoft. If it is not, add the employer to the Address List.
2. Check the Insurance Carrier List to see if the patient's primary and secondary insurance carrier is already listed in Medisoft. Remember the insurance carrier address must be **exactly the same** as what is written on the patient information form. If the carrier is not listed, add the carrier(s) to the Insurance Carrier List.
3. Check to see if the patient has a Referring Physician (or PCP) listed on the patient information form. If one is listed, check the Referring Provider List to see if the physician is already listed in Medisoft. If the provider is not listed, add the provider.
4. Add the patient to the Patient/Guarantor List if the patient is new. If the patient is not the guarantor, add the guarantor to the Patient/Guarantor List.
5. Make a new Case for the patient. Entering the employer, insurance carrier, and referring provider **prior** to making a patient case allows you to have all the data already entered when you come to the drop down menus (in the case and the patient/guarantor list) for employer, insurance carrier, etc. This saves the hassle of closing the patient case, opening the Address Book (or Insurance Carrier List, etc.), adding the data, saving and closing the window and then opening the patient case again.

Before beginning the simulation, you will need to enter your physician's information into the Medisoft database. Open the **Provider List** (accessed either by shortcut button or Lists menu) and click **New.**

Enter the following information in the *Address* folder in the window:

Your Name
1933 E. Frankford Rd. #110   office telephone: 972-555-5482
Carrollton, TX 12345   home phone: 214-555-8888
                          cell phone: 469-555-3657   fax: 972-555-5416

Medicare Participating, Signature on File   License no.: B1740
Specialty: General Practice

In the *Default PINs* folder enter: 75-1234567 for Federal Tax ID Indicator
Medicare PIN: B94765   Medicaid: K89J2   UPIN: B94765
NPI: 1234569860

Be sure to save any data entered. All of the patients you enter during the simulation will be seeing you.

There are two more things to do before you begin. Open the File menu in Medisoft and Click on Practice Information. Click in the Practice name box. Enter your name as Your Name Medical Clinic.

Click the Save button on the right side of the window.

Go the Address List and enter a new Facility. The facility will be Your Name Medical Clinic, with the address on Frankford Road that you entered for the Practice Name. Click Save and exit the Address List.

You are ready to begin the simulation.

Answers to Practice Exercises

Chapter 2: Managed Care Terminology

Practice Exercise 2-1

1. Discount amount = $23.00; Carrier pays provider = $77.00
2. Discount amount = $424.33; Carrier pays provider = $1,580.98
3. Discount amount = $0; Carrier pays provider = $0
4. Discount amount = $225.00; Carrier pays provider = $800.00
5. Discount amount = $30.00; Carrier pays provider = $95.00
6. Discount amount = $160.00; Carrier pays provider = $162.75

Practice Exercise 2-2

1. Inform Ms. Miller that her carrier states her coverage is not active. Allow her the option of rescheduling her appointment or explain that she may be seen today but will have to pay for the visit herself, out of her own pocket.
2. $32.60

Chapter 3: Understanding Managed Care: Medical Contracts and Ethics

Practice Exercise 3-1

1. The administrative requirements of submitting claims and the timing of receiving payment.
2. The particular forms used to submit claims must be identified by name.
3. All arrangements with regards to the coordination of benefits and late payments must be carefully spelled out in the contract.

Chapter 4: ICD-9 Medical Coding

Practice Exercise 4-1

1. True
2. True
3. False

In the following answers, the main term is listed first, then the subterm.

1. Syndrome; restless leg 333.94
2. Arthritis; rheumatoid 714.0
3. Asthma; spasmodic 493.9
4. Otitis media; acute, serous 381.01
5. Stenosis; aortic valve, congenital 746.3
6. Narrowing; artery vertebral, with cerebral infarction 433.2

7. Donor; bone marrow V59.3
8. Disorder; gastrointestinal 536.9
9. Test; pregnancy, positive result V72.42
10. Ulcer; with gangrene 707.9
11. Examination; follow-up V67.9
12. Pneumopathy; due to dust 504
13. Keratitis; sclerosing 370.54
14. Malocclusion; due to missing teeth 524.30
15. Apnea; sleep, organic 327.20

Practice Exercise 4-2

1. 272.7, 330.2
2. 737.40
3. 117.5, 321.0

Practice Exercise 4-3

The alphabetic index is where the search begins; once the code is found, the tabular list is used to code to the highest level of specificity.

1. Cramps; abdominal
2. 789.0
3. 789.00 (Code to the fifth-digit subclassification.)
4. No
5. Fifth digit required; unspecified site.

Practice Exercise 4-4

1. 784.0

Practice Exercise 4-5

1. 564.02
2. 780.50
3. 345.10
4. 493.22
5. 707.04

Practice Exercise 4-6

1. Preoperative diagnosis: 611.72
   Postoperative diagnosis: 174.9
2. The postoperative report should be reported.

Practice Exercise 4-7

1. 787.2, 438.82
2. 719.01, 905.2
3. 787.02, 909.2
4. 728.87, 905.7

Practice Exercise 4-8

1. 584.9
2. 585.9

Practice Exercise 4-9

1. Functional disorders of stomach specified as psychogenic (306.4).
2. Athyroidism (acquired); hypothyroidism (acquired); myxedema (adult) (juvenile); thyroid (gland) insufficiency (acquired).
3. Acute nasophyaryngitis is the main term and the supplementary term is common cold.
4. Code first any associated obstructed labor (660.1).
5. 250.4 (fifth-digit requirement); Diabetes Mellitus, then the nephropathy–583.81.

Practice Exercise 4-10

1. V57.21
2. V70.0
3. V01.82

Practice Exercise 4-11

1. E908.0
2. E925.1
3. E919.0

Practice Exercise 4-12

1. 198.3
2. 198.4
3. 193

Practice Exercise 4-13

1. 405.19
2. 405.99
3. 401.9

Practice Exercise 4-14

796.2

Practice Exercise 4-15

780.01, 967.0, E980.1

Practice Exercise 4-16

945.34, 943.21, 948.31

Practice Exercise 4-17

1. 0
2. 250.42, 581.81

Practice Exercise 4-18

1. 807.03
2. 815.11
3. 806.02

Chapter 5: Introduction to CPT® and Place of Service Coding

Practice Exercise 5-1

1. Problem Focused
2. Expanded Problem Focused

Practice Exercise 5-2

1. 99214
2. 99211; 99363 (new code for 2007) for Anticoagulant Management
3. 99221
4. 99347

Chapter 6: Coding Procedures and Services

Practice Exercise 6-1

1. 00500
2. 47
3. 01472
4. P2
5. 00142, 99100

Practice Exercise 6-2

1. Facial Nerve; Injection, Anesthetic–64402
2. Clavicle; Fracture, Closed Treatment, without manipulation–23500
3. Excision; Gallbladder–47600

Practice Exercise 6-3

1. 64831, 64832
2. 15400, 15401
3. 26860, 26861(2)

Practice Exercise 6-4

1. TC
2. 26
3. 73592
4. 75554-26
5. 72132-TC

Practice Exercise 6-5

1. 87169
2. 80162
3. 80101
4. 81001
5. 80438

CPT is a registered trademark of the American Medical Association.

Chapter 9: Physician Medical Billing

Practice Exercise 9-1. See completed form in chapter (page 234)

Practice Exercise 9-2

CMS-1500 Health Insurance Claim Form completed for Practice Exercise 9-2. Insurance: BMA INSURANCE, P O BOX 7459, MEMPHIS TN 12345.

- 1a. INSURED'S I.D. NUMBER: 7881508007000
- 2. PATIENT'S NAME: SMITH LIZ M
- 3. BIRTH DATE: 07 01 1996, Sex: F
- 4. INSURED'S NAME: SMITH HARRY L
- 5. ADDRESS: 4591 EXPLORER DRIVE, PLANO TX 12345, (214) 5552984
- 6. RELATIONSHIP: Child
- 7. INSURED'S ADDRESS: 5419 W 8TH ST APT 306, NORMAN OK 12345
- 8. STATUS: Single, Full-Time Student
- 11. POLICY GROUP: G123456
- 11a. INSURED'S DOB: 08 05 1950, M
- 11b. EMPLOYER: VINES LUMBER CO
- 11c. PLAN: BMA
- 12. DATE: 01/03/20XX, SIGNATURE ON FILE

Practice Exercise 9-3

Practice Exercise 9-4

1500
HEALTH INSURANCE CLAIM FORM
APPROVED BY NATIONAL UNIFORM CLAIM COMMITTEE 08/05

PICA

1. MEDICARE (Medicare #) MEDICAID (Medicaid #) TRICARE CHAMPUS (Sponsor's SSN) CHAMPVA (Member ID#) GROUP HEALTH PLAN (SSN or ID) FECA BLK LUNG (SSN) OTHER (ID)	1a. INSURED'S I.D. NUMBER (For Program in Item 1)

2. PATIENT'S NAME (Last Name, First Name, Middle Initial)
3. PATIENT'S BIRTH DATE MM DD YY   SEX M☐ F☐
4. INSURED'S NAME (Last Name, First Name, Middle Initial)

5. PATIENT'S ADDRESS (No, Street)
6. PATIENT RELATIONSHIP TO INSURED Self☐ Spouse☐ Child☐ Other☐
7. INSURED'S ADDRESS (No, Street)

CITY   STATE
8. PATIENT STATUS Single☐ Married☐ Other☐ Employed☐ Full-Time Student☐ Part-Time Student☐
CITY   STATE

ZIP CODE   TELEPHONE (Include Area Code) ( )
ZIP CODE   TELEPHONE (Include Area Code) ( )

9. OTHER INSURED'S NAME (Last Name, First Name, Middle Initial)
10. IS PATIENT'S CONDITION RELATED TO:
11. INSURED'S POLICY GROUP OR FECA NUMBER

a. OTHER INSURED'S POLICY OR GROUP NUMBER
a. EMPLOYMENT? (Current or Previous) ☐YES ☐NO
a. INSURED'S DATE OF BIRTH MM DD YY SEX M☐ F☐

b. OTHER INSURED'S DATE OF BIRTH MM DD YY SEX M☐ F☐
b. AUTO ACCIDENT? PLACE (State) ☐YES ☐NO
b. EMPLOYER'S NAME OR SCHOOL NAME

c. EMPLOYER'S NAME OR SCHOOL NAME
c. OTHER ACCIDENT? ☐YES ☐NO
c. INSURANCE PLAN NAME OR PROGRAM NAME

d. INSURANCE PLAN NAME OR PROGRAM NAME
10d. RESERVED FOR LOCAL USE
d. IS THERE ANOTHER HEALTH BENEFIT PLAN? ☐YES ☐NO If yes, return to and complete item 9 a-d

READ BACK OF FORM BEFORE COMPLETING & SIGNING THIS FORM.
12. PATIENT'S OR AUTHORIZED PERSON'S SIGNATURE I authorize the release of any medical or other information necessary to process this claim. I also request payment of government benefits either to myself or to the party who accepts assignment below.
SIGNED ___ DATE ___
13. INSURED'S OR AUTHORIZED PERSON'S SIGNATURE I authorize payment of medical benefits to the undersigned physician or supplier for services described below.
SIGNED ___

14. DATE OF CURRENT MM XX DD XX YY XXXX ILLNESS (First symptom) OR INJURY (Accident) OR PREGNANCY (LMP)
15. IF PATIENT HAS HAD SAME OR SIMILAR ILLNESS, GIVE FIRST DATE MM DD YY
16. DATES PATIENT UNABLE TO WORK IN CURRENT OCCUPATION FROM MM DD YY TO MM DD YY

17. NAME OF REFERRING PHYSICIAN OR OTHER SOURCE 17a. 17b. NPI
18. HOSPITALIZATION DATES RELATED TO CURRENT SERVICES FROM MM DD YY TO MM DD YY

19. RESERVED FOR LOCAL USE
20. OUTSIDE LAB? ☐YES ☒NO $ CHARGES

21. DIAGNOSIS OR NATURE OF ILLNESS OR INJURY (Relate Items 1,2,3 or 4 to Item 24E by Line)
1. 843 . 9   3. 413 . 9
2. 401 . 9   4.
22. MEDICAID RESUBMISSION CODE   ORIGINAL REF. NO.
23. PRIOR AUTHORIZATION NUMBER

24. A. DATE(S) OF SERVICE From MM DD YY	To MM DD YY	B. PLACE OF SERVICE	C. EMG	D. PROCEDURES, SERVICES, OR SUPPLIES CPT/HCPCS	MODIFIER	E. DIAGNOSIS POINTER	F. $ CHARGES	G. DAYS OR UNITS	H. EPSDT Family Plan	I. ID. QUAL.	J. RENDERING PROVIDER ID. #
1 XX XX XX	XX XX XX	11	Y	99214		1,2	80 00	1		NPI	
2 XX XX XX	XX XX XX	11	Y	36415		2	18 00	1		NPI	
3 XX XX XX	XX XX XX	11	Y	73510		1	90 00	1		NPI	
4 XX XX XX	XX XX XX	11	Y	90782		1	12 00	1		NPI	
5 XX XX XX	XX XX XX	11	Y	93000		2	55 00	1		NPI	
6 XX XX XX	XX XX XX	11		99212		2,3	35 00	1		NPI	

25. FEDERAL TAX ID NUMBER SSN EIN 52-9753211 ☐ ☒
26. PATIENT'S ACCOUNT NO. BUTMAO
27. ACCEPT ASSIGNMENT? (For govt. claims, see back) ☒YES ☐NO
28. TOTAL CHARGE $ 290 00
29. AMOUNT PAID $
30. BALANCE DUE $

31. SIGNATURE OF PHYSICIAN OR SUPPLIER INCLUDING DEGREES OR CREDENTIALS (I certify that the statements on the reverse apply to this bill and are made a part thereof)
SIGNED SIGNATURE ON FILE   DATE XXXXXXXX
32. SERVICE FACILITY LOCATION INFORMATION SHERWOOD, FOREST MD 325 NICHOLS RD SUITE 20B BROOKFIELD, WI 12345 a. 1226449762 b. 1GS985621
33. BILLING PROVIDER INFO & PH. # (414) 555-6790 SHERWOOD, FOREST MD 325 NICHOLS RD SUITE 20B BROOKFIELD, WI 12345 a. 1226449762 b. 1GS985621

NUCC Instruction Manual available at: www.nucc.org   WCMS-1500CS
APPROVED OMB 0938-0999 FORM CMS-1500 (08/05)

Practice Exercise 9-5

(1500)	

HEALTH INSURANCE CLAIM FORM
APPROVED BY NATIONAL UNIFORM CLAIM COMMITTEE 08/05

PICA

☐☐ PICA	

1. MEDICARE ☐ (Medicare #) **MEDICAID** ☐ (Medicaid #) **TRICARE CHAMPUS** ☐ (Sponsor's SSN) **CHAMPVA** ☐ (Member ID#) **GROUP HEALTH PLAN** ☐ (SSN or ID) **FECA BLK LUNG** ☐ (SSN) **OTHER** ☐ (ID)

1a. INSURED'S I.D. NUMBER (For Program in Item 1)

2. PATIENT'S NAME (Last Name, First Name, Middle Initial)

3. PATIENT'S BIRTH DATE MM DD YY   **SEX** M☐ F☐

4. INSURED'S NAME (Last Name, First Name, Middle Initial)

5. PATIENT'S ADDRESS (No, Street)

6. PATIENT RELATIONSHIP TO INSURED Self☐ Spouse☐ Child☐ Other☐

7. INSURED'S ADDRESS (No, Street)

CITY — **STATE**

8. PATIENT STATUS Single☐ Married☐ Other☐
Employed☐ Full-Time Student☐ Part-Time Student☐

CITY — **STATE**

ZIP CODE — **TELEPHONE (Include Area Code)** ( )

ZIP CODE — **TELEPHONE (Include Area Code)** ( )

9. OTHER INSURED'S NAME (Last Name, First Name, Middle Initial)

10. IS PATIENT'S CONDITION RELATED TO:

11. INSURED'S POLICY GROUP OR FECA NUMBER

a. OTHER INSURED'S POLICY OR GROUP NUMBER

a. EMPLOYMENT? (Current or Previous) ☐YES ☐NO

a. INSURED'S DATE OF BIRTH MM DD YY   **SEX** M☐ F☐

b. OTHER INSURED'S DATE OF BIRTH MM DD YY   **SEX** M☐ F☐

b. AUTO ACCIDENT? PLACE (State) ☐YES ☐NO

b. EMPLOYER'S NAME OR SCHOOL NAME

c. EMPLOYER'S NAME OR SCHOOL NAME

c. OTHER ACCIDENT? ☐YES ☐NO

c. INSURANCE PLAN NAME OR PROGRAM NAME

d. INSURANCE PLAN NAME OR PROGRAM NAME

10d. RESERVED FOR LOCAL USE

d. IS THERE ANOTHER HEALTH BENEFIT PLAN? ☐YES ☐NO *If yes,* return to and complete item 9 a-d

READ BACK OF FORM BEFORE COMPLETING & SIGNING THIS FORM.
12. PATIENT'S OR AUTHORIZED PERSON'S SIGNATURE I authorize the release of any medical or other information necessary to process this claim. I also request payment of government benefits either to myself or to the party who accepts assignment below.

SIGNED _____ DATE _____

13. INSURED'S OR AUTHORIZED PERSON'S SIGNATURE I authorize payment of medical benefits to the undersigned physician or supplier for services described below.

SIGNED _____

14. DATE OF CURRENT MM DD YY XX XX XXXX   **ILLNESS (First symptom) OR INJURY (Accident) OR PREGNANCY (LMP)**

15. IF PATIENT HAS HAD SAME OR SIMILAR ILLNESS, GIVE FIRST DATE MM DD YY

16. DATES PATIENT UNABLE TO WORK IN CURRENT OCCUPATION FROM MM DD YY TO MM DD YY

17. NAME OF REFERRING PHYSICIAN OR OTHER SOURCE

17a.
17b. NPI

18. HOSPITALIZATION DATES RELATED TO CURRENT SERVICES FROM MM DD YY TO MM DD YY

19. RESERVED FOR LOCAL USE

20. OUTSIDE LAB? ☐YES ☒NO   **$ CHARGES**

21. DIAGNOSIS OR NATURE OF ILLNESS OR INJURY (Relate Items 1,2,3 or 4 to Item 24E by Line)

1. V 70 . 0
2. 796 . 2
3. 401 . 9
4. _____

22. MEDICAID RESUBMISSION CODE — ORIGINAL REF. NO.

23. PRIOR AUTHORIZATION NUMBER

24. A. DATE(S) OF SERVICE		B. PLACE OF SERVICE	C. EMG	D. PROCEDURES, SERVICES, OR SUPPLIES (Explain Unusual Circumstances)		E. DIAGNOSIS POINTER	F. $ CHARGES	G. DAYS OR UNITS	H. EPSDT Family Plan	I. ID. QUAL.	J. RENDERING PROVIDER ID. #
From MM DD YY	To MM DD YY			CPT/HCPCS	MODIFIER						
1 XX XX XX XX XX XX		11		99386		1	125 00	1		NPI	
2 XX XX XX XX XX XX		11		71020		1,2	45 00	1		NPI	
3 XX XX XX XX XX XX		11		93000		1,2	55 00	1		NPI	
4 XX XX XX XX XX XX		11		81000		1	15 00	1		NPI	
5 XX XX XX XX XX XX		11		99212		2	35 00	1		NPI	
6 XX XX XX XX XX XX		11		99213		3	60 00	1		NPI	

25. FEDERAL TAX ID NUMBER SSN EIN
529753211 ☐ ☒

26. PATIENT'S ACCOUNT NO.
SMIAU

27. ACCEPT ASSIGNMENT? (For govt. claims, see back) ☒YES ☐NO

28. TOTAL CHARGE $ 335 00

29. AMOUNT PAID $

30. BALANCE DUE $

31. SIGNATURE OF PHYSICIAN OR SUPPLIER INCLUDING DEGREES OR CREDENTIALS (I certify that the statements on the reverse apply to this bill and are made a part thereof)
XXXXXX
SIGNED SIGNATURE ON FILE DATE

32. SERVICE FACILITY LOCATION INFORMATION
FORREST M. SHERWOOD MD
325 NICHOLAS RD SUITE 20B
BROOKFIELD, WI 12345
a. 122644972   b. N5 17FMS 53

33. BILLING PROVIDER INFO & PH. # (414) 555-6790
FORREST M. SHERWOOD MD
325 NICHOLS ROAD SUITE 20B
BROOKFIELD, WI 12345
a. 1226449762   b. N5 17FMS 53

NUCC Instruction Manual available at: www.nucc.org
WCMS-1500CS

APPROVED OMB 0938-0999 FORM CMS-1500 (08/05)

CARRIER

PATIENT AND INSURED INFORMATION

PHYSICIAN OR SUPPLIER INFORMATION

SECOND FOLD

FIRST FOLD   WHCF-10-ENV / WHCF-10-ENV-SS

Practice Exercise 9-6

Practice Exercise 9-7

1500

HEALTH INSURANCE CLAIM FORM
APPROVED BY NATIONAL UNIFORM CLAIM COMMITTEE 08/05

☐☐ PICA

PICA ☐☐☐

1. MEDICARE ☐ (Medicare #)	MEDICAID ☐ (Medicaid #)	TRICARE CHAMPUS ☐ (Sponsor's SSN)	CHAMPVA ☐ (Member ID#)	GROUP HEALTH PLAN ☒ (SSN or ID)	FECA BLK LUNG ☐ (SSN)	OTHER ☐ (ID)

1a. INSURED'S I.D. NUMBER (For Program in Item 1)
75300865

2. PATIENT'S NAME (Last Name, First Name, Middle Initial)
TILLMAN RANDALL J

3. PATIENT'S BIRTH DATE   SEX
MM 02 DD 19 YY 1989   M ☒   F ☐

4. INSURED'S NAME (Last Name, First Name, Middle Initial)
TILLMAN THERESA M

5. PATIENT'S ADDRESS (No, Street)
1212 FRY STREET

6. PATIENT RELATIONSHIP TO INSURED
Self ☐ Spouse ☐ Child ☒ Other ☐

7. INSURED'S ADDRESS (No, Street)
4225 BENTON AVE APT 6

CITY   DES PLAINES   STATE IL

8. PATIENT STATUS
Single ☒   Married ☐   Other ☐
Employed ☐   Full-Time Student ☒   Part-Time Student ☐

CITY   DES PLAINES   STATE IL

ZIP CODE 12345   TELEPHONE (Include Area Code) (312) 5554993

ZIP CODE 12345   TELEPHONE (Include Area Code) (312) 5554993

9. OTHER INSURED'S NAME (Last Name, First Name, Middle Initial)

10. IS PATIENT'S CONDITION RELATED TO:

11. INSURED'S POLICY GROUP OR FECA NUMBER
DP 139

a. OTHER INSURED'S POLICY OR GROUP NUMBER

a. EMPLOYMENT? (Current or Previous)
☐ YES   ☒ NO

a. INSURED'S DATE OF BIRTH   SEX
MM 01 DD 03 YY 1958   M ☐   F ☒

b. OTHER INSURED'S DATE OF BIRTH   SEX
MM DD YY   M ☐   F ☐

b. AUTO ACCIDENT?   PLACE (State)
☐ YES   ☒ NO

b. EMPLOYER'S NAME OR SCHOOL NAME
DES PLAINES CHEVROLET

c. EMPLOYER'S NAME OR SCHOOL NAME

c. OTHER ACCIDENT?
☐ YES   ☒ NO

c. INSURANCE PLAN NAME OR PROGRAM NAME
CIGNA

d. INSURANCE PLAN NAME OR PROGRAM NAME

10d. RESERVED FOR LOCAL USE

d. IS THERE ANOTHER HEALTH BENEFIT PLAN?
☐ YES   ☒ NO   If yes, return to and complete item 9 a-d

READ BACK OF FORM BEFORE COMPLETING & SIGNING THIS FORM.
12. PATIENT'S OR AUTHORIZED PERSON'S SIGNATURE I authorize the release of any medical or other information necessary to process this claim. I also request payment of government benefits either to myself or to the party who accepts assignment below.

SIGNED   SIGNATURE ON FILE   DATE

13. INSURED'S OR AUTHORIZED PERSON'S SIGNATURE I authorize payment of medical benefits to the undersigned physician or supplier for services described below.

SIGNED   SIGNATURE ON FILE

14. DATE OF CURRENT   ILLNESS (First symptom) OR
MM XX DD XX YY XXXX   INJURY (Accident) OR PREGNANCY (LMP)

15. IF PATIENT HAS HAD SAME OR SIMILAR ILLNESS, GIVE FIRST DATE MM DD YY

16. DATES PATIENT UNABLE TO WORK IN CURRENT OCCUPATION
FROM MM DD YY   TO MM DD YY

17. NAME OF REFERRING PHYSICIAN OR OTHER SOURCE

17a.
17b. NPI

18. HOSPITALIZATION DATES RELATED TO CURRENT SERVICES
FROM MM DD YY   TO MM DD YY

19. RESERVED FOR LOCAL USE

20. OUTSIDE LAB? $ CHARGES
☐ YES   ☒ NO

21. DIAGNOSIS OR NATURE OF ILLNESS OR INJURY (Relate Items 1,2,3 or 4 to Item 24E by Line)
1. |48 . 71
2. |____
3. |____
4. |____

22. MEDICAID RESUBMISSION
CODE   ORIGINAL REF. NO.

23. PRIOR AUTHORIZATION NUMBER

24. A. DATE(S) OF SERVICE From MM DD YY	To MM DD YY	B. PLACE OF SERVICE	C. EMG	D. PROCEDURES, SERVICES, OR SUPPLIES (Explain Unusual Circumstances) CPT/HCPCS	MODIFIER	E. DIAGNOSIS POINTER	F. $ CHARGES	G. DAYS OR UNITS	H. EPSDT Family Plan	I. ID. QUAL.	J. RENDERING PROVIDER ID. #
1	XX XX XX	XX XX XX	11		99202		1	50 00	1		N5 NPI	3266113 5524998733
2											NPI	
3											NPI	
4											NPI	
5											NPI	
6											NPI	

25. FEDERAL TAX ID NUMBER   SSN EIN
563342560   ☐ ☒

26. PATIENT'S ACCOUNT NO.
TILLRA

27. ACCEPT ASSIGNMENT? (For govt. claims, see back)
☒ YES   ☐ NO

28. TOTAL CHARGE
$ 50 00

29. AMOUNT PAID
$

30. BALANCE DUE
$

31. SIGNATURE OF PHYSICIAN OR SUPPLIER INCLUDING DEGREES OR CREDENTIALS (I certify that the statements on the reverse apply to this bill and are made a part thereof)

SIGNED   SIGNATURE ON FILE   DATE

32. SERVICE FACILITY LOCATION INFORMATION
YOUNG BLOOD AND ASSOC
2128 EAST 144TH ST STE 15
CHICAGO IL 12345

a. 6625897130   b. N506 55872

33. BILLING PROVIDER INFO & PH. # (312) 555-7690
YOUNG BLOOD AND ASSOC
2128 EAST 144TH ST STE 15
CHICAGO IL 12345

a. 6625897130   b. N506 55872

NUCC Instruction Manual available at: www.nucc.org
WCMS-1500CS

APPROVED OMB 0938-0999 FORM CMS-1500 (08/05)

Practice Exercise 9-8

(1500)

HEALTH INSURANCE CLAIM FORM
APPROVED BY NATIONAL UNIFORM CLAIM COMMITTEE 08/05

☐☐☐ PICA

1. MEDICARE	MEDICAID	TRICARE CHAMPUS	CHAMPVA	GROUP HEALTH PLAN	FECA BLK LUNG	OTHER	1a. INSURED'S I.D. NUMBER	(For Program in Item 1)
☐ (Medicare #)	☐ (Medicaid #)	☐ (Sponsor's SSN)	☐ (Member ID#)	☐ (SSN or ID)	☐ (SSN)	☒ (ID)	512539751	

2. PATIENT'S NAME (Last Name, First Name, Middle Initial)
LYNCH AMY LOUISE

3. PATIENT'S BIRTH DATE   SEX
MM 01 DD 09 YY 1999   M☐ F☒

4. INSURED'S NAME (Last Name, First Name, Middle Initial)
LYNCH FRED K

5. PATIENT'S ADDRESS (No, Street)
893 BAY STREET

6. PATIENT RELATIONSHIP TO INSURED
Self ☐ Spouse ☐ Child ☒ Other ☐

7. INSURED'S ADDRESS (No, Street)
1776 LIBERTY ROAD

CITY PHILADELPHIA   STATE PA

8. PATIENT STATUS
Single ☒ Married ☐ Other ☐
Employed ☐ Full-Time Student ☒ Part-Time Student ☐

CITY PHILADELPHIA   STATE PA

ZIP CODE 12345   TELEPHONE (Include Area Code) (214) 555-0081

ZIP CODE 12345   TELEPHONE (Include Area Code) (214) 555-0704

9. OTHER INSURED'S NAME (Last Name, First Name, Middle Initial)
LYNCH, JESSIE M

10. IS PATIENT'S CONDITION RELATED TO:

11. INSURED'S POLICY GROUP OR FECA NUMBER
W45980

a. OTHER INSURED'S POLICY OR GROUP NUMBER
491510003A

a. EMPLOYMENT? (Current or Previous)
☐ YES ☒ NO

a. INSURED'S DATE OF BIRTH
MM 06 DD 15 YY 1947   SEX M☒ F☐

b. OTHER INSURED'S DATE OF BIRTH   SEX
MM 08 DD 05 YY 1950   M☐ F☒

b. AUTO ACCIDENT?   PLACE (State)
☐ YES ☒ NO

b. EMPLOYER'S NAME OR SCHOOL NAME
WDAF RADIO

c. EMPLOYER'S NAME OR SCHOOL NAME
SOUTHERLAND LUMBER

c. OTHER ACCIDENT?
☐ YES ☒ NO

c. INSURANCE PLAN NAME OR PROGRAM NAME
BCBS OF PA

d. INSURANCE PLAN NAME OR PROGRAM NAME
METROPOLITAN FAMILY

10d. RESERVED FOR LOCAL USE

d. IS THERE ANOTHER HEALTH BENEFIT PLAN?
☒ YES ☐ NO   If yes, return to and complete item 9 a-d

READ BACK OF FORM BEFORE COMPLETING & SIGNING THIS FORM.

12. PATIENT'S OR AUTHORIZED PERSON'S SIGNATURE I authorize the release of any medical or other information necessary to process this claim. I also request payment of government benefits either to myself or to the party who accepts assignment below.

SIGNED ___ SOF ___   DATE XX XX XXXX

13. INSURED'S OR AUTHORIZED PERSON'S SIGNATURE I authorize payment of medical benefits to the undersigned physician or supplier for services described below.

SIGNED ___ SIGNATURE ON FILE

14. DATE OF CURRENT   ILLNESS (First symptom) OR INJURY (Accident) OR PREGNANCY (LMP)
MM XX DD XX YY XXXX

15. IF PATIENT HAS HAD SAME OR SIMILAR ILLNESS, GIVE FIRST DATE   MM   DD   YY

16. DATES PATIENT UNABLE TO WORK IN CURRENT OCCUPATION
FROM MM DD YY   TO MM DD YY

17. NAME OF REFERRING PHYSICIAN OR OTHER SOURCE
17a.
17b. NPI

18. HOSPITALIZATION DATES RELATED TO CURRENT SERVICES
FROM MM DD YY   TO MM DD YY

19. RESERVED FOR LOCAL USE

20. OUTSIDE LAB?   ☐ YES ☒ NO $ CHARGES

21. DIAGNOSIS OR NATURE OF ILLNESS OR INJURY (Relate Items 1,2,3 or 4 to Item 24E by Line)
1. 382 . 00
2.
3.
4.

22. MEDICAID RESUBMISSION CODE   ORIGINAL REF. NO.

23. PRIOR AUTHORIZATION NUMBER

24. A. DATE(S) OF SERVICE From / To						B. PLACE OF SERVICE	C. EMG	D. PROCEDURES, SERVICES, OR SUPPLIES (Explain Unusual Circumstances) CPT/HCPCS	MODIFIER	E. DIAGNOSIS POINTER	F. $ CHARGES	G. DAYS OR UNITS	H. EPSDT Family Plan	I. ID. QUAL.	J. RENDERING PROVIDER ID. #
MM	DD	YY	MM	DD	YY										
XX	XX	XX	XX	XX	XX	11		99212		1	40 00	1		IB	49552978
														NPI	9998755667
														NPI	
														NPI	
														NPI	
														NPI	
														NPI	

25. FEDERAL TAX ID NUMBER   SSN EIN
51-4290642   ☐ ☒

26. PATIENT'S ACCOUNT NO.
LYNAM

27. ACCEPT ASSIGNMENT? (For govt. claims, see back)
☒ YES ☐ NO

28. TOTAL CHARGE
$ 40 00

29. AMOUNT PAID
$

30. BALANCE DUE
$

31. SIGNATURE OF PHYSICIAN OR SUPPLIER INCLUDING DEGREES OR CREDENTIALS
(I certify that the statements on the reverse apply to this bill and are made a part thereof)
SIGNED SIGNATURE ON FILE   DATE XX XX XXXX

32. SERVICE FACILITY LOCATION INFORMATION
PCL MEDICAL ASSOCIATES
1720 FRONT STREET
PHILADELPHIA, PA 12345
a. 6666455522   b. IBB50862

33. BILLING PROVIDER INFO & PH. # (214) 555-3000
PCL MEDICAL ASSOCIATES
1720 FRONT STREET
PHILADELPHIA, PA 12345
a. 6666455522   b. IBB50862

NUCC Instruction Manual available at: www.nucc.org
WCMS-1500CS

APPROVED OMB 0938-0999 FORM CMS-1500 (08/05)

Practice Exercise 9-9 a

Practice Exercise 9-9 b

(1500)

HEALTH INSURANCE CLAIM FORM
APPROVED BY NATIONAL UNIFORM CLAIM COMMITTEE 08/05

☐☐☐ PICA

1. MEDICARE ☐ (Medicare #) MEDICAID ☐ (Medicaid #) TRICARE CHAMPUS ☐ (Sponsor's SSN) CHAMPVA ☐ (Member ID#) GROUP HEALTH PLAN ☒ (SSN or ID) FECA BLK LUNG ☐ (SSN) OTHER ☐ (ID)	1a. INSURED'S I.D. NUMBER (For Program in Item 1)
	2630254

| 2. PATIENT'S NAME (Last Name, First Name, Middle Initial) BOWMAN VERONICA LEE | 3. PATIENT'S BIRTH DATE MM 06 DD 07 YY 1961   SEX M☐ F☒ | 4. INSURED'S NAME (Last Name, First Name, Middle Initial) SAME |

| 5. PATIENT'S ADDRESS (No, Street) 25 ELM STREET | 6. PATIENT RELATIONSHIP TO INSURED Self ☒ Spouse ☐ Child ☐ Other ☐ | 7. INSURED'S ADDRESS (No, Street) |

| CITY GARDNER   STATE KS | 8. PATIENT STATUS Single ☒ Married ☐ Other ☐ | CITY   STATE |

| ZIP CODE 12345   TELEPHONE (Include Area Code) (913) 5557779 | Employed ☒ Full-Time Student ☐ Part-Time Student ☐ | ZIP CODE   TELEPHONE (Include Area Code) (   ) |

| 9. OTHER INSURED'S NAME (Last Name, First Name, Middle Initial) | 10. IS PATIENT'S CONDITION RELATED TO: | 11. INSURED'S POLICY GROUP OR FECA NUMBER FR 2856 |

| a. OTHER INSURED'S POLICY OR GROUP NUMBER | a. EMPLOYMENT? (Current or Previous) ☐YES ☒NO | a. INSURED'S DATE OF BIRTH MM DD YY   SEX M☐ F☐ |

| b. OTHER INSURED'S DATE OF BIRTH MM DD YY   SEX M☐ F☐ | b. AUTO ACCIDENT?   PLACE (State) ☐YES ☒NO | b. EMPLOYER'S NAME OR SCHOOL NAME FRITO LAY |

| c. EMPLOYER'S NAME OR SCHOOL NAME | c. OTHER ACCIDENT? ☐YES ☒NO | c. INSURANCE PLAN NAME OR PROGRAM NAME CIGNA |

| d. INSURANCE PLAN NAME OR PROGRAM NAME | 10d. RESERVED FOR LOCAL USE | d. IS THERE ANOTHER HEALTH BENEFIT PLAN? ☐YES ☒NO   If yes, return to and complete item 9 a-d |

READ BACK OF FORM BEFORE COMPLETING & SIGNING THIS FORM.
12. PATIENT'S OR AUTHORIZED PERSON'S SIGNATURE I authorize the release of any medical or other information necessary to process this claim. I also request payment of government benefits either to myself or to the party who accepts assignment below.

SIGNED   SOF   DATE XX XX XX

13. INSURED'S OR AUTHORIZED PERSON'S SIGNATURE I authorize payment of medical benefits to the undersigned physician or supplier for services described below.

SIGNED   SIGNATURE ON FILE

| 14. DATE OF CURRENT   ILLNESS (First symptom) OR MM XX DD XX YY XX   INJURY (Accident) OR PREGNANCY (LMP) | 15. IF PATIENT HAS HAD SAME OR SIMILAR ILLNESS, GIVE FIRST DATE   MM DD YY | 16. DATES PATIENT UNABLE TO WORK IN CURRENT OCCUPATION FROM MM DD YY   TO MM DD YY |

| 17. NAME OF REFERRING PHYSICIAN OR OTHER SOURCE | 17a. 17b. NPI | 18. HOSPITALIZATION DATES RELATED TO CURRENT SERVICES FROM MM DD YY   TO MM DD YY |

| 19. RESERVED FOR LOCAL USE | 20. OUTSIDE LAB? ☒YES ☐NO $ CHARGES 12.00 | 10.00 |

21. DIAGNOSIS OR NATURE OF ILLNESS OR INJURY (Relate Items 1,2,3 or 4 to Item 24E by Line)
1. 487 . 0
2.
3.
4.

22. MEDICAID RESUBMISSION CODE   ORIGINAL REF. NO.

23. PRIOR AUTHORIZATION NUMBER

24. A. DATE(S) OF SERVICE From To MM DD YY MM DD YY	B. PLACE OF SERVICE	C. EMG	D. PROCEDURES, SERVICES, OR SUPPLIES (Explain Unusual Circumstances) CPT/HCPCS MODIFIER	E. DIAGNOSIS POINTER	F. $ CHARGES	G. DAYS OR UNITS	H. EPSDT Family Plan	I. ID. QUAL.	J. RENDERING PROVIDER ID. #
1 XX XX XX XX XX XX	11		87015	1	18 00	1		NS NPI	045657 4531118907
2 XX XX XX XX XX XX	11		85025	1	17 00	1		NS NPI	045657 4531118907
3								NPI	
4			.					NPI	
5								NPI	
6								NPI	

| 25. FEDERAL TAX ID NUMBER   SSN EIN 531919011   ☐ ☒ | 26. PATIENT'S ACCOUNT NO. BOWVEI | 27. ACCEPT ASSIGNMENT? (For govt. claims, see back) ☒YES ☐NO | 28. TOTAL CHARGE $ 35 00 | 29. AMOUNT PAID $ | 30. BALANCE DUE $ |

| 31. SIGNATURE OF PHYSICIAN OR SUPPLIER INCLUDING DEGREES OR CREDENTIALS (I certify that the statements on the reverse apply to this bill and are made a part thereof) XX XX XX SIGNED SIGNATURE ON FILE DATE | 32. SERVICE FACILITY LOCATION INFORMATION JOHNSON COUNTY LAB 15107 SOUTH LOCUST OLATHE, KS 12345 | 33. BILLING PROVIDER INFO & PH. # (913) 555-2700 FAMILY MEDICINE PC 2500 EAST AVENUE OLATHE, KS 12345 |
| | a. 032564444321   b. G2 528761 | a. 7221160934   b. N5 567203 |

NUCC Instruction Manual available at: www.nucc.org
WCMS-1500CS

APPROVED OMB 0938-0999 FORM CMS-1500 (08/05)

Practice Exercise 9-10

(1500)

HEALTH INSURANCE CLAIM FORM
APPROVED BY NATIONAL UNIFORM CLAIM COMMITTEE 08/05

PICA   PICA

1. MEDICARE	MEDICAID	TRICARE CHAMPUS	CHAMPVA	GROUP HEALTH PLAN	FECA BLK LUNG	OTHER	1a. INSURED'S I.D. NUMBER	(For Program in Item 1)
☐ (Medicare #)	☐ (Medicaid #)	☐ (Sponsor's SSN)	☐ (Member ID#)	☒ (SSN or ID)	☐ (SSN)	☐ (ID)	60923	

2. PATIENT'S NAME (Last Name, First Name, Middle Initial)
BLACK KATHY A

3. PATIENT'S BIRTH DATE   SEX
MM 01 | DD 20 | YY 1949   M☐   F☒

4. INSURED'S NAME (Last Name, First Name, Middle Initial)
BLACK JASON D

5. PATIENT'S ADDRESS (No, Street)
79 NORTH WEST TERRACE

6. PATIENT RELATIONSHIP TO INSURED
Self☐   Spouse☒   Child☐   Other☐

7. INSURED'S ADDRESS (No, Street)
SAME

CITY   KANSAS CITY   STATE KS

8. PATIENT STATUS
Single☐   Married☒   Other☐
Employed☐   Full-Time Student☐   Part-Time Student☐

CITY   STATE

ZIP CODE 12345   TELEPHONE (Include Area Code) (913) 5551560

ZIP CODE   TELEPHONE (Include Area Code) ( )

9. OTHER INSURED'S NAME (Last Name, First Name, Middle Initial)

10. IS PATIENT'S CONDITION RELATED TO:

11. INSURED'S POLICY GROUP OR FECA NUMBER
2222

a. OTHER INSURED'S POLICY OR GROUP NUMBER

a. EMPLOYMENT? (Current or Previous)
☐YES ☒NO

a. INSURED'S DATE OF BIRTH   SEX
MM 04 | DD 01 | YY 1945   M☒   F☐

b. OTHER INSURED'S DATE OF BIRTH   SEX
MM | DD | YY   M☐   F☐

b. AUTO ACCIDENT?   PLACE (State)
☐YES ☒NO

b. EMPLOYER'S NAME OR SCHOOL NAME
EDS

c. EMPLOYER'S NAME OR SCHOOL NAME

c. OTHER ACCIDENT?
☐YES ☒NO

c. INSURANCE PLAN NAME OR PROGRAM NAME
FORTIS INS CO

d. INSURANCE PLAN NAME OR PROGRAM NAME

10d. RESERVED FOR LOCAL USE

d. IS THERE ANOTHER HEALTH BENEFIT PLAN?
☐YES ☒NO   If yes, return to and complete item 9 a-d

READ BACK OF FORM BEFORE COMPLETING & SIGNING THIS FORM.
12. PATIENT'S OR AUTHORIZED PERSON'S SIGNATURE I authorize the release of any medical or other information necessary to process this claim. I also request payment of government benefits either to myself or to the party who accepts assignment below.

SIGNED   SIGNATURE ON FILE   DATE   09/15/20XX

13. INSURED'S OR AUTHORIZED PERSON'S SIGNATURE I authorize payment of medical benefits to the undersigned physician or supplier for services described below.

SIGNED   SIGNATURE ON FILE

14. DATE OF CURRENT ILLNESS (First symptom) OR INJURY (Accident) OR PREGNANCY (LMP)
MM XX | DD XX | YY XX

15. IF PATIENT HAS HAD SAME OR SIMILAR ILLNESS, GIVE FIRST DATE MM | DD | YY

16. DATES PATIENT UNABLE TO WORK IN CURRENT OCCUPATION
FROM MM DATES GO HERE DD YY   TO MM DD YY HERE

17. NAME OF REFERRING PHYSICIAN OR OTHER SOURCE
HENDERSON CHARLES MD

17a. 1G | 08623
17b. NPI | 0815094410

18. HOSPITALIZATION DATES RELATED TO CURRENT SERVICES
FROM MM DATES GO HERE DD YY   TO MM DD YY HERE

19. RESERVED FOR LOCAL USE

20. OUTSIDE LAB? ☐YES ☒NO $ CHARGES

21. DIAGNOSIS OR NATURE OF ILLNESS OR INJURY (Relate Items 1,2,3 or 4 to Item 24E by Line)
1. 611 . 72
2. 174 . 9
3.
4.

22. MEDICAID RESUBMISSION CODE   ORIGINAL REF. NO.

23. PRIOR AUTHORIZATION NUMBER
52521212

24. A. DATE(S) OF SERVICE From MM DD YY To MM DD YY	B. PLACE OF SERVICE	C. EMG	D. PROCEDURES, SERVICES, OR SUPPLIES (Explain Unusual Circumstances) CPT/HCPCS	MODIFIER	E. DIAGNOSIS POINTER	F. $ CHARGES	G. DAYS OR UNITS	H. EPSDT Family Plan	I. ID. QUAL.	J. RENDERING PROVIDER ID. #
1	XX XX XX XX XX XX	11		99204		1	150 00	1		NPI	
2	XX XX XX XX XX XX	11		19100	50	1	350 00	2		NPI	
3	XX XX XX XX XX XX	11		99214		2	40 00	1		NPI	
4	XX XX XX XX XX XX	21		99221		2	150 00	1		NPI	
5	XX XX XX XX XX XX	21		19200	50	2	3700 00	2		NPI	
6	XX XX XX XX XX XX	21		99238		2	50 00	1		NPI	

25. FEDERAL TAX ID NUMBER   SSN EIN
551530016   ☐☒

26. PATIENT'S ACCOUNT NO.
BLAKA

27. ACCEPT ASSIGNMENT? (For govt. claims, see back)
☒YES ☐NO

28. TOTAL CHARGE
$ 4440 00

29. AMOUNT PAID
$

30. BALANCE DUE
$

31. SIGNATURE OF PHYSICIAN OR SUPPLIER INCLUDING DEGREES OR CREDENTIALS
(I certify that the statements on the reverse apply to this bill and are made a part thereof)

SIGNED   SIGNATURE ON FILE   DATE

32. SERVICE FACILITY LOCATION INFORMATION
METROPOLITAN MEDICAL CTR
153 SLATER RD
LEA WOOD KS 12345

a. 0066677889   b.

33. BILLING PROVIDER INFO & PH. #   (913) 5559706
TINA HARRIS MD
16670 WEST 95 TERRACE
OVERLAND PARK KS 12345

a. 8954433148   b.

NUCC Instruction Manual available at: www.nucc.org   WCMS-1500CS

APPROVED OMB 0938-0999 FORM CMS-1500 (08/05)

Practice Exercise 9-11

(1500)

HEALTH INSURANCE CLAIM FORM
APPROVED BY NATIONAL UNIFORM CLAIM COMMITTEE 08/05

| | | PICA | | | | | | | PICA | |

1. MEDICARE ☐ (Medicare #) **MEDICAID** ☐ (Medicaid #) **TRICARE CHAMPUS** ☐ (Sponsor's SSN) **CHAMPVA** ☐ (Member ID#) **GROUP HEALTH PLAN** ☒ (SSN or ID) **FECA BLK LUNG** ☐ (SSN) **OTHER** ☐ (ID)

1a. INSURED'S I.D. NUMBER (For Program in Item 1)
622648701

2. PATIENT'S NAME (Last Name, First Name, Middle Initial)
WARD BARBARA

3. PATIENT'S BIRTH DATE MM 08 DD 02 YY 1956 **SEX** M ☐ F ☒

4. INSURED'S NAME (Last Name, First Name, Middle Initial)
WARD CHARLES

5. PATIENT'S ADDRESS (No, Street)
214 BAND RD

6. PATIENT RELATIONSHIP TO INSURED
Self ☐ Spouse ☒ Child ☐ Other ☐

7. INSURED'S ADDRESS (No, Street)
SAME

CITY FRISCO **STATE** TX

8. PATIENT STATUS
Single ☐ Married ☒ Other ☐
Employed ☒ Full-Time Student ☐ Part-Time Student ☐

CITY **STATE**

ZIP CODE 12345 **TELEPHONE (Include Area Code)** (972) 5558943

ZIP CODE **TELEPHONE (Include Area Code)** (   )

9. OTHER INSURED'S NAME (Last Name, First Name, Middle Initial)
WARD BARBARA

10. IS PATIENT'S CONDITION RELATED TO:

11. INSURED'S POLICY GROUP OR FECA NUMBER
2223389

a. OTHER INSURED'S POLICY OR GROUP NUMBER
214689852

a. EMPLOYMENT? (Current or Previous)
☐ YES ☒ NO

a. INSURED'S DATE OF BIRTH MM 10 DD 09 YY 1953 **SEX** M ☒ F ☐

b. OTHER INSURED'S DATE OF BIRTH MM 08 DD 02 YY 1956 **SEX** M ☐ F ☒

b. AUTO ACCIDENT? **PLACE (State)**
☐ YES ☒ NO

b. EMPLOYER'S NAME OR SCHOOL NAME
DALMETH ENTERPRISES

c. EMPLOYER'S NAME OR SCHOOL NAME
ALLIED CAREER CENTER

c. OTHER ACCIDENT?
☐ YES ☒ NO

c. INSURANCE PLAN NAME OR PROGRAM NAME
AETNA HEALTH

d. INSURANCE PLAN NAME OR PROGRAM NAME
OXFORD HEALTH

10d. RESERVED FOR LOCAL USE

d. IS THERE ANOTHER HEALTH BENEFIT PLAN?
☒ YES ☐ NO *If yes*, return to and complete item 9 a-d

READ BACK OF FORM BEFORE COMPLETING & SIGNING THIS FORM.

12. PATIENT'S OR AUTHORIZED PERSON'S SIGNATURE I authorize the release of any medical or other information necessary to process this claim. I also request payment of government benefits either to myself or to the party who accepts assignment below.

SIGNED   SIGNATURE ON FILE   DATE XXXXXXXX

13. INSURED'S OR AUTHORIZED PERSON'S SIGNATURE I authorize payment of medical benefits to the undersigned physician or supplier for services described below.

SIGNED   SIGNATURE ON FILE

14. DATE OF CURRENT MM XX DD XX YY XXXX ILLNESS (First symptom) OR INJURY (Accident) OR PREGNANCY (LMP)

15. IF PATIENT HAS HAD SAME OR SIMILAR ILLNESS, GIVE FIRST DATE MM DD YY

16. DATES PATIENT UNABLE TO WORK IN CURRENT OCCUPATION FROM MM DD YY TO MM DD YY

17. NAME OF REFERRING PHYSICIAN OR OTHER SOURCE

17a.
17b. NPI

18. HOSPITALIZATION DATES RELATED TO CURRENT SERVICES FROM MM DD YY TO MM DD YY

19. RESERVED FOR LOCAL USE

20. OUTSIDE LAB? ☐ YES ☒ NO **$ CHARGES**

21. DIAGNOSIS OR NATURE OF ILLNESS OR INJURY (Relate Items 1,2,3 or 4 to Item 24E by Line)

1. 401 . 1
2.
3.
4.

22. MEDICAID RESUBMISSION CODE ORIGINAL REF. NO.

23. PRIOR AUTHORIZATION NUMBER

24. A. DATE(S) OF SERVICE From MM DD YY	To MM DD YY	B. PLACE OF SERVICE	C. EMG	D. PROCEDURES, SERVICES, OR SUPPLIES (Explain Unusual Circumstances) CPT/HCPCS MODIFIER	E. DIAGNOSIS POINTER	F. $ CHARGES	G. DAYS OR UNITS	H. EPSDT Family Plan	I. ID. QUAL.	J. RENDERING PROVIDER ID. #
1 XX XX XX	XX XX XX	11		99203	1	150 00	1		NPI	
2									NPI	
3									NPI	
4									NPI	
5									NPI	
6									NPI	

25. FEDERAL TAX ID NUMBER 168749532 **SSN EIN** ☐ ☒

26. PATIENT'S ACCOUNT NO. WARBA

27. ACCEPT ASSIGNMENT? (For govt. claims, see back) ☒ YES ☐ NO

28. TOTAL CHARGE $ 150 00

29. AMOUNT PAID $ 100 00

30. BALANCE DUE $ 50 00

31. SIGNATURE OF PHYSICIAN OR SUPPLIER INCLUDING DEGREES OR CREDENTIALS (I certify that the statements on the reverse apply to this bill and are made a part thereof)

SIGNED   SIGNATURE ON FILE   XXXXXXXX DATE

32. SERVICE FACILITY LOCATION INFORMATION
JAMES BROWN MD
1400 LAST STREET
DALLAS TX 12345
a. 5598565422   b. N5AET06

33. BILLING PROVIDER INFO & PH. # (555) 3457654
JAMES BROWN MD
1400 LAST STREET
DALLAS TX 12345
a. 5598565422   b. N5AET06

NUCC Instruction Manual available at: www.nucc.org
WCMS-1500CS

APPROVED OMB 0938-0999 FORM CMS-1500 (08/05)

For Student Use Only

Payer's Name and Address

| Oxford Health |
| 12030 Plano Parkway |
| Plano, Virginia 43098 |

Today's Date:

CHECK #287613

Provider's Name and Address

| Dr. James Brown |
| 1400 Last Street |
| Dallas, TX 12345 |

This statement covers payments for the following patient(s):

Claim Detail Section

Patient Name: Ward, Barbara **Patient Account #:** 0654
Patient ID#: 214689852   **Insured's Name:** Same   **Group #:** 54790012
Provider Name: Dr. Brown   **Inventory #:** 33782   **Claim Control #:** 55502

Service Date(s)	Procedure	Total Billed	Allowed Charges	Contract Adjust	Deduct	Coins	Paid Amt.	Total Paid	
Claim Date	99203	$150.00	$125.00	$25.00	$0.00	$25.00	80%	$100.00	
TOTALS									

BALANCE DUE FROM PATIENT: PT'S DED/NOT COV $ 0
PT'S COINSURANCE $ 25.00

PAYMENT SUMMARY SECTION (Totals)

Charges	Adjustment	Allowed	Copay	Deduct/Not Covered	Coins	Total Paid
$150.00	$25.00	$125.00	$0.00	$0.00	$25.00	$100.00

Practice Exercise 9-12

(1500)

HEALTH INSURANCE CLAIM FORM
APPROVED BY NATIONAL UNIFORM CLAIM COMMITTEE 08/05

PICA

1. MEDICARE ☐ (Medicare #) MEDICAID ☐ (Medicaid #) TRICARE CHAMPUS ☐ (Sponsor's SSN) CHAMPVA ☐ (Member ID#) GROUP HEALTH PLAN ☒ (SSN or ID) FECA BLK LUNG ☐ (SSN) OTHER ☐ (ID)

1a. INSURED'S I.D. NUMBER (For Program in Item 1): ASD56987

2. PATIENT'S NAME (Last Name, First Name, Middle Initial): WAGNER JAY

3. PATIENT'S BIRTH DATE: MM 02 DD 19 YY 1989 SEX M☒ F☐

4. INSURED'S NAME (Last Name, First Name, Middle Initial): WAGNER HOWARD

5. PATIENT'S ADDRESS (No, Street): 265 FIRST STREET CITY ITHACA STATE NY ZIP CODE 12345 TELEPHONE (312) 5554993

6. PATIENT RELATIONSHIP TO INSURED: Self☐ Spouse☐ Child☒ Other☐

7. INSURED'S ADDRESS (No, Street): SAME

8. PATIENT STATUS: Single☒ Married☐ Other☐ Employed☐ Full-Time Student☐ Part-Time Student☐

9. OTHER INSURED'S NAME: WAGNER THERESA
a. OTHER INSURED'S POLICY OR GROUP NUMBER: 75300865
b. OTHER INSURED'S DATE OF BIRTH MM 01 DD 03 YY 1958 SEX M☐ F☒
c. EMPLOYER'S NAME OR SCHOOL NAME: THE FAMOUS GOURMET
d. INSURANCE PLAN NAME OR PROGRAM NAME: CIGNA

10. IS PATIENT'S CONDITION RELATED TO:
a. EMPLOYMENT? ☐YES ☒NO
b. AUTO ACCIDENT? ☐YES ☒NO PLACE (State)
c. OTHER ACCIDENT? ☐YES ☒NO
10d. RESERVED FOR LOCAL USE

11. INSURED'S POLICY GROUP OR FECA NUMBER: 1256893
a. INSURED'S DATE OF BIRTH MM 09 DD 21 YY 1958 SEX M☒ F☐
b. EMPLOYER'S NAME OR SCHOOL NAME: THE PRINT SHOP
c. INSURANCE PLAN NAME OR PROGRAM NAME: ALLMERICA INS
d. IS THERE ANOTHER HEALTH BENEFIT PLAN? ☒YES ☐NO If yes, return to and complete item 9 a-d

12. PATIENT'S OR AUTHORIZED PERSON'S SIGNATURE: SIGNED SIGNATURE ON FILE DATE XXXXXXXX
13. INSURED'S OR AUTHORIZED PERSON'S SIGNATURE: SIGNED SIGNATURE ON FILE

14. DATE OF CURRENT: MM XX DD XX YY XXXX
15. IF PATIENT HAS HAD SAME OR SIMILAR ILLNESS
16. DATES PATIENT UNABLE TO WORK
17. NAME OF REFERRING PHYSICIAN: 17a. 17b. NPI
18. HOSPITALIZATION DATES
19. RESERVED FOR LOCAL USE
20. OUTSIDE LAB? ☐YES ☒NO

21. DIAGNOSIS: 1. 490 .0

24.
DATE(S) OF SERVICE From MM DD YY To MM DD YY	B. PLACE	C. EMG	D. CPT/HCPCS MOD	E. DX PTR	F. $ CHARGES	G. UNITS	H.	I.	J. RENDERING ID
XX XX XX XX XX XX	11		99203	1	150 00	1		NPI	

25. FEDERAL TAX ID NUMBER: 563342560 ☒ EIN
27. ACCEPT ASSIGNMENT? ☒YES ☐NO
28. TOTAL CHARGE $ 150 00
29. AMOUNT PAID $ 115 00
30. BALANCE DUE $ 35 00
31. SIGNED SIGNATURE ON FILE DATE XXXXXXXX
32. SERVICE FACILITY: FRANCIS J BOYER MD 916 E FRISCO RD ITHACA NY 12345 a.5562811442 b.N5 123266
33. BILLING PROVIDER INFO & PH # (555) 8882233 FRANCIS J BOYER MD 916 E FRISCO RD ITHACA NY 12345 a.5562811442 b.N5 123266

NUCC Instruction Manual available at: www.nucc.org WCMS-1500CS APPROVED OMB 0938-0999 FORM CMS-1500 (08/05)

For Student Use Only

Payer's Name and Address

Cigna Health Insurance Company
243 Harrison Avenue
Hartford, CT 12345

Today's Date:

CHECK #8822469

Provider's Name and Address

Francis J. Boyer, M.D.
916 E. Frisco Road
Ithaca, NY 12345

Patient Name: Jay Wagner   **Patient Account #:** WAGJ00
Patient ID#: 753-00865   **Insured's Name:** Theresa Wagner   **Group #:** DP139
Provider: Francis J. Boyer, M.D.   **Inventory Control #:** 3987540

Service Date(s)	Procedure	Total Charges	Contract Amount	Copay	Deduct/Not Covered	Coins	Paid Amt.	Total Paid	Remarks
Claim Date	99203	$150.00	$125.00	$10.00	$0.00	$0.00	100%	$115.00	
TOTALS									

BALANCE DUE FROM PATIENT: PT'S DED/NOT COV $ __0__

PT'S COINSURANCE $ __0__

PAYMENT SUMMARY SECTION (Totals)

Charges	Adjustment	Allowed	Copay	Deduct/Not Covered	Coins	Total Paid
$150.00	$25.00	$125.00	$10.00	$0.00	$0.00	$115.00

Practice Exercise 9-13

(1500)

HEALTH INSURANCE CLAIM FORM
APPROVED BY NATIONAL UNIFORM CLAIM COMMITTEE 08/05

☐☐☐ PICA

1. MEDICARE	MEDICAID	TRICARE CHAMPUS	CHAMPVA	GROUP HEALTH PLAN	FECA BLK LUNG	OTHER	1a. INSURED'S I.D. NUMBER	PICA ☐☐ (For Program in Item 1)

☐ (Medicare #) ☐ (Medicaid #) ☐ (Sponsor's SSN) ☐ (Member ID#) ☒ (SSN or ID) ☐ (SSN) ☐ (ID)   323542234

2. PATIENT'S NAME (Last Name, First Name, Middle Initial)
GROSS STEPHANIE

3. PATIENT'S BIRTH DATE   SEX
MM 08 DD 02 YY 1956   M ☐ F ☒

4. INSURED'S NAME (Last Name, First Name, Middle Initial)
GROSS JOHN J

5. PATIENT'S ADDRESS (No, Street)
310 FARM ROAD

6. PATIENT RELATIONSHIP TO INSURED
Self ☐ Spouse ☒ Child ☐ Other ☐

7. INSURED'S ADDRESS (No, Street)
SAME

CITY TOLEDO   STATE OH

8. PATIENT STATUS
Single ☐ Married ☒ Other ☐
Full-Time Student ☐ Part-Time Student ☐
Employed ☒

CITY   STATE

ZIP CODE 12345   TELEPHONE (Include Area Code) (789) 5553641

ZIP CODE   TELEPHONE (Include Area Code) (   )

9. OTHER INSURED'S NAME (Last Name, First Name, Middle Initial)
GROSS STEPHANIE

10. IS PATIENT'S CONDITION RELATED TO:

11. INSURED'S POLICY GROUP OR FECA NUMBER
JC 7843

a. OTHER INSURED'S POLICY OR GROUP NUMBER
78235606

a. EMPLOYMENT? (Current or Previous)
☐ YES ☒ NO

a. INSURED'S DATE OF BIRTH
MM 09 DD 04 YY 1953   SEX M ☒ F ☐

b. OTHER INSURED'S DATE OF BIRTH   SEX
MM 08 DD 02 YY 1956   M ☐ F ☒

b. AUTO ACCIDENT?   PLACE (State)
☐ YES ☒ NO

b. EMPLOYER'S NAME OR SCHOOL NAME
STEWART'S TUXEDOS

c. EMPLOYER'S NAME OR SCHOOL NAME
EDS COMPANY

c. OTHER ACCIDENT?
☐ YES ☒ NO

c. INSURANCE PLAN NAME OR PROGRAM NAME
CIGNA

d. INSURANCE PLAN NAME OR PROGRAM NAME
BCBS

10d. RESERVED FOR LOCAL USE

d. IS THERE ANOTHER HEALTH BENEFIT PLAN?
☒ YES ☐ NO   If yes, return to and complete item 9 a-d

READ BACK OF FORM BEFORE COMPLETING & SIGNING THIS FORM.
12. PATIENT'S OR AUTHORIZED PERSON'S SIGNATURE I authorize the release of any medical or other information necessary to process this claim. I also request payment of government benefits either to myself or to the party who accepts assignment below.

SIGNED SIGNATURE ON FILE   DATE XXXXXXXX

13. INSURED'S OR AUTHORIZED PERSON'S SIGNATURE I authorize payment of medical benefits to the undersigned physician or supplier for services described below.

SIGNED SIGNATURE ON FILE

14. DATE OF CURRENT   ILLNESS (First symptom) OR INJURY (Accident) OR PREGNANCY (LMP)
MM XX DD XX YY XXXX

15. IF PATIENT HAS HAD SAME OR SIMILAR ILLNESS. GIVE FIRST DATE   MM DD YY

16. DATES PATIENT UNABLE TO WORK IN CURRENT OCCUPATION
FROM MM DD YY   TO MM DD YY

17. NAME OF REFERRING PHYSICIAN OR OTHER SOURCE

17a.
17b. NPI

18. HOSPITALIZATION DATES RELATED TO CURRENT SERVICES
FROM MM DD YY   TO MM DD YY

19. RESERVED FOR LOCAL USE

20. OUTSIDE LAB?
☐ YES ☒ NO $ CHARGES

21. DIAGNOSIS OR NATURE OF ILLNESS OR INJURY (Relate Items 1,2,3 or 4 to Item 24E by Line)
1. 465 . 9
2.
3.
4.

22. MEDICAID RESUBMISSION
CODE   ORIGINAL REF. NO.

23. PRIOR AUTHORIZATION NUMBER

24. A. DATE(S) OF SERVICE From MM DD YY To MM DD YY	B. PLACE OF SERVICE	C. EMG	D. PROCEDURES, SERVICES, OR SUPPLIES (Explain Unusual Circumstances) CPT/HCPCS MODIFIER	E. DIAGNOSIS POINTER	F. $ CHARGES	G. DAYS OR UNITS	H. EPSDT Family Plan	I. ID. QUAL.	J. RENDERING PROVIDER ID. #
1 XX XX XX XX XX XX	11		99213	1	75 00	1		NPI	
2								NPI	
3								NPI	
4								NPI	
5								NPI	
6								NPI	

25. FEDERAL TAX ID NUMBER   SSN EIN
161246791   ☐ ☒

26. PATIENT'S ACCOUNT NO.

27. ACCEPT ASSIGNMENT? (For govt. claims, see back)
☒ YES ☐ NO

28. TOTAL CHARGE
$ 75 00

29. AMOUNT PAID
$ 51 25

30. BALANCE DUE
$ 23 75

31. SIGNATURE OF PHYSICIAN OR SUPPLIER INCLUDING DEGREES OR CREDENTIALS (I certify that the statements on the reverse apply to this bill and are made a part thereof)

SIGNED SIGNATURE ON FILE   XXXXXXXX DATE

32. SERVICE FACILITY LOCATION INFORMATION
DAVID ROSENBERG MD
1400 WEST CENTER ST
TOLEDO OH 12345

a. 5556214735   b. 1G 1001239

33. BILLING PROVIDER INFO & PH. # (999) 555-2121
DAVID ROSENBERG MD
1400 WEST CENTER ST
TOLEDO OH 12345

a. 5556214735   b. 1G 1001239

NUCC Instruction Manual available at: www.nucc.org
WCMS-1500CS

APPROVED OMB 0938-0999 FORM CMS-1500 (08/05)

For Student Use Only

Payer's Name and Address

| Blue Cross Blue Shield |
| P.O. Box 810 |
| Columbus, Ohio 12345 |

Today's Date:

CHECK #19562

Provider's Name and Address

| David Rosenberg, MD |
| 1400 West Center Street |
| Toledo, Ohio 12345 |

This statement covers payments for the following patient(s):
Claim Detail Section (if there are numbers in the 'SEE REMARKS' column, see the Remarks Section for explanation.)

Patient Name: Gross, Stephanie   **Patient Account #:** GROST
Patient ID#: 78235606
Provider Name: David Rosenberg, MD   **Claim Control #** 002456

Service Date(s)	Procedure	Charges	Adjustment	Allowed	Copay	Deduct/Not Covered	Coins	Paid Amt.	Total Paid
Claim Date	99213	$75.00	$8.75	$66.25	$15.00	$0.00	$0.00	100%	$51.25
TOTALS									

BALANCE DUE FROM PATIENT: PT'S DED/NOT COV $ 0
                                 PT'S COINSURANCE $ 0

PAYMENT SUMMARY SECTION (Totals)

Charges	Adjustment	Allowed	Copay	Deduct/Not Covered	Coins	Total Paid
$75.00	$8.75	$66.25	$15.00	$0.00	$0.00	$51.25

Practice Exercise 9-14

(1500)

HEALTH INSURANCE CLAIM FORM
APPROVED BY NATIONAL UNIFORM CLAIM COMMITTEE 08/05

☐☐☐ PICA   PICA ☐☐☐

1. MEDICARE MEDICAID TRICARE CHAMPVA GROUP FECA OTHER	1a. INSURED'S I.D. NUMBER (For Program in Item 1)

1. MEDICARE ☐(Medicare #) MEDICAID ☐(Medicaid #) TRICARE CHAMPUS ☐(Sponsor's SSN) CHAMPVA ☐(Member ID#) GROUP HEALTH PLAN ☒(SSN or ID) FECA BLK LUNG ☐(SSN) OTHER ☐(ID)

1a. INSURED'S I.D. NUMBER (For Program in Item 1)
5076241

2. PATIENT'S NAME (Last Name, First Name, Middle Initial)
HENDERSON SANDRA

3. PATIENT'S BIRTH DATE   SEX
MM 06 DD 05 YY 1966   M☐ F☒

4. INSURED'S NAME (Last Name, First Name, Middle Initial)
HENDERSON CHARLES

5. PATIENT'S ADDRESS (No, Street)
15 MAIN STREET

6. PATIENT RELATIONSHIP TO INSURED
Self☐ Spouse☒ Child☐ Other☐

7. INSURED'S ADDRESS (No, Street)
SAME

CITY WADSWORTH   STATE OH

8. PATIENT STATUS
Single☐ Married☒ Other☐

CITY   STATE

ZIP CODE 12345   TELEPHONE (Include Area Code) (703) 5556969

Employed☒ Full-Time Student☐ Part-Time Student☐

ZIP CODE   TELEPHONE (Include Area Code) (   )

9. OTHER INSURED'S NAME (Last Name, First Name, Middle Initial)
HENDERSON SANDRA

10. IS PATIENT'S CONDITION RELATED TO:

11. INSURED'S POLICY GROUP OR FECA NUMBER
K2565

a. OTHER INSURED'S POLICY OR GROUP NUMBER
931

a. EMPLOYMENT? (Current or Previous)
☐YES ☒NO

a. INSURED'S DATE OF BIRTH   SEX
MM 08 DD 22 YY 1960   M☒ F☐

b. OTHER INSURED'S DATE OF BIRTH   SEX
MM 06 DD 05 YY 1966   M☐ F☒

b. AUTO ACCIDENT?   PLACE (State)
☐YES ☒NO

b. EMPLOYER'S NAME OR SCHOOL NAME
DELL COMPUTER

c. EMPLOYER'S NAME OR SCHOOL NAME
COMPAQ COMPUTERS

c. OTHER ACCIDENT?
☐YES ☒NO

c. INSURANCE PLAN NAME OR PROGRAM NAME
PHYSICIANS CHOICE SERVICES

d. INSURANCE PLAN NAME OR PROGRAM NAME
US LIFE

10d. RESERVED FOR LOCAL USE

d. IS THERE ANOTHER HEALTH BENEFIT PLAN?
☒YES ☐NO   If yes, return to and complete item 9 a-d

READ BACK OF FORM BEFORE COMPLETING & SIGNING THIS FORM.

12. PATIENT'S OR AUTHORIZED PERSON'S SIGNATURE I authorize the release of any medical or other information necessary to process this claim. I also request payment of government benefits either to myself or to the party who accepts assignment below.

SIGNED SIGNATURE ON FILE   DATE

13. INSURED'S OR AUTHORIZED PERSON'S SIGNATURE I authorize payment of medical benefits to the undersigned physician or supplier for services described below.

SIGNED SIGNATURE ON FILE

14. DATE OF CURRENT ILLNESS (First symptom) OR INJURY (Accident) OR PREGNANCY (LMP)
MM XX DD XX YY XXXX

15. IF PATIENT HAS HAD SAME OR SIMILAR ILLNESS, GIVE FIRST DATE   MM DD YY

16. DATES PATIENT UNABLE TO WORK IN CURRENT OCCUPATION
FROM MM DD YY   TO MM DD YY

17. NAME OF REFERRING PHYSICIAN OR OTHER SOURCE

17a.
17b. NPI

18. HOSPITALIZATION DATES RELATED TO CURRENT SERVICES
FROM MM DD YY   TO MM DD YY

19. RESERVED FOR LOCAL USE

20. OUTSIDE LAB? $ CHARGES
☐YES ☒NO

21. DIAGNOSIS OR NATURE OF ILLNESS OR INJURY (Relate Items 1,2,3 or 4 to Item 24E by Line)
1. 726 . 32   3.
2.   4.

22. MEDICAID RESUBMISSION
CODE   ORIGINAL REF. NO.

23. PRIOR AUTHORIZATION NUMBER

24. A. DATE(S) OF SERVICE					B. PLACE OF SERVICE	C. EMG	D. PROCEDURES, SERVICES, OR SUPPLIES		E. DIAGNOSIS POINTER	F. $ CHARGES	G. DAYS OR UNITS	H. EPSDT Family Plan	I. ID. QUAL.	J. RENDERING PROVIDER ID. #
From MM DD YY			To MM DD YY				CPT/HCPCS	MODIFIER						
1	XX XX XX	XX XX XX		11		99203		1	150 00	1		NPI		
2				11		73070		1	50 00	1		NPI		
3				11		73090		1	50 00	1		NPI		
4												NPI		
5												NPI		
6												NPI		

25. FEDERAL TAX ID NUMBER   SSN EIN
34086541   ☐☒

26. PATIENT'S ACCOUNT NO.

27. ACCEPT ASSIGNMENT? (For govt. claims, see back)
☒YES ☐NO

28. TOTAL CHARGE
$ 250 00

29. AMOUNT PAID
$ 120 00

30. BALANCE DUE
$ 130 00

31. SIGNATURE OF PHYSICIAN OR SUPPLIER INCLUDING DEGREES OR CREDENTIALS (I certify that the statements on the reverse apply to this bill and are made a part thereof)
XXXXXXXX
SIGNED SIGNATURE ON FILE   DATE

32. SERVICE FACILITY LOCATION INFORMATION
CHRISTOPHER M BROWN MD
234 HAVERFORD RD
HAVERFORD OH 12345
a. 8903789447   b. N5 B4321

33. BILLING PROVIDER INFO & PH. # (999) 555-3111
CHRISTOPHER M BROWN MD
234 HAVERFORD RD
HAVERFORD OH 12345
a. 8903789447   b. N5B4321

NUCC Instruction Manual available at: www.nucc.org
WCMS-1500CS

APPROVED OMB 0938-0999 FORM CMS-1500 (08/05)

For Student Use Only

Payer's Name and Address

U.S. Life
2788 Broadway
New York, NY 12345

Today's Date:

CHECK #21763

Provider's Name and Address

Christopher M. Brown, MD
234 Haverford Road
Haverford, Ohio 12345

This statement covers payments for the following patient(s):
Claim Detail Section (If there are numbers in the 'SEE REMARKS' column, see the Remarks Section for explanation.)

Patient Name: Henderson, Sandra   **Patient Account #:** Hen03
Patient ID#: 331779183   **Insured's Name:** Sandra Henderson
Provider Name: Christopher M. Brown, MD   **Inventory #:** 25133   **Claim Control #** 55614

Service Date(s)	Procedure	Charges	Adjustment	Allowed	Copay	Deduct/Not Covered	Coins	Paid Amt.	Remarks
Claim Date	99203	$150.00	$0.00	$150.00	$0.00	$100.00	$10.00	80%	01
Claim Date	73070	$50.00	$0.00	$ 50.00	$0.00	$ 0.00	$10.00	80%	
Claim Date	73070	$50.00	$0.00	$ 50.00	$0.00	$ 0.00	$10.00	80%	
TOTALS									

BALANCE DUE FROM PATIENT: PT'S DED/NOT COV $ 100.00
PT'S COINSURANCE $ 30.00

PAYMENT SUMMARY SECTION (Totals)

Charges	Adjustment	Allowed	Copay	Deduct/Not Covered	Coins	Total Paid
$250.00	$0.00	$250.00	$0.00	$100.00	$30.00	$120.00

REMARKS SECTION: 01 Deductible

Practice Exercise 9-15

(1500)

HEALTH INSURANCE CLAIM FORM

APPROVED BY NATIONAL UNIFORM CLAIM COMMITTEE 08/05

☐☐☐ PICA	PICA ☐☐☐

1. MEDICARE ☐ (Medicare #)   MEDICAID ☐ (Medicaid #)   TRICARE CHAMPUS ☐ (Sponsor's SSN)   CHAMPVA ☐ (Member ID#)   GROUP HEALTH PLAN ☒ (SSN or ID)   FECA BLK LUNG ☐ (SSN)   OTHER ☐ (ID)

1a. INSURED'S I.D. NUMBER   (For Program in Item 1)
512539751

2. PATIENT'S NAME (Last Name, First Name, Middle Initial)
LYNCH AMY L

3. PATIENT'S BIRTH DATE   SEX
MM 01 DD 09 YY 1998   M☐ F☒

4. INSURED'S NAME (Last Name, First Name, Middle Initial)
LYNCH FRED K

5. PATIENT'S ADDRESS (No, Street)
1776 LIBERTY ROAD

6. PATIENT RELATIONSHIP TO INSURED
Self ☐ Spouse ☐ Child ☒ Other ☐

7. INSURED'S ADDRESS (No, Street)
SAME

CITY PHILADELPHIA   STATE PA

8. PATIENT STATUS
Single ☒ Married ☐ Other ☐
Employed ☐ Full-Time Student ☐ Part-Time Student ☒

CITY   STATE

ZIP CODE 12345   TELEPHONE (Include Area Code) (215) 5559632

ZIP CODE   TELEPHONE (Include Area Code) (   )

9. OTHER INSURED'S NAME (Last Name, First Name, Middle Initial)
LYNCH JESSIE M

10. IS PATIENT'S CONDITION RELATED TO:

11. INSURED'S POLICY GROUP OR FECA NUMBER
W 45980

a. OTHER INSURED'S POLICY OR GROUP NUMBER
7989

a. EMPLOYMENT? (Current or Previous)
☐ YES ☒ NO

a. INSURED'S DATE OF BIRTH
MM 07 DD 15 YY 1967   SEX M☒ F☐

b. OTHER INSURED'S DATE OF BIRTH
MM 05 DD 06 YY 1969   SEX M☐ F☒

b. AUTO ACCIDENT?   PLACE (State)
☐ YES ☒ NO

b. EMPLOYER'S NAME OR SCHOOL NAME
WDAF RADIO

c. EMPLOYER'S NAME OR SCHOOL NAME
SOUTHERLAND LUMBER

c. OTHER ACCIDENT?
☐ YES ☒ NO

c. INSURANCE PLAN NAME OR PROGRAM NAME
BCBS OF PA

d. INSURANCE PLAN NAME OR PROGRAM NAME
METROPOLITAN FAMILY

10d. RESERVED FOR LOCAL USE

d. IS THERE ANOTHER HEALTH BENEFIT PLAN?
☒ YES ☐ NO   If yes, return to and complete item 9 a-d

READ BACK OF FORM BEFORE COMPLETING & SIGNING THIS FORM.

12. PATIENT'S OR AUTHORIZED PERSON'S SIGNATURE I authorize the release of any medical or other information necessary to process this claim. I also request payment of government benefits either to myself or to the party who accepts assignment below.

SIGNED SIGNATURE ON FILE   DATE XXXXXXXX

13. INSURED'S OR AUTHORIZED PERSON'S SIGNATURE I authorize payment of medical benefits to the undersigned physician or supplier for services described below.

SIGNED SIGNATURE ON FILE

14. DATE OF CURRENT   ILLNESS (First symptom) OR INJURY (Accident) OR PREGNANCY (LMP)
MM XX DD XX YY XXXX

15. IF PATIENT HAS HAD SAME OR SIMILAR ILLNESS, GIVE FIRST DATE MM DD YY

16. DATES PATIENT UNABLE TO WORK IN CURRENT OCCUPATION
FROM MM DD YY   TO MM DD YY

17. NAME OF REFERRING PHYSICIAN OR OTHER SOURCE

17a.

17b. NPI

18. HOSPITALIZATION DATES RELATED TO CURRENT SERVICES
FROM MM DD YY   TO MM DD YY

19. RESERVED FOR LOCAL USE

20. OUTSIDE LAB? ☐ YES ☒ NO $ CHARGES

21. DIAGNOSIS OR NATURE OF ILLNESS OR INJURY (Relate Items 1,2,3 or 4 to Item 24E by Line)
1. V70 . 0
2.
3.
4.

22. MEDICAID RESUBMISSION
CODE   ORIGINAL REF. NO.

23. PRIOR AUTHORIZATION NUMBER

24. A. DATE(S) OF SERVICE						B. PLACE OF SERVICE	C. EMG	D. PROCEDURES, SERVICES, OR SUPPLIES (Explain Unusual Circumstances)		E. DIAGNOSIS POINTER	F. $ CHARGES	G. DAYS OR UNITS	H. EPSDT Family Plan	I. ID. QUAL.	J. RENDERING PROVIDER ID. #
From MM	DD	YY	To MM	DD	YY			CPT/HCPCS	MODIFIER						
XX	XX	XX	XX	XX	XX	11		99385		1	85 00	1		NPI	
														NPI	
														NPI	
														NPI	
														NPI	
														NPI	

25. FEDERAL TAX ID NUMBER   SSN EIN
514290642   ☐ ☒

26. PATIENT'S ACCOUNT NO.

27. ACCEPT ASSIGNMENT? (For govt. claims, see back)
☒ YES ☐ NO

28. TOTAL CHARGE
$ 85 00

29. AMOUNT PAID
$ 68 00

30. BALANCE DUE
$ 17 00

31. SIGNATURE OF PHYSICIAN OR SUPPLIER INCLUDING DEGREES OR CREDENTIALS (I certify that the statements on the reverse apply to this bill and are made a part thereof)

SIGNED SIGNATURE ON FILE   DATE XXXXXXXX

32. SERVICE FACILITY LOCATION INFORMATION
MARY ANN BROCK MD
1547 SAMPSON ST
PHILADELPHIA PA 12345
a. 6632588874   b. 1B495529

33. BILLING PROVIDER INFO & PH. # (215) 555-3000
MARY ANN BROCK MD
1547 SAMPSON ST
PHILADELPHIA PA 12345
a. 6632588874   b. 1B495529

NUCC Instruction Manual available at: www.nucc.org
WCMS-1500CS

APPROVED OMB 0938-0999 FORM CMS-1500 (08/05)

For Student Use Only

The charges are being paid at 80%.

Payer's Name and Address

| Metropolitan Family |
| 414 E Franklin RD |
| Philadelphia PA 19111 |
| 800-555-4141 |

Today's Date:

CHECK #24466

Provider's Name and Address

| Mary Ann Brock, MD |
| 1547 Sampson Street |
| Philadelphia, PA 12345 |

This statement covers payments for the following patient(s): Lynch, Amy
Claim Detail Section (If there are numbers in the 'SEE REMARKS' column, see the
Remarks Section for explanation.)

Patient Name: Lynch, Amy	**Patient Account #:** Lyncham1
Patient ID#: 491.51.0003	**Insured's Name:** Lynch Jessie M
Group #: 7989	
Provider Name: Mary Ann Brock, MD	**Inventory #:** 44562 **Claim Control #:** 28081

Service Date(s)	Procedure	Charges	Adjustment	Allowed	Copay	Deduct/Not Covered	Coins	Paid Amt.	Remarks
Claim Date	99385	$85.00	$0.00	$85.00	$0.00	$0.00	$17.00	80%	
TOTALS									

BALANCE DUE FROM PATIENT: PT'S DED/NOT COV $___0_____

PT'S COINSURANCE $___17.00_____

PAYMENT SUMMARY SECTION (Totals)

Charges	Adjustment	Allowed	Copay	Deduct/Not Covered	Coins	Total Paid
$85.00	$0.00	$85.00	$0.00	$0.00	$17.00	$68.00

Chapter 10: Medicare Medical Billing

Practice Exercise 10-1

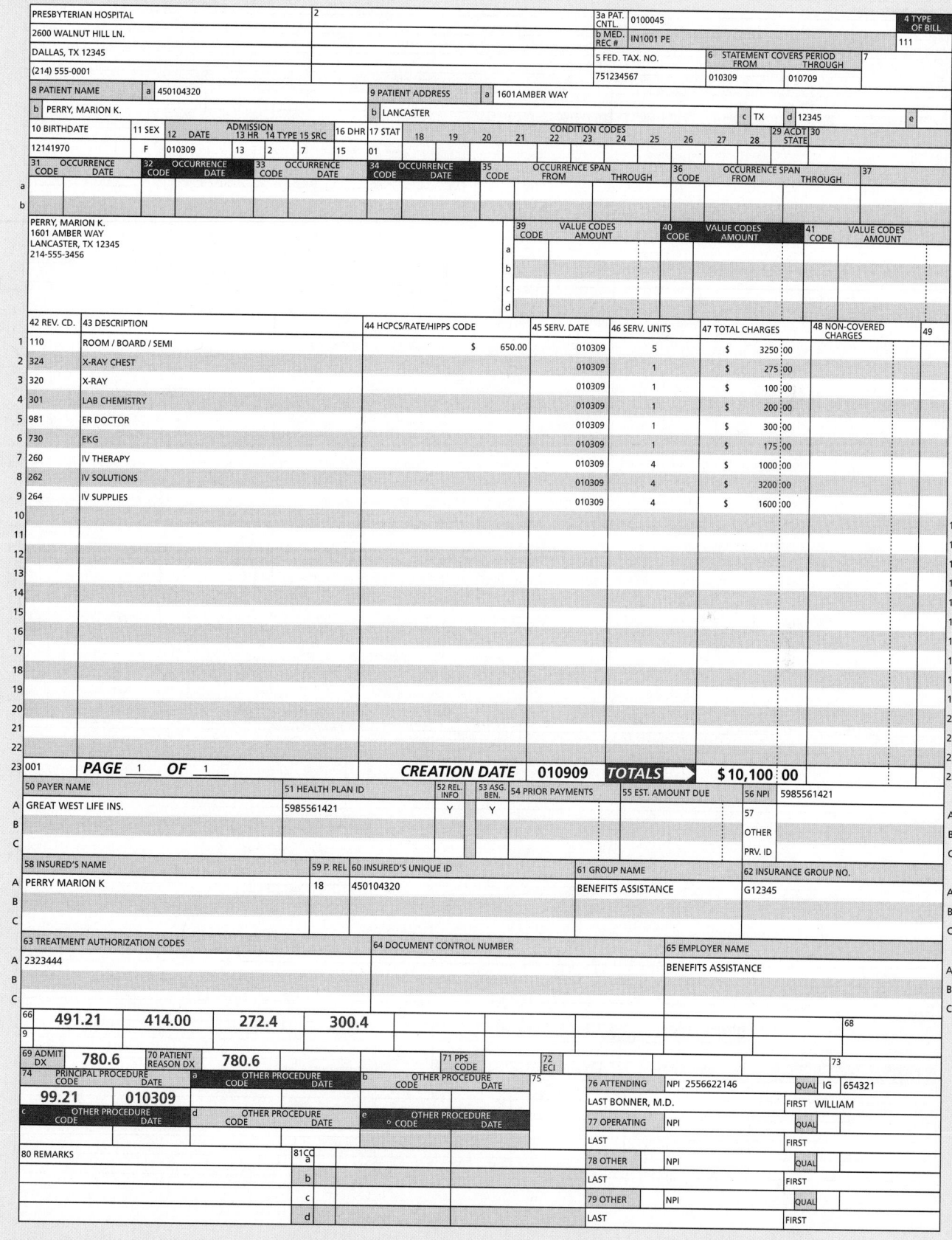

Practice Exercise 10-2

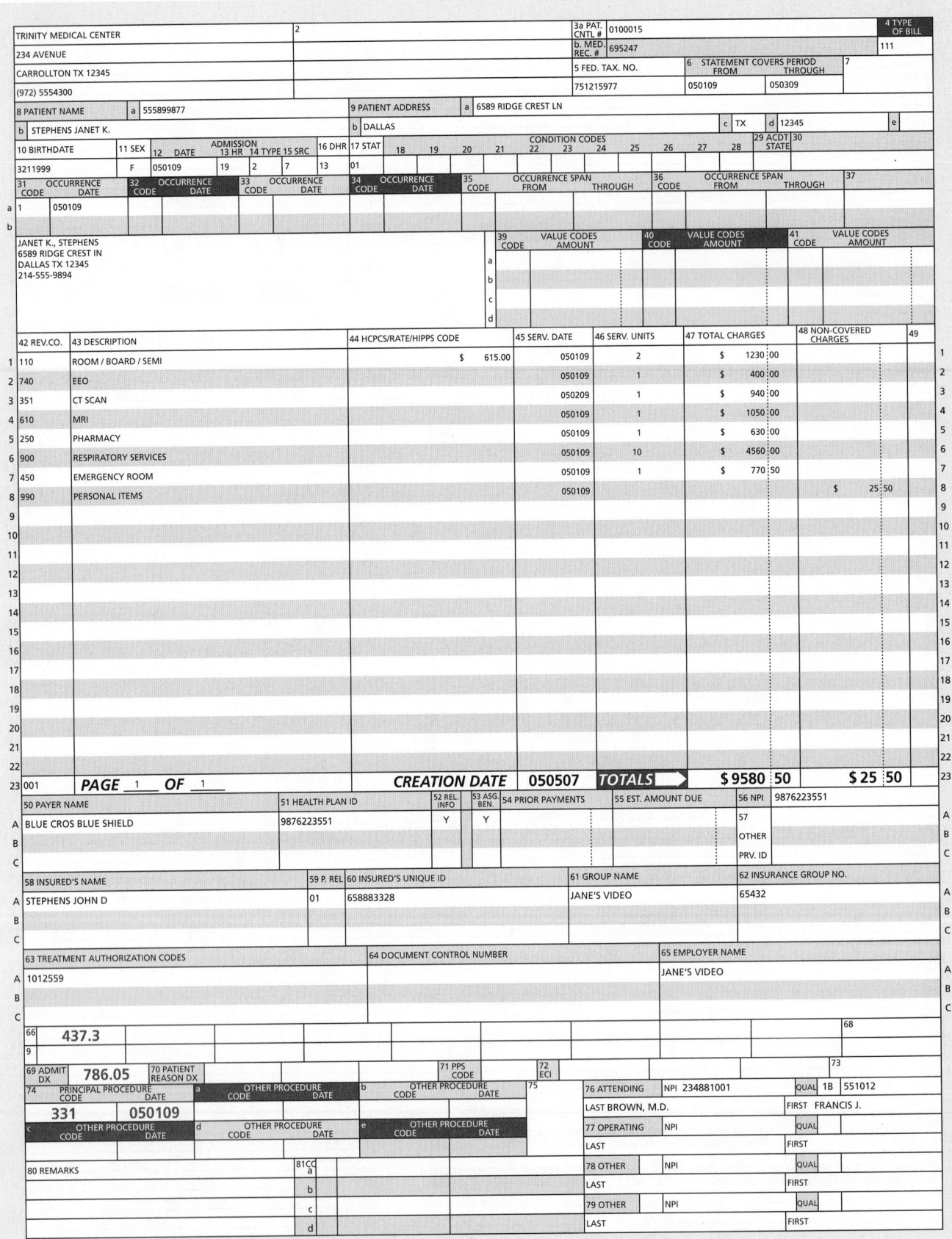

Practice Exercise 10-3

UNIVERSITY MEDICAL CENTER	2		3a PAT. CNTL # 0030087	4 TYPE OF BILL
700 JOSE LANE			b. MED. REC. # 232774	111
CARROLLTON, TX 12345			5 FED. TAX. NO.	6 STATEMENT COVERS PERIOD FROM / THROUGH 7
(972) 5554400			75251487	012109 / 012309

8 PATIENT NAME	a 555555544	9 PATIENT ADDRESS	a 5489 SLOW BEND DR.			
b JAMES MICHAEL R		b DALLAS		c TX	d 12345	e

10 BIRTHDATE	11 SEX	12 DATE	ADMISSION 13 HR 14 TYPE 15 SRC	16 DHR	17 STAT	CONDITION CODES 18 19 20 21 22 23 24 25 26 27 28	29 ACDT STATE	30
07011968	M	012109	23 2 7	10	01			

31 OCCURRENCE CODE DATE	32 OCCURRENCE CODE DATE	33 OCCURRENCE CODE DATE	34 OCCURRENCE CODE DATE	35 OCCURRENCE SPAN CODE FROM THROUGH	36 OCCURRENCE SPAN CODE FROM THROUGH	37
a 1						
b						

MICHAEL R. JAMES 5489 SLOW BEND DR. DALLAS TX, 12345 (214) 555-9458		39 CODE VALUE CODES AMOUNT	40 CODE VALUE CODES AMOUNT	41 CODE VALUE CODES AMOUNT
	a			
	b			
	c			
	d			

	42 REV.CD.	43 DESCRIPTION	44 HCPCS/RATE/HIPPS CODE	45 SERV. DATE	46 SERV. UNITS	47 TOTAL CHARGES	48 NON-COVERED CHARGES	49	
1	110	ROOM / BOARD PRIVATE	$ 615.00	012109	2	$ 1230 00			1
2	320	X-RAY		012109	1	$ 275 00			2
3	305	LAB / CHEMISTRY		012209	1	$ 180 00			3
4	260	IV THERAPY		012209	1	$ 125 00			4
5	250	PHARMACY		012309	1	$ 208 00			5
6	730	EKG / ECG		012309	1	$ 210 00			6
7									7
8									8
9									9
10									10
11									11
12									12
13									13
14									14
15									15
16									16
17									17
18									18
19									19
20									20
21									21
22									22
23	01	PAGE 1 OF 1	CREATION DATE 012509	TOTALS		$ 2228 00			23

50 PAYER NAME	51 HEALTH PLAN ID	52 REL. INFO	53 ASG. BEN.	54 PRIOR PAYMENTS	55 EST. AMOUNT DUE	56 NPI 5874446521	
A CIGNA PPO	5874446521	Y	Y			57	A
B						OTHER	B
C						PRV. ID	C

58 INSURED'S NAME	59 P. REL	60 INSURED'S UNIQUE ID	61 GROUP NAME	62 INSURANCE GROUP NO.	
A JAMES JENNIFER M	01	555666548	NASTEC	8488	A
B					B
C					C

63 TREATMENT AUTHORIZATION CODES	64 DOCUMENT CONTROL NUMBER	65 EMPLOYER NAME	
A 551478		NASTEC	A
B			B
C			C

66 531.00				68
9				

69 ADMIT DX 789.09	70 PATIENT REASON DX	71 PPS CODE	72 ECI	73		76 ATTENDING NPI 4589854428	QUAL N5 27069
74 PRINCIPAL PROCEDURE CODE DATE 44.41 012109	a OTHER PROCEDURE CODE DATE	b OTHER PROCEDURE CODE DATE	75			LAST OCONNOR H.D.	FIRST DENNIS J.
c OTHER PROCEDURE CODE DATE	d OTHER PROCEDURE CODE DATE	e OTHER PROCEDURE CODE DATE				77 OPERATING NPI	QUAL
						LAST	FIRST

80 REMARKS	81CC a		78 OTHER NPI	QUAL
	b		LAST	FIRST
	c		79 OTHER NPI	QUAL
	d		LAST	FIRST

Practice Exercise 10-4

PRESBYTERIAN HOSPITAL DALLAS	2	3a PAT. CNTL # 987625941		4 TYPE OF BILL
2600 WALNUT HILL LANE		b. MED. REC. # OLIWES0226		111
DALLAS, TX 12345		5 FED. TAX. NO.	6 STATEMENT COVERS PERIOD FROM THROUGH	7
(214) 5550001		751234567	022609 022809	

8 PATIENT NAME	a 144401442	9 PATIENT ADDRESS	a 5 APPLE LANE			
b WESTCOT, OLIVE		b WEST HARTFORD		c CT	d 12345	e

10 BIRTHDATE	11 SEX	12 DATE	ADMISSION 13 HR 14 TYPE 15 SRC	16 DHR	17 STAT	CONDITION CODES 18 19 20 21 22 23 24 25 26 27 28	29 ACDT STATE	30
03021949	F	022607	13 2 7	09	01			

31 OCCURRENCE CODE DATE	32 OCCURRENCE CODE DATE	33 OCCURRENCE CODE DATE	34 OCCURRENCE CODE DATE	35 OCCURRENCE SPAN CODE FROM THROUGH	36 OCCURRENCE SPAN CODE FROM THROUGH	37
a						
b						

OLIVE WESTCOT
5 APPLE LANE
WEST HARTFORD, CT 12345
(860) 555-2269

	39 VALUE CODES CODE AMOUNT	40 VALUE CODES CODE AMOUNT	41 VALUE CODES CODE AMOUNT
a			
b			
c			
d			

	42 REV. CD.	43 DESCRIPTION	44 HCPCS/RATE/HIPPS CODE	45 SERV. DATE	46 SERV. UNITS	47 TOTAL CHARGES	48 NON-COVERED CHARGES	49	
1	110	SEMI PRIVATE ROOM	$ 340.00	022609	2	$ 680 00			1
2	730	ECG		022709	1	$ 95 00			2
3	997	ADMISSION KIT		022609	1	$ 25 00			3
4	351	CT SCAN		022709	1	$ 1536 00			4
5	300	LAB		022609	1	$ 356 00			5
6	981	ER DOCTOR		022609	1	$ 300 00			6
7									7
8									8
9									9
10									10
11									11
12									12
13									13
14									14
15									15
16									16
17									17
18									18
19									19
20									20
21									21
22									22
23	001	PAGE 1 OF 1	CREATION DATE 023009	TOTALS ➤		$ 2992 00			23

	50 PAYER NAME	51 HEALTH PLAN ID	52 REL INFO	53 ASG BEN.	54 PRIOR PAYMENTS	55 EST. AMOUNT DUE	56 NPI 5985561421	
A	AETNA	5985561421	Y	Y			57	A
B							OTHER	B
C							PRV. ID	C

	58 INSURED'S NAME	59 P. REL	60 INSURED'S UNIQUE ID	61 GROUP NAME	62 INSURANCE GROUP NO.	
A	WESTCOT OLIVE	18	005598JA	JAMISON CASKET	JAM908	A
B						B
C						C

	63 TREATMENT AUTHORIZATION CODES	64 DOCUMENT CONTROL NUMBER	65 EMPLOYER NAME	
A	900 ASC		JAMISON CASKET	A
B				B
C				C

66 574.50				68
9				

69 ADMIT DX 789.09	70 PATIENT REASON DX		71 PPS CODE	72 ECI	75	76 ATTENDING NPI 0006667999	QUAL N5 5689IT

74 PRINCIPAL PROCEDURE CODE DATE	a OTHER PROCEDURE CODE DATE	b OTHER PROCEDURE CODE DATE		LAST HENDERSON MD	FIRST CHARLES W
51.41 022609					
c OTHER PROCEDURE CODE DATE	d OTHER PROCEDURE CODE DATE	e OTHER PROCEDURE CODE DATE		77 OPERATING NPI	QUAL
				LAST	FIRST

80 REMARKS	81CC a		78 OTHER NPI	QUAL
	b		LAST	FIRST
	c		79 OTHER NPI	QUAL
	d		LAST	FIRST

Practice Exercise 10-5

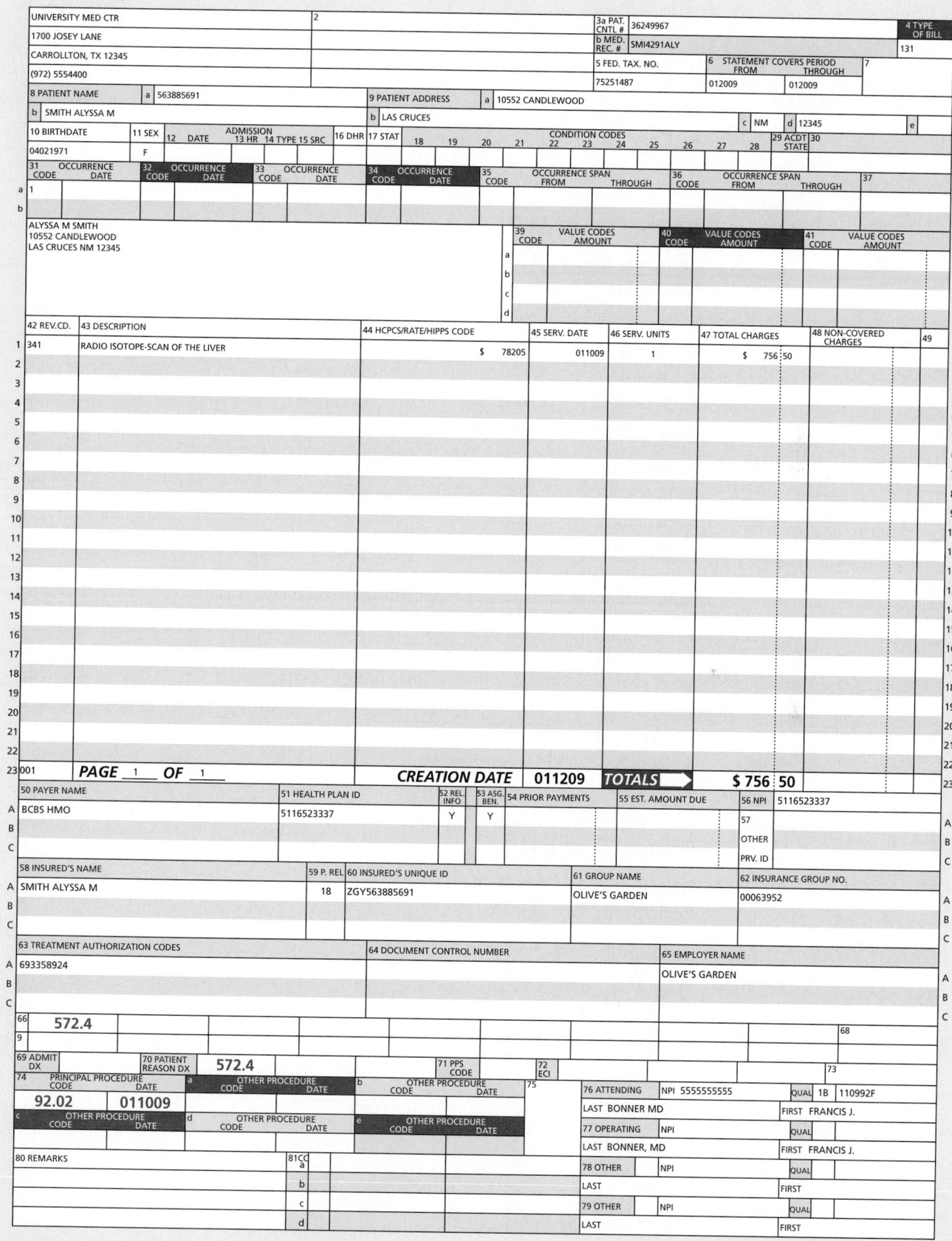

UNIVERSITY MED CTR		2		3a PAT. CNTL # 36249967					4 TYPE OF BILL
1700 JOSEY LANE				b MED. REC. # SMI4291ALY					
CARROLLTON, TX 12345				5 FED. TAX. NO.		6 STATEMENT COVERS PERIOD FROM THROUGH		7	131
(972) 5554400				75251487		012009	012009		

8 PATIENT NAME	a 563885691		9 PATIENT ADDRESS	a 10552 CANDLEWOOD				
b SMITH ALYSSA M			b LAS CRUCES			c NM	d 12345	e

10 BIRTHDATE	11 SEX	12 DATE	ADMISSION 13 HR 14 TYPE 15 SRC	16 DHR	17 STAT	18 19 20 21	CONDITION CODES 22 23 24 25 26 27 28	29 ACDT STATE	30
04021971	F								

31 OCCURRENCE CODE DATE	32 OCCURRENCE CODE DATE	33 OCCURRENCE CODE DATE	34 OCCURRENCE CODE DATE	35 OCCURRENCE CODE	OCCURRENCE SPAN FROM THROUGH	36 OCCURRENCE SPAN CODE FROM THROUGH	37
a 1							
b							

ALYSSA M SMITH 10552 CANDLEWOOD LAS CRUCES NM 12345			39 CODE VALUE CODES AMOUNT	40 CODE VALUE CODES AMOUNT	41 CODE VALUE CODES AMOUNT
		a			
		b			
		c			
		d			

	42 REV.CD.	43 DESCRIPTION	44 HCPCS/RATE/HIPPS CODE	45 SERV. DATE	46 SERV. UNITS	47 TOTAL CHARGES	48 NON-COVERED CHARGES	49	
1	341	RADIO ISOTOPE-SCAN OF THE LIVER	$ 78205	011009	1	$ 756:50			1
2									2
3									3
4									4
5									5
6									6
7									7
8									8
9									9
10									10
11									11
12									12
13									13
14									14
15									15
16									16
17									17
18									18
19									19
20									20
21									21
22									22
23	001	PAGE 1 OF 1	CREATION DATE 011209	TOTALS		$ 756:50			23

50 PAYER NAME	51 HEALTH PLAN ID	52 REL. INFO	53 ASG. BEN.	54 PRIOR PAYMENTS	55 EST. AMOUNT DUE	56 NPI 5116523337	
A BCBS HMO	5116523337	Y	Y			57	A
B						OTHER	B
C						PRV. ID	C

58 INSURED'S NAME	59 P. REL	60 INSURED'S UNIQUE ID	61 GROUP NAME	62 INSURANCE GROUP NO.	
A SMITH ALYSSA M	18	ZGY563885691	OLIVE'S GARDEN	00063952	A
B					B
C					C

63 TREATMENT AUTHORIZATION CODES	64 DOCUMENT CONTROL NUMBER	65 EMPLOYER NAME	
A 693358924		OLIVE'S GARDEN	A
B			B
C			C

66 572.4						68
9						

69 ADMIT DX	70 PATIENT REASON DX 572.4		71 PPS CODE	72 ECI		73

74 PRINCIPAL PROCEDURE CODE DATE	a OTHER PROCEDURE CODE DATE	b OTHER PROCEDURE CODE DATE	75	76 ATTENDING NPI 5555555555	QUAL 1B 110992F
92.02 011009				LAST BONNER MD	FIRST FRANCIS J.
c OTHER PROCEDURE CODE DATE	d OTHER PROCEDURE CODE DATE	e OTHER PROCEDURE CODE DATE		77 OPERATING NPI	QUAL
				LAST BONNER, MD	FIRST FRANCIS J.

80 REMARKS	81CC a		78 OTHER NPI	QUAL
	b		LAST	FIRST
	c		79 OTHER NPI	QUAL
	d		LAST	FIRST

Chapter 11: Medicare Medical Billing

Practice Exercise 11-1

1. False
2. True
3. True
4. True

Practice Exercise 11-2

Physicians Standard fee: $175.00; Medicare fee: $140.00
Participating Provider

1. $112.00
2. $28.00
3. $35.00

Nonparticipating Provider Accepting Assignment

1. $133.00
2. $106.40
3. $26.60
4. $42.00

Nonparticipating Provider Not Accepting Assignment

1. $133.00
2. $152.95
3. $152.95
4. $106.40
5. $152.95
6. $46.55

Practice Exercise 11-3

Standard fee: $75.00; Medicare fee: $38.32
Participating Provider

1. $75.00
2. $38.32
3. $30.66
4. $7.66
5. $36.68

Nonparticipating Provider Accepting Assignment

1. $75.00
2. $36.40
3. $29.12
4. $7.28
5. $38.60

Nonparticipating Provider Not Accepting Assignment

1. $75.00
2. $36.40
3. $41.86
4. $41.86
5. $29.12
6. $41.86
7. $12.74
8. $5.46
9. $33.14

Practice Exercise 11-4

Standard fee: $100.00; Medicare fee: $52.12
Participating Provider

1. $100.00
2. $52.12
3. $41.70
4. $10.42
5. $47.88

Nonparticipating Provider Accepting Assignment

1. $100.00
2. $49.51
3. $39.61
4. $9.90
5. $50.49

Nonparticipating Provider Not Accepting Assignment

1. $100.00
2. $49.51
3. $56.94
4. $56.94
5. $39.61
6. $56.94
7. $43.06

Practice Exercise 11-5

Standard fee: $150.00; Medicare fee: $95.75
Participating Provider

1. $150.00
2. $95.75
3. $76.60
4. $19.15
5. $54.25

Nonparticipating Provider Accepting Assignment

1. $150.00
2. $90.96
3. $72.77
4. $18.19
5. $59.04

Nonparticipating Not Accepting Assignment

1. $150.00
2. $90.96
3. $104.60
4. $104.60
5. $72.77
6. $104.60
7. $45.40

Practice Exercise 11-6

1. False
2. False
3. True

Practice Exercise 11-7 Medicare

CMS-1500 Health Insurance Claim Form

1500
HEALTH INSURANCE CLAIM FORM
APPROVED BY NATIONAL UNIFORM CLAIM COMMITTEE 08/05

☐☐☐ PICA | | | | | PICA ☐☐☐

1. MEDICARE   MEDICAID   TRICARE   CHAMPVA   GROUP   FECA   OTHER
CHAMPUS   HEALTH PLAN   BLK LUNG
☒ (Medicare #)   ☐ (Medicaid #)   ☐ (Sponsor's SSN)   ☐ (Member ID#)   ☐ (SSN or ID)   ☐ (SSN)   ☐ (ID)

1a. INSURED'S I.D. NUMBER (For Program in Item 1)
145875988A

2. PATIENT'S NAME (Last Name, First Name, Middle Initial)
NAME YOUR

3. PATIENT'S BIRTH DATE   SEX
MM 06 | DD 25 | YY 1944   M☐ F☒

4. INSURED'S NAME (Last Name, First Name, Middle Initial)

5. PATIENT'S ADDRESS (No, Street)
1884 DALLAS WAY

6. PATIENT RELATIONSHIP TO INSURED
Self ☒ Spouse ☐ Child ☐ Other ☐

7. INSURED'S ADDRESS (No, Street)

CITY   DALLAS   STATE TX

8. PATIENT STATUS
Single ☒   Married ☐   Other ☐
Employed ☒   Full-Time Student ☐   Part-Time Student ☐

CITY   STATE

ZIP CODE 12345   TELEPHONE (Include Area Code) (912) 555 4572

ZIP CODE   TELEPHONE (Include Area Code) ( )

9. OTHER INSURED'S NAME (Last Name, First Name, Middle Initial)

10. IS PATIENT'S CONDITION RELATED TO:

11. INSURED'S POLICY GROUP OR FECA NUMBER
NONE

a. OTHER INSURED'S POLICY OR GROUP NUMBER
MG 223546721

a. EMPLOYMENT? (Current or Previous)
☐ YES   ☒ NO

a. INSURED'S DATE OF BIRTH   SEX
MM | DD | YY   M☐ F☐

b. OTHER INSURED'S DATE OF BIRTH   SEX
MM | DD | YY   M☐ F☐

b. AUTO ACCIDENT?   PLACE (State)
☐ YES   ☒ NO

b. EMPLOYER'S NAME OR SCHOOL NAME

c. EMPLOYER'S NAME OR SCHOOL NAME

c. OTHER ACCIDENT?
☐ YES   ☒ NO

c. INSURANCE PLAN NAME OR PROGRAM NAME

d. INSURANCE PLAN NAME OR PROGRAM NAME
UNITED HEALTH CARE

10d. RESERVED FOR LOCAL USE

d. IS THERE ANOTHER HEALTH BENEFIT PLAN?
☐ YES   ☐ NO   *If yes,* return to and complete item 9 a-d

READ BACK OF FORM BEFORE COMPLETING & SIGNING THIS FORM.
12. PATIENT'S OR AUTHORIZED PERSON'S SIGNATURE I authorize the release of any medical or other information necessary to process this claim. I also request payment of government benefits either to myself or to the party who accepts assignment below.

SIGNED SOF   DATE

13. INSURED'S OR AUTHORIZED PERSON'S SIGNATURE I authorize payment of medical benefits to the undersigned physician or supplier for services described below.

SIGNED SOF

14. DATE OF CURRENT ILLNESS (First symptom) OR INJURY (Accident) OR PREGNANCY (LMP)
MM | DD | YY 2 DAYS AGO

15. IF PATIENT HAS HAD SAME OR SIMILAR ILLNESS, GIVE FIRST DATE MM | DD | YY

16. DATES PATIENT UNABLE TO WORK IN CURRENT OCCUPATION
MM | DD | YY   FROM   TO   MM | DD | YY

17. NAME OF REFERRING PHYSICIAN OR OTHER SOURCE
BONNER, MD WILLIAM F

17a. | IG | 465922113
17b. | NPI | 1111199999

18. HOSPITALIZATION DATES RELATED TO CURRENT SERVICES
MM | DD | YY   FROM   TO   MM | DD | YY

19. RESERVED FOR LOCAL USE

20. OUTSIDE LAB? $ CHARGES
☐ YES   ☒ NO

21. DIAGNOSIS OR NATURE OF ILLNESS OR INJURY (Relate Items 1,2,3 or 4 to Item 24E by Line)
1. 789 . 00   3. |
2. 401 . 9   4. |

22. MEDICAID RESUBMISSION
CODE   ORIGINAL REF. NO.

23. PRIOR AUTHORIZATION NUMBER

24. A. DATE(S) OF SERVICE		B. PLACE OF SERVICE	C. EMG	D. PROCEDURES, SERVICES, OR SUPPLIES (Explain Unusual Circumstances)		E. DIAGNOSIS POINTER	F. $ CHARGES	G. DAYS OR UNITS	H. EPSDT Family Plan	I. ID. QUAL.	J. RENDERING PROVIDER ID. #
From MM DD YY	To MM DD YY			CPT/HCPCS	MODIFIER						
										1G	234665212
1 XX XX XX	XX XX XX	11	N	99203		1	80 00	1		NPI	8888877777
										1G	234665212
2 XX XX XX	XX XX XX	11	N	71020		1	75 00	1		NPI	8888877777
										1G	234665212
3 XX XX XX	XX XX XX	11	N	93000		2	65 00	1		NPI	8888877777
4										NPI	
5										NPI	
6										NPI	

25. FEDERAL TAX ID NUMBER   SSN EIN
725727222   ☐ ☒

26. PATIENT'S ACCOUNT NO.
NAMYO

27. ACCEPT ASSIGNMENT?
(For govt. claims, see back)
☒ YES   ☐ NO

28. TOTAL CHARGE
$ 220 00

29. AMOUNT PAID
$

30. BALANCE DUE
$ 220 00

31. SIGNATURE OF PHYSICIAN OR SUPPLIER INCLUDING DEGREES OR CREDENTIALS
(I certify that the statements on the reverse apply to this bill and are made a part thereof)

SIGNED SIGNATURE ON FILE   TODAY'S DATE

32. SERVICE FACILITY LOCATION INFORMATION
MALLARD AND ASSOCIATES PA
19333 FORREST HAVEN
DALLAS TX 123452222

a. 7777788888   b. 1CM23548711

33. BILLING PROVIDER INFO & PH. # (214) 555-5040
MALLARD AND ASSOCIATES PA
19333 FORREST HAVEN
DALLAS TX 12345

a. 7777788888   b. 1CM23548711

NUCC Instruction Manual available at: www.nucc.org
WCMS-1500CS

APPROVED OMB 0938-0999 FORM CMS-1500 (08/05)

Side margins: CARRIER — PATIENT AND INSURED INFORMATION — PHYSICIAN OR SUPPLIER INFORMATION

Left margin: SECOND FOLD — WHCF-10-ENV / WHCF-10-ENV-SS — FIRST FOLD

Practice Exercise 11-8

1. Upcoding
2. Fraud
3. Fraud
4. Noncovered
5. Misrepresents as medically necessary
6. Misrepresents as medically necessary
7. Choice C—Services/items not furnished to a patient but billed to Medicare.

Chapter 12: Medicaid Medical Billing

Practice Exercise 12-1

	1500	

HEALTH INSURANCE CLAIM FORM
APPROVED BY NATIONAL UNIFORM CLAIM COMMITTEE 08/05

MEDICAID
PO BOX 200555
AUSTIN TX 78705

CARRIER

□ PICA   PICA □□

1. MEDICARE MEDICAID TRICARE CHAMPUS CHAMPVA GROUP HEALTH PLAN FECA BLK LUNG OTHER	1a. INSURED'S I.D. NUMBER (For Program in Item 1)
□ (Medicare #) ☒ (Medicaid #) □ (Sponsor's SSN) □ (Member ID#) □ (SSN or ID) □ (SSN) □ (ID)	558479630

2. PATIENT'S NAME (Last Name, First Name, Middle Initial)	3. PATIENT'S BIRTH DATE SEX	4. INSURED'S NAME (Last Name, First Name, Middle Initial)
SHELTON MARGARET	MM 03 DD 25 YY 2007 M□ F☒	

5. PATIENT'S ADDRESS (No, Street)	6. PATIENT RELATIONSHIP TO INSURED	7. INSURED'S ADDRESS (No, Street)
12 BONNIE LANE	Self ☒ Spouse □ Child □ Other □	

CITY	STATE	8. PATIENT STATUS	CITY	STATE
DALLAS	TX	Single ☒ Married □ Other □		

ZIP CODE	TELEPHONE (Include Area Code)		ZIP CODE	TELEPHONE (Include Area Code)
12345	(214) 5551212	Employed □ Full-Time Student □ Part-Time Student □		( )

9. OTHER INSURED'S NAME (Last Name, First Name, Middle Initial)	10. IS PATIENT'S CONDITION RELATED TO:	11. INSURED'S POLICY GROUP OR FECA NUMBER — NONE
a. OTHER INSURED'S POLICY OR GROUP NUMBER	a. EMPLOYMENT? (Current or Previous) □ YES ☒ NO	a. INSURED'S DATE OF BIRTH MM DD YY SEX M□ F□
b. OTHER INSURED'S DATE OF BIRTH SEX MM DD YY M□ F□	b. AUTO ACCIDENT? PLACE (State) □ YES ☒ NO	b. EMPLOYER'S NAME OR SCHOOL NAME
c. EMPLOYER'S NAME OR SCHOOL NAME	c. OTHER ACCIDENT? □ YES ☒ NO	c. INSURANCE PLAN NAME OR PROGRAM NAME
d. INSURANCE PLAN NAME OR PROGRAM NAME	10d. RESERVED FOR LOCAL USE	d. IS THERE ANOTHER HEALTH BENEFIT PLAN? □ YES □ NO If yes, return to and complete item 9 a-d

READ BACK OF FORM BEFORE COMPLETING & SIGNING THIS FORM.

12. PATIENT'S OR AUTHORIZED PERSON'S SIGNATURE I authorize the release of any medical or other information necessary to process this claim. I also request payment of government benefits either to myself or to the party who accepts assignment below.	13. INSURED'S OR AUTHORIZED PERSON'S SIGNATURE I authorize payment of medical benefits to the undersigned physician or supplier for services described below.
SIGNED SIGNATURE ON FILE DATE _____	SIGNED SIGNATURE ON FILE

14. DATE OF CURRENT ILLNESS (First symptom) OR INJURY (Accident) OR PREGNANCY (LMP) MM DD YY	15. IF PATIENT HAS HAD SAME OR SIMILAR ILLNESS, GIVE FIRST DATE MM DD YY	16. DATES PATIENT UNABLE TO WORK IN CURRENT OCCUPATION FROM MM DD YY TO MM DD YY
17. NAME OF REFERRING PHYSICIAN OR OTHER SOURCE	17a. 17b. NPI	18. HOSPITALIZATION DATES RELATED TO CURRENT SERVICES FROM MM DD YY TO MM DD YY
19. RESERVED FOR LOCAL USE		20. OUTSIDE LAB? □ YES ☒ NO $ CHARGES

21. DIAGNOSIS OR NATURE OF ILLNESS OR INJURY (Relate Items 1,2,3 or 4 to Item 24E by Line)	22. MEDICAID RESUBMISSION CODE ORIGINAL REF. NO.
1. V20 . 2 3.	23. PRIOR AUTHORIZATION NUMBER
2. 4.	

24. A. DATE(S) OF SERVICE						B. PLACE OF SERVICE	C. EMG	D. PROCEDURES, SERVICES, OR SUPPLIES (Explain Unusual Circumstances)		E. DIAGNOSIS POINTER	F. $ CHARGES	G. DAYS OR UNITS	H. EPSDT Family Plan	I. ID. QUAL.	J. RENDERING PROVIDER ID. #
From MM	DD	YY	To MM	DD	YY			CPT/HCPCS	MODIFIER						
														10	51750
1 XX	XX	XX	XX	XX	XX	11		99214		1	95 00	1		NPI	1234567890
2														NPI	
3														NPI	
4														NPI	
5														NPI	
6														NPI	

25. FEDERAL TAX ID NUMBER SSN EIN	26. PATIENT'S ACCOUNT NO.	27. ACCEPT ASSIGNMENT? (For govt. claims, see back)	28. TOTAL CHARGE	29. AMOUNT PAID	30. BALANCE DUE
751234567 □ ☒	SHEMA 000 10	☒ YES □ NO	$ 95 00	$	$

31. SIGNATURE OF PHYSICIAN OR SUPPLIER INCLUDING DEGREES OR CREDENTIALS (I certify that the statements on the reverse apply to this bill and are made a part thereof)	32. SERVICE FACILITY LOCATION INFORMATION	33. BILLING PROVIDER INFO & PH. # (972) 5555482
	ALLIED MEDICAL CENTER 1933 E FRANKFORD RD CARROLLTON TX 12345	SAMANTHA E SMITH MD 1933 E FRANKFORD RD CARROLLTON TX 12345
SIGNED SIGNATURE ON FILE DATE	a. 1234567890 b. 1D S1750	a. 1234567890 b. 1D S1750

Practice Exercise 12-2

(1500)

HEALTH INSURANCE CLAIM FORM
APPROVED BY NATIONAL UNIFORM CLAIM COMMITTEE 08/05

MEDICAID
PO BOX 200555
AUSTIN TX 78705

PICA							PICA

1. MEDICARE ☐ (Medicare #)   MEDICAID ☒ (Medicaid #)   TRICARE CHAMPUS ☐ (Sponsor's SSN)   CHAMPVA ☐ (Member ID#)   GROUP HEALTH PLAN ☐ (SSN or ID)   FECA BLK LUNG ☐ (SSN)   OTHER ☐ (ID)

1a. INSURED'S I.D. NUMBER   (For Program in Item 1)
599630014

2. PATIENT'S NAME (Last Name, First Name, Middle Initial)
CHURCHILL, SHAWN, L

3. PATIENT'S BIRTH DATE   MM 07 | DD 29 | YY 2005   SEX M ☒ F ☐

4. INSURED'S NAME (Last Name, First Name, Middle Initial)

5. PATIENT'S ADDRESS (No, Street)
6580 BELT LINE ROAD 12B

6. PATIENT RELATIONSHIP TO INSURED
Self ☒ Spouse ☐ Child ☐ Other ☐

7. INSURED'S ADDRESS (No, Street)

CITY   PLANO   STATE TX

8. PATIENT STATUS
Single ☒ Married ☐ Other ☐
Employed ☐ Full-Time Student ☐ Part-Time Student ☐

CITY   STATE

ZIP CODE 12345   TELEPHONE (Include Area Code) (469) 5557406

ZIP CODE   TELEPHONE (Include Area Code) (   )

9. OTHER INSURED'S NAME (Last Name, First Name, Middle Initial)

10. IS PATIENT'S CONDITION RELATED TO:

11. INSURED'S POLICY GROUP OR FECA NUMBER
NONE

a. OTHER INSURED'S POLICY OR GROUP NUMBER

a. EMPLOYMENT? (Current or Previous) ☐ YES ☒ NO

a. INSURED'S DATE OF BIRTH MM | DD | YY   SEX M ☐ F ☐

b. OTHER INSURED'S DATE OF BIRTH MM | DD | YY   SEX M ☐ F ☐

b. AUTO ACCIDENT?   PLACE (State) ☐ YES ☒ NO

b. EMPLOYER'S NAME OR SCHOOL NAME

c. EMPLOYER'S NAME OR SCHOOL NAME

c. OTHER ACCIDENT? ☐ YES ☒ NO

c. INSURANCE PLAN NAME OR PROGRAM NAME

d. INSURANCE PLAN NAME OR PROGRAM NAME

10d. RESERVED FOR LOCAL USE

d. IS THERE ANOTHER HEALTH BENEFIT PLAN?
☐ YES ☐ NO   If yes, return to and complete item 9 a-d

READ BACK OF FORM BEFORE COMPLETING & SIGNING THIS FORM.

12. PATIENT'S OR AUTHORIZED PERSON'S SIGNATURE I authorize the release of any medical or other information necessary to process this claim. I also request payment of government benefits either to myself or to the party who accepts assignment below.

SIGNED   SIGNATURE ON FILE   DATE

13. INSURED'S OR AUTHORIZED PERSON'S SIGNATURE I authorize payment of medical benefits to the undersigned physician or supplier for services described below.

SIGNED   SIGNATURE ON FILE

14. DATE OF CURRENT MM | DD | YY   ILLNESS (First symptom) OR INJURY (Accident) OR PREGNANCY (LMP)

15. IF PATIENT HAS HAD SAME OR SIMILAR ILLNESS, GIVE FIRST DATE MM | DD | YY

16. DATES PATIENT UNABLE TO WORK IN CURRENT OCCUPATION FROM MM | DD | YY   TO MM | DD | YY

17. NAME OF REFERRING PHYSICIAN OR OTHER SOURCE

17a.
17b. NPI

18. HOSPITALIZATION DATES RELATED TO CURRENT SERVICES FROM MM | DD | YY   TO MM | DD | YY

19. RESERVED FOR LOCAL USE

20. OUTSIDE LAB? ☐ YES ☒ NO $ CHARGES

21. DIAGNOSIS OR NATURE OF ILLNESS OR INJURY (Relate Items 1,2,3 or 4 to Item 24E by Line)
1. V04 . 81
2.
3.
4.

22. MEDICAID RESUBMISSION CODE   ORIGINAL REF. NO.

23. PRIOR AUTHORIZATION NUMBER

24. A. DATE(S) OF SERVICE						B. PLACE OF SERVICE	C. EMG	D. PROCEDURES, SERVICES, OR SUPPLIES (Explain Unusual Circumstances) CPT/HCPCS	MODIFIER	E. DIAGNOSIS POINTER	F. $ CHARGES	G. DAYS OR UNITS	H. EPSDT Family Plan	I. ID. QUAL.	J. RENDERING PROVIDER ID. #
From MM	DD	YY	To MM	DD	YY										
XX	XX	XX	XX	XX	XX	11		90658		1	15 00	1		1D NPI	S1750 1234567890
XX	XX	XX	XX	XX	XX	11		90471		1	5 00	1		1D NPI	S1750 1234567890
														NPI	
														NPI	
														NPI	
														NPI	

25. FEDERAL TAX ID NUMBER SSN EIN
751234567   ☐ ☒

26. PATIENT'S ACCOUNT NO.
CHUSH000   12

27. ACCEPT ASSIGNMENT? (For govt. claims, see back) ☒ YES ☐ NO

28. TOTAL CHARGE $ 20 00

29. AMOUNT PAID $

30. BALANCE DUE $

31. SIGNATURE OF PHYSICIAN OR SUPPLIER INCLUDING DEGREES OR CREDENTIALS (I certify that the statements on the reverse apply to this bill and are made a part thereof)

SIGNED   SIGNATURE ON FILE   DATE

32. SERVICE FACILITY LOCATION INFORMATION
ALLIED MEDICAL CENTER
1933 E FRANKFORD RD
CARROLLTON TX 12345
a. 1234567890   b. 1D S1750

33. BILLING PROVIDER INFO & PH. # (972) 555-5482
SAMANTHA E SMITH MD
1933 E FRANKFORD RD
CARROLLTON TX 12345
a. 1234567890   b. 1D S1750

NUCC Instruction Manual available at: www.nucc.org
WCMS-1500CS

APPROVED OMB 0938-0999 FORM CMS-1500 (08/05)

Practice Exercise 12-3

(1500)		AMERICAID
HEALTH INSURANCE CLAIM FORM		**PO BOX 61117**
APPROVED BY NATIONAL UNIFORM CLAIM COMMITTEE 08/05		**VIRGINIA BEACH VA 23466-1117**

☐☐ PICA						PICA ☐☐☐

1. MEDICARE MEDICAID TRICARE CHAMPVA GROUP FECA OTHER	1a. INSURED'S I.D. NUMBER (For Program in Item 1)
CHAMPUS HEALTH PLAN BLK LUNG	515301607
☐(Medicare #) ☒(Medicaid #) ☐(Sponsor's SSN) ☐(Member ID#) ☐(SSN or ID) ☐(SSN) ☐(ID)	

2. PATIENT'S NAME (Last Name, First Name, Middle Initial)	3. PATIENT'S BIRTH DATE SEX	4. INSURED'S NAME (Last Name, First Name, Middle Initial)
BRADFORD, LUELLA	MM DD YY 03 17 1988 M☐ F☒	

5. PATIENT'S ADDRESS (No, Street)	6. PATIENT RELATIONSHIP TO INSURED	7. INSURED'S ADDRESS (No, Street)
2594B LOVERS LANE	Self☒ Spouse☐ Child☐ Other☐	
CITY DALLAS STATE TX	8. PATIENT STATUS Single☒ Married☐ Other☐	CITY STATE
ZIP CODE 12345 TELEPHONE (Include Area Code) (214) 5550147	Full-Time Part-Time Employed☐ Student☐ Student☐	ZIP CODE TELEPHONE (Include Area Code) ( )

9. OTHER INSURED'S NAME (Last Name, First Name, Middle Initial)	10. IS PATIENT'S CONDITION RELATED TO:	11. INSURED'S POLICY GROUP OR FECA NUMBER NONE
a. OTHER INSURED'S POLICY OR GROUP NUMBER	a. EMPLOYMENT? (Current or Previous) ☐YES ☒NO	a. INSURED'S DATE OF BIRTH SEX MM DD YY M☐ F☐
b. OTHER INSURED'S DATE OF BIRTH SEX MM DD YY M☐ F☐	b. AUTO ACCIDENT? PLACE (State) ☐YES ☒NO	b. EMPLOYER'S NAME OR SCHOOL NAME
c. EMPLOYER'S NAME OR SCHOOL NAME	c. OTHER ACCIDENT? ☐YES ☒NO	c. INSURANCE PLAN NAME OR PROGRAM NAME
d. INSURANCE PLAN NAME OR PROGRAM NAME	10d. RESERVED FOR LOCAL USE	d. IS THERE ANOTHER HEALTH BENEFIT PLAN? ☐YES ☐NO If yes, return to and complete item 9 a-d

READ BACK OF FORM BEFORE COMPLETING & SIGNING THIS FORM.	13. INSURED'S OR AUTHORIZED PERSON'S SIGNATURE I authorize payment of medical benefits to the undersigned physician or supplier for services described below.
12. PATIENT'S OR AUTHORIZED PERSON'S SIGNATURE I authorize the release of any medical or other information necessary to process this claim. I also request payment of government benefits either to myself or to the party who accepts assignment below.	
SIGNED SIGNATURE ON FILE DATE	SIGNED SIGNATURE ON FILE

14. DATE OF CURRENT ILLNESS (First symptom) OR MM DD YY INJURY (Accident) OR PREGNANCY (LMP)	15. IF PATIENT HAS HAD SAME OR SIMILAR ILLNESS, GIVE FIRST DATE MM DD YY	16. DATES PATIENT UNABLE TO WORK IN CURRENT OCCUPATION MM DD YY MM DD YY FROM TO
17. NAME OF REFERRING PHYSICIAN OR OTHER SOURCE	17a. 17b. NPI	18. HOSPITALIZATION DATES RELATED TO CURRENT SERVICES MM DD YY MM DD YY FROM TO
19. RESERVED FOR LOCAL USE		20. OUTSIDE LAB? ☐YES ☒NO $ CHARGES
21. DIAGNOSIS OR NATURE OF ILLNESS OR INJURY (Relate Items 1,2,3 or 4 to Item 24E by Line) 1. V72 . 40 3. 2. 4.		22. MEDICAID RESUBMISSION CODE ORIGINAL REF. NO. 23. PRIOR AUTHORIZATION NUMBER

24. A. DATE(S) OF SERVICE		B. PLACE OF SERVICE	C. EMG	D. PROCEDURES, SERVICES, OR SUPPLIES (Explain Unusual Circumstances) CPT/HCPCS MODIFIER	E. DIAGNOSIS POINTER	F. $ CHARGES	G. DAYS OR UNITS	H. EPSDT Family Plan	I. ID. QUAL.	J. RENDERING PROVIDER ID. #
From MM DD YY	To MM DD YY									
1 XX XX XX	XX XX XX	11		81025	1	20 00	1		1D NPI	S1750 1234567890
2									NPI	
3									NPI	
4									NPI	
5									NPI	
6									NPI	

25. FEDERAL TAX ID NUMBER SSN EIN	26. PATIENT'S ACCOUNT NO.	27. ACCEPT ASSIGNMENT? (For govt. claims, see back)	28. TOTAL CHARGE	29. AMOUNT PAID	30. BALANCE DUE
751234567 ☐☒	BRALU000 11	☒YES ☐NO	$ 20 00	$	$

31. SIGNATURE OF PHYSICIAN OR SUPPLIER INCLUDING DEGREES OR CREDENTIALS (I certify that the statements on the reverse apply to this bill and are made a part thereof)	32. SERVICE FACILITY LOCATION INFORMATION ALLIED MEDICAL CENTER 1933 E FRANKFORD RD CARROLLTON TX 12345	33. BILLING PROVIDER INFO & PH. # (972) 5555482 SAMANTHA E SMITH MD 1933 E FRANKFORD RD CARROLLTON TX 12345
SIGNED SIGNATURE ON FILE DATE	a. 1234567890 b. 1D S1750	a. 1234567890 b. 1D S1750

NUCC Instruction Manual available at: www.nucc.org   APPROVED OMB 0938-0999 FORM CMS-1500 (08/05)

WCMS-1500CS

Side markings: CARRIER →   PATIENT AND INSURED INFORMATION   PHYSICIAN OR SUPPLIER INFORMATION   SECOND FOLD   FIRST FOLD WHCF-10-ENV / WHCF-10-ENV-SS

Practice Exercise 12-4

(1500)		
HEALTH INSURANCE CLAIM FORM		**MEDICAID**
APPROVED BY NATIONAL UNIFORM CLAIM COMMITTEE 08/05		**PO BOX 200555**
		AUSTIN TX 78705

PICA

1. MEDICARE MEDICAID TRICARE CHAMPUS CHAMPVA GROUP HEALTH PLAN FECA BLK LUNG OTHER

☐ (Medicare #) ☒ (Medicaid #) ☐ (Sponsor's SSN) ☐ (Member ID#) ☐ (SSN or ID) ☐ (SSN) ☐ (ID)

1a. INSURED'S I.D. NUMBER (For Program in Item 1)
999528741

2. PATIENT'S NAME (Last Name, First Name, Middle Initial)
NGUYEN, THUY

3. PATIENT'S BIRTH DATE   SEX
MM 05 DD 01 YY 2007   M☐ F☒

4. INSURED'S NAME (Last Name, First Name, Middle Initial)

5. PATIENT'S ADDRESS (No, Street)
7619 CHATTINGTON LANE

6. PATIENT RELATIONSHIP TO INSURED
Self ☒ Spouse ☐ Child ☐ Other ☐

7. INSURED'S ADDRESS (No, Street)

CITY DALLAS   **STATE** TX

8. PATIENT STATUS
Single ☒ Married ☐ Other ☐
Employed ☐ Full-Time Student ☐ Part-Time Student ☐

CITY   **STATE**

ZIP CODE 12345   **TELEPHONE (Include Area Code)** (214) 5556488

ZIP CODE   **TELEPHONE (Include Area Code)** ( )

9. OTHER INSURED'S NAME (Last Name, First Name, Middle Initial)

10. IS PATIENT'S CONDITION RELATED TO:

11. INSURED'S POLICY GROUP OR FECA NUMBER
NONE

a. OTHER INSURED'S POLICY OR GROUP NUMBER

a. EMPLOYMENT? (Current or Previous)
☐ YES ☒ NO

a. INSURED'S DATE OF BIRTH   SEX
MM DD YY   M☐ F☐

b. OTHER INSURED'S DATE OF BIRTH   SEX
MM DD YY   M☐ F☐

b. AUTO ACCIDENT?   PLACE (State)
☐ YES ☒ NO

b. EMPLOYER'S NAME OR SCHOOL NAME

c. EMPLOYER'S NAME OR SCHOOL NAME

c. OTHER ACCIDENT?
☐ YES ☒ NO

c. INSURANCE PLAN NAME OR PROGRAM NAME

d. INSURANCE PLAN NAME OR PROGRAM NAME

10d. RESERVED FOR LOCAL USE

d. IS THERE ANOTHER HEALTH BENEFIT PLAN?
☐ YES ☐ NO   If yes, return to and complete item 9 a-d

READ BACK OF FORM BEFORE COMPLETING & SIGNING THIS FORM.

12. PATIENT'S OR AUTHORIZED PERSON'S SIGNATURE I authorize the release of any medical or other information necessary to process this claim. I also request payment of government benefits either to myself or to the party who accepts assignment below.

SIGNED SIGNATURE ON FILE   DATE

13. INSURED'S OR AUTHORIZED PERSON'S SIGNATURE I authorize payment of medical benefits to the undersigned physician or supplier for services described below.

SIGNED SIGNATURE ON FILE

14. DATE OF CURRENT MM DD YY ILLNESS (First symptom) OR INJURY (Accident) OR PREGNANCY (LMP)

15. IF PATIENT HAS HAD SAME OR SIMILAR ILLNESS, GIVE FIRST DATE MM DD YY

16. DATES PATIENT UNABLE TO WORK IN CURRENT OCCUPATION FROM MM DD YY TO MM DD YY

17. NAME OF REFERRING PHYSICIAN OR OTHER SOURCE   17a.   17b. NPI

18. HOSPITALIZATION DATES RELATED TO CURRENT SERVICES FROM MM DD YY TO MM DD YY

19. RESERVED FOR LOCAL USE

20. OUTSIDE LAB? ☐ YES ☒ NO $ CHARGES

21. DIAGNOSIS OR NATURE OF ILLNESS OR INJURY (Relate Items 1,2,3 or 4 to Item 24E by Line)
1. V21 . 35
2.
3.
4.

22. MEDICAID RESUBMISSION CODE   ORIGINAL REF. NO.

23. PRIOR AUTHORIZATION NUMBER

24. A. DATE(S) OF SERVICE						B. PLACE OF SERVICE	C. EMG	D. PROCEDURES, SERVICES, OR SUPPLIES (Explain Unusual Circumstances) CPT/HCPCS MODIFIER	E. DIAGNOSIS POINTER	F. $ CHARGES	G. DAYS OR UNITS	H. EPSDT Family Plan	I. ID. QUAL.	J. RENDERING PROVIDER ID. #
From MM	DD	YY	To MM	DD	YY									
XX	XX	XX	XX	XX	XX	11		99382	1	175 00	1		1D NPI	S1750 1234567890
													NPI	
													NPI	
													NPI	
													NPI	
													NPI	

25. FEDERAL TAX ID NUMBER   SSN EIN
751234567   ☐ ☒

26. PATIENT'S ACCOUNT NO.
NGUTH000   13

27. ACCEPT ASSIGNMENT? (For govt. claims, see back)
☒ YES ☐ NO

28. TOTAL CHARGE
$ 175 00

29. AMOUNT PAID
$

30. BALANCE DUE
$

31. SIGNATURE OF PHYSICIAN OR SUPPLIER INCLUDING DEGREES OR CREDENTIALS (I certify that the statements on the reverse apply to this bill and are made a part thereof)

SIGNED SIGNATURE ON FILE   DATE

32. SERVICE FACILITY LOCATION INFORMATION
ALLIED MEDICAL CENTER
1933 E FRANKFORD RD
CARROLLTON TX 12345
a. 1234567890   b. 1D S1750

33. BILLING PROVIDER INFO & PH. # (972) 5555482
SAMANTHA E SMITH MD
1933 E FRANKFORD RD
CARROLLTON TX 12345
a. 1234567890   b. 1D S1750

NUCC Instruction Manual available at: www.nucc.org
WCMS-1500CS

APPROVED OMB 0938-0999 FORM CMS-1500 (08/05)

Chapter 13: Tricare Medical Billing

Practice Exercise 13-1

(1500)

HEALTH INSURANCE CLAIM FORM
APPROVED BY NATIONAL UNIFORM CLAIM COMMITTEE 08/05

☐☐ PICA

PICA ☐☐☐

1. MEDICARE	MEDICAID	TRICARE CHAMPUS	CHAMPVA	GROUP HEALTH PLAN	FECA BLK LUNG	OTHER	1a. INSURED'S I.D. NUMBER (For Program in Item 1)
☐ (Medicare #)	☐ (Medicaid #)	☒ (Sponsor's SSN)	☐ (Member ID#)	☐ (SSN or ID)	☐ (SSN)	☐ (ID)	603879521

2. PATIENT'S NAME (Last Name, First Name, Middle Initial)	3. PATIENT'S BIRTH DATE	SEX	4. INSURED'S NAME (Last Name, First Name, Middle Initial)
COOK BARBARA	MM 06 DD 18 YY 1972	M ☐ F ☒	COOK CHRISTOPHER F

5. PATIENT'S ADDRESS (No, Street)	6. PATIENT RELATIONSHIP TO INSURED	7. INSURED'S ADDRESS (No, Street)
8742 FAIRVIEW RD	Self ☐ Spouse ☒ Child ☐ Other ☐	PO BOX 5431

CITY	STATE	8. PATIENT STATUS	CITY	STATE
DALLAS	TX	Single ☐ Married ☒ Other ☐	FORT DIX	NJ

ZIP CODE	TELEPHONE (Include Area Code)		ZIP CODE	TELEPHONE (Include Area Code)
12345	(999) 5553457	Employed ☐ Full-Time Student ☐ Part-Time Student ☐	12345	(555) 1248947

9. OTHER INSURED'S NAME (Last Name, First Name, Middle Initial)	10. IS PATIENT'S CONDITION RELATED TO:	11. INSURED'S POLICY GROUP OR FECA NUMBER

a. OTHER INSURED'S POLICY OR GROUP NUMBER	a. EMPLOYMENT? (Current or Previous) ☐ YES ☒ NO	a. INSURED'S DATE OF BIRTH MM DD YY SEX M ☐ F ☐

b. OTHER INSURED'S DATE OF BIRTH SEX MM DD YY M ☐ F ☐	b. AUTO ACCIDENT? PLACE (State) ☐ YES ☒ NO	b. EMPLOYER'S NAME OR SCHOOL NAME

c. EMPLOYER'S NAME OR SCHOOL NAME	c. OTHER ACCIDENT? ☐ YES ☒ NO	c. INSURANCE PLAN NAME OR PROGRAM NAME TRICARE

d. INSURANCE PLAN NAME OR PROGRAM NAME	10d. RESERVED FOR LOCAL USE	d. IS THERE ANOTHER HEALTH BENEFIT PLAN? ☐ YES ☒ NO If yes, return to and complete item 9 a-d

READ BACK OF FORM BEFORE COMPLETING & SIGNING THIS FORM.

12. PATIENT'S OR AUTHORIZED PERSON'S SIGNATURE I authorize the release of any medical or other information necessary to process this claim. I also request payment of government benefits either to myself or to the party who accepts assignment below.

SIGNED SIGNATURE ON FILE   DATE TODAY'S DATE

13. INSURED'S OR AUTHORIZED PERSON'S SIGNATURE I authorize payment of medical benefits to the undersigned physician or supplier for services described below.

SIGNED SIGNATURE ON FILE

14. DATE OF CURRENT MM DD YY ILLNESS (First symptom) OR INJURY (Accident) OR PREGNANCY (LMP)	15. IF PATIENT HAS HAD SAME OR SIMILAR ILLNESS, GIVE FIRST DATE MM DD YY	16. DATES PATIENT UNABLE TO WORK IN CURRENT OCCUPATION FROM MM DD YY TO MM DD YY

17. NAME OF REFERRING PHYSICIAN OR OTHER SOURCE	17a.	18. HOSPITALIZATION DATES RELATED TO CURRENT SERVICES
	17b. NPI	FROM MM DD YY TO MM DD YY

19. RESERVED FOR LOCAL USE	20. OUTSIDE LAB? ☐ YES ☒ NO $ CHARGES

21. DIAGNOSIS OR NATURE OF ILLNESS OR INJURY (Relate Items 1,2,3 or 4 to Item 24E by Line)

1. 487 . 1   3.
2.   4.

22. MEDICAID RESUBMISSION CODE   ORIGINAL REF. NO.
23. PRIOR AUTHORIZATION NUMBER

24. A. DATE(S) OF SERVICE From MM DD YY To MM DD YY	B. PLACE OF SERVICE	C. EMG	D. PROCEDURES, SERVICES, OR SUPPLIES (Explain Unusual Circumstances) CPT/HCPCS MODIFIER	E. DIAGNOSIS POINTER	F. $ CHARGES	G. DAYS OR UNITS	H. EPSDT Family Plan	I. ID. QUAL.	J. RENDERING PROVIDER ID. #
1	XX XX XX XX XX XX	11		99213	1	85 00	1		NPI	
2									NPI	
3									NPI	
4									NPI	
5									NPI	
6									NPI	

25. FEDERAL TAX ID NUMBER SSN EIN	26. PATIENT'S ACCOUNT NO.	27. ACCEPT ASSIGNMENT? (For govt. claims, see back)	28. TOTAL CHARGE	29. AMOUNT PAID	30. BALANCE DUE
229872767 ☐ ☒	COOBA 11	☒ YES ☐ NO	$ 85 00	$	$

31. SIGNATURE OF PHYSICIAN OR SUPPLIER INCLUDING DEGREES OR CREDENTIALS (I certify that the statements on the reverse apply to this bill and are made a part thereof) SIGNED SIGNATURE ON FILE DATE	32. SERVICE FACILITY LOCATION INFORMATION CHARLES H BORDEN MD 980 FREDERICK RD DALLAS TX 12345	33. BILLING PROVIDER INFO & PH. # (899) 5552276 CHARLES H BORDEN MD 980 FREDERICK RD DALLAS TX 12345
	a. 7536982014 b. 1H9856471	a. 7536982014 b. 1H9856471

NUCC Instruction Manual available at: www.nucc.org

APPROVED OMB 0938-0999 FORM CMS-1500 (08/05)

WCMS-1500CS

Chapter 14: Explanation of Benefits and Payment Adjudication

Practice Exercise 14-1

	Dallas	Houston	Fort Worth
99203:	$100.67	$ 97.27	$ 96.57
99213:	$ 55.41	$ 53.10	$ 52.93
23500:	$239.04	$228.72	$226.60

Practice Exercise 14-2

	Dallas	Houston	Fort Worth
99203:	$ 99.18	$ 95.84	$ 95.14
99213:	$ 54.59	$ 52.31	$ 52.14
23500:	$235.50	$225.34	$223.25

Practice Exercise 14-3

1. Usual charge _____ $315.00 _____
   Allowed charge _____ $175.00 _____
   Deductible _____ $ 0.00 _____
   Policy pays ___70%___ of the allowed charge, which is ___$122.50___.
   Patient responsible for ___30%___ of the allowed charge, which is ___$52.50___.
   Provider writes off the difference between the usual and allowed charge: ___$140.00___.

___$52.50___	___$140.00___	___$122.50___
Patient's responsibility	Write-off	Carrier pays

2. Usual charge _____ $200.00 _____
   Allowed charge _____ $135.00 _____
   Deductible _____ $100.00 _____
   Policy pays ___75%___ of the allowed charge, which is ___$26.25___.
   Patient responsible for ___25%___ of the allowed charge, which is ___$8.75___.
   Provider writes off the difference between the usual and allowed charge: ___$65.00___.

___$108.75___	___$65.00___	___$26.25___
Patient's responsibility	Write-off	Carrier pays

3. Usual charge _____ $200.00 _____
   Allowed charge _____ $ 0.00 _____
   Deductible _____ $ 0.00 _____

(continued)

Practice Exercise 14-3 (continued)

Policy pays _____0%_____ of the allowed charge, which is _____$0.00_____.

Patient responsible for __100%__ of the allowed charge, which is __200.00__.

Provider writes off the difference between the usual and allowed charge: _____$0.00_____.

$200.00	$0.00	$0.00
Patient's responsibility	Write-off	Carrier pays

4. Usual charge   _____$1,489.32_____

   Allowed charge   _____$1,489.32_____

   Deductible   _____$ 250.00_____

   Policy pays _____80%_____ of the allowed charge, which is _____$991.46_____.

   Patient responsible for _20%_ of the allowed charge, which is __$247.86__.

   Provider writes off the difference between the usual and allowed charge: _____$0.00_____.

$497.86	$0.00	$991.46
Patient's responsibility	Write-off	Carrier pays

Practice Exercise 14-4

1. Usual charge $215.00
    Allowed charge $175.00
    Deductible $150.00
    Policy pays ___100%___ of the allowed charge, which is _____$5.00_____.
    Patient responsible for the _copay_ of the allowed charge, which is _$20.00_.
    Provider writes off the difference between the usual and allowed charge:
    _____$40.00_____.

    _____$170.00_____   _____$40.00_____   _____$5.00_____
    Patient's responsibility   Write-off   Carrier pays

2. Usual charge $217.00
    Allowed charge $125.00
    Deductible $500.00
    Policy pays ___0%___ of the allowed charge, which is _____$0.00_____.
    Patient responsible for _100%_ of the allowed charge, which is _$125.00_.
    Provider writes off the difference between the usual and allowed charge:
    ___$92.00___.

    _____$125.00_____   _____$92.00_____   _____$0.00_____
    Patient's responsibility   Write-off   Carrier pays

3. Usual charge $3,895.56
    Allowed charge $2,956.18
    Deductible $ 500.00
    Policy pays ___90%___ of the allowed charge, which is ___$2210.56___.
    Patient responsible for _10%_ of the allowed charge, which is _$245.62_.
    Provider writes off the difference between the usual and allowed charge:
    ___$939.38___.

    _____$745.62_____   _____$939.38_____   _____$2,210.56_____
    Patient's responsibility   Write-off   Carrier pays

4. Usual charge $85 office, $175 lab
    Allowed charge $65 office, $125 lab
    Deductible $100.00 lab
    Policy pays _100% ofc, 80% lab_ of the allowed charge, which is _$45.00 ofc, $20.00 lab_.
    Patient responsible for _20%_ (lab) of the allowed charge, which is _$5.00_.
    Provider writes off the difference between the usual and allowed charge:
    $20.00 ofc, $50.00 lab .

    _____$125.00_____   _____$70.00_____   _____$65.00_____
    Patient's responsibility   Write-off   Carrier pays

Practice Exercise 14-5

1. Usual charge $175.00
   Allowed charge $125.00
   Deductible $ 0.00
   Policy pays 100% of the allowed charge, less copay which is 105.00.
   Patient responsible for the copay of the allowed charge, which is 20.00.
   Provider writes off the difference between the usual and allowed charge: $50.00.

$20.00	$50.00	$105.00
Patient's responsibility	Write-off	Carrier pays

2. Usual charge $726.25
   Allowed charge $558.16
   Deductible $250.00
   Policy pays 80% of the allowed charge, which is $246.53.
   Patient responsible for 20% of the allowed charge, which is $61.63.
   Provider writes off the difference between the usual and allowed charge: $168.09.

$311.63	$168.09	$246.53
Patient's responsibility	Write-off	Carrier pays

3. Usual charge $576.00
   Allowed charge $576.00
   Deductible $250.00
   Policy pays 80% of the allowed charge, which is $260.80.
   Patient responsible for the 20% of the allowed charge, which is $65.20.
   Provider writes off the difference between the usual and allowed charge: $0.00.

$315.20	$0.00	$260.80
Patient's responsibility	Write-off	Carrier pays

4. Usual charge $175.00
   Allowed charge $175.00
   Deductible $100.00
   Policy pays 90% of the allowed charge, which is $67.50.
   Patient responsible for 10% of the allowed charge, which is $7.50.
   Provider writes off the difference between the usual and allowed charge: $0.00.

$107.50	$0.00	$67.50
Patient's responsibility	Write-off	Carrier pays

Practice Exercise 14-6

1. Patient #1 charges 99213, 73630, and 97110. No deductible applies. Plan pays @ 80/20.

   Payer payment to provider _____ $122.40 _____

   Coinsurance _____ $30.60 _____

   Discount amount _____ $70.00 _____

2. Patient #2 charges 99212 and 73630. Deductible of $100.00 applies. Plan pays @ 80/20.

   Payer payment to provider _____ $20.80 _____

   Coinsurance _____ $5.20 (20%) _____

   Discount amount _____ $28.00 _____

3. Patient #3 charges 93040 and 97032. Deductible of $100.00 applies. Plan pays @ 90/10.

   Payer payment to provider _____ $0.00 _____

   Coinsurance $0.00 ($65.00 is applied to ded.)(Patient responsibility)

   Discount amount _____ $24.00 _____

4. Patient #4 charge 99201. Copay of $20 applies. Plan pays @ 100% after copay.

   Payer payment to provider _____ $42.00 _____

   Copayment _____ $20.00 _____

   Discount amount _____ $26.00 _____

5. Patient #5 charge 99204. Copay of $25.00 applies. Plan pays 100% after copay.

   Payer payment to provider _____ $50.00 _____

   Copayment _____ $25.00 _____

   Discount amount _____ $33.00 _____

Practice Exercise 14-7

Physician Charges	Allowed Amounts	Insurance Pays	Deductible
$ 88.00	$66.00	80%	$150.00*
$120.00	$99.00		
$ 90.00	$81.00		

	Charge	Adjustment	Allowed	Deductible	Copay	Ins. Pays	Coinsurance
	$88.00	$22.00	$66.00	$66.00	$0.00	$0.00	$0.00
	$120.00	$21.00	$99.00	$84.00	$0.00	$12.00	$3.00
	$90.00	$9.00	$81.00	$0	$0.00	$64.80	$16.20
TOTALS	$298.00	$52.00	246.00	$150.00	$0.00	$76.80	$19.20

*Deductible not met.

BALANCE DUE FROM PATIENT:

Patient's Deductible: $_____ 150.00 _____
Patient's Coinsurance: $_____ 19.20 _____

TOTAL INSURANCE PAYMENT: $_____ 76.80 _____

TOTAL PHYSICIAN WRITE-OFF: $_____ 52.00 _____

Practice Exercise 14-8

Physician Charges	Allowed Amounts	Insurance Pays	Deductible
$2,000.00	85%	70%	$200.00*

	Charge	Adjustment	Allowed	Deductible	Copay	Ins. Pays	Coinsurance
	$2000.00	$300.00	$1700.00	$155.00	$0.00	$1081.50	$463.50
TOTALS	$2000.00	$300.00	$1700.00	$155.00	$0.00	$1081.50	$463.50

*$45.00 of deductible has been met.

BALANCE DUE FROM PATIENT:

Patient's Deductible: $_____ 155.00 _____
Patient's Coinsurance: $_____ 463.50 _____

TOTAL INSURANCE PAYMENT: $_____ 1081.50 _____

TOTAL PROVIDER WRITE-OFF: $_____ 300.00 _____

Practice Exercise 14-9

Physician Charges	Allowed Amounts	Insurance Pays	Deductible
$3875.00	80%	90%	$250.00*

	Charge	Adjustment	Allowed	Deductible	Copay	Ins. Pays	Coinsurance
	$3875.00	$775.00	$3100.00	$250.00	$0.00	$2565.00	$285.00
TOTALS	$3875.00	$775.00	$3100.00	$250.00	$0.00	$2565.00	$285.00

*Deductible has not been met.

BALANCE DUE FROM PATIENT:

Patient's Deductible:	$	250.00
Patient's Coinsurance:	$	285.00
TOTAL INSURANCE PAYMENT	$	2,565.00
TOTAL PROVIDER WRITE-OFF:	$	775.00

Practice Exercise 14-10

For Student Use Only

EXPLANATION OF BENEFITS

Today's Date

Payer's Name and Address

| Aetna Insurance Company |
| P.O. Box 15999 |
| New York, NY 12345 |

Provider's Name and Address

| J.D. Mallard, M.D. |
| 1933 East Frankford Road |
| Carrollton, TX 12345 |

This statement covers payments for the following patient(s): Lynch, Amy
Claim Detail Section (If there are numbers in the "SEE REMARKS" column, see the Remarks Section for explanation.)

Patient Name: Hughes, Patsy **Patient Account Number:** Hugan0
Patient ID Number: **Insured's Name:** Andrew Hughes
Group Number: 55216
Provider Name: J.D. Mallard, M.D. **Inventory Number:** 44562 **Claim Control Number:** 28971

Service Date(s)	Procedure	Charges	Adjustment	Allowed	Copay	Deduct/Not Covered	Coins	Paid At.	Provider Paid/Remarks
02/16/2008	97039	$50.00	$ 1.00	$49.00	$0.00	$ 0.00	$ 9.80	80%	$39.20
02/16/2008	97042	$65.00	$65.00	$ 0.00	$0.00	$ 0.00	$ 0.00		$ 0.00
02/19/2008	97039	$50.00	$ 0.00	$50.00	$0.00	$ 0.00	$10.00	80%	$40.00
02/21/2008	97039	$50.00	$ 0.00	$50.00		$ 50.00	$ 0.00	80%	031*
TOTALS			$66.00			$50.00	$19.80		$79.20

BALANCE DUE FROM PATIENT: PT'S DED/NOT COV $_____ 50.00 _____
PT'S COINS. $_____ 19.80 _____

031 Met Maximum Limit

PAYMENT SUMMARY SECTION (TOTALS)

Charges	Adjustment	Allowed	Copay	Deduct/Not Covered	Coins	Total Paid
$215.00	$66.00	$149.00	$0	$50.00	$19.80	$79.20

Practice Exercise 14-11

For Student Use Only

EXPLANATION OF BENEFITS

Today's Date

Payer's Name and Address

Aetna Insurance Company
P.O. Box 15999
New York, NY 12345

Provider's Name and Address

J.D. Mallard, M.D.
1933 East Frankford Road
Carrollton, TX 12345

This statement covers payments for the following patient(s):
Claim Detail Section (If there are numbers in the "SEE REMARKS" column, see the Remarks Section for explanation.)

Patient Name: Hughes, Patsy   **Patient Account Number:** Hugan0
Patient ID Number: **Insured's Name:** Andrew Hughes
Group Number: 55216
Provider Name: J.D. Mallard, M.D.   **Inventory Number:** 44562   **Claim Control Number:** 28971

Service Date(s)	Procedure	Charges	Adjustment	Allowed	Copay	Deduct/Not Covered	Coins	Paid At.	Provider Paid/Remarks
01/02/2008	65542	$1500.00	$300.00	$1,200.00	$0.00	$300.00	$180.00	80%	$720.00
TOTALS		$1,500.00	$300.00	$1,200.00	$0.00	$300.00	$180.00		$720.00

BALANCE DUE FROM PATIENT: PT'S DED/NOT COV $_____300.00_____

PT'S COINS. $_____180.00_____

PAYMENT SUMMARY SECTION (TOTALS)

Charges	Adjustment	Allowed	Copay	Deduct/Not Covered	Coins	Total Paid
$1500.00	$300.00	$1200.00	$0.00	$300.00	$180.00	$720.00

Practice Exercise 14-12

For Student Use Only

EXPLANATION OF BENEFITS

Today's Date

Payer's Name and Address

Aetna Insurance Company
P.O. Box 15999
New York, NY 12345

Provider's Name and Address

J.D. Mallard, M.D.
1933 East Frankford Road
Carrollton, TX 12345

This statement covers payments for the following patient(s):
Claim Detail Section (If there are numbers in the "SEE REMARKS" column, see the Remarks Section for explanation.)

Patient Name: Hughes, Patsy   **Patient Account Number:** Hugan0
Patient ID Number: **Insured's Name:** Andrew Hughes
Group Number: 55216
Provider Name: J.D. Mallard, M.D.   **Inventory Number:** 44562   **Claim Control Number:** 28971

Service Date(s)	Procedure	Charges	Adjustment	Allowed	Copay	Deduct/Not Covered	Coins	Paid At.	Provider Paid/Remarks
04/09/2008	99213	$100.00	$22.00	$ 78.00	$ 25.00	$0.00	$0.00	100%	$ 53.00
04/09/2008	80048	$150.00	$50.00	$100.00	$ 0.00	$0.00		100%	$100.00
04/09/2008	71020	$ 78.00	$22.00	$ 56.00	$ 0.00	$0.00		100%	$ 56.00
		$328.00	$94.00	$234.00	$25.00				$209.00

BALANCE DUE FROM PATIENT: PT'S DED/NOT COV $_____0.00_____

                                   PT'S COINS. $_____0.00_____

PAYMENT SUMMARY SECTION (TOTALS)

Charges	Adjustment	Allowed	Copay	Deduct/Not Covered	Coins	Total Paid
$328.00	$94.00	$234.00	$25.00	$0.00	$0.00	$209.00

Practice Exercise 14-13

For Student Use Only

EXPLANATION OF BENEFITS

Today's Date

Payer's Name and Address

Aetna Insurance Company
P.O. Box 15999
New York, NY 12345

Provider's Name and Address

J.D. Mallard, M.D.
1933 East Frankford Road
Carrollton, TX 12345

This statement covers payments for the following patient(s):
Claim Detail Section (If there are numbers in the "SEE REMARKS" column, see the Remarks Section for explanation.)

Patient Name: Hughes, Patsy   **Patient Account Number:** Hugan0
Patient ID Number: **Insured's Name:** Andrew Hughes
Group Number: 55216
Provider Name: J.D. Mallard, M.D.   **Inventory Number:** 44562   **Claim Control Number:** 28971

Service Date(s)	Procedure	Charges	Adjustment	Allowed	Copay	Deduct/Not Covered	Coins	Paid At.	Provider Paid/Remarks
05/02/2008	72149	$1,300.00	$350.00	$ 950.00	$0.00	$500.00	$ 90.00	80%	$360.00
05/02/2008	94010	$ 325.00	$ 80.00	$ 245.00	$0.00		$ 49.00	80%	$196.00
05/02/2008	99214	$ 150.00	$ 25.00	$ 125.00	$0.00		$ 25.00	80%	$100.00
TOTALS		$1,775.00	$455.00	$1,320.00		$500.00	$164.00		$656.00

BALANCE DUE FROM PATIENT:

PT'S DED/NOT COV $_____500.00_____

PT'S COINS. $_____164.00_____

PAYMENT SUMMARY SECTION (TOTALS)

Charges	Adjustment	Allowed	Copay	Deduct/Not Covered	Coins	Total Paid
$1775.00	$455.00	$1320.00	$0.00	$500.00	$164.00	$656.00

Practice Exercise 14-14

Physician Charges	Allowed Amounts	Insurance Pays	Deductible
$200.00	$169.43	90%	$0.00
$ 25.00	$ 23.69		

	Charge	Adjustment	Allowed	Deductible	Copay	Ins. Pays	Coinsurance
	$200.00	$30.57	$169.43	$	$	$152.49	$16.94
	$ 25.00	$ 1.31	$ 23.69	$	$	$ 21.32	$ 2.37
TOTALS	$225.00	$31.88	$193.12	$	$	$173.81	$19.31

BALANCE DUE FROM PATIENT:

Patient's Deductible: $_____0.00_____

Patient's Coinsurance: $_____19.31_____

TOTAL INSURANCE PAYS: $_____173.81_____

TOTAL PHYSICIAN WRITE-OFF: $_____31.88_____

Practice Exercise 14-15

Physician Charges	Allowed Amounts	Insurance Pays	Deductible
$1,750.00	$1,750.00	95%	$150.00*
$ 925.00	$ 925.00		
$ 400.00	$ 400.00		
$ 108.00	$ 108.00		

	Charge	Adjustment	Allowed	Deductible	Copay	Ins. Pays	Coinsurance
	$1,750.00	$	$1750.00	$150.00	$	$1520.00	$ 80.00
	$ 925.00	$	$ 925.00	$ 00.00	$	$ 878.75	$ 46.25
	$ 400.00	$	$ 400.00	$ 00.00	$	$ 380.00	$ 20.00
	$ 108.00	$	$ 108.00	$ 00.00	$	$ 102.60	$ 5.40
TOTALS	$3,183.00	$	$3,183.00	$150.00	$	$2,881.35	$151.65

*Deductible not met.

BALANCE DUE FROM PATIENT:

Patient's Deductible: $_____150.00_____

Patient's Coinsurance: $_____151.65_____

TOTAL INSURANCE PAYS: $_____2,881.35_____

TOTAL PHYSICIAN WRITE-OFF: $_____0.00_____

Practice Exercise 14-16

Physician Charges	Allowed Amounts	Insurance Pays	Deductible
$1,650.00	$123.70	90%	$250.00*
$1,650.00	$412.50		

	Charge	Adjustment	Allowed	Deductible	Copay	Ins. Pays	Coinsurance
	$1,650.00	$1,526.30	$123.70	$115.00	$0.00	$ 7.83	$ 0.87
	$1,650.00	$1,237.50	$412.50	$ 00.00	$0.00	$371.25	$41.25
TOTALS	$3,300.00	$2,763.80	$536.20	$115.00	$0.00	$379.08	$42.12

*$115.00 of deductible not met.

BALANCE DUE FROM PATIENT:

Patient's Deductible: $_____115.00_____

Patient's Coinsurance: $_____42.12_____

TOTAL INSURANCE PAYMENT: $_____379.08_____

TOTAL PHYSICIAN WRITE-OFF: $_____2,763.80_____

Practice Exercise 14.17

Insurance company name: Health Insurance Company

Patient's name: Pam White

Patient's ID: 633-33-3333

Provider's name: Medical Center Subsidiary

Date of service: 12/12/08

Total charge: $5,363.50

Procedure(s): Hosp exp

Copay: $0.00

Deductible: $0.00

Coinsurance due from patient: $0.00

Allowed amount: $3,261.10

Discount amount: $2,102.40

Noncovered items: $0.00

Rate of benefit (%): 100%

Amount paid: $3,261.10

Remarks: 0054

Outcome: ▦ Bill patient balance
            ▦ Appeal
            ▦ Call carrier
            ⊠ Claim paid in full

Practice Exercise 14.18

Insurance company name: Medical Care

Patient's name: Joe Smith

Patient's ID: 555-66-4444

Provider's name: Surgical Associates of Texas

Date of service: 01/02/2009

Total charge: $550.00

Procedure(s): 93880

Copay: $0.00

Deductible: $0.00

Coinsurance due from patient: $0.00

Allowed amount: $190.13

Discount amount: $359.87

Noncovered items: $359.87

Rate of benefit (%): 100%

Amount paid: $190.13

Remarks: Contractual adjustment of billed amount

Outcome: ▨ Bill patient balance
             ▨ Appeal
             ▨ Call carrier
             ☒ Claim paid in full

(continued)

Practice Exercise 14.18 (Continued)

Insurance company name: Medical Care

Patient's name: Kelly Jones

Patient's ID: 444-55-6666

Provider's name: Surgical Associates of Texas

Date of service: 01/02/2009

Total charge: $162.00

Procedure(s): 93880

Copay: $0.00

Deductible: $0.00

Coinsurance due from patient: $0.00

Allowed amount: $41.30

Discount amount: $120.70

Noncovered items: $120.70

Rate of benefit (%): 100%

Amount paid: $41.30

Remarks: Contractual adjustment of billed amount

Outcome: ■   Bill patient balance
              ■   Appeal
              ☒   Call carrier
              ■   Claim paid in full

Practice Exercise 14.18 (Continued)

Insurance company name: Medical Care

Patient's name: Mary Young

Patient's ID: 454-55-5555

Provider's name: Surgical Associates of Texas

Date of service: 01/01/2009–01/02/2009

Total charge: $358.00

Procedure(s): 99203, 72100

Copay: $10.00

Deductible: $0.00

Coinsurance due from patient: $0.00

Allowed amount: $278.00

Discount amount: $80.00

Noncovered items: $80.00

Rate of benefit (%): 100%

Amount paid: $268.00

Remarks: Contractual adjustment of billed amount

Outcome: ■ Bill patient balance
            ■ Appeal
            ■ Call carrier
            ☒ Claim paid in full

Practice Exercise 14.19

Insurance company name: TOTALS ONLY

Patient's name: N/A

Patient's ID: N/A

Provider's name: Allied Medical Center

Date of service: N/A

Total charge: $856.00

Procedure(s): N/A

Total Copay: $125.00

Total deductible: $12.82

Total coinsurance due from patients: $0.00

Total allowed amount: $488.54

Total discount amount: $367.46

Total noncovered items: $0.00

Rate of benefit (%): N/A

Total amount paid to provider: $350.72

Remarks: 001 SERVICES PROVIDED ARE COVERED UP TO AN ALLOWED AMOUNT. SINCE THIS AMOUNT HAS BEEN PAID, NO ADDITIONAL PAYMENT CAN BE MADE.

Practice Exercise 14.20

Insurance company name: Insurance Company of America

Patient's name: Jeff Staubach

Patient's ID: N/A

Provider's name: Allied Medical Center

Date of service: 10/13/2008

Total charge: $148.00

Procedure(s): 99214

Copay: $0.00

Deductible: $0.00

Coinsurance due from patient: $0.00

Allowed amount: $0.00

Discount amount: $0.00

Noncovered items: $148.00

Rate of benefit (%): $0.00

Amount paid: $0.00

Remarks: ab   This claim was previously processed.

Outcome: ▨ Bill patient balance
          ▨ Appeal
          ☒ Call carrier
          ▨ Claim paid in full

Chapter 15: Refunds and Appeals

Practice Exercise 15.1

1. W
2. W
3. T
4. W
5. T
6. W
7. T
8. T

Practice Exercise 15.2

Answers will vary.

Practice Exercise 15.3

1. Yes
2. $89.00
3. Positive
4. Yes
5. $89.00 (to Patient)

Practice Exercise 15.4

1. Yes
2. $32
3. Positive
4. Yes
5. $32.00 (to Patient)

Practice Exercise 15.5

1. Yes
2. $6.20
3. Positive
4. Yes
5. $6.20 (to Patient)

Practice Exercise 15.6

1. Yes
2. $25.30
3. Positive
4. Yes
5. $25.30 (to Patient)

Practice Exercise 15.3

(1500)

HEALTH INSURANCE CLAIM FORM
APPROVED BY NATIONAL UNIFORM CLAIM COMMITTEE 08/05

CARRIER

☐☐☐ PICA   PICA ☐☐☐

| 1. MEDICARE ☐ (Medicare #) MEDICAID ☐ (Medicaid #) TRICARE CHAMPUS ☐ (Sponsor's SSN) CHAMPVA ☐ (Member ID#) GROUP HEALTH PLAN ☒ (SSN or ID) FECA BLK LUNG ☐ (SSN) OTHER ☐ (ID) | 1a. INSURED'S I.D. NUMBER (For Program in Item 1) 581144448 |

| 2. PATIENT'S NAME (Last Name, First Name, Middle Initial) BROWN SANDRA | 3. PATIENT'S BIRTH DATE MM 09 DD 06 YY 1975   SEX M☐ F☒ | 4. INSURED'S NAME (Last Name, First Name, Middle Initial) SAME |

| 5. PATIENT'S ADDRESS (No, Street) 1658 N LOVERS LANE | 6. PATIENT RELATIONSHIP TO INSURED Self☒ Spouse☐ Child☐ Other☐ | 7. INSURED'S ADDRESS (No, Street) |

| CITY DALLAS | STATE TX | 8. PATIENT STATUS Single☒ Married☐ Other☐ | CITY | STATE |

| ZIP CODE 12345 | TELEPHONE (Include Area Code) (214) 555 8288 | Employed☒ Full-Time Student☐ Part-Time Student☐ | ZIP CODE | TELEPHONE (Include Area Code) (   ) |

| 9. OTHER INSURED'S NAME (Last Name, First Name, Middle Initial) | 10. IS PATIENT'S CONDITION RELATED TO: | 11. INSURED'S POLICY GROUP OR FECA NUMBER 1274 |

| a. OTHER INSURED'S POLICY OR GROUP NUMBER | a. EMPLOYMENT? (Current or Previous) ☐YES ☒NO | a. INSURED'S DATE OF BIRTH MM DD YY   SEX M☐ F☐ |

| b. OTHER INSURED'S DATE OF BIRTH MM DD YY   SEX M☐ F☐ | b. AUTO ACCIDENT?   PLACE (State) ☐YES ☒NO | b. EMPLOYER'S NAME OR SCHOOL NAME CENTRAL MARKET |

| c. EMPLOYER'S NAME OR SCHOOL NAME | c. OTHER ACCIDENT? ☐YES ☒NO | c. INSURANCE PLAN NAME OR PROGRAM NAME AETNA |

| d. INSURANCE PLAN NAME OR PROGRAM NAME | 10d. RESERVED FOR LOCAL USE | d. IS THERE ANOTHER HEALTH BENEFIT PLAN? ☐YES ☒NO If yes, return to and complete item 9 a-d |

PATIENT AND INSURED INFORMATION

READ BACK OF FORM BEFORE COMPLETING & SIGNING THIS FORM.

12. PATIENT'S OR AUTHORIZED PERSON'S SIGNATURE I authorize the release of any medical or other information necessary to process this claim. I also request payment of government benefits either to myself or to the party who accepts assignment below.

SIGNED __SIGNATURE ON FILE__   DATE_____

13. INSURED'S OR AUTHORIZED PERSON'S SIGNATURE I authorize payment of medical benefits to the undersigned physician or supplier for services described below.

SIGNED __SIGNATURE ON FILE__

| 14. DATE OF CURRENT MM XX DD XX YY XX ILLNESS (First symptom) OR INJURY (Accident) OR PREGNANCY (LMP) | 15. IF PATIENT HAS HAD SAME OR SIMILAR ILLNESS, GIVE FIRST DATE MM DD YY | 16. DATES PATIENT UNABLE TO WORK IN CURRENT OCCUPATION FROM MM DD YY   TO MM DD YY |

| 17. NAME OF REFERRING PHYSICIAN OR OTHER SOURCE | 17a. | 18. HOSPITALIZATION DATES RELATED TO CURRENT SERVICES |
| | 17b. NPI | FROM MM DD YY   TO MM DD YY |

| 19. RESERVED FOR LOCAL USE | 20. OUTSIDE LAB? ☐YES ☒NO $ CHARGES |

21. DIAGNOSIS OR NATURE OF ILLNESS OR INJURY (Relate Items 1,2,3 or 4 to Item 24E by Line)

1. | 487 . 1   3. |_____
2. |_____   4. |_____

| 22. MEDICAID RESUBMISSION CODE   ORIGINAL REF. NO. |
| 23. PRIOR AUTHORIZATION NUMBER |

24. A. DATE(S) OF SERVICE				B. PLACE OF SERVICE	C. EMG	D. PROCEDURES, SERVICES, OR SUPPLIES (Explain Unusual Circumstances)		E. DIAGNOSIS POINTER	F. $ CHARGES	G. DAYS OR UNITS	H. EPSDT Family Plan	I. ID. QUAL.	J. RENDERING PROVIDER ID. #
From MM DD YY	To MM DD YY					CPT/HCPCS	MODIFIER						
1 XX XX XX	XX XX XX			11		99204		1	180 00	1		1G NPI	234665212 8888877777
2 XX XX XX	XX XX XX			11		87081		1	54 00	1		1G NPI	234665212 8888877777
3												NPI	
4												NPI	
5												NPI	
6												NPI	

| 25. FEDERAL TAX ID NUMBER SSN EIN 725727222 ☐ ☒ | 26. PATIENT'S ACCOUNT NO. BROSA | 27. ACCEPT ASSIGNMENT? (For govt. claims, see back) ☒YES ☐NO | 28. TOTAL CHARGE $ 234 00 | 29. AMOUNT PAID $ | 30. BALANCE DUE $ |

| 31. SIGNATURE OF PHYSICIAN OR SUPPLIER INCLUDING DEGREES OR CREDENTIALS (I certify that the statements on the reverse apply to this bill and are made a part thereof) SIGNED SIGNATURE ON FILE DATE | 32. SERVICE FACILITY LOCATION INFORMATION MALLARD & ASSOCIATES PA 19333 FORREST HAVEN DALLAS TX 12345 a. 7777788888   b. 1GM23548711 | 33. BILLING PROVIDER INFO & PH. # (215) 555 5040 MALLARD & ASSOCIATES PA 19333 FORREST HAVEN DALLAS TX 12345 a. 7777788888   b. 1GM23548711 |

PHYSICIAN OR SUPPLIER INFORMATION

Practice Exercise 15.4

(1500)

HEALTH INSURANCE CLAIM FORM

APPROVED BY NATIONAL UNIFORM CLAIM COMMITTEE 08/05

PICA

| | | | | | | | | PICA |

1. MEDICARE [ ] (Medicare #) **MEDICAID** [ ] (Medicaid #) **TRICARE CHAMPUS** [ ] (Sponsor's SSN) **CHAMPVA** [ ] (Member ID#) **GROUP HEALTH PLAN** [X] (SSN or ID) **FECA BLK LUNG** [ ] (SSN) **OTHER** [ ] (ID)

1a. INSURED'S I.D. NUMBER (For Program in Item 1)
625148544

2. PATIENT'S NAME (Last Name, First Name, Middle Initial)
OCONNOR ELIZABETH

3. PATIENT'S BIRTH DATE MM 04 DD 08 YY 1982   **SEX** M [ ] F [X]

4. INSURED'S NAME (Last Name, First Name, Middle Initial)
SAME

5. PATIENT'S ADDRESS (No, Street)
1900 LEMON LANE

6. PATIENT RELATIONSHIP TO INSURED
Self [X] Spouse [ ] Child [ ] Other [ ]

7. INSURED'S ADDRESS (No, Street)

CITY
DALLAS   **STATE** TX

8. PATIENT STATUS
Single [X] Married [ ] Other [ ]
Employed [X] Full-Time Student [ ] Part-Time Student [ ]

CITY   **STATE**

ZIP CODE 12345   **TELEPHONE (Include Area Code)** (214) 5551589

ZIP CODE   **TELEPHONE (Include Area Code)** ( )

9. OTHER INSURED'S NAME (Last Name, First Name, Middle Initial)

10. IS PATIENT'S CONDITION RELATED TO:

11. INSURED'S POLICY GROUP OR FECA NUMBER
11158

a. OTHER INSURED'S POLICY OR GROUP NUMBER

a. EMPLOYMENT? (Current or Previous) [ ] YES [X] NO

a. INSURED'S DATE OF BIRTH MM DD YY   **SEX** M [ ] F [ ]

b. OTHER INSURED'S DATE OF BIRTH MM DD YY   **SEX** M [ ] F [ ]

b. AUTO ACCIDENT? PLACE (State) [ ] YES [X] NO

b. EMPLOYER'S NAME OR SCHOOL NAME
CVS PHARMACY

c. EMPLOYER'S NAME OR SCHOOL NAME

c. OTHER ACCIDENT? [ ] YES [X] NO

c. INSURANCE PLAN NAME OR PROGRAM NAME
UNITED HEALTH CARE

d. INSURANCE PLAN NAME OR PROGRAM NAME

10d. RESERVED FOR LOCAL USE

d. IS THERE ANOTHER HEALTH BENEFIT PLAN? [ ] YES [X] NO   *If yes, return to and complete item 9 a-d*

READ BACK OF FORM BEFORE COMPLETING & SIGNING THIS FORM.
12. PATIENT'S OR AUTHORIZED PERSON'S SIGNATURE I authorize the release of any medical or other information necessary to process this claim. I also request payment of government benefits either to myself or to the party who accepts assignment below.

SIGNED SIGNATURE ON FILE   DATE XX XX XXXX

13. INSURED'S OR AUTHORIZED PERSON'S SIGNATURE I authorize payment of medical benefits to the undersigned physician or supplier for services described below.

SIGNED SIGNATURE ON FILE

14. DATE OF CURRENT MM XX DD XX YY XX   ILLNESS (First symptom) OR INJURY (Accident) OR PREGNANCY (LMP)

15. IF PATIENT HAS HAD SAME OR SIMILAR ILLNESS, GIVE FIRST DATE MM DD YY

16. DATES PATIENT UNABLE TO WORK IN CURRENT OCCUPATION FROM MM DD YY TO MM DD YY

17. NAME OF REFERRING PHYSICIAN OR OTHER SOURCE
17a.
17b. NPI

18. HOSPITALIZATION DATES RELATED TO CURRENT SERVICES FROM MM DD YY TO MM DD YY

19. RESERVED FOR LOCAL USE

20. OUTSIDE LAB? [ ] YES [X] NO $ CHARGES

21. DIAGNOSIS OR NATURE OF ILLNESS OR INJURY (Relate Items 1,2,3 or 4 to Item 24E by Line)
1. 737 . 30
2. |___
3. |___
4. |___

22. MEDICAID RESUBMISSION CODE   ORIGINAL REF. NO.

23. PRIOR AUTHORIZATION NUMBER

24. A. DATE(S) OF SERVICE From MM DD YY To MM DD YY	B. PLACE OF SERVICE	C. EMG	D. PROCEDURES, SERVICES, OR SUPPLIES (Explain Unusual Circumstances) CPT/HCPCS MODIFIER	E. DIAGNOSIS POINTER	F. $ CHARGES	G. DAYS OR UNITS	H. EPSDT Family Plan	I. ID. QUAL.	J. RENDERING PROVIDER ID. #
1 XX XX XX XX XX XX	11		99214	1	65 00	1		1G NPI	234665212 8888877777
2 XX XX XX XX XX XX	11		97260	1	30 00	1		1G NPI	234665212 8888877777
3								NPI	
4								NPI	
5								NPI	
6								NPI	

25. FEDERAL TAX ID NUMBER SSN EIN
725727222 [ ] [X]

26. PATIENT'S ACCOUNT NO.
OCOEL

27. ACCEPT ASSIGNMENT? (For govt. claims, see back) [X] YES [ ] NO

28. TOTAL CHARGE $ 95 00

29. AMOUNT PAID $

30. BALANCE DUE $

31. SIGNATURE OF PHYSICIAN OR SUPPLIER INCLUDING DEGREES OR CREDENTIALS (I certify that the statements on the reverse apply to this bill and are made a part thereof)

SIGNED SIGNATURE ON FILE   DATE XXXXXX

32. SERVICE FACILITY LOCATION INFORMATION
MALLARD & ASSOCIATES PA
19333 FORREST HAVEN
DALLAS TX 12345
a. 7777788888   b. 1GM23548711

33. BILLING PROVIDER INFO & PH. # (215) 5555040
MALLARD & ASSOCIATES PA
19333 FORREST HAVEN
DALLAS TX 12345
a. 7777788888   b. 1GM23548711

NUCC Instruction Manual available at: www.nucc.org
WCMS-1500CS

APPROVED OMB 0938-0999 FORM CMS-1500 (08/05)

Practice Exercise 15.5

(1500)

HEALTH INSURANCE CLAIM FORM

APPROVED BY NATIONAL UNIFORM CLAIM COMMITTEE 08/05

☐☐☐PICA   PICA☐☐☐

1. MEDICARE ☐ (Medicare #) **MEDICAID** ☐ (Medicaid #) **TRICARE CHAMPUS** ☐ (Sponsor's SSN) **CHAMPVA** ☐ (Member ID#) **GROUP HEALTH PLAN** ☒ (SSN or ID) **FECA BLK LUNG** ☐ (SSN) **OTHER** ☐ (ID)

1a. INSURED'S I.D. NUMBER (For Program in Item 1)
514258522

2. PATIENT'S NAME (Last Name, First Name, Middle Initial)
BLAKE NORBERT

3. PATIENT'S BIRTH DATE MM 05 DD 07 YY 1984   **SEX** M☒ F☐

4. INSURED'S NAME (Last Name, First Name, Middle Initial)
SAME

5. PATIENT'S ADDRESS (No, Street)
1721 ELM STREET

6. PATIENT RELATIONSHIP TO INSURED
Self ☒ Spouse ☐ Child ☐ Other ☐

7. INSURED'S ADDRESS (No, Street)

CITY RICHARDSON   **STATE** TX

8. PATIENT STATUS
Single ☒ Married ☐ Other ☐
Employed ☒ Full-Time Student ☐ Part-Time Student ☐

CITY   **STATE**

ZIP CODE 12345   **TELEPHONE** (Include Area Code) (912) 4148544

ZIP CODE   **TELEPHONE** (Include Area Code) ( )

9. OTHER INSURED'S NAME (Last Name, First Name, Middle Initial)

10. IS PATIENT'S CONDITION RELATED TO:

11. INSURED'S POLICY GROUP OR FECA NUMBER
58999

a. OTHER INSURED'S POLICY OR GROUP NUMBER

a. EMPLOYMENT? (Current or Previous) ☐YES ☒NO

a. INSURED'S DATE OF BIRTH MM DD YY   **SEX** M☐ F☐

b. OTHER INSURED'S DATE OF BIRTH MM DD YY   **SEX** M☐ F☐

b. AUTO ACCIDENT?   PLACE (State) ☐YES ☒NO

b. EMPLOYER'S NAME OR SCHOOL NAME
LIZIS CHICKEN

c. EMPLOYER'S NAME OR SCHOOL NAME

c. OTHER ACCIDENT? ☐YES ☒NO

c. INSURANCE PLAN NAME OR PROGRAM NAME
CIGNA HEALTH CARE

d. INSURANCE PLAN NAME OR PROGRAM NAME

10d. RESERVED FOR LOCAL USE

d. IS THERE ANOTHER HEALTH BENEFIT PLAN?
☐YES ☒NO   *If yes*, return to and complete item 9 a-d

READ BACK OF FORM BEFORE COMPLETING & SIGNING THIS FORM.
12. PATIENT'S OR AUTHORIZED PERSON'S SIGNATURE I authorize the release of any medical or other information necessary to process this claim. I also request payment of government benefits either to myself or to the party who accepts assignment below.

SIGNED   SIGNATURE ON FILE   DATE   XX XX XXXX

13. INSURED'S OR AUTHORIZED PERSON'S SIGNATURE I authorize payment of medical benefits to the undersigned physician or supplier for services described below.

SIGNED   SIGNATURE ON FILE

14. DATE OF CURRENT MM XX DD XX YY XXXX **ILLNESS** (First symptom) OR **INJURY** (Accident) OR **PREGNANCY** (LMP)

15. IF PATIENT HAS HAD SAME OR SIMILAR ILLNESS, GIVE FIRST DATE MM DD YY

16. DATES PATIENT UNABLE TO WORK IN CURRENT OCCUPATION FROM MM DD YY TO MM DD YY

17. NAME OF REFERRING PHYSICIAN OR OTHER SOURCE
17a.
17b. NPI

18. HOSPITALIZATION DATES RELATED TO CURRENT SERVICES FROM MM DD YY TO MM DD YY

19. RESERVED FOR LOCAL USE

20. OUTSIDE LAB? ☐YES ☒NO $ CHARGES

21. DIAGNOSIS OR NATURE OF ILLNESS OR INJURY (Relate Items 1,2,3 or 4 to Item 24E by Line)
1. 959 . 4
2.
3.
4.

22. MEDICAID RESUBMISSION CODE   ORIGINAL REF. NO.

23. PRIOR AUTHORIZATION NUMBER

24. A. DATE(S) OF SERVICE						B. PLACE OF SERVICE	C. EMG	D. PROCEDURES, SERVICES, OR SUPPLIES (Explain Unusual Circumstances)		E. DIAGNOSIS POINTER	F. $ CHARGES	G. DAYS OR UNITS	H. EPSDT Family Plan	I. ID. QUAL.	J. RENDERING PROVIDER ID. #
From MM	DD	YY	To MM	DD	YY			CPT/HCPCS	MODIFIER						
1 XX	XX	XX	XX	XX	XX	11		99213		1	60 00	1		1G NPI	234665212 8888877777
2 XX	XX	XX	XX	XX	XX	11		73130		1	45 00	1		1G NPI	234665212 8888877777
3														NPI	
4														NPI	
5														NPI	
6														NPI	

25. FEDERAL TAX ID NUMBER   SSN EIN
725727222   ☐ ☒

26. PATIENT'S ACCOUNT NO.
BLANO

27. ACCEPT ASSIGNMENT? (For govt. claims, see back) ☒YES ☐NO

28. TOTAL CHARGE $ 105 00

29. AMOUNT PAID $

30. BALANCE DUE $

31. SIGNATURE OF PHYSICIAN OR SUPPLIER INCLUDING DEGREES OR CREDENTIALS (I certify that the statements on the reverse apply to this bill and are made a part thereof)

SIGNED   SIGNATURE ON FILE   DATE XXXXXX

32. SERVICE FACILITY LOCATION INFORMATION
MALLARD & ASSOCIATES PA
19333 FORREST HAVEN
DALLAS TX 12345

a. 7777788888   b. 1GM 23548711

33. BILLING PROVIDER INFO & PH. # (215) 5555040
MALLARD & ASSOCIATES PA
19333 FORREST HAVEN
DALLAS TX 12345

a. 7777788888   b. 1GM23548711

NUCC Instruction Manual available at: www.nucc.org
WCMS-1500CS

APPROVED OMB 0938-0999 FORM CMS-1500 (08/05)

Left margin: SECOND FOLD   FIRST FOLD   WHCF-10-ENV / WHCF-10-ENV-SS

Right margin: CARRIER   PATIENT AND INSURED INFORMATION   PHYSICIAN OR SUPPLIER INFORMATION

Practice Exercise 15.6

```
(1500)
```

HEALTH INSURANCE CLAIM FORM
APPROVED BY NATIONAL UNIFORM CLAIM COMMITTEE 08/05

	PICA						PICA	

1. MEDICARE   MEDICAID   TRICARE CHAMPUS   CHAMPVA   GROUP HEALTH PLAN   FECA BLK LUNG   OTHER

☐ (Medicare #) ☐ (Medicaid #) ☐ (Sponsor's SSN) ☐ (Member ID#) ☒ (SSN or ID) ☐ (SSN) ☐ (ID)

1a. INSURED'S I.D. NUMBER (For Program in Item 1)
411658744

2. PATIENT'S NAME (Last Name, First Name, Middle Initial)
SESSIONS ROBERT

3. PATIENT'S BIRTH DATE   SEX
MM 02 DD 04 YY 1975   M ☒   F ☐

4. INSURED'S NAME (Last Name, First Name, Middle Initial)
SAME

5. PATIENT'S ADDRESS (No, Street)
1221 HIGH COUNTRY

6. PATIENT RELATIONSHIP TO INSURED
Self ☒   Spouse ☐   Child ☐   Other ☐

7. INSURED'S ADDRESS (No, Street)

CITY CARROLLTON   **STATE** TX

8. PATIENT STATUS
Single ☒   Married ☐   Other ☐
Employed ☒   Full-Time Student ☐   Part-Time Student ☐

CITY   **STATE**

ZIP CODE 12345   **TELEPHONE (Include Area Code)** (972) 9398244

ZIP CODE   **TELEPHONE (Include Area Code)** ( )

9. OTHER INSURED'S NAME (Last Name, First Name, Middle Initial)

10. IS PATIENT'S CONDITION RELATED TO:

11. INSURED'S POLICY GROUP OR FECA NUMBER
15555

a. OTHER INSURED'S POLICY OR GROUP NUMBER

a. EMPLOYMENT? (Current or Previous)
☐ YES   ☒ NO

a. INSURED'S DATE OF BIRTH   SEX
MM DD YY   M ☐   F ☐

b. OTHER INSURED'S DATE OF BIRTH   SEX
MM DD YY   M ☐   F ☐

b. AUTO ACCIDENT?   PLACE (State)
☐ YES   ☒ NO

b. EMPLOYER'S NAME OR SCHOOL NAME
TONY'S TIRE SHOP

c. EMPLOYER'S NAME OR SCHOOL NAME

c. OTHER ACCIDENT?
☐ YES   ☒ NO

c. INSURANCE PLAN NAME OR PROGRAM NAME
ALL HEALTH CARE

d. INSURANCE PLAN NAME OR PROGRAM NAME

10d. RESERVED FOR LOCAL USE

d. IS THERE ANOTHER HEALTH BENEFIT PLAN?
☐ YES   ☒ NO   If yes, return to and complete item 9 a-d

READ BACK OF FORM BEFORE COMPLETING & SIGNING THIS FORM.

12. PATIENT'S OR AUTHORIZED PERSON'S SIGNATURE I authorize the release of any medical or other information necessary to process this claim. I also request payment of government benefits either to myself or to the party who accepts assignment below.

SIGNED   SIGNATURE ON FILE   DATE   XX XX XXXX

13. INSURED'S OR AUTHORIZED PERSON'S SIGNATURE I authorize payment of medical benefits to the undersigned physician or supplier for services described below.

SIGNED   SIGNATURE ON FILE

14. DATE OF CURRENT   ILLNESS (First symptom) OR INJURY (Accident) OR PREGNANCY (LMP)
MM XX DD XX YY XXXX

15. IF PATIENT HAS HAD SAME OR SIMILAR ILLNESS, GIVE FIRST DATE   MM DD YY

16. DATES PATIENT UNABLE TO WORK IN CURRENT OCCUPATION
FROM MM DD YY   TO MM DD YY

17. NAME OF REFERRING PHYSICIAN OR OTHER SOURCE

17a.
17b. NPI

18. HOSPITALIZATION DATES RELATED TO CURRENT SERVICES
FROM MM DD YY   TO MM DD YY

19. RESERVED FOR LOCAL USE

20. OUTSIDE LAB? $ CHARGES
☐ YES   ☒ NO

21. DIAGNOSIS OR NATURE OF ILLNESS OR INJURY (Relate Items 1,2,3 or 4 to Item 24E by Line)
1. 465 . 9
2.
3.
4.

22. MEDICAID RESUBMISSION
CODE   ORIGINAL REF. NO.

23. PRIOR AUTHORIZATION NUMBER

24. A. DATE(S) OF SERVICE						B. PLACE OF SERVICE	C. EMG	D. PROCEDURES, SERVICES, OR SUPPLIES (Explain Unusual Circumstances) CPT/HCPCS	MODIFIER	E. DIAGNOSIS POINTER	F. $ CHARGES		G. DAYS OR UNITS	H. EPSDT Family Plan	I. ID. QUAL.	J. RENDERING PROVIDER ID. #
From MM	DD	YY	To MM	DD	YY											
XX	XX	XX	XX	XX	XX	11		99213		1	60	00	1		1G NPI	234665212 8888877777
XX	XX	XX	XX	XX	XX	11		71040		1	50	00	1		1G NPI	234665212 8888877777
XX	XX	XX	XX	XX	XX	11		81000		1	11	00	1		1G NPI	234665212 8888877777
															NPI	
															NPI	
															NPI	

25. FEDERAL TAX ID NUMBER   SSN EIN
725727222   ☐ ☒

26. PATIENT'S ACCOUNT NO.
SESRO   11

27. ACCEPT ASSIGNMENT? (For govt. claims, see back)
☒ YES   ☐ NO

28. TOTAL CHARGE
$ 121 00

29. AMOUNT PAID
$

30. BALANCE DUE
$

31. SIGNATURE OF PHYSICIAN OR SUPPLIER INCLUDING DEGREES OR CREDENTIALS (I certify that the statements on the reverse apply to this bill and are made a part thereof)

SIGNED   SIGNATURE ON FILE   DATE

32. SERVICE FACILITY LOCATION INFORMATION
MALLARD & ASSOCIATES PA
19333 FORREST HAVEN
DALLAS TX 12345

a. 7777788888   b. 1GM23548711

33. BILLING PROVIDER INFO & PH. # (215) 555-5040
MALLARD & ASSOCIATES PA
19333 FORREST HAVEN
DALLAS TX 12345

a. 7777788888   b. 1GM23548711

NUCC Instruction Manual available at: www.nucc.org
WCMS-1500CS

APPROVED OMB 0938-0999 FORM CMS-1500 (08/05)

Chapter 16: Workers' Compensation

Practice Exercise 16.1

1. Not WC covered
2. WC covered
3. Not WC covered
4. Not WC covered
5. WC covered
6. Not WC covered
7. WC covered
8. Not WC covered

Practice Exercise 16.2

	Workers' Compensation Fees					
CPT Code	Dallas County 2005		Dallas County 2006		Dallas County 2007	
	MFS	WC	MFS	WC	MFS	WC
95861	$121.38	$151.73	$120.86	$151.08	$117.97	$147.46
95900	$ 68.44	$ 85.55	$ 68.38	$ 85.48	$ 63.69	$ 79.61
95904	$ 58.53	$ 73.16	$ 58.48	$ 73.10	$ 54.97	$ 68.71
99201	$ 38.17	$ 47.71	$ 38.13	$ 47.66	$ 37.05	$ 46.31
99202	$ 67.52	$ 84.40	$ 67.46	$ 84.33	$ 64.45	$ 80.56
99203	$100.43	$125.54	$100.34	$125.43	$ 95.39	$119.24
99204	$141.81	$177.26	$141.67	$177.09	$144.39	$180.49

Practice Exercise 16.3

<table>
<tr><td colspan="3">1500</td></tr>
</table>

HEALTH INSURANCE CLAIM FORM
APPROVED BY NATIONAL UNIFORM CLAIM COMMITTEE 08/05

☐☐☐ PICA   PICA ☐☐☐

1. MEDICARE MEDICAID TRICARE CHAMPUS CHAMPVA GROUP HEALTH PLAN FECA BLK LUNG OTHER	1a. INSURED'S I.D. NUMBER (For Program in Item 1)
☐(Medicare #) ☐(Medicaid #) ☐(Sponsor's SSN) ☐(Member ID#) ☐(SSN or ID) ☐(SSN) ☒(ID)	968449876

2. PATIENT'S NAME (Last Name, First Name, Middle Initial) MOORE KENNEDY	3. PATIENT'S BIRTH DATE SEX MM 04 DD 25 YY 1944 M☐ F☒	4. INSURED'S NAME (Last Name, First Name, Middle Initial) DATA MATIC INC

5. PATIENT'S ADDRESS (No, Street) 346 AUSTIN BLVD	6. PATIENT RELATIONSHIP TO INSURED Self☐ Spouse☐ Child☐ Other☒	7. INSURED'S ADDRESS (No, Street) 644 SAN JUAN ST
CITY DALLAS STATE TX	8. PATIENT STATUS Single☐ Married☒ Other☐	CITY DALLAS STATE TX
ZIP CODE 12345 TELEPHONE (Include Area Code) (972) 5550087	Employed☒ Full-Time Student☐ Part-Time Student☐	ZIP CODE 12345 TELEPHONE (Include Area Code) (214) 5558674

9. OTHER INSURED'S NAME (Last Name, First Name, Middle Initial)	10. IS PATIENT'S CONDITION RELATED TO:	11. INSURED'S POLICY GROUP OR FECA NUMBER 0856
a. OTHER INSURED'S POLICY OR GROUP NUMBER	a. EMPLOYMENT? (Current or Previous) ☒YES ☐NO	a. INSURED'S DATE OF BIRTH SEX MM DD YY M☐ F☐
b. OTHER INSURED'S DATE OF BIRTH SEX MM DD YY M☐ F☐	b. AUTO ACCIDENT? PLACE (State) ☐YES ☒NO	b. EMPLOYER'S NAME OR SCHOOL NAME
c. EMPLOYER'S NAME OR SCHOOL NAME	c. OTHER ACCIDENT? ☐YES ☒NO	c. INSURANCE PLAN NAME OR PROGRAM NAME
d. INSURANCE PLAN NAME OR PROGRAM NAME	10d. RESERVED FOR LOCAL USE	d. IS THERE ANOTHER HEALTH BENEFIT PLAN? ☐YES ☒NO If yes, return to and complete item 9 a-d

READ BACK OF FORM BEFORE COMPLETING & SIGNING THIS FORM.

12. PATIENT'S OR AUTHORIZED PERSON'S SIGNATURE I authorize the release of any medical or other information necessary to process this claim. I also request payment of government benefits either to myself or to the party who accepts assignment below. SIGNED _____ DATE _____	13. INSURED'S OR AUTHORIZED PERSON'S SIGNATURE I authorize payment of medical benefits to the undersigned physician or supplier for services described below. SIGNED _____

14. DATE OF CURRENT MM XX DD XX YY XXXX ◄ ILLNESS (First symptom) OR INJURY (Accident) OR PREGNANCY (LMP)	15. IF PATIENT HAS HAD SAME OR SIMILAR ILLNESS, GIVE FIRST DATE MM DD YY	16. DATES PATIENT UNABLE TO WORK IN CURRENT OCCUPATION FROM MM DD YY TO MM DD YY
17. NAME OF REFERRING PHYSICIAN OR OTHER SOURCE	17a. 17b. NPI	18. HOSPITALIZATION DATES RELATED TO CURRENT SERVICES FROM MM DD YY TO MM DD YY
19. RESERVED FOR LOCAL USE		20. OUTSIDE LAB? $ CHARGES ☐YES ☒NO
21. DIAGNOSIS OR NATURE OF ILLNESS OR INJURY (Relate Items 1,2,3 or 4 to Item 24E by Line) 1. 354 . 0 3. ⌐___ 2. ⌐___ 4. ⌐___		22. MEDICAID RESUBMISSION CODE _____ ORIGINAL REF. NO. _____ 23. PRIOR AUTHORIZATION NUMBER

24. A. DATE(S) OF SERVICE					B. PLACE OF SERVICE	C. EMG	D. PROCEDURES, SERVICES, OR SUPPLIES (Explain Unusual Circumstances) CPT/HCPCS MODIFIER	E. DIAGNOSIS POINTER	F. $ CHARGES	G. DAYS OR UNITS	H. EPSDT Family Plan	I. ID. QUAL.	J. RENDERING PROVIDER ID. #
From MM	DD	YY	To MM	DD									
1	XX	XX	XX	XX	XX	XX	11	99203	1	119 24	1		NPI
2											1		NPI
3													NPI
4													NPI
5													NPI
6													NPI

25. FEDERAL TAX ID NUMBER SSN EIN 575562147 ☐☒	26. PATIENT'S ACCOUNT NO.	27. ACCEPT ASSIGNMENT? (For govt. claims, see back) ☒YES ☐NO	28. TOTAL CHARGE $ 119 24	29. AMOUNT PAID $	30. BALANCE DUE $
31. SIGNATURE OF PHYSICIAN OR SUPPLIER INCLUDING DEGREES OR CREDENTIALS (I certify that the statements on the reverse apply to this bill and are made a part thereof) SIGNED SIGNATURE ON FILE DATE	32. SERVICE FACILITY LOCATION INFORMATION DENNIS J BONNER MD 980 FREDERICK RD DALLAS TX 12345 a. 7536982100 b. 0BTX5529		33. BILLING PROVIDER INFO & PH. # (800) 5555000 DENNIS J BONNER MD 980 FREDERICK RD DALLAS TX 12345 a. 7536982100 b. 0BTX5529		

NUCC Instruction Manual available at: www.nucc.org
WCMS-1500CS

APPROVED OMB 0938-0999 FORM CMS-1500 (08/05)

Practice Exercise 16.4

(1500)

HEALTH INSURANCE CLAIM FORM

APPROVED BY NATIONAL UNIFORM CLAIM COMMITTEE 08/05

☐☐☐PICA   PICA☐☐

1. MEDICARE MEDICAID TRICARE CHAMPVA GROUP FECA OTHER	1a. INSURED'S I.D. NUMBER (For Program in Item 1)
CHAMPUS HEALTH PLAN BLK LUNG	968340025
☐(Medicare #) ☐(Medicaid #) ☐(Sponsor's SSN) ☐(Member ID#) ☐(SSN or ID) ☐(SSN) ☒(ID)	

2. PATIENT'S NAME (Last Name, First Name, Middle Initial)	3. PATIENT'S BIRTH DATE SEX	4. INSURED'S NAME (Last Name, First Name, Middle Initial)
DALEY CATHERINE	MM DD YY 04 25 1969 M☐ F☒	COCA COLA CORP

5. PATIENT'S ADDRESS (No, Street)	6. PATIENT RELATIONSHIP TO INSURED	7. INSURED'S ADDRESS (No, Street)
346 HIGHPOINT DRIVE	Self☐ Spouse☐ Child☐ Other☒	6345 HARVEY DRIVE

CITY STATE	8. PATIENT STATUS	CITY STATE
DALLAS TX	Single☐ Married☒ Other☐	DALLAS TX

ZIP CODE TELEPHONE (Include Area Code)	Full-Time Part-Time	ZIP CODE TELEPHONE (Include Area Code)
12345 (999) 5550756	Employed☒ Student☐ Student☐	12345 (998) 5556785

9. OTHER INSURED'S NAME (Last Name, First Name, Middle Initial)	10. IS PATIENT'S CONDITION RELATED TO:	11. INSURED'S POLICY GROUP OR FECA NUMBER
		81526

a. OTHER INSURED'S POLICY OR GROUP NUMBER	a. EMPLOYMENT? (Current or Previous) ☒YES ☐NO	a. INSURED'S DATE OF BIRTH SEX MM DD YY M☐ F☐

b. OTHER INSURED'S DATE OF BIRTH SEX MM DD YY M☐ F☐	b. AUTO ACCIDENT? PLACE (State) ☐YES ☒NO	b. EMPLOYER'S NAME OR SCHOOL NAME

c. EMPLOYER'S NAME OR SCHOOL NAME	c. OTHER ACCIDENT? ☐YES ☒NO	c. INSURANCE PLAN NAME OR PROGRAM NAME AETNA TX

d. INSURANCE PLAN NAME OR PROGRAM NAME	10d. RESERVED FOR LOCAL USE	d. IS THERE ANOTHER HEALTH BENEFIT PLAN? ☐YES ☒NO If yes, return to and complete item 9 a-d

READ BACK OF FORM BEFORE COMPLETING & SIGNING THIS FORM.

12. PATIENT'S OR AUTHORIZED PERSON'S SIGNATURE I authorize the release of any medical or other information necessary to process this claim. I also request payment of government benefits either to myself or to the party who accepts assignment below.	13. INSURED'S OR AUTHORIZED PERSON'S SIGNATURE I authorize payment of medical benefits to the undersigned physician or supplier for services described below.
SIGNED _____ DATE_____	SIGNED SIGNATURE ON FILE _____

14. DATE OF CURRENT ILLNESS (First symptom) OR MM DD YY INJURY (Accident) OR XX XX XXXX PREGNANCY (LMP)	15. IF PATIENT HAS HAD SAME OR SIMILAR ILLNESS, GIVE FIRST DATE MM DD YY	16. DATES PATIENT UNABLE TO WORK IN CURRENT OCCUPATION MM DD YY MM DD YY FROM TO

17. NAME OF REFERRING PHYSICIAN OR OTHER SOURCE	17a.	18. HOSPITALIZATION DATES RELATED TO CURRENT SERVICES MM DD YY MM DD YY FROM TO
	17b. NPI	

19. RESERVED FOR LOCAL USE	20. OUTSIDE LAB? $ CHARGES ☐YES ☒NO

21. DIAGNOSIS OR NATURE OF ILLNESS OR INJURY (Relate Items 1,2,3 or 4 to Item 24E by Line)	22. MEDICAID RESUBMISSION CODE ORIGINAL REF. NO.
1. 847 . 2 3.	23. PRIOR AUTHORIZATION NUMBER
2. 4.	

24. A. DATE(S) OF SERVICE		B. PLACE OF	C.	D. PROCEDURES, SERVICES, OR SUPPLIES		E. DIAGNOSIS	F.	G. DAYS OR	H. EPSDT Family	I. ID.	J. RENDERING
From	To	SERVICE	EMG	CPT/HCPCS	MODIFIER	POINTER	$ CHARGES	UNITS	Plan	QUAL.	PROVIDER ID. #
MM DD YY MM DD YY											
XX XX XX XX XX XX		11		99202		1	80 56	1		NPI	
XX XX XX XX XX XX		11		95861		1	147 46	1		NPI	
XX XX XX XX XX XX		11		95900		1	477 66	6		NPI	
XX XX XX XX XX XX		11		95904		1	206 13	3		NPI	
										NPI	
										NPI	

25. FEDERAL TAX ID NUMBER SSN EIN	26. PATIENT'S ACCOUNT NO.	27. ACCEPT ASSIGNMENT? (For govt. claims, see back) ☒YES ☐NO	28. TOTAL CHARGE $ 986 81	29. AMOUNT PAID $	30. BALANCE DUE $
229872767 ☐☒					

31. SIGNATURE OF PHYSICIAN OR SUPPLIER INCLUDING DEGREES OR CREDENTIALS (I certify that the statements on the reverse apply to this bill and are made a part thereof)	32. SERVICE FACILITY LOCATION INFORMATION CHARLES H. HESS MD 980 FREDERICK ROAD DALLAS TX 12345	33. BILLING PROVIDER INFO & PH. # (899) 5552276 CHARLES H. HESS MD 980 FREDERICK ROAD DALLAS TX 12345
SIGNED SIGNATURE ON FILE DATE	a. 1471236545 b. 0BTX2056	a. 1471236545 b. 0BTX2056

NUCC Instruction Manual available at: www.nucc.org   APPROVED OMB 0938-0999 FORM CMS-1500 (08/05)

WCMS-1500CS

Books and Manuals

American Medical Association, (2007). *CPT 2007 Professional Edition.* Chicago, IL: Author

Berry, M. J. (1999). *Collections made easy.* Los Angeles: PMIC.

Boyd, P. M., and Boyd, B. D. (1999). *Office procedures in managed health care.* Westerville, OH: Glencoe/McGraw-Hill.

Brown, J. L. (2006). *Medical insurance made easy.* St. Louis, MO: Saunders.

Brown, S. E. (1999). *Exercises for coding and reimbursement.* Los Angeles: Insurance Career Development Center.

Chabner, D. (2004). *The language of medicine.* St. Louis, MO: Saunders.

Davis, J. B. (2004). *Reimbursement manual for the medical office.* Los Angeles: PMIC.

Dennerll, J. T., and Davis, P. E. (2005). *Medical terminology—a programmed systems approach.* Clifton Park, NY: Thomson Delmar Learning.

Falen, T. J., and Libesman, A. (2005). *Learning to code with ICD-9-CM for health information management and health services administration.* Philadelphia, PA: Lippincott Williams & Wilkins.

Ingenix Publishing . (2007). *ICD-9-CM.* Salt Lake City, UT: Author.

Keene, R. D., and Naus, F. F. (1994). *Negotiating managed care contracts.* Los Angeles: PMIC.

Marshall, J. R. (2004). *Being a medical clerical worker.* Upper Saddle River, NJ: Pearson Prentice Hall.

Meyer, J. M., and Schiff, M. (2004). *HIPAA: The questions you didn't know to ask.* Upper Saddle River, NJ: Pearson Prentice Hall.

Moini, J. (2005). *Medical assisting review.* New York

National Health Insurance Company. (2006). *Texas Medicaid provider procedures manual.* Austin, TX: Author.

Sanderson, S. (2005). *Capstone billing simulation.* New York: McGraw-Hill.

Internet-Based Newsletters and Articles

Fierce Health IT, www.fiercehealthit.com

Kelly Montgomery, About Health Insurance, http://healthinsurance.about.com

MDLinx Communication Network, www.mdlinx.com

Quality Management Consulting Group, Ltd., www.qmcg.com/Publications/Newsletters

abuse: Improper billing practices that result in financial benefit to the provider but are not fraudulent.

addenda: An addition made to a book or publication normally at the end to document a change or revision.

add-on code: A CPT code with a + symbol in front of it, used to specify a procedure in addition to the primary procedure. An add-on code cannot be used alone.

adjudication: The insurance carrier's process of evaluating a claim for payment, which includes investigating the details of the claim to determine which items should be paid and how much should be paid on each.

adjustment: A positive or negative change to a patient's account balance. This is done to make changes, corrections, or discount write-offs.

administrative law judge (ALJ) hearing: The third level of appeal for physician claims with Medicare. Physicians have 60 days to file an appeal. Medicare must make a decision within 90 days.

Admission of Liability: Acknowledgment to an employee that the worker's compensation claim has been accepted or approved.

admitting clerk: Clerk who enters patient's demographical information into a computer and obtains signed statement(s) from patients to protect hospitals' interests. Responsibilities of the admitting clerk may also include general filing of patient charts.

admitting physician: The doctor responsible for admitting a patient to a hospital or other inpatient health facility.

advanced beneficiary notice (ABN): A written notification that must be signed by the patient or guardian prior to the provider rendering a service to a Medicare beneficiary that could be potentially denied or deemed "not medically necessary."

adverse affect: An undesired condition that results from use of a medication or drug given in the correct dosage.

advisory opinion: An opinion issued by legal counsel that advises a healthcare professional on the legal rights of the facility.

Aid to Families with Dependent Children (AFDC): A cash assistance program of Medicaid that was repealed in 1996 with the implementation of Temporary Assistance to Needy Families (TANF) that limited the amount and duration of cash assistance.

allowed amount: Maximum amount an insurance payer considers reasonable for medical services. Participating providers agree by contract to accept the allowed amount for services they provide. The allowed amount is often paid in part by the insurance company and in part by the patient's co-insurance or co-payment.

Ambulatory Payment Classification (APC) system: Prospective payment system patterned after that of ambulatory patient groups. APCs are used for outpatient services, certain Medicare Part B services, and partial hospitalization. This payment method is based on procedures rather than diagnosis.

ambulatory surgical center (ASC): Facility designed for patients receiving minor surgical procedures who are expected to be discharged the same day.

ambulatory surgical unit (ASU): Facility within a hospital designed for patients receiving minor surgical procedures who are expected to be discharged the same day.

American Medical Association (AMA): Professional society that assists patients and physicians by creating a sense of unity in the medical industry. It implemented the first of standard terms and descriptors to document procedures in the medical record.

appeal: The process used by a provider to ask an insurance carrier to reconsider a denied claim. The provider bases an appeal on documentation that backs up the medical necessity of the medical treatment.

assignment of benefits: Request made by a patient to allow the insurance carrier to pay the healthcare professional directly rather than issuing monies to the patient.

assumption coding: Billing for reasonable undocumented services presumably preformed by the healthcare professional as part of the documented procedure.

attending physician: Physician primarily responsible for the medical care of a patient; supervises medical students and residents.

audit: A formal examination of patients' medical records and accounts.

audit/edit report: Feedback from the insurance company documenting the progress of individual claims that have been submitted. This report documents changes to be made or additional information to be submitted on a claim.

balance billing: BIlling patients for the dollar amount left over after the insurance carrier has paid. If the provider has a contract with the third party payer, balance billing may be prohibited.

batch out: The process used by a medical office specialist to calculate all monies received, tally all cash on hand, and compare the totals with the Patient Day Sheet report.

beneficiary: A person eligible to receive benefits under an insurance policy.

benefit period: A period of time during which medical benefits are available to an insurance beneficiary.

billing services: A third-party agency outside of the hospital or physician's practice that is responsible for submitting claims for the hospital or physician's practice.

birthday rule: Determines which insurance is primary when two policies are valid for a child. The plan of the parent whose birthday month comes first in the calendar year is usually primary.

bundled code: A group of related procedures covered by a single code.

burial benefits: Benefits paid to the person who pays a deceased worker's funeral expenses.

capitation plan: Contract that a provider signs with a carrier agreeing to treat a certain number of members in the carrier's plan. The carrier then pays the provider based on a designated fee each month for each member in that plan.

carrier: The responsible party issuing an insurance policy.

catastrophic cap: Limits the amount of out-of-pocket expenses a family will have to pay for TRICARE-covered medical services.

categorically needy: The Medicaid eligibility group that includes cash recipients of Aid to Families with Dependent Children (AFDC), now known as Temporary Assistance to Needy Families (TANF), most cash recipients of Social Security Income (SSI), and certain other groups of low income, aged, and disabled persons.

Centers for Medicare and Medicaid Services (CMS): The department of the federal government responsible for administering Medicare and Medicaid. Formerly the Health Care Financing Administration (HCFA).

centralized billing office (CBO): Specializes in maintaining patient accounting records, filing health insurance claims, working with insurance carriers to receive reimbursement on insurance claims filed, and appealing denied claims.

certification: Training received in a particular field that acknowledges a medical office specialist's expertise.

CHAMPVA: (The Civilian Health and Medical Program of the Department of Veterans Affairs) Healthcare for veterans with 100% service-related disabilities and their families.

charge: Amount a practice charges for medical services rendered.

charge description master (CDM): A database that contains a detailed narrative of each procedure, service, dollar amount and revenue code that is used in inpatient facilities. This information is transferred to the patient bill or UB-04 after the patient is discharged.

charge-based fees: Fees providers routinely charge for medical procedures performed. Providers reference the nationwide fee database to determine if their fees will be at the high, low, or midpoint range to be competitive with other providers of their specialty.

chief complaint (CC): A concise statement describing the symptom, problem, condition, diagnosis, or other factor that is the reason for the patient encounter.

Civilian Health and Medical Program of the Uniformed Services (CHAMPUS): Comprehensive health benefit program designed by Congress for military personnel and their families. Now called TRICARE.

claim attachment: Additional documentation or information necessary when submitting a claim.

clean claim: A claim that has no data errors when submitted to an insurance carrier.

clearinghouse: A company that receives claims from multiple providers, evaluates them, and batches them for electronic submission to multiple insurance carriers.

Clinical Laboratory Improvement Amendment of 1988 (CLIA): An act passed by Congress establishing quality standards for all laboratory testing to ensure the accuracy, reliability, and timeliness of patient test results regardless of where the test was performed.

CMS-1500 claim form: Standard claim form used by physicians and other health care professionals to bill for services rendered.

code edits: Computer program function which screens for improperly or incorrectly reported procedure codes.

code linkage: The process of joining a diagnosis code and a procedure code for the purpose of justifying medical necessity.

coinsurance: Percentage of the allowed amount that is the patient's responsibility.

combination code: A single code that classifies more than one condition, such as both the etiology and the manifestation of an illness or injury.

commercial health insurance (CHI): Any type of health insurance not paid for by a government agency. The policy can be based on fee for service or managed care. Also know as private health insurance.

comorbidity: One or more diseases or disorders that presents in addition to the primary disease or disorder.

compliance officer: Individual responsible for reviewing office policies and procedures to ensure that all applicable HIPAA laws, rules, and regulations are being followed.

complication: The disease or condition that arises during the course of treatment or during a medical procedure.

Consolidated Omnibus Budget Reconciliation Act of 1985 (COBRA): Contains provisions giving former employees, retirees, spouses, and dependent children the right to temporary continuation of health coverage for 18 months after employment has ended. Group health coverage for COBRA participants is usually more expensive than health coverage for active employees, because the COBRA participant usually has to pay the part of the premium that was formerly paid by the employer.

consultation: Service by a physician whose opinion or advice regarding a patient's condition and or treatment is requested by another physician. The consulting physician must communicate the findings, results, and recommendations in a written report to the requesting physician.

conventions: Formatting used in coding books that is exclusive to each volume and publisher.

conversion factor: A dollar amount used to multiply relative value units (RVU) in order to arrive at the price for a service.

coordination of benefits (COB): When a patient has more than one insurance policy, insurance carriers work together to coordinate the insurance benefit so that the maximum payment does not exceed 100% of the charge.

copayment: A fixed dollar amount the patient pays at each office visit or hospital encounter, as specified in the patient's insurance policy.

cost outlier: Medical services rendered for extenuating circumstances that cannot be assigned to a Diagnosis Related Group (DRG). Reimbursement is based on the DRG rate, plus an additional payment for services rendered.

cost share: The amount of healthcare charges that are the responsibility of the sponsor or family member.

counseling: A method of providing advice and guidance to a patient by a healthcare professional. This could include physician discussion with a patient and/or family regarding the diagnosis, diagnostic testing results, prognosis, and treatment options.

crossover: Reassignment of gaps in coverage that eliminates the need for a beneficiary to file a separate claim with his or her Medigap insurer. It usually requires the beneficiary to sign release of information and assignment of benefit forms with their providers.

cross-reference: Reference to information found elsewhere; directs the reader where to search for additional information.

crosswalk: A reference aid that compares information in one system to information in another system. A crosswalk between the ICD-9 and ICD-10 will allow a coder to look up an ICD-9 code and see what the corresponding code is in the new ICD-10 system.

Current Procedural Terminology (CPT) code: A five-digit code used to describe what procedures were performed.

death benefits: Benefits that can replace a portion of lost family income for eligible family members of workers killed on the job.

deductible: Amount a beneficiary is responsible for before the insurance company pays as stated in the insurance policy.

Defense Enrollment Eligibility Reporting System (DEERS): A support office for TRICARE. Sponsors and family members can contact DEERS to check the status of enrollment or inquire about plan benefits.

descriptor: All Current Procedural Terminology codes are five digits followed by a descriptor, which is a brief description of the procedure.

designated doctor: 1. Treating physician chosen by the employer for initial treatment of injured employees. 2. An independent physician who has not seen the patient chosen by the Workers' Compensation Insurance Board to examine the patient for an independent medical review.

diagnosis: The process of determining by examination the nature and circumstances of a diseased condition.

Diagnosis Related Group (DRG): A patient classification method that categorizes patients, for reimbursement purposes, who are medically related with respect to diagnosis and treatment and who are statistically similar in terms of their length of hospital stay.

diagnostic statement: The main reason for the patient encounter along with the descriptions of additional conditions or symptoms that have been treated or related to the patient's current illness.

dirty claim: A claim that is incorrect or is missing information when submitted.

disability compensation programs: Programs that reimburse a covered individual for lost wages that occur due to a disability that prevents the individual from working.

District of Columbia Workers' Compensation Act: Provides benefits for any employee performing work on a regular basis in the District of Columbia.

documentation: A consistent, medical record format, often in chronological order, that records facts and observations regarding a patient's health status.

downcode: Occurs when the procedure code billed is for a procedure that is less involved than the procedure actually documented in the chart. Carriers will downcode or deny payment when the documentation fails to justify the level of service billed.

durable medical equipment (DME): Any medical device, equipment, or instrument used in the care of a patient.

durable medical equipment number (DMEN): A number assigned to a medical device or piece of equipment or instrument for billing purposes.

early and periodic screening, diagnosis, and treatment (EPSDT): Medicaid's comprehensive and preventive child health program for individuals under the age of 21; includes periodic screening, vision, dental, and hearing services.

Electronic Remittance Advice (ERA): An electronic notification sent to the provider who accepts assignment. The ERA lists the dates of service, type of service, and charges filed on the claim.

electronic media claim (EMC): An insurance claim submitted to the carrier in a flat file format via electronic means, such as tape, diskette, direct wire, direct data entry, or telephone lines.

emergency care: Medical care necessary to sustain life and limbs.

Employee Retirement Income Security Act (ERISA) of 1974: Act that set standards for administering health insurance plans. It protects the interests of beneficiaries who depend on benefits from private employee benefit plans.

employer identification number (EIN): A number issued by the Internal Revenue Service to any medical facility, provider, or business for tax purposes.

Employer's First Report of Injury or Illness: Form filled out by the employer and sent to the insurance company in workers' compensation cases. A case number will not be assigned to workers' compensation injury or illness until this form has been filled out and received by the insurance carrier.

end-stage renal disease (ESRD): Total or nearly complete failure of the kidneys.

Energy Employees Occupational Illness Compensation Program Act (EEOICP): Act that provides benefits to eligible and former employees of the U.S. Department of Energy, its contractors and subcontractors, and certain survivors of such individuals.

enrollee: An individual who takes out an insurance policy in his or her name.

eponym: A procedure or diagnosis name derived from the name of a person.

established patient: One who has received professional services from a physician or another physician of the same specialty who belongs to the same group practice within the past three years.

etiology: The cause or origin of a disease.

evaluation and management (E&M) codes: CPT code numbers 99201 to 99499. These codes are used to report encounters in which the physician evaluates the patient's problem or complaint, considers treatment options, and recommends a plan of treatment. The most common E&M visits are "office visits" and "hospital visits." Codes are categorized by place of service and subdivided based on the complexity of the problem and treatment options. Three to five levels of codes are available for reporting purposes. The number of levels in a category varies and is dependent on the types of services that might be provided.

examination: An evaluation performed by a physician who is involved in a patient's care for the purpose of establishing a medical diagnosis and treatment.

excluded services: Services not covered by an insurance payer as stated in the insurance policy.

Explanation of Benefits (EOB): Hardcopy notification sent by an insurance carrier to a patient and provider (if provider accepts assignment) indicating the disposition of a claim. It shows the dates of service, type of service, and charges filed on the claim, as well as what was paid and the reason(s) for any denials.

external audit: An investigation performed by an external party to review patient documentation and records.

facility provider number (FPN): Number issued to a facility and used by a physician to report services provided at a particular location.

Federal Coal Mine Health and Safety Act (Black Lung Benefits Reform Act): Act that provides benefits to current coal mine employees as well as monthly payments to surviving dependents of deceased workers.

Federal Employees' Compensation Act (FECA): Provides benefits to millions of civilian employees of the United States, members of the Peace Corp, and Vista volunteers.

Federal Medical Assistance Percentages (FMAP) program: Specifies the formula for calculating federal medical assistance percentages. This program is available to certain children who qualify for medical assistance.

final report: Report filed by the treating physician in a state's workers' compensation case when the patient is released from medical care and is fit to return to work.

form locators: The boxes located on the UB-04 and CMS-1500 claim forms. Each form locator is assigned a number and requires designated information to be entered into that field.

fragmented billing: Occurs when procedures are reported separately that should have been included under a bundled code.

fraud: An intentional deception or misrepresentation that an individual knows, or should know, to be false, or does not believe to be true, and makes, knowing the deception could result in some unauthorized benefit to himself or some other person(s).

fraud indicators: In regards to worker's compensation, unusual events or circumstances that sometimes mean an employer, employee, or attorney is attempting to falsify facts for financial gain.

Geographic Practice Cost Index (GPCI): An adjustment that accounts for geographic variations in the costs of practicing medicine in different areas of the country. This adjustment factor is applied to each component (work, practice expense, and malpractice) used in calculating a physician payment.

global period: The number of days surrounding a surgical procedure during which all services relating to the procedure—preoperative, during the surgery, and postoperative—are considered part of the surgical package.

global surgical concept: A surgical package that includes specific services in addition to the operation.

group insurance: An insurance policy offered to groups of employees and often their dependents covered under a single policy and issued by an employer or other group.

group provider number (GPN): A number assigned to a group for billing purposes.

grouper: A computer software program that abstracts data from a medical record and assigns the DRG payment group.

guarantor: The person who is ultimately responsible for paying for the healthcare services rendered.

Health Insurance Portability and Accountability Act (HIPAA): Act that required the Department of Health and Human Services to establish national standards for electronic healthcare transactions and national identifiers for providers, health plans, and employers. It also addressed the security and privacy of health data.

health maintenance organization (HMO): A medical center or a designated group of medical professionals that provide medical services to subscribers for a fixed monthly or annual rate of pay.

Health Care Common Procedure Coding System (HCPCS): Standard code set for reporting professional services, procedures, and supplies.

history: Information gained by a healthcare professional by asking the patient specific questions with the aim of obtaining information useful in formulating a diagnosis and providing medical care to the patient.

history of present illness (HPI): A chronological description of the development of the patient's present illness from the first sign or symptom to the present.

hospice: Pallative care for a person who is dying that is given at home, in day care, or in a hospice facility. Services may include pain control, symptom relief, skilled nursing care, and counseling but not active treatment of the terminal condition.

ICD-9-CM: Abbreviation for International Classification of Diseases, Ninth Revision, Clinical Modification. A coding system used to code signs, symptoms, injuries, diseases, and conditions.

impairment: With regard to workers' compensation claims, permanent physical damage to a worker's body from a work-related injury or illness.

impairment income benefits: Benefits paid to an injured worker if the injured worker is found to have permanent impairment from a work-related injury or illness

impairment rating: With regard to workers' compensation claims, describes the degree, in percentages, of permanent damage done to a worker's body as a whole.

income benefits: With regard to workers' compensation claims, benefits that replace a portion of any wages a worker loses because of a work-related injury or illness.

independent review organization (IRO): A company that provides a third party assessment of a treatment plan and patient's status when the insurance carrier has denied treatment or considers the services medically unnecessary or inappropriate. The injured worker must request an appeal process before an IRO is called in.

inpatient: A patient who has been admitted to the hospital and is expected to stay 24 hours or more.

inpatient care: Care provided to a patient whose hospital stay is expected to be for 24 hours or more; usually requires approval by a patient's insurance carrier to prove medical necessity.

insurance commissioner: An elected official in each state charged with consumer protection and regulation of the state's insurance industry.

insurance verification representative: Coordinates all financial aspects of patient visits and admissions, including insurance verification, precertification information, follow-up of third-party payment denials, and financial counseling.

insured: An individual listed as the policyholder under an insurance agreement.

intermediaries: A private company that has a contract with Medicare to pay Part A and some Part B bills.

internal audit: An review of claims that is performed by a facility to protect against submitting dirty claims.

late effect: A condition that remains after a patient's acute illness or injury.

Level I (HCPCS coding level): CPT codes published by the American Medical Association that are made up of five numeric digits. These codes are used to report services and procedures when billing insurance carriers.

Level II (HCPCS coding level): Alphanumeric codes published by CMS that consist of one letter followed by four numbers. These codes are used to report certain medical services not included in the CPT manual, services by non-physician providers and ambulances, and durable medical equipment and supplies when billing insurance carriers.

Level III (HCPCS coding level): Local codes used to electronically process claims for services where a Level I or Level II code has not yet been established. These codes were originally developed by Medicaid and Medicare state contractors and were discontinued in 2004.

lifetime income benefits: Benefits that an injured worker becomes eligible for from the date of disability if the injury is the loss of both feet at or above the ankle; the loss of both hands at or above the wrist; or the loss of one foot at or above the ankle; the loss of one hand at or above the wrist; and other injuries of permanent damage.

lifetime maximum: As stated in the insurance policy, the maximum amount of money a plan will pay toward healthcare services over the lifetime of the insured. Once this amount has been met, no more benefits will be paid.

limiting charge (LC): The maximum amount a non-participating physician can charge a Medicare patient on a non-assigned claim. The limiting charge is 115% of the nonparticipating Medicare fee.

Local Coverage Determination (LCD): A decision by a Medicare fiscal intermediary or carrier on whether to cover a particular service on an intermediary-wide or carrier-wide basis in accordance with Section 1862(a)(1)(A) of the Social Security Act (i.e., a determination as to whether the service is reasonable and necessary).

Longshore and Harbor Workers' Compensation Act (LHWCA): Act that covers maritime workers injured or killed on navigable waters of the United States and those working on or adjoining piers, docks, and terminals.

main term: The term used when searching for a specific diagnosis code. Is usually the chief complaint (CC).

managed care: A system of health care delivery aimed at controlling costs by shifting utilization risk to the provider. Usually requires a gatekeeper or primary care physician to approve tests, surgeries, and visits to specialists.

managed care organization (MCO): Organization designed to provide quality health care that is cost effective. Through supervision, monitoring, and advising, managed care plans seek to ensure a certain standard of care, measure performance, and control costs. Additionally, some managed care plans seek to assist members in staying healthy through prevention.

manifestations: Symptoms related to the patient's condition.

manual review: Occurs when a claim is removed from an automated claims processing system and sent to a claims examiner to request additional information in order to complete the processing of the claim.

master patient index: Identifies all patients who have been treated in a facility or hospital and lists the medical record or identification number associated with each patient.

maximum medical improvement: With regard to workers' compensation claims, the point in time at which an injured worker's injury or illness has improved as much as it is likely to improve.

medical benefits: In the context of worker's compensation, medical care that is reasonable and necessary to treat a work-related injury or illness.

medical biller: Submits and tracks all insurance claims and ensures that insurance companies correctly reimburse the healthcare provider.

medical coder: Assigns numerical codes to diagnoses and procedures using the ICD-9-CM and CPT manuals.

medical decision making (MDM): The process of establishing a diagnosis and selecting a management option as measured by the number of diagnoses or treatment options, the amount and complexity of data (medical records, test result, or other information) to be reviewed, and the risk of complications, morbidity, or mortality.

medical practice management (MPM) software: Medical software database used in medical practices that stores physician's charges, patient data, adjustment information, and demographical and other information within a medical practice.

medically needy: An optional Medicaid program that allows states to extend Medicaid eligibility to additional qualified persons who may have too much income to qualify under the mandatory or optional categorically needy groups. Generally, those qualifying under the medically needy program receive medical services, but not cash assistance.

Medicare abuse: Includes improper payments for items or services when there was no legal entitlement to that payment; may directly or indirectly result in costs to the Medicare or Medicaid programs.

Medicare Advantage (MA): Offers expanded benefits for a fee through private health insurance programs such as health maintenance organizations and preferred provider organizations that have contracts with Medicare. Also known as Medicare Part C.

Medicare conversion factor (MCF): Determined by Centers for Medicare and Medicaid Services, the MCF is a national value that converts the total relative value units into a payment amount to reimburse providers for medical services.

Medicare Development Letter: A letter sent to a provider by Medicare requesting additional information or documentation to process a claim.

Medicare Fee Schedule (MFS): Based on the resource-based relative value scale (RBRVS) fees. This amount is the most Medicare will allow to be paid for a procedure.

Medicare fraud: Knowingly and intentionally executing a plan to scheme or defraud any healthcare benefit program in order to obtain, by means of false or fraudulent pretenses, any money or property.

Medicare Part A: The U.S. government's health insurance program for the elderly, individuals with disabilities, and individuals with qualifying end-stage renal disease. This portion covers hospital fees.

Medicare Part B: Medical insurance that helps pay for physicians' services, outpatient hospital care, durable medical equipment, and some medical services that are not covered by Medicare Part A.

Medicare Part C: Offers expanded benefits for a fee through private health insurance programs such as health maintenance organizations and preferred provider organizations that have contracts with Medicare. Also called Medicare Advantage.

Medicare Part D: Medicare prescription drug coverage program.

Medicare Remittance Notice (MRN): Notice sent to providers by Medicare contractors on assigned claims; details how a claim was processed.

Medicare secondary payer (MSP): Any situation in which a payer is required by federal law, to pay before Medicare pays. There are several instances where another payer could be primary to Medicare.

Medicare Summary Notice (MSN): An easy-to-read document that clearly lists the health insurance claim information. The MSN lists the details of the services rendered by a provider and shows amounts paid and beneficiaries' responsibilities.

Medigap: A privately offered, Medicare-supplemental health insurance policy designed to provide additional coverage for services that Medicare does not pay for and for noncovered services.

Medi-Medi: Term used to refer to a beneficiary who is covered under the Medicare program, but is also eligible for coverage through the Medicaid program.

military treatment facility (MTF): A clinic, hospital, or provider within the military or armed forces. Some TRICARE plans require that sponsors and their families go to a MTF.

modifier: A two-digit number placed after the five-digit CPT code to indicate that the description of the service or procedure has been altered.

morphology: The study of the structure of words.

National Committee for Quality Assurance (NCQA): Promotes quality in the delivery of health care in managed care organizations by rating their performance from information obtained from Healthcare Effectiveness Data and Information Set (HEDIS). NCQA works with managed care organizations to help them in their efforts to improve the delivery of quality health care to their members.

National Correct Coding Initiative (NCCI): Coding policies to standardize bundled codes and control improper coding that would lead to inappropriate payment for Medicare claims for physician services.

National Provider Identifier (NPI): A unique 10-digit number for HIPAA-covered health care providers to be used in the administrative and financial transactions adopted under HIPAA.

nationally uniform relative value: A standardized scale, based on three cost elements: the physician's effort or amount of work to account for each service; the practice cost associated with delivering the service; and the professional liability insurance to cover the procedure being performed. Used as a basis for establishing Medicare fees for physicians.

network: An organization of members contracted with a managed care organization.

new patient: A person who has not received any professional services from the physician or another physician of the same specialty who belongs to the same group practice within the past three years.

nomenclature: A listing of descriptive terms, guidelines, and identifying codes for reporting medical services and procedures.

nonavailability statement (NAS): Document that must be obtained through the DEERS office in order for a sponsor or family member to see a civilian provider or be treated in a nonmilitary facility.

Non-PAR MFS: Amount that applies to unassigned services performed by physicians and suppliers who choose not to participate in the Medicare program, which is 5% less than the MFS for participating providers. Providers who are non-PAR and not accepting assignment may charge a limiting charge of 115% of the nonparticipating fee amount.

nonparticipating provider: A provider who does not have a contract with a designated insurance carrier and is not obligated to offer discounted rates.

not elsewhere classified (NEC): A designation used in the ICD-9-CM coding manual that indicates a more specific code is not available to describe the condition, even though there is more detailed information in the medical record.

not otherwise specified (NOS): A designation used in the ICD-9-CM coding manual that indicates there is lack of sufficient details in the medical record to assign a more specific code.

Notice of Contest: With regard to workers' compensation claims, notice issued to an employee if his or her employer denies a workers' compensation claim.

occupational diseases and illnesses: Health problems that are the direct result of a workplace health hazard, such as dust, gas, and radiation. These can come on rapidly or develop over time.

Occupational Safety and Health Act: Act that gave the federal government the authority to set and enforce safety and health standards for most employees in the United States; administered by the Occupational Safety and Health Administration.

Office of Inspector General Fraud Alert (OIGFA): Alerts that are periodically issued and posted on the Centers for Medicare and Medicaid Services website to advise providers of problematic actions that have come to the Office of Inspector General's attention.

Office of Inspector General Work Plan (OIGWP): Plan that lists the year's planned projects for sampling types of billing to determine if there are any problems.

Office of Workers' Compensation Programs (OWCP): Office that administers work-related injuries and illness for civilian employees of federal agencies, which is also part of the U.S. Department of Labor.

ombudsman: A representative of workers' compensation insurance plans who can assist the injured worker with the workers' compensation claim at no charge. The ombudsman is not a lawyer but knows the law as it pertains to workers' compensation claims.

operating physician: A physician who performed the surgical procedure being billed on a specific claim.

optical character recognition (OCR): The mechanical or electronic translation of images of typewritten text into machine-editable text. Software used with a scanner allows for the transfer of printed or typed text and bar codes to an insurance company's computer memory.

out-of-pocket expenses: Amount of healthcare expenses a policyholder or patient is responsible for. The amount is determined by the payer and listed in the insured's policy. The payer reimburses services at 100% once the out-of-pocket expenses are met in a calendar year.

outpatient: A patient who is treated at a hospital or other medical facility during a stay of less than 24 hours.

outpatient (ambulatory) care: Care that is usually provided in less than 24 hours and may not need preauthorization for the insured's insurance carrier, depending on the particular carrier.

Palmetto Government Benefits Administrators (PGBA): Claim processor for TRICARE's northern region of the United States.

panel: A group of tests ordered together to detect particular diseases or malfunctioning organs.

participating provider: A provider who signs a contract with an insurance carrier agreeing to see patients at a discounted rate. They are usually listed in a provider book given to beneficiaries at enrollment.

past, family, and social history (PFSH): A review of the past medical experiences of the patient and the patient's family as well as an age appropriate review of past and current social activities such as marital status, employment, sexual history, and use of drugs, alcohol, and tobacco..

patient account services (PAS): A facility that centralizes the process of billing patients and carriers for treatment received at an inpatient facility.

patient control number (PCN): Unique alphanumeric identifier assigned by a provider to facilitate retrieval of individual case records and posting of payments. Found on the UB-04.

patient information form (PIF): Form that contains demographic, employment, and insurance information about a patient. The form varies from one practice to another.

payer of last resort: Under the Medicaid program, if an insured person has any other insurance in addition to Medicaid, then those insurance carriers will be approached first for payment and Medicaid will be approached last.

payment: Money received in a physician's practice. Includes insurance payments attached to an Explanation of Benefits or patient payments by check, money order, or cash.

peer review: An objective unbiased review by a group of physicians employed by an insurance carrier to determine what payment is adequate for the services provided. This review is used by a physician as a last attempt to resolve an appeal dispute when all other efforts at resolution have failed.

pending claim: A claim that has been received by the carrier but has not yet been processed. Usually additional information is requested from the provider to continue processing of the claim.

per member per month (PMPM): Refers to the fees paid on a capitation plan. The rate is based on a list with a number of members sent to the provider at the beginning of the month. The provider is paid up front for medical services rendered whether the patients are treated or not.

Performing Provider Identification Number (PPIN): A unique number assigned by Medicare when the performing provider of a service is a member of a group and billing under the group name. This number was replaced with the NPI in 2007.

physical status modifier: A 2-character code beginning with "P", required after a CPT code for anesthesia to indicate the patient's health status at the time anesthesia is administered. Established by the American Society of Anesthesiologists.

physician of record: With regard to workers' compensation claims, physician who treats a patient's injury or illness; also known as the treating doctor.

Physician Quality Reporting Initiative (PQRI): A voluntary reporting system implemented by the Centers for Medicare and Medicaid Services that offers participating professionals the opportunity to earn a bonus payment for prospectively entering codes related to specific quality performance measures.

point of service (POS): A type of managed healthcare plan that allows the member to choose between an HMO, PPO or indemnity plan at the time of service.

policyholder: Owner of an insurance policy.

preauthorization: Authorization from an insurance company that allows a patient to receive treatment using their benefits. Some insurance companies require this prior to admission for a hospital stay or outpatient surgery.

preexisting condition: A diagnosis or condition for which a beneficiary is treated prior to the effective date of coverage with his or her insurance carrier.

preferred provider organization (PPO): Organization that contracts with physicians and facilities to perform services for preferred provider members for specified rates.

premium: A dollar amount a person pays for an insurance policy. Often deducted from an employee's paycheck.

presenting problem: A disease, condition, illness, injury, symptom, sign, complaint, or other reason for encounter with or without a diagnosis being established at the time of the encounter

primary care manager (PCM): Physician who coordinates and manages a TRICARE Prime patient's care. This can be a civilian or military provider.

primary care physician (PCP): A provider who coordinates a patient's care.

primary diagnosis: The patient's main reason for the outpatient visit or encounter.

primary procedure: The most resource-intensive CPT procedure done during a patient encounter.

principal diagnosis: The condition established, after all tests and procedures are completed, to be chiefly responsible for the admission of a patient to a hospital for care.

professional component: The part of the relative value associated with a procedure that represents a physician's skill, time, and expertise used in performing the procedure.

Programs for All-Inclusive Care for the Elderly (PACE): Features a comprehensive service delivery system and integrated Medicare and Medicaid financing. The PACE program was developed to address the needs of long-term care clients, providers, and payers. For most participants, the comprehensive service package permits them to continue living at home while receiving services rather than be institutionalized.

prospective audit: Completed before the claim is submitted for payment.

prospective payment system: A method of reimbursement in which third party payment is made based on a predetermined, fixed amount, based on the classification of type of service. Medicare DRGs are a major example.

provider: An individual or facility providing medical care.

provider identification number (PIN): Unique identification number given to providers for billing purposes.

qualified independent contractors (QICs): Companies that contract with Medicare to conduct all second-level appeals (reconsiderations) for Medicare, Medicaid, and SCHIP (State Children's Health Insurance Plan).

reason code/remark code: Numeric or alphabetic digits that indicate the reason why a claim was not paid in full, how the claim was calculated, or why the claim was denied.

redetermination: The first level of appeal for physician claims with Medicare. The provider has 120 days to file this request from the date of denial. Medicare carriers must process these requests with 30 days.

referral: The transfer of total care or a specific portion of care of a patient from one physician to another.

registered health information technician (RHIT): Coordinates services related to inpatient medical coding, medical documentation, abstracting, data collection, and reimbursement requirements; supervises inpatient medical coding.

registration: The process of collecting a patient's personal information, including insurance information, and entering it into the hospital's computer system. Includes scheduling the hospital stay, completing preadmission testing, receiving and following all of the appropriate preadmission instructions, completing all consent forms, and verifying insurance benefits.

relative value unit (RVU): Unit of measure assigned to a medical procedure based on the time required to perform it. This system is composed of three elements: work, practice expense, and liability insurance.

release of information form: Specifies which information from a patient's medical chart may be released and to whom it may be released.

residual effect: A condition that remains after a patient's acute injury or illness.

resource-based fees: Fees based on resource-based relative value scale (RBRVS).

resource-based relative value scale (RBRVS): A payment schedule system that represents the resources used to perform a procedure or service by assigning a relative value for each procedure.

restricted status: Status that requires a beneficiary to see a designated physician or pharmacy for eligible persons covered under the Medicaid program.

retention schedule: Determines how long patient records must be stored. This determination is based on state regulations and federal laws.

retrospective audit: Audit completed after payment has been received from a carrier.

review of systems (ROS): An inventory of body systems obtained through a series of questions asked by the physician, who seeks to identify signs or symptoms that the patient may be experiencing.

rule out (r/o): A designation for an uncertain diagnosis that the provider orders tests or studies for in an attempt to eliminate it as the cause of the patient's complaint. When coding outpatient services, rule out diagnoses are not to be coded; rather, the presenting signs and symptoms should be coded.

schedule of benefits (SOB): A list of medical services covered under an insurance policy and the amount paid for each treatment.

secondary insurance: Any insurance a patient may have in addition to his or her primary insurance. Claims can be submitted to secondary insurance carriers for the balance of a medical claim not paid by the primary insurer.

secondary procedure: A procedure performed in addition to the primary procedure.

separate procedure: A descriptor used in coding for a procedure that is sometimes part of a surgical package, but can be performed separately and billed separately.

sign: An indication of a particular disorder that can be observed or measured by a physician.

skilled nursing facility (SNF): A nursing facility with the staff and equipment to give skilled nursing care or skilled rehabilitation services and other related health services.

SOAP format: A documentation method that records the patient's Subjective complaint, the provider's Objective evaluation and examination, the Assessment or diagnosis, and the Plan for treatment

Social Security Disability Insurance (SSDI): Federal disability compensation program that pays benefits to employed or self-employed individuals with disabilities who are under age 65 and have paid Social Security taxes for a minimum number of calendar year quarters. The number of quarters worked varies depending on the age of the individual. Pays benefits to people who cannot work because they have a medical condition that is expected to last at least 1 year or result in death.

special report: A report to detail the reason for a new, variable, or unlisted procedure or service; it explains the patient's condition and justifies the procedure's medical necessity.

special risk insurance (SRI): Insurance that an individual can purchase to protect against a certain type of accident or illness.

spend-down program: Program that allows patients to pay a portion of their medical expenses each month and Medicaid will be available to assist with the remaining medical expenses. This program is for persons who are at or below the state income level. Medicaid eligibility is then determined month to month.

sponsor: The beneficiary or policyholder of a TRICARE plan.

State Children's Health Insurance Program (SCHIP): Health insurance for children through the Medicaid program. SCHIP is jointly financed by the state and federal governments and administered by the states. Each state determines the guidelines for its own program, eligibility groups, benefit packages, payment levels for coverage, and administrative and operating procedures.

state license number (SLN): Unique identification number issued by the state for billing purposes.

subscriber: Person responsible for payment of insurance premiums or person whose employment or group affiliation is the basis for membership in a health plan.

subterms: Coding terms that provide more specific information than the main term. They also provide the anatomic site affected by the disease or injury.

superbills: Document that contains ICD-9 and CPT codes for the diagnoses and services that the office routinely uses. Also referred to as an encounter form, charge slip, or routing slip.

supplemental income benefits: With regard to workers' compensation claims, benefits that may be issued to an injured worker due to the percent of impairment rating, or if the worker has not been able to find employment that matches his or her ability to work.

supplemental insurance: Provides coverage for medical services not covered by the primary plan. An example of supplemental insurance would be a Medigap policy that pays the insured's coinsurance and items not covered by Medicare.

Supplemental Security Income (SSI): Government program funded by general taxes that helps pay living expenses for low-income older people and those who are blind or have disabilities. May be issued to an injured worker due to the percent of impairment rating, or if the worker has not been able to find employment that matches his or her ability to work.

supplementary term: A nonessential word or phrase that helps to define a code in the ICD-9-CM; it is usually enclosed in parentheses or brackets.

surgical package: The services before and after a surgical procedure that are considered to be part of the CPT code billed and should not be billed separately. The CPT manual defines the "CPT surgical package" but payers may vary this to suit their needs. Also called a global package.

symbol: Used in the CPT book to show changes and alert the reader to new codes, deletions, or alterations to a code. The symbol is located before the code number for one year, after which it becomes part of the next annual printing.

symptom: An indication of a disorder or disease that the patient reports to the physician, but that the physician cannot observe or measure.

tax identification number (TIN): Identification number used by the Internal Revenue Service in the administration of tax laws.

Tax Relief and Health Care Act (TRHCA): Act that helps to maintain key tax reforms, expand our commitment to renewable energy resources, make it easier for Americans to afford health insurance, and open markets overseas for farmers and small businesses.

technical component: Part of the relative value associated with a procedure that reflects the technologist, the equipment, and processing including pre-injection and post-injection services.

Temporary Assistance for Needy Families (TANF): A time-limited (5 years) cash assistance benefit for families that qualify based on the state income or poverty level. TANF replaced Aid to Families with Dependent Children (AFDC) in 1996.

temporary income benefits: With regard to workers' compensation claims, benefits a worker may receive if an injury or illness caused the worker to lose some or all income for 7 days.

transaction: The task of entering a charge, payment, or adjustment on a patient's account.

treating doctor: With regard to workers' compensation claims, doctor who treats the injured worked; also known as the physician of record.

TRICARE: The civilian health and medical program of the uniformed services for qualified family members of military personnel. (Note that the name changed from CHAMPUS to TRICARE in January 1994, but it continues to be listed as CHAMPUS on the CMS-1500 form.)

TRICARE Extra: A PPO type of managed care plan that allows TRICARE beneficiaries who do not have priority at a military treatment facility to receive services primarily from a civilian provider at a reduced fee.

TRICARE Prime: A voluntary HMO-style plan for TRICARE beneficiaries that offers preventive care and routine physical examinations. Each individual on this plan is assigned a primary care manager.

TRICARE Prime Remote (TPR): A healthcare plan that is available to active duty members who are stationed more than 50 miles from a military treatment facility, enabling them to receive treatment from a civilian provider.

TRICARE Prime Remote for Active Duty Family Members (TPRADFM): Healthcare plan for family members of active duty service personnel who are assigned a permanent station (active duty for a certain period of time). There are no out-of-pocket expenses for this plan.

TRICARE Senior Prime: Healthcare coverage for Medicare-eligible beneficiaries ages 65 and older.

TRICARE Standard: A fee-for-service health plan for families of active duty personnel and retirees that goes into effect when treated by a civilian provider. Most enrollees pay an annual deductible. In addition to the deductible, families of active duty members pay 20% of out-of-pocket expenses, while retirees and their families and former spouses pay 25% of out-of-pocket expenses for medical services.

turnaround time: Length of time an insurance carrier takes to process a claim from the time it is received in their office.

UB-04 claim form: Standard health insurance claim form used by institutional providers, such as hospital, skilled nursing facility, and rehabilitation centers, to file insurance claims with Medicare Part A and other health insurance companies. The UB-04 replaced the UB-92 and was mandatory beginning in 2007.

unbundling: Occurs when separate procedures are reported that should have been included under a bundled code.

Unique Provider Identification Number (UPIN): A number assigned by Medicare to physicians, doctors of osteopathy, limited licensed practitioners, and some non-physician practitioners who are enrolled in the Medicare program. In 2007 the UPIN was replaced with the NPI.

unlisted procedure: A service or procedure that does not have a unique code listed in the CPT codebook. Each section's guidelines have codes for unlisted procedures.

upcode: Occurs when the procedure code stated is for a procedure that is more involved than the one actually documented in the chart.

urgent care: Immediate medical care for a condition that requires prompt attention, but does not pose an immediate, serious health threat.

usual, customary, and reasonable (UCR): A fee determined by third-party payers to reimburse providers based on the provider's normal fee, the range of fees charged by providers of the same specialty in the same geographic area, and other factors to determine appropriate fees in unusual situations.

utilization: A review process that compares requests for medical services to treatment guidelines that are deemed appropriate for such services and includes the preparation of a recommendation based on that comparison.

verification of benefits (VOB) form: Form used to identify and record the benefits a patient has with the insurance company, before service is rendered, to ensure that the patient is eligible.

Veteran's Disability Compensation: Benefits paid to a veteran because of injury or disease that happened while on active duty, or were made worse because of active military service.

Veteran's Disability Pension Benefits: Benefits paid to wartime veterans with limited income who are no longer able to work.

vocational rehabilitation: The retraining of an employee so he or she can return to the workforce.

walkout receipt: A printed statement, given to the patient at the end of a visit that lists the patient's charges for that day.

welfare reform bill: Term used for a policy change in state-administered social welfare systems that reduced dependence on welfare, as demanded by political conservatives. It made restrictive changes regarding eligibility for SSI benefits.

Wisconsin Physicians Services (WPS): Claims processor for all TRICARE Senior Prime claims

withhold: Under a capitation plan, this is a percentage of the provider's payment that is deducted from the check to offset any additional costs. At the end of the year, any withhold not used is distributed as a bonus.

Work Status Report (progress report, supplemental report): Form issued by the state for transmission of information between the employee and the employer's insurance carrier and the treating physician.

write-off: A negative adjustment to a patient's account. Usually when the provider has a contract with a carrier, the difference between the billed amount and the allowed amount is written off.

11) accept code as stated
12) A & B
+13) always billed seperately over labove
14) all of the above
15) (b)
16) (A)
17) surgical
18) ~~medically~~ advanced Ben notice
19) clean claim
20) Fraud